A Guide to Physical Examination

A Guide to
PHYSICAL
EXAMINATION
Third Edition

BARBARA BATES, M.D.,

Lecturer in Medicine, Department of Medicine
University of Pennsylvania School of Medicine
and
Lecturer in Nursing
University of Pennsylvania School of Nursing
Philadelphia, Pennsylvania

WITH A SECTION ON THE PEDIATRIC EXAMINATION
by
Robert A. Hoekelman, M.D.,

Professor and Associate Chairman
Department of Pediatrics
University of Rochester
School of Medicine and Dentistry
and
Professor of Nursing
University of Rochester School of Nursing
Rochester, New York

Illustrations by
Robert Wabnitz and Staff
University of Rochester School of Medicine
and
Susan Shapiro Brenman, M.S., Medical Illustrator

J.B. Lippincott Company • Philadelphia
London   Mexico City   New York   St. Louis   São Paulo   Sydney

Sponsoring Editor: David T. Miller
Manuscript Editor: Delois Patterson
Indexer: Norman Duren
Art Director: Tracy Baldwin
Designer: Arlene Putterman
Production Supervisor: N. Carol Kerr
Production Coordinator: Susan A. Caldwell
Compositor: Waldman Graphics, Inc.
Printer/Binder: The Murray Printing Company

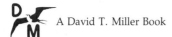 A David T. Miller Book

3rd Edition

6 5

Library of Congress Cataloging in Publication Data

Bates, Barbara.
  A guide to physical examination.
  Bibliography
  Includes index.
  1. Physical diagnosis.   2. Children—Medical
examination.   I. Hoekelman,
Robert A.   II. Title. III. Title: Physical
examination. [DNLM: 1. Physical
examination. WB 205 B329g]
RC76.B37 1983   616.07′54   82-10005
ISBN 0-397-54399-9   AACR2

Acknowledgments

Good colleagues are a great delight, and we are pleased to acknowledge their contributions. Susan Shapiro Brenman, M.S., medical illustrator, created the new artwork in this edition, adding importantly to previous work by Robert Wabnitz and his staff and by Pamela Rowles. Art Siegel and Jordan Denner, both of the Biomedical Communications Facility, School of Medicine, University of Pennsylvania, produced the new photographs. Photographs from the Second Edition were done by William L. Chisholm of the University of Missouri–Kansas City School of Medicine.

Ruth M. Ouimette, R.N., M.S.N., among other nurses, encouraged us to expand this edition by including changes with age. She also reviewed and criticized early versions of the sections on puberty. Mathy D. Mezey, R.N., Ed.D., graciously enabled one of us (B.B.) to attend her lectures on changes in the elderly.

Milton N. Luria, M.D., William R. Harlan, M.D., and Mohammad Amin, M.D., responded helpfully to specific inquiries, and James L. Stinnett, M.D., reviewed the chapter on mental status.

Students, as usual, have had an important influence in shaping the new edition. We hope they will identify and enjoy some of their contributions.

In Pennsylvania, Elizabeth Popper prepared the manuscript in its many permutations, while in Rochester, Sydney Sutherland provided editorial assistance and Kathy Schafer prepared the manuscript. The skill of Mary W. Norris, copy editor, has added both form and clarity to the final version. The staff of J.B. Lippincott Company has contributed in countless ways, with competence, patience, and hard work.

Contents

List of Tables   *xi*

Introduction   *xv*

Chapter 1   **INTERVIEWING AND THE HEALTH HISTORY**   **1**
THE INFORMATION NEEDED, 1   SETTING THE STAGE FOR THE INTERVIEW, 8   APPROACH TO THE PRESENT ILLNESS, 10   THE REST OF THE STORY, 14   PATIENTS AT DIFFERENT AGES, 16 SPECIAL PROBLEMS, 20   A FINAL NOTE, 27

Chapter 2   **PHYSICAL EXAMINATION: APPROACH AND OVERVIEW**   **28**

Chapter 3   **THE GENERAL SURVEY**   **35**

Anatomy and Physiology, 35

Techniques of Examination, 39

Chapter 4   **THE SKIN**   **43**

Anatomy and Physiology, 43
CHANGES WITH AGE, 44

Techniques of Examination, 46

Tables of Related Abnormalities, 48

Chapter 5   **THE HEAD AND NECK**   **54**

Anatomy and Physiology, 54
THE HEAD, 54   THE EYE, 55   THE EAR, 60   THE NOSE AND PARANASAL SINUSES, 62 THE MOUTH AND THE PHARYNX, 64   THE NECK, 65   CHANGES WITH AGE, 68

Techniques of Examination, 70
THE HEAD, 70   THE EYES, 70   THE EARS, 83   THE NOSE AND SINUSES, 85 THE MOUTH AND PHARYNX, 89   THE NECK, 91

Tables of Related Abnormalities, 95

Chapter 6   **THE THORAX AND LUNGS**   **125**

Anatomy and Physiology, 125
CHANGES WITH AGE, 135

Techniques of Examination, 136

GENERAL APPROACH, 136   EXAMINATION OF THE POSTERIOR CHEST, 136   Inspection, 136
Palpation, 137   Percussion, 139   Auscultation, 143   EXAMINATION OF THE ANTERIOR CHEST, 144
Inspection, 144   Palpation, 145   Percussion, 146   Auscultation, 148
CLINICAL ASSESSMENT OF PULMONARY FUNCTION, 148

Tables of Related Abnormalities, 149

Chapter 7   THE HEART, PRESSURES, AND PULSES   157

Anatomy and Physiology, 157

SURFACE PROJECTIONS OF THE HEART AND GREAT VESSELS, 157
CARDIAC CHAMBERS, VALVES, AND CIRCULATION, 160   EVENTS IN THE CARDIAC CYCLE, 161
RELATION OF HEART SOUNDS TO THE CHEST WALL, 164   THE CONDUCTION SYSTEM, 165
ARTERIAL PULSES AND BLOOD PRESSURE, 166   JUGULAR VENOUS PRESSURE AND PULSES, 168
CHANGES WITH AGE, 169

Techniques of Examination, 172

THE HEART, 172   Inspection and Palpation, 172   Auscultation, 176   THE ARTERIAL PULSE, 180
BLOOD PRESSURE, 182   JUGULAR VENOUS PRESSURE AND PULSES, 187
A NOTE ON CARDIOVASCULAR ASSESSMENT, 189

Tables of Related Abnormalities, 191

Chapter 8   THE BREASTS AND AXILLAE   210

Anatomy and Physiology, 210
CHANGES WITH AGE, 212   LYMPHATICS, 214

Techniques of Examination, 216
THE FEMALE BREAST, 216   General Approach, 216   Inspection, 216   Palpation, 219   THE MALE BREAST, 222
THE AXILLAE, 222   Inspection, 222   Palpation, 222

Tables of Related Abnormalities, 224

Chapter 9   THE ABDOMEN   228

Anatomy and Physiology, 228
CHANGES WITH AGE, 231

Techniques of Examination, 232
GENERAL APPROACH, 232   Inspection, 232   Auscultation, 234   Percussion, 235   Light Palpation, 238
Deep Palpation, 239   Palpating the Liver, Spleen, Kidneys, and Aorta, 240   Special Maneuvers, 246

Tables of Related Abnormalities, 250

Chapter 10   MALE GENITALIA AND HERNIAS   258

Anatomy and Physiology, 258
CHANGES WITH AGE, 260

Techniques of Examination, 263
GENERAL APPROACH, 263   ASSESSMENT OF SEXUAL DEVELOPMENT, 263   PENIS, 264
Inspection, 264   Palpation, 265   SCROTUM, 265   Inspection, 265   Palpation, 265   HERNIAS, 266   Inspection, 266
Palpation, 266

Tables of Related Abnormalities, 268

Chapter 11   FEMALE GENITALIA   273

Anatomy and Physiology, 273
CHANGES WITH AGE, 275

Techniques of Examination, 277
GENERAL APPROACH, 277   EXTERNAL EXAMINATION, 279   INTERNAL EXAMINATION, 280

Tables of Related Abnormalities, 286

Chapter 12   THE ANUS AND RECTUM   296

Anatomy and Physiology, 296

Techniques of Examination, 298
MALE, 298   FEMALE, 300

Tables of Related Abnormalities, 301

Chapter 13   THE PERIPHERAL VASCULAR SYSTEM   304

Anatomy and Physiology, 304
ARTERIES, 304   VEINS, 305   THE LYMPHATIC SYSTEM AND LYMPH NODES, 307
FLUID EXCHANGE AND THE CAPILLARY BED, 309   CHANGES WITH AGE, 309

Techniques of Examination, 310
ARMS, 310   LEGS, 312   SPECIAL EXAMINATION OF THE BED PATIENT, 316

Tables of Related Abnormalities, 318

Chapter 14   THE MUSCULOSKELETAL SYSTEM   324

Anatomy and Physiology, 324
STRUCTURE AND FUNCTION OF JOINTS, 324   SPECIFIC JOINTS, 325   CHANGES WITH AGE, 338

Techniques of Examination, 340
GENERAL APPROACH, 340   HEAD AND NECK, 341   HANDS AND WRISTS, 342   ELBOWS, 344
SHOULDERS AND ENVIRONS, 344   FEET AND ANKLES, 345   KNEES AND HIPS, 347   THE SPINE, 350
SPECIAL MANEUVERS, 352

Tables of Related Abnormalities, 355

Chapter 15   THE NERVOUS SYSTEM   370

Anatomy and Physiology, 370
THE REFLEX ARC, 370   MOTOR PATHWAYS, 373   SENSORY PATHWAYS, 374
THE CRANIAL NERVES, 378   THE BRAIN, 380   CHANGES WITH AGE, 381

Techniques of Examination, 382
GENERAL APPROACH, 382   SURVEY OF MENTAL STATUS AND SPEECH, 382
THE CRANIAL NERVES, 383   THE MOTOR SYSTEM, 387   THE SENSORY SYSTEM, 397
REFLEXES, 401   SPECIAL MANEUVERS, 408

Tables of Related Abnormalities, 413

Chapter 16   MENTAL STATUS   428

Components of Mental Function, 428
CHANGES WITH AGE, 429

Techniques of Examination, 430
APPEARANCE AND BEHAVIOR, 431   MOOD, 432
THOUGHT PROCESSES, THOUGHT CONTENT, AND PERCEPTIONS, 432
COGNITIVE FUNCTIONS, 434   A NOTE ON MENTAL ASSESSMENT, 446

Tables of Related Abnormalities, 438

Chapter 17 **THE PHYSICAL EXAMINATION OF INFANTS AND CHILDREN   447**
Robert A. Hoekelman

APPROACH TO THE PATIENT, 448   Infancy, 448   Early Childhood, 452   Late Childhood, 455
THE GENERAL SURVEY, 456   Temperature, 456   Pulse, 457   Respiratory Rate, 458   Blood Pressure, 458
Somatic Growth, 460   THE SKIN, 462   Infancy, 462   Early and Late Childhood, 465   THE HEAD AND NECK, 465
Infancy, 465   Early and Late Childhood, 470   THE EYE, 471   Infancy, 471   Early Childhood, 474
Late Childhood, 477   THE EAR, 478   Infancy, 478   Early Childhood, 479   Late Childhood, 482
THE NOSE AND THROAT, 482   Infancy, 482   Early and Late Childhood, 483   THE THORAX AND LUNGS, 487
Infancy, 487   Early and Late Childhood, 488   THE HEART, 489   THE ABDOMEN, 492   Infancy, 492
Early and Late Childhood, 494   THE GENITALIA AND RECTUM, 496   Infancy, 496
Early and Late Childhood, 497   THE MUSCULOSKELETAL SYSTEM, 498   Infancy, 498   Early and Late Childhood, 502
THE NERVOUS SYSTEM, 503   Infancy, 503   Early and Late Childhood, 510   At All Ages, 512

Tables, 450, 457, 468, 469, 491, 495

Chapter 18 **CLINICAL THINKING: FROM DATA TO PLAN   513**

From Data Base to Plan, 513

Assessment: The Process of Clinical Thinking, 515

Difficulties and Variations, 517

The Interplay of Assessment and Data Collection, 522

Developing a Problem List and Plan, 522

Chapter 19 **THE PATIENT'S RECORD   524**

Bibliography   537

Index   549

List of Tables

Chapter 4   **THE SKIN**

     Table 4–1   *Variations in Skin Color, 48*
     Table 4–2   *Vascular and Purpuric Lesions of the Skin, 50*
     Table 4–3   *Basic Types of Skin Lesions, 51*
     Table 4–4   *Abnormalities and Variations of the Nails, 53*

Chapter 5   **THE HEAD AND THE NECK**

     Table 5–1   *Selected Facies, 95*
     Table 5–2   *Visual Field Defects Produced by Selected Lesions in the Visual Pathways, 96*
     Table 5–3   *Abnormalities of the Eyelids, 97*
     Table 5–4   *Lumps and Swellings In and Around the Eyes, 98*
     Table 5–5   *Red Eyes, 99*
     Table 5–6   *Opacities of the Cornea and Lens, 100*
     Table 5–7   *Pupillary Abnormalities, 101*
     Table 5–8   *Deviations of the Eyes, 103*
     Table 5–9   *Normal Variations of the Optic Disc, 104*
     Table 5–10   *Abnormalities of the Optic Disc, 105*
     Table 5–11   *Retinal Arterioles and Arteriovenous Crossings: Normal and Hypertensive, 106*
     Table 5–12   *Red Spots in the Retina, 107*
     Table 5–13   *Light-Colored Spots in the Retina, 108*
     Table 5–14   *Ocular Fundi, 109*
     Table 5–15   *Nodules in and Around the Ears, 113*
     Table 5–16   *Abnormalities of the Eardrum, 114*
     Table 5–17   *Patterns of Hearing Loss, 115*
     Table 5–18   *Common Abnormalities of the Nose, 116*
     Table 5–19   *Abnormalities of the Lips, 117*
     Table 5–20   *Abnormalities of the Buccal Mucosa and Hard Palate, 119*
     Table 5–21   *Abnormalities of the Gums and Teeth, 120*
     Table 5–22   *Abnormalities of the Tongue, 122*
     Table 5–23   *Abnormalities of the Pharynx, 123*
     Table 5–24   *Thyroid Enlargement and Nodules, 124*

Chapter 6   **THE THORAX AND LUNGS**

    Table 6–1   *Abnormalities in Rate and Rhythm of Breathing, 149*
    Table 6–2   *Deformities of the Thorax, 150*
    Table 6–3   *Alterations in Breath and Voice Sounds, 151*
    Table 6–4   *Added Lung Sounds: Crackles, Wheezes, and Rubs, 152*
    Table 6–5   *Physical Signs in Selected Abnormalities of Bronchi and Lungs, 154*

Chapter 7   **THE HEART, PRESSURES, AND PULSES**

    Table 7–1   *Comparison of the Apical Impulse in Normal People and in Those with Left Ventricular Enlargement, 191*
    Table 7–2   *Approach to the Differentiation of Selected Heart Rates and Rhythms, 192*
    Table 7–3   *Differentiation of Selected Regular Rhythms, 193*
    Table 7–4   *Differentiation of Selected Irregular Rhythms, 195*
    Table 7–5   *Variations in the First Heart Sound, 196*
    Table 7–6   *Variations in the Second Heart Sound, 197*
    Table 7–7   *Extra Heart Sounds in Systole, 198*
    Table 7–8   *Extra Heart Sounds in Diastole, 199*
    Table 7–9   *Three Causes of an Apparently Split First Heart Sound, 200*
    Table 7–10   *Mechanisms of Heart Murmurs, 201*
    Table 7–11   *Midsystolic Ejection Murmurs, 202*
    Table 7–12   *Pansystolic Regurgitant Murmurs, 204*
    Table 7–13   *Diastolic Murmurs, 205*
    Table 7–14   *Differentiation of Cardiovascular Sounds with Both Systolic and Diastolic Components, 207*
    Table 7–15   *Abnormalities of the Arterial Pulse, 209*

Chapter 8   **THE BREASTS AND AXILLAE**

    Table 8–1   *Visible Signs of Breast Cancer, 224*
    Table 8–2   *Abnormalities of Nipple and Areola, 225*
    Table 8–3   *Differentiation of Common Breast Nodules, 226*
    Table 8–4   *Abnormalities of the Male Breast, 227*

Chapter 9   **THE ABDOMEN**

    Table 9–1   *Abdominal Hernias and Bulges, 250*
    Table 9–2   *Protuberant Abdomens, 251*
    Table 9–3   *Sounds in the Abdomen, 252*
    Table 9–4   *Tender Abdomens, 253*
    Table 9–5   *Liver Enlargement: Apparent and Real, 255*
    Table 9–6   *Steps in Splenic Enlargement, 257*

Chapter 10   **MALE GENITALIA AND HERNIAS**

    Table 10–1   *Abnormalities of the Penis, 268*
    Table 10–2   *Abnormalities in the Scrotum, 269*
    Table 10–3   *Course and Presentation of Hernias in the Groin, 271*
    Table 10–4   *Differentiation of Hernias in the Groin, 272*

Chapter 11   **FEMALE GENITALIA**

    Table 11–1   *Lesions of the Vulva, 286*
    Table 11–2   *Bulges and Swellings of Vulva and Vagina, 287*
    Table 11–3   *Variations and Abnormalities of the Cervix, 288*
    Table 11–4   *Inflammations of and Around the Vagina, 290*

Color tabs identify
tables at the end of
respective chapters

4

5

6

7

8

9

10

11

12

13

14

15

16

17

Table 11–5   Changes in Pregnancy, 292
Table 11–6   Abnormalities and Displacements of the Uterus, 293
Table 11–7   Adnexal Masses, 295

Chapter 12   **THE ANUS AND RECTUM**

Table 12–1   Abnormalities of the Anus, Surrounding Skin, and Rectum, 301
Table 12–2   Abnormalities of the Prostate, 303

Chapter 13   **THE PERIPHERAL VASCULAR SYSTEM**

Table 13–1   Chronic Insufficiency of Arteries and Veins, 318
Table 13–2   Common Ulcers of the Feet and Ankles, 319
Table 13–3   Mechanisms and Patterns of Edema, 320
Table 13–4   Some Peripheral Causes of Edema, 322
Table 13–5   The Retrograde Filling Test for Incompetent Venous Valves, 323

Chapter 14   **THE MUSCULOSKELETAL SYSTEM**

Table 14–1   Problems in the Neck, 355
Table 14–2   Swellings and Deformities of the Hands, 357
Table 14–3   Swollen or Tender Elbows, 360
Table 14–4   Painful Shoulders, 361
Table 14–5   Abnormalities of the Feet and Toes, 363
Table 14–6   Swellings of the Knee, 365
Table 14–7   Local Tenderness in the Knee, 366
Table 14–8   Abnormal Spinal Curvatures, 368

Chapter 15   **THE NERVOUS SYSTEM**

Table 15–1   Abnormalities of Speech, 413
Table 15–2   Abnormalities of Consciousness, 413
Table 15–3   Nystagmus, 414
Table 15–4   Types of Facial Paralysis, 416
Table 15–5   Abnormalities of Gait and Posture, 418
Table 15–6   Involuntary Movements, 420
Table 15–7   Differentiation of Motor Dysfunctions, 423
Table 15–8   Patterns of Sensory Loss, 425
Table 15–9   Abnormal Postures in the Comatose Patient, 427

Chapter 16   **MENTAL STATUS**

Table 16–1   Distinguishing Features of Depressive Disorders, 438
Table 16–2   Variations and Abnormalities in Thought Processes, 439
Table 16–3   Irrational Anxiety and Avoidance Behaviors, 440
Table 16–4   Distinguishing Features of Psychotic Disorders, 442
Table 16–5   Distinguishing Features of Organic Brain Syndromes, 444

Chapter 17   **THE PHYSICAL EXAMINATION OF INFANTS AND CHILDREN**

Table 17–1   The Apgar Scoring System, 450
Table 17–2   Average Heart Rate of Infants and Children at Rest, 457
Table 17–3   Abnormal Enlargement of the Head in Infancy, 468
Table 17–4   Diagnostic Facies in Childhood, 469
Table 17–5   Cyanosis and Congenital Heart Disease, 491
Table 17–6   Expected Liver Span of Infants, Children, and Adolescents by Percussion, 495

Introduction

A GUIDE TO PHYSICAL EXAMINATION is designed for practitioners and students in health care who are learning to talk with and examine patients. It deals first with interviewing and the health history. Then, in chapters devoted to body regions or body systems, it reviews the relevant anatomy and physiology, describes the sequence and techniques of examination, and helps the student to identify selected abnormalities. Two final chapters deal with clinical thinking and organizing the patient's record.

THE THIRD EDITION

Important alterations have been made in the Third Edition. The anatomy and physiology section of almost every chapter has been expanded to include changes with age, with emphasis on adolescence and the aging years. Knowledge of these bodily changes not only helps the clinician to assess growth, development, and aging, but also helps him or her to distinguish normal from pathologic states. A section analogous to anatomy and physiology, entitled "Components of Mental Function," has been added to the chapter on mental status; and five new tables in that chapter deal with the differentiation of mental disorders. A new table on the mechanisms and patterns of edema has been added; the table on involuntary movements has been helpfully illustrated; additional abnormalities have been added to other tables; and a new color plate of ocular fundi provides a simulated ophthalmoscopic exercise. In some chapters, most notably those on the breasts, genitalia, and mental status, we have tried to address some of the common concerns and anxieties of beginning students. A new chapter, which follows those on physical examination, discusses clinical thinking—the thought processes involved as the clinician moves from data collection through assessment to plan.

Two chapters from the Second Edition—on recording the health history and the physical examination—have been combined and revised to form the new and final chapter, The Patient's Record. Materials on the heart, pressures, and pulses have been brought together into a single chapter to facilitate their intercorrelations. Almost every chapter has been revised or completely rewritten in an effort to clarify, explain more fully, and bring content up to date. Many new illustrations, photographs, and diagrams have been added throughout the book.

We have also made a few deletions. We have dropped Homans's sign as diagnostically misleading, desirable body weights as insufficiently substantiated, and cremasteric reflexes as unnecessary in the usual neurologic examination. Some clinicians may mourn the loss of these materials just as they regret the omission of cardiac percussion. Weeding hurts and judgments differ.

STRUCTURE AND PHILOSOPHY OF THE TEXT

The basic structure and philosophy of the book have not changed. While we assume that the learners have had basic courses in human anatomy and physiology, we also recognize the need for a bridge between these classic basic sciences and their application to examining patients. Accordingly, most chapters begin with sections on anatomy and physiology that are intended to fill this gap.

The sections on techniques are presented systematically, without interruption, so that the student may use them easily when practicing on a laboratory partner. We strongly encourage supervised practice of this kind before examining patients.

Abnormalities are presented in two places: parallel to the techniques and in tabular form at the ends of chapters. While learning techniques, students may wish to survey some of these abnormalities quickly, but they should not try to memorize them. The best time to learn about an abnormality is when a patient presents with one. The student should then try to analyze it with *A GUIDE TO PHYSICAL EXAMINATION* and subsequently pursue the subject in other clinical texts.

We have selected specific abnormalities for inclusion primarily because of their frequency or importance. An occasional physical sign has been included despite its rarity because it enjoys a solid niche in classic physical diagnosis. We have tried *not* to present an encyclopedic array of abnormalities, but have attempted to guide the learner toward the common and important in contrast to the infrequent or esoteric.

In designing the text we assume that student clinicians will learn their examination skills by first practicing on other adults. Most of the anatomy and physiology, some of the techniques, and many of the abnormalities are common to both adults and children. Dr. Hoekelman's chapter on the physical examination of infants and children describes variations as they occur in the younger age groups and those that are unique to them.

As students proceed systematically through specific chapters on physical examination, they may find it helpful to review at least briefly Chapter 2, *"Physical Examination: Approach and Overview"*; Chapter 18, *"Clinical Thinking: From Data to Plan"*; and Chapter 19, *"The Patient's Record."* These three chapters, together with the first chapter on interviewing, introduce the student to the basic skills underlying patient assessment: gathering, thinking about, and organizing data. They also provide a framework into which students may fit their new learning.

A VISUAL GUIDE TO PHYSICAL EXAMINATION

A series of 12 sound motion pictures, now available in a second edition, demonstrates the examination procedures outlined in this book. The *VISUAL GUIDE* is available from J. B. Lippincott Company.

EQUIPMENT

Equipment necessary for a physical examination includes the following:

1. An otoscope and ophthalmoscope. If the otoscope does not include a short wide speculum, a separate nasal speculum is required.
2. A flashlight
3. Tongue depressors
4. A ruler and flexible tape measure, preferably marked in centimeters
5. A thermometer
6. A watch with a second hand
7. A sphygmomanometer
8. A stethoscope with the following characteristics:
   a. Snugly fitting and comfortable ear tips, achieved through properly sized tips, an angle that approximates that of the ear canal, and an appropriately tight spring in the connecting metal band
   b. Thick-walled double tubes, each about 30 cm (12 inches) in length
   c. A large bell, about 2.5 cm (1 inch) in diameter
   d. A diaphragm about 3.7 cm (1½ inches) in diameter (2.5 cm or 1 inch in diameter for those specializing in pediatrics)
9. Gloves ⎫ For vaginal and rectal examination
10. Lubricant ⎬
11. Vaginal specula
12. A reflex hammer
13. Tuning forks, one of 128 cps and one of 512 cps or possibly 1024 cps
14. Safety pins
15. Cotton
16. Two test tubes (needed only for selected neurologic examinations)
17. Paper and pen or pencil

A Guide to Physical Examination

Chapter 1

INTERVIEWING AND THE HEALTH HISTORY

Barbara Bates and Robert A. Hoekelman

Talking with the patient and obtaining his health history are usually the first and often the most important parts of the health care process. Here you *gather the information necessary* to form a tentative diagnosis. You *begin a relationship* with the patient that will help him trust and confide in you. By talking with you *the patient may learn something about himself,* such as how his illness relates to his life situation. You share in that learning. Finally both you and the patient can *start to define your therapeutic goals.* You have made an implicit contract.

The relative importance of these four objectives varies, as do the time and effort they require. When a patient comes to the emergency room with severe chest pain, for example, you must usually concentrate on the acute problem. A psychosocial exploration may be deferred for the time being. When a patient comes to the clinic with poorly controlled diabetes, however, diagnostic data will not suffice. Here both you and the patient need to examine the problem in relation to the patient's eating patterns, life situation, and emotional reactions, among other factors, and try to reach a tentative agreement on therapeutic goals. You must modify your interviewing style according to the needs of the patient as they unfold.

THE INFORMATION NEEDED

No person can ever fully comprehend another, nor can any history be truly complete. Yet with practice, guidance, and self-awareness, you can learn to talk with a patient and obtain the comprehensive, organized set of data that constitutes the traditional health history. You must know (1) what information to get and (2) how to get it, while building a relationship as you proceed.

On pages 2 to 5 are outlined the components of a *comprehensive history* suitable when an adult patient makes a first visit. Pages 5 to 8 give a suggested format for the comprehensive evaluation of a child. Review these outlines to get an overview of their content and organization. The items listed, however, are neither mandatory nor all-inclusive. As your knowledge and experience grow, you will limit your questions in some areas and expand them in others, depending on such variables as the patient's age, sex, and symptoms. In making these judgments you will draw on all the clinical knowledge and human experience you have accumulated. Skilled clinicians may demonstrate a disconcerting ability to ask the one additional question that unlocks the door to understanding and to do so in a tenth of the time that you have spent. Let this be a stimulus rather than a discouragement!

COMPREHENSIVE HISTORY: ADULT PATIENT

Date of History

Identifying Data, including at least age, sex, race, place of birth, marital status, occupation, and perhaps religion

Source of Referral, if any

Source of History, which may be the patient or relative or friend, for example, together with the practitioner's judgment of the validity of his reporting. Other possible sources include the patient's medical record or a referral letter.

Chief Complaints, when possible in the patient's own words

Present Illness. This is a clear, chronological narrative account of the problems for which the patient is seeking care. It should include the onset of the problem, the setting in which it developed, its manifestations, its treatments, its impact upon the patient's life, and its meaning to the patient. The principal symptoms should be described in terms of their (1) location, (2) quality, (3) quantity or severity, (4) timing (*i.e.,* onset, duration, and frequency), (5) setting, (6) factors that have aggravated or relieved these symptoms, and (7) associated manifestations. Relevant data from the patient's chart, such as laboratory reports, also belong in the present illness, as do significant negatives (*i.e.,* the absence of certain symptoms that will aid in differential diagnosis).

Past Medical History

General State of Health

Childhood Illnesses, such as measles, rubella, mumps, whooping cough, chicken pox, rheumatic fever, scarlet fever, polio

Immunizations, such as tetanus, pertussis, diphtheria, polio, measles, rubella, mumps

Adult Illnesses

Psychiatric Illnesses

Operations

Injuries

Hospitalizations, not already described

Allergies

Current Medications, including home remedies, nonprescription drugs, and medicines borrowed from family or friends. When a patient seems likely to be taking one or more medications, survey one 24-hour period in detail: "Take yesterday, for example. Starting from when you woke up, what was the first medicine you took? How much? How often in the day did you take it? What are you taking it for? What other medicines . . .?"

Diet. Use a similar line of questioning: "Let's look at yesterday. Starting from when you woke up, what did you eat or drink first? . . . Then what? . . . And then?"

Sleep Patterns, including times that the person goes to bed and awakens, difficulties in falling asleep or staying asleep, and daytime naps

Habits, including exercise and the use of coffee, alcohol, other drugs, and tobacco

Family History

The age and health, or age and cause of death, of each immediate family member (*i.e.*, parents, siblings, spouse, and children). Data on grandparents or grandchildren may also be useful.

The occurrence within the family of any of the following conditions: diabetes, tuberculosis, heart disease, high blood pressure, stroke, kidney disease, cancer, arthritis, anemia, headaches, mental illness, or symptoms like those of the patient

Psychosocial History

This is an outline or narrative description that captures the important and relevant information about the patient as a person:

His lifestyle, home situation, significant others
A typical day—how he spends his time from when he gets up to when he goes to bed
Important experiences, including upbringing, schooling, military service, job history, financial situation, marriage, recreation, retirement

Religious beliefs relevant to perceptions of health, illness, and treatment

His view of the present and outlook for the future

Review of Systems

General. Usual weight, recent weight change, weakness, fatigue, fever

Skin. Rashes, lumps, itching, dryness, color change, changes in hair or nails

Head. Headache, head injury

Eyes. Vision, glasses or contact lenses, last eye examination, pain, redness, excessive tearing, double vision, glaucoma, cataracts

Ears. Hearing, tinnitus, vertigo, earaches, infection, discharge

Nose and Sinuses. Frequent colds, nasal stuffiness, hay fever, nosebleeds, sinus trouble

Mouth and Throat. Condition of teeth and gums, bleeding gums, last dental examination, sore tongue, frequent sore throats, hoarseness

Neck. Lumps in neck, "swollen glands," goiter, pain in the neck

Breasts. Lumps, pain, nipple discharge, self-examination

Respiratory. Cough, sputum (color, quantity), hemoptysis, wheezing, asthma, bronchitis, emphysema, pneumonia, tuberculosis, pleurisy, tuberculin test; last chest x-ray film

Cardiac. Heart trouble, high blood pressure, rheumatic fever, heart murmurs; dyspnea, orthopnea, paroxysmal nocturnal dyspnea, edema; chest pain, palpitations; past electrocardiogram or other heart tests

Gastrointestinal. Trouble swallowing, heartburn, appetite, nausea, vomiting, vomiting of blood, indigestion, frequency of bowel movements, change in bowel habits, rectal bleeding or black tarry stools, constipation, diarrhea; abdominal pain, food intolerance, excessive belching or passing of gas, hemorrhoids; jaundice, liver or gall bladder trouble, hepatitis

Urinary. Frequency of urination, polyuria, nocturia, dysuria, hematuria, urgency, hesitancy, incontinence; urinary infections, stones

Genito-reproductive
Male. Discharge from or sores on penis, history of venereal disease and its treatment, hernias, testicular pain or masses; frequency of intercourse, libido, sexual difficulties
Female. Age at menarche; regularity, frequency, and duration of periods;

amount of bleeding, bleeding between periods or after intercourse, last menstrual period; dysmenorrhea; age of menopause, menopausal symptoms, post-menopausal bleeding. Discharge, itching, venereal disease and its treatment; last Pap smear. Number of pregnancies, number of deliveries, number of abortions (spontaneous and induced); complications of pregnancy; birth control methods; frequency of intercourse, libido, sexual difficulties

Musculoskeletal. Joint pains or stiffness, arthritis, gout, backache. If present, describe location and symptoms (for example, swelling, redness, pain, stiffness, weakness, limitation of motion or activity). Muscle pains or cramps

Peripheral Vascular. Intermittent claudication, cramps, varicose veins, thrombophlebitis

Neurologic. Fainting, blackouts, seizures, paralysis, local weakness, numbness, tingling, tremors, memory

Psychiatric. Nervousness, tension, mood, depression

Endocrine. Thyroid trouble, heat or cold intolerance, excessive sweating, diabetes, excessive thirst, hunger, or urination

Hematologic. Anemia, easy bruising or bleeding, past transfusions and possible reactions

COMPREHENSIVE HISTORY: CHILD PATIENT

In addition to the obvious age-related differences between histories obtained on children and adults, there are present and past historical data specifically pertinent to the assessment of infants, children, and adolescents. These relate particularly to the patient's chronological age and stage of development. The child's history, then, follows the same outline as the adult's history, with certain additions which are presented here.

Identifying Data. Date of birth for patients less than 3 years of age. Nickname, particularly for those between 2 and 10 years of age. First names of parents (and last name of each, if different) and where they may be reached during work hours

Chief Complaints. It should be made clear whether these are concerns of the patient, the parent(s), or both. In some instances it may be a third party, such as a schoolteacher, who has expressed concerns about the child.

Present Illness. Should include how each member of the family responds to the patient's symptoms, their concerns about them, and whether the patient achieves any secondary gains from the illness

Past Medical History

Birth History. Particularly important during the first 2 years of life and for neurological and developmental problems. Hospital records should be reviewed if preliminary information from the parent(s) indicates significant difficulties before, during, or after delivery.

Prenatal. Maternal health before and during pregnancy, including nutrition and specific illnesses related to or complicated by pregnancy; doses and duration of all drugs taken during pregnancy; weight gain; vaginal bleeding; duration of pregnancy; parental attitudes concerning the pregnancy and parenthood in general and for this child in particular

Natal. Nature of labor and delivery, including degree of difficulty, analgesia used, and complications encountered; birth order if a multiple birth; birth weight

Neonatal. Onset of respirations; resuscitation efforts; Apgar scores (see pp. 449–450) and estimation of gestational age; specific problems with feeding, respiratory distress, cyanosis, jaundice, anemia, convulsions, congenital anomalies, or infection; mother's health postpartum; separation of mother and infant and reasons for; initial maternal reaction to her baby and the nature of bonding; patterns of crying and sleeping, and of urination and defecation

Feeding History. Particularly important during the first 2 years of life and in dealing with problems of under- and overnutrition

Infancy. *Breast feeding*—frequency and duration of feeds, use of complementary or supplementary artificial feedings, difficulties encountered, timing and method of weaning. *Artificial feeding*—type, concentration, amount, and frequency of feeds, difficulties (regurgitation, colic, diarrhea) encountered, timing and method of weaning. *Vitamin and iron supplements*—type, amount given, frequency, and duration. *Solid foods*—types and amounts of baby foods given, when introduced, infant's response, introduction of junior and table foods, self-feeding, maternal and infant responses to feeding process

Childhood. *Eating habits*—likes and dislikes, specific types and amounts of food eaten, parental attitudes toward eating in general and toward this child's under- or overeating, parental response to feeding problems (if present). A *diet diary* kept over a 7- to 14-day period may be required for an accurate assessment of food intake in childhood feeding problems.

Growth and Developmental History. Particularly important during infancy and childhood and in dealing with problems of delayed physical growth, psychomotor and intellectual retardation, and behavioral disturbances

Physical Growth. Actual (or approximate) weight and height at birth and at 1, 2, 5, and 10 years; history of any slow or rapid gains or losses; tooth eruption and loss pattern

Developmental Milestones. Ages at which patient held up head while in a prone position, rolled over from front to back and back to front, sat with support and alone, stood with support and alone, walked with support and alone, said first word, combinations of words, and sentences, tied own shoes, dressed without help

Social Development. *Sleep*—amount and patterns during day and at night; bedtime routines; type of bed and its location; nightmares, terrors, and somnambulation. *Toileting*—methods of training used, when bladder and bowel control attained, occurrence of accidents or of enuresis or encopresis, parental attitudes, terms used within the family for urination and defecation (important to know when a young child is admitted to hospital). *Speech*—hesitation, stuttering, baby talk, lisping, estimate of number of words in vocabulary. *Habits*—bed rocking, head banging, tics, thumb sucking, nailbiting, pica, ritualistic behavior. *Discipline*—parental assessment of child's temperament and response to discipline; methods used, success or failure, negativism, temper tantrums, withdrawal, aggressive behavior. *Schooling*—experience with day care, nursery school, and kindergarten; age and adjustment upon entry; current parental and child satisfaction; academic achievement; school's concerns. *Sexuality*—relations with members of opposite sex; inquisitiveness regarding conception, pregnancy, and girl–boy differences; parental responses to child's questions and the sex education they have offered regarding masturbation, menstruation, nocturnal emissions, development of secondary sexual characteristics, and sexual urges; dating patterns. *Personality*—degree of independence, relationship with parents, siblings, and peers; group and independent activities and interests; congeniality; special friends (real or imaginary); major assets and skills; self-image

Childhood Illnesses. Specific illnesses experienced, such as measles, chicken pox, or mumps. Mention of any recent exposures to childhood illnesses should be made here.

Immunizations. Specific dates of administration of each vaccine should be recorded so that an ongoing booster program can be maintained throughout childhood and adolescence. Any untoward reactions to specific vaccines should also be recorded.

Screening Procedures. The dates and results of any screening tests performed should be recorded. For example, vision, hearing, tuberculin, urinalysis, hematocrit, sickle cell, blood lead, phenylketonuria, galactosemia and other genetic–metabolic disorders, alpha$_1$-antitrypsin deficiency, and others that may be indicated for certain high-risk populations

Operations
Injuries } The reactions of the child and his parents to these
Hospitalizations } events should be ascertained.

Allergies. Particular attention should be given to those allergies that are more prevalent during infancy and childhood—eczema, urticaria, perennial allergic rhinitis, and insect hypersensitivity.

Family History. The education attained, job history, emotional health, and family background of each parent or parent substitute; the family socioeconomic circumstances, including income, type of dwelling, and neighborhood in which the family lives; parental work schedules; family cohesiveness and interdependence; support available from relatives, friends, and neighbors; the ethnic and cultural milieu in which the family lives; parental expectations of the patient and attitudes toward him in relation to his siblings. (All or portions of this information may be recorded in the present illness section, if pertinent to it, or under psychosocial history.) Consanguinity of the parents should be ascertained (by inquiring if they are "related by blood").

Some patients may not need a comprehensive evaluation or you may lack the time to do one. Under these circumstances you should obtain a short history appropriate to a *limited* visit. In addition to the routine identifying data, a history of the present illness is usually all that is indicated. You must remain alert, however, to the need for a somewhat broader line of inquiry. When seeing a patient with an acute sore throat, for example, you may need to inquire about similar illnesses in the family, past rheumatic fever, or possible penicillin allergy.

Still another pattern of history is appropriate to a *follow-up* visit. Here you need to find out how the patient thinks he is doing, how his symptoms have changed, what he understands about his condition and treatment, and what therapeutic measures he has taken or perhaps not taken.

You can enhance your understanding of the patient's concerns on any visit if you keep in mind three questions: *why he has come* ("I have a pain in my stomach"), *what is worrying him* ("I think I may have appendicitis"), and *why that is a worry* ("My Uncle Charlie died of a ruptured appendix"). The answers to these questions must be determined directly or indirectly at some point during the visit, since the patient is not likely to be satisfied if they are not addressed. Patients often need to know what they do *not* have as much as or more than what they *do* have, especially if they believe they may be suffering from a serious or potentially fatal disease.

Once you know what information to get, it is time, paradoxically, to lay that knowledge temporarily aside lest it come between you and the patient, for the course of the interview should be guided primarily by what the patient says and does. At least at the start you should be following his cues, not the printed form.

SETTING THE STAGE FOR THE INTERVIEW

Reviewing the Chart. Before seeing the patient, quickly review his chart. Note the identifying data. His age, sex, race, marital status, address, occupation, and religion give you important glimpses into his likely life experiences and may even guide your diagnostic hypotheses. If the patient has been referred from elsewhere, you should know both the source and goals of referral. Reviewing the medical chart will give you invaluable information about past diagnoses and treatments, although it should not prevent you from developing new approaches or ideas. In a complex medical setting this review might even remind you that you have seen the patient before and help to avoid an awkward interaction.

The Environment. Although you may have to talk with the patient under difficult circumstances—for example, in a four-bed room or in the corridor of a busy emergency department—a proper environment will improve communication. Your relationship with the patient may begin with his first telephone call to clinic or office. If the response projects courtesy, interest, and a desire to be helpful, if he can be seen reasonably promptly, if you are punctual for his appointment, you are setting the stage for a trusting relationship.

These early stages in the patient–clinician communication, including the proper use of names and titles, are the critical determinants of the patient's "reflexive self-concept" (what he thinks you think of him). If this is high, the patient is more likely to be satisfied and more likely to be compliant with your diagnostic and therapeutic recommendations. If it is low, it may not matter what you say or do later in the visit in terms of gaining the patient's trust and cooperation.

The environment itself tells the patient something about your interest in him. Is it quiet? Does it afford privacy? Are you free from interruptions? There should be places where both you and the patient can sit down in clear view of each other, preferably at eye level. Leaning against the far wall, inching toward the door, or shifting around uncomfortably from foot to foot discourage the patient's attempts at communication. So do arrangements that indicate inequality of power or even disrespect, such as greeting and interviewing a woman while she is lying supine, positioned for a pelvic examination.

Your distance from the patient should probably be several feet, not so close as to be uncomfortably intimate nor too distant for easy conversation. Patients may be able to talk with you more easily when sitting next to your desk, rather than peering over it as if over a barrier. When patients prefer greater social distance they are telling you something about themselves, psychologically or perhaps culturally. Lighting also makes a difference. Beware of sitting between the patient and a bright light or window. Although you can see him well, he must squint uncomfortably toward your silhouette. You unwittingly conduct an interrogation, not a helping interview.

Finally, your clothing may also affect the ease with which you establish a relationship. There are few rules here except that you should be clean, reasonably neat, and dressed appropriately for the patients you wish to serve. Conservative dress and white coat, for example, are suitable for talking with most adults, whereas casual dress without uniform may be preferable when dealing with children or young people. You may feel that you should dress to express yourself rather than to respond to the wishes of others. You should be aware of the effects of your own appearance, however, and not blame the patient for adverse consequences. Compromises are usually possible.

APPROACH TO THE PRESENT ILLNESS

Greeting the Patient. You are now ready to approach the patient, greet him by name, and give him your undivided attention. Shake hands if you feel comfortable doing so. Unless you are talking with a child or adolescent or unless you already know the patient well, use the appropriate title—for example, Mr. O'Neill or Mrs. Washington. Use of first names or terms of endearment with unfamiliar adults, use of "Granny" for an aged woman or "Mother" for a child's parent, tend to depersonalize and demean. Introduce yourself by name. If there is any ambiguity in your role, such as your status as a student, explain your relation to the patient's care.

The Patient's Comfort. Be alert to the patient's comfort. In office or clinic, there should be a place for his coat and belongings other than his own lap. In the hospital inquire how the patient is feeling and whether it is convenient for him to see you now. Watch for signs of discomfort such as poor positioning, evidence of pain or anxiety, or the need to urinate. An improved position in bed or a short delay so that he can say goodbye to his family or make a trip to the bathroom may be the shortest route to a good history.

Opening Questions. Now you are ready to find out why the patient is here—his chief complaints, if any, and the present illness. (Occasionally a patient may come for a checkup or may wish to discuss a health-related matter without having either complaint or illness.) Begin your interview with a general question that allows full freedom of response—for example, "What brings you here?" or "What seems to be the trouble?" After he answers, inquire again, or even several times, "Anything else?" When he has finished, encourage him to amplify by saying, "Tell me about it," or, if there seems to be more than one problem, ask about one of them: "Tell me about the headaches" or ". . . about what bothers you most." As he answers, pick up the thread of his history and follow wherever it leads.

Following the Patient's Leads. Not all histories are complicated. Many patients want help with relatively straightforward medical problems. Others, however, have illnesses with complex psychosocial and pathophysiologic causes; they have complicated feelings about themselves, their illnesses, potential treatments, and those who are trying to help them. At the start you cannot tell one kind of patient from another. In order to do so your interviewing technique must allow each patient to recount his own story spontaneously. If you intervene verbally too soon, if you ask specific questions prematurely, you risk trampling on the very evidence you are seeking. Your role, however, is not passive. You should listen actively and watch for clues to important symptoms, emotions, events, and relationships. You can then guide the patient into telling you more about these areas. Methods of helping and guiding the patient without diverting him from his own account include facilitation, reflection, clarification, empathic responses, confrontation, interpretation, and questions that elicit feelings. Your demeanor throughout is also important.

Facilitation. You use facilitation when by posture, actions, or words you encourage the patient to say more but do not specify his topic. Silence itself, when attentive yet relaxed, is facilitative. Leaning forward, making eye contact, saying "Mm-hmm" or "Go on" or "I'm listening," all help the patient to continue.

Reflection. Closely akin to facilitation is reflection, a repetition of the patient's words that encourages him to give you more details. Reflection may be useful in eliciting both facts and feelings, as in the following example:

Patient:	The pain got worse and began to spread. (Pause)
Response:	It spread?
Patient:	Yes, it went to my shoulder and down my left arm to the fingers. It was so bad that I thought I was going to die. (Pause)
Response:	You thought you were going to die?
Patient:	Yes. It was just like the pain my father had when he had his heart attack, and I was afraid the same thing was happening to me.

Here a reflective technique has helped to discover not only the location and severity of the patient's pain, but also its meaning to the patient. There was no risk of biasing the patient's story or interrupting his train of thought.

Clarification. Sometimes the patient's words are ambiguous or his associations are unclear. If you are to understand what he is saying, you must request clarification. For example, "Tell me what you meant by a 'cold'," or "You said you were behaving just like your mother. What did you mean?"

Empathic Responses. As a patient talks with you, he may express—with or without words—feelings about which he is embarrassed, ashamed, or otherwise reticent. These feelings may well be crucial to understanding his illness or planning treatment. If you can recognize and respond to them in a way that shows understanding and acceptance, you show empathy for the patient, make him feel more secure, and encourage him to continue. Empathic responses may be as simple as "I understand." Other examples include, "You must have been very upset," or "That must have been very depressing for you." Empathic responses may also be nonverbal—for example, offering a tissue to a crying patient or gently placing your hand on his arm to convey understanding. In using an empathic response, be sure that you are responding correctly to what the patient has already expressed. If you have acknowledged how upset a patient must have been at the death of a parent, when in fact he was relieved to be freed from a long-standing financial and emotional burden, you have seriously misunderstood your patient and probably blocked further communication on the subject.

Confrontation. While an empathic response acknowledges expressed feelings, confrontation points out to the patient something about his own words or behavior. If you observe clues of anger, anxiety, or depression, for example, confrontation may help to bring these feelings out in the open: "Your hands are trembling whenever you talk about that," or "You say you don't care but there are tears in your eyes." Confrontation may also be useful when the patient's story has been inconsistent: "You say you don't know what brings on your stomach pains; yet whenever you've had them, you were feeling picked on."

Interpretation. Interpretation goes a step beyond confrontation. Here you make an inference, rather than a simple observation: "Nothing has been right for you today. You seem fed up with the hospital." "You are asking a lot of questions about the x-rays. Are you worried about them?" In interpreting a patient's words or behavior, you take some risk of making the wrong inference and impeding further communication. When used wisely, however, an interpretation can both demonstrate empathy and increase understanding.

Asking about Feelings. Rather than making an inference or reflecting a feeling, you may simply ask the patient how he feels, or felt, about something such as his symptoms or an event. Unless you let him know that you are interested in his feelings as well as in facts, he may withhold them and you may miss important insights.

Your General Demeanor. Just as you have been observing the patient throughout the early portions of the interview, so too has he been watching you. Consciously or not, you have been sending him messages through both your words and your behavior. You should be sensitive to those messages and control them insofar as you can. Posture, gestures, eye contact, and words can all express interest, attention, acceptance, and understanding. The skilled interviewer seems calm and unhurried, even when his time is limited. Reactions that betray disgust, disapproval, embarrassment, impatience, or boredom block communication, as do behaviors that condescend, stereotype, or make sport of the patient. Although negative reactions such as these are normal and often quite understandable, they should not be expressed. Guard against them not only when talking with the patient but also when discussing the patient with your colleagues or instructors, either at the bedside or in the hall.

Beginning practitioners may have special problems in dealing with their own limited knowledge; all practitioners confront this problem at least occasionally. When you do not know the answer to a patient's direct question, it is usually best to be honest about it and say so, but also add that you will try to find out the answer. Clearly acknowledging your status as a student may help you out of otherwise awkward situations.

Direct Questions. Using the nondirective techniques described thus far, you will usually be able to obtain a general idea of the patient's principal problems. You can encourage a chronologic account by such questions as "What then?" or "What happened next?" Most of the time, however, you will need further specific information. Fill in the details with direct questions. If the patient's present illness involves pain, for example, you must determine the following: (1) Its location. Where is it? Does it radiate? (2) Its quality. What is it like? (3) Its quantity or severity. How bad is it? (4) Its timing. When did it start? How long does it last? How often does it come? (5) The setting in which it occurs. (6) Factors that make it better or worse. (7) Associated manifestations. Most other symptoms can be described in the same terms.

Several principles apply to the use of direct questions. They should *proceed from the general to the specific.* A possible sequence, for example, might be "What was your chest pain like? . . . Where did you feel it? . . . Show me. . . . Did it stay right there or did it travel anywhere? . . . To which fingers?"

Direct questions *should not be leading questions.* If a patient says "yes" to "Did your stools look like tar?" you must always wonder if the description is his or yours. A better wording is "What color were your stools?" Leading questions often give misleading answers. A classic example, "Is everything all right at home?"

When possible, ask questions that *require a graded response* rather than a yes or no answer. "How many stairs can you climb before stopping for breath?" is better than "Do you get short of breath climbing stairs?"

Sometimes patients seem quite unable to describe their symptoms without help. To minimize bias here, *offer multiple choice answers:* "Is your pain aching, sharp, pressing, burning, shooting, or what?" Almost any specific question can have at least two choices: "Do you bring up any phlegm with your cough, or not?"

Ask one question at a time. "Any tuberculosis, pleurisy, asthma, bronchitis, pneumonia?" may lead to a negative answer out of sheer confusion.

Finally, *use language that is understandable and appropriate* to the patient. Although you might ask a trained health professional about dyspnea, the more customary term is shortness of breath. When talking with an Appalachian coal miner, on the other hand, it may help to use the colloquial "smothering spells." Words in the history outlines are not intended for verbatim use. They need appropriate translations.

THE REST OF THE STORY

By now you should be able to synthesize a chronologic narrative of the patient's illness, using both his spontaneous account and his answers to direct questions. You are ready to proceed to past medical history, family history, psychosocial history, and the review of systems. Except in the psychosocial history, specific questions will constitute your major technique. Stay alert, however, for important medical or emotional material, and be prepared to revert to a nondirective style whenever indicated. While taking a family history, for example, you may learn of a parent's death or a child's illness. Here is a good opportunity to find out what it meant to the patient. "How was it for you then?" or "What were your feelings at the time?" The review of systems may also uncover material that requires as full an exploration as the present illness. Keep your technique flexible.

Two sections of history beyond the present illness seem particularly troublesome to many interviewers: the psychosocial and the sexual histories. These are discussed in somewhat more detail.

Psychosocial History. Earlier in the interview the patient may already have told you much of his psychosocial history. Some further clues, as yet unexplored, can be followed now. Try to use words or ideas that the patient himself has expressed before. At times you may still know relatively little about the patient and will be entering new territory. Open-ended questions can give you some leads. You should vary these questions, of course, according to the patient's age and life situation.

> Who lives at home with you?
> What is a typical day like?
> Where were you born? . . . raised? What was your childhood like?
> How is it going for you in school?
> What is your job like?
> What do you think of your boss?
> How is your financial situation? How much money do you have coming in now? How about expenses? Do you have any problems with your medical bills? . . . Any insurance? . . . Medicare? . . . Medicaid?
> What do you do for recreation or fun?
> What do you think about retirement?
> What do you see for yourself in the future?

Sexual History. Like other parts of the history, a sexual history should be obtained where it seems most relevant, perhaps in the present illness or psychosocial history but most probably in the review of systems. Because of our social taboos, both practitioner and patient may find this difficult. With a female patient, questions about sexual function follow naturally after the menstrual and obstetrical histories. Here are some useful questions to open the discussion:

> Are you having sex, or intercourse, now?
> About how often?
> Is that more or less often than in previous years?
> How often do you reach a climax (or have an orgasm)?
> Do you have any pain or discomfort during intercourse?
> Has your interest in sex changed recently?
> How satisfied are you with your sex life as it is now?
> How satisfied do you think your partner is (or, your partners are)?

For male patients, here is a similar group of questions, which logically follow the urinary history:

> Are you having intercourse now?
> About how often?
> Is that more or less often than in previous years?
> Do you have any trouble getting an erection?
> Do you have any trouble coming (ejaculating) too soon?
> Has your interest in sex changed recently?
> How satisfied are you with your sex life as it is now?
> How satisfied do you think your partner is (or, your partners are)?

Note the use of the term "partner(s)" here. It assumes neither a marital nor a heterosexual relationship and leaves other kinds of relationships open for possible discussion.

The possible impact of a person's present illness on his or her sex life offers another valuable and natural line of inquiry. When a person has shortness of breath, chest pain, back pain, fatigue, an unsightly skin rash, or indeed almost any other symptom of consequence, it can influence his sexual function and pleasure. Ask about it just as you would ask about the effects of illness on a person's ability to work or participate in social activities: "Does the pain affect your sex life?" Or, better, "In what ways does the pain affect your sex life?"

When approaching a sexual history, it may be helpful to make some introductory remarks that let the patient know that his experiences, feelings, or problems are common, not rare, wrong, or bizarre. For example,

> Many teenagers are trying to figure out whether they should use
> birth control or when they should have sex. What are your
> thoughts about these things?
> Most young people know that they can get VD but don't know
> what it's like or what to do about it. What has your experience
> been?

Not only may questions about sexual function give you important diagnostic insights; they also let patients know that they can discuss these problems with you in the future. Although patients are occasionally unwilling to talk about this subject (and should not be pushed), most are willing and some quite relieved. As in other parts of the history, your demeanor is important: calm, unembarrassed, yet sensitive. Use words that the patient can understand, preferably his or her own, as long as both of you know what they mean. Further reading, discussion, and interviewing experience will help you improve your skills and confidence in this area.

Transitions. As you move from one part of the history to another, it helps to orient the patient with brief transitional phrases: "Now I'd like to ask some questions about your past health," or ". . . about your family's health."

Closing. After you have completed your questions, return the initiative briefly to the patient: "Is there anything else we should talk about?" or "Have we omitted anything?" You may want to recapitulate part of the present illness to be sure of a common understanding. Finally, make clear to the patient what he is to do or what he is to expect next. "I will step out for a few minutes. Please get completely undressed and put on this gown. I would like to examine you."

Note-taking. Since no one can remember all the details of a comprehensive history, you need to take notes. Most patients are accustomed to note-taking but some may seem uncomfortable with it. If so, explore their concerns and explain your desire to make an accurate record. With practice you may be able to record most of the past medical history, family history, and review of systems in final form as you talk with the patient, especially if you have the help of a written questionnaire. Note-taking should not divert your attention from the patient, however, nor should a written form prevent you from following a patient's leads. While eliciting the present illness, the psychosocial history, or other complex portions of the patient's account, do not attempt to write your final report. Instead, jot down short phrases, words, dates, and so forth, that will aid your memory later. When the patient is talking about sensitive or disturbing material, it is best not to take notes at all.

PATIENTS AT DIFFERENT AGES

As people develop, have families, and age, they provide you with special opportunities and require certain adaptations in your interviewing style.

Talking with Parents. In obtaining histories on infants and children, for example, you gather all or at least part of your information from a third party, the parent(s) or legal guardian. Children under 5 years of age usually add no relevant historical data. As children grow older, however, you can get information of increasing value and reliability by interviewing them directly. Special ways of enhancing your interviews with children and adolescents are described in subsequent sections. This section deals with parents. Here your techniques are basically the same as in interviewing adult patients, with some special modifications.

Parents, of course, are speaking about their children and describing what they have observed as well as what they perceive to be their child's symptoms. Although these observations and perceptions can generally be considered accurate, they are subject to parental biases and needs. This is especially the case with the mother who, in our society, is usually responsible for the immediate care of the children. A mother includes her ability to keep her children well as part of her concept of adequate mothering. When you ask her questions concerning her child's health or ill health, you are in a sense testing her capabilities as a mother. Her responses to those questions may be accordingly biased. Mothers need health practitioners who are supportive rather than judgmental or critical. Comments like, "You mean you *didn't* give him aspirin for the fever?" "Why didn't you bring him in sooner?" or "Why, in heaven's name, did you do that?" will not improve your rapport with a worried and distraught mother whose infant or child is acutely ill.

Refer to the infant or child by his name rather than "him" or "the baby." When the mother's marital status is not immediately clear, you may avoid embarrassment in asking about the father by saying, "Is Jane's father in good health?" rather than, "Is your husband in good health?" Address the parents as "Mr. or Mrs. Smith" rather than by their first names or, heaven forbid, "Mother" or "Father." First names may be used with permission when you have established a reasonably longstanding relationship. You should be prepared, however, for the parent who calls you by your first name.

In interviewing parents, open-ended questions are usually more productive than direct questions. In the realm of psychosocial issues and problems, however, you must more often than not use explicit direct questions, since mothers rarely introduce these subjects spontaneously, even when given the opportunity with open-ended approaches. This may be especially likely for mothers of lower socioeconomic status.

Finally, you need to recognize that the chief complaint may not relate at all to the apparent reason the mother has brought the child to see you. The complaint may serve as a "ticket of admission" to care, through which, if the circumstances are right, she may bring up another concern that, by itself, is not viewed as a "legitimate" reason for seeking care. Try to create an atmosphere that will allow the mother to express all of her concerns. If necessary, ask questions that will allow easier expression of those concerns.

Are there any other problems with Johnny that you would like to tell me about?

What did you hope that I would be able to do for you when you came today?

Is there anything special you would like me to explain to you about Jody?

Is there anything else bothering you about the other children, your husband, or yourself that you'd like to talk about?

Talking with Children. For the most part, pediatric practitioners conduct interviews with both the parent and the child present. This is a matter of convenience that presents some disadvantages as well as some distinct advantages. The history you obtain in the child's presence may be less accurate and couched in more limited terms than when you interview the parent(s) alone. When sensitive areas are not fully explored because the child is present, you will need to interview the parent at a later time (often at the end of the visit when the child has left the room) to clarify certain points or to fill in missing data.

The interview with the child present offers an opportunity to observe parent–child interactions and the child's ability to amuse himself while his mother is engaged in conversation. These observations may provide a clearer picture of the relationship between mother and child (or, if the father is present, father and child and the parents themselves) than can the answers to any number of questions.

For the younger child, this interlude may help to dispel fears of the practitioner or of the visit and allow for a smooth transition from the interview to the examination.

The older child will be able to add significantly to his history and can describe more accurately the severity of his symptoms and his level of concern regarding them. You can sometimes improve the accuracy of your information by interviewing the child without the parent.

Take care to avoid "talking down" to children, for they are sensitive to affectations of speech and condescending behaviors.

Talking with Adolescents. Many adults find talking with an adolescent difficult and frustrating because the adolescent often does not answer questions in an "adult" manner and may appear laconic and disdainful. This need not be the case. The adolescent, like most other people, will usually respond positively to anyone who demonstrates a genuine interest in him, not as a "case" but as a person. That interest must be established early and sustained if communication is to be effective. Adolescents tend to "open up" when the focus of the interview is on themselves and not on their problems. Thus, a good way to begin the interview with an adolescent is to chat informally about his friends, school, hobbies, and family.

Adolescents seek health care on their own initiative or at the suggestion or insistence of their parents. They may come alone or with at least one parent. In the latter case, it is best to explain to both parent and adolescent that health care at this stage of one's individual development requires some degree of confidentiality. This requires speaking to the adolescent alone after obtaining past medical and social information from the parent(s). A confidential relationship is not based on "keeping secrets"; it is based on mutual respect. If it becomes necessary for the adolescent's own sake or for the sake of others to share confidential information, it is important to include the adolescent in that process.

In a preceding section of this chapter, certain techniques of promoting good communication are discussed. For the adolescent, some of these approaches may be threatening. Reflection is a technique that should be avoided with the younger, cognitively immature adolescent, since it requires thinking skills that he has not yet acquired. The use of silence in an attempt to get the patient to talk is rarely successful with adolescents, who usually do not have sufficient self-assurance to respond appropriately to this form of facilitation. Confrontation, rather than "bringing feelings out in the open," may cause an anxious adolescent to retreat into silence. Closely related to this is the technique of asking about feelings. Adolescents often find discussing their feelings with adults very difficult.

These caveats need not deter you from talking with adolescents. Most adolescents will talk to someone they respect and accept when given the opportunity in a friendly, informal atmosphere. Acceptance is more likely for the professional who "plays it straight," acts his age, and does not stretch too far in trying to bridge the generation gap.

Aging Patients. At the other end of the life cycle, aging patients also pose special opportunities and special problems. They face relatively high risks for a number of conditions, such as decreased vision and hearing, memory loss, and depression. They often have chronic illness, with its associated discomforts and difficulties in getting about, and have usually experienced important losses including the deaths of family members or friends and diminutions in vigor, physical attractiveness, status, power, or income. Be especially alert for problems such as these, but be sure not to stereotype the aging patient. Many older persons adapt well to change, continue to grow and learn, and maintain a high morale.

From middle age on people become increasingly aware of their personal aging and begin to measure their lives in terms of the years left rather than the years lived. It is normal for older people to reminisce about the past and to reflect upon previous experience, including its joys, regrets, and conflicts. Listening to this process of life review can give you important insights into a person and may help him work through some of his painful feelings.

Try to determine the patient's priorities and goals. Learn how he has handled crises. Since he may pursue similar adaptive patterns in the present situation, this knowledge will help you plan with him. Because aging patients have longer histories and may tell them more slowly, they often require extra time. Do not try to accomplish everything in one visit.

Many interviewers face special problems within themselves in relating to older patients. They may feel helpless in curing the ills of the aged, and their views toward aging people may be distorted by their own feelings toward parents and grandparents. They may fear their own old age and want to avoid reminders of it. Be alert to your own feelings.

SPECIAL PROBLEMS

Regardless of patient age, certain behaviors and special situations may particularly vex the practitioner.

Silence. Neophyte interviewers may grow uncomfortable during periods of silence, feeling somehow obligated to keep the conversation going. They need not feel so. Silences have many meanings and many uses. When recounting their present illnesses, patients frequently fall silent for short periods in order to collect their thoughts or remember details. An attentive silence on the interviewer's part is usually the best response here, sometimes followed by brief encouragement to continue. During periods of silence be particularly alert to nonverbal signs of distress. Patients may fall silent because they are having difficulty controlling their emotions. If so, these are almost invariably significant feelings that are best expressed. A gentle confrontation may help: "You seem to be having trouble talking about this." Depressed patients or those with organic brain syndrome may have lost their usual spontaneity of expression, give short answers to questions, and fall silent quickly after each one. If you sense one of these problems, shift your inquiry to an exploratory mental status examination (see pp. 431–446).

At times, a patient's silence results from interviewer error or insensitivity. Are you asking too many direct questions in rapid sequence? The patient may simply have yielded the initiative to you and taken the passive role he thinks you expect. Have you offended the patient in any way—for example, by signs of disapproval or criticism? Have you failed to recognize an overwhelming symptom such as pain, nausea, dyspnea, the need to urinate or defecate? If so, you may need to abbreviate the interview considerably or return after the patient has been relieved.

Overtalkative Patients. The garrulous, rambling patient may be just as difficult as the silent one, possibly more so. Faced with limited time and the perceived need to "get the whole story," the interviewer may grow impatient, even exasperated. Although there are no perfect solutions for this problem, several techniques are helpful. First, you may need to lower your own goals and accept less than a comprehensive history. It may be unobtainable. Second, give the patient free rein for the first 5 or 10 minutes of the interview. You will then have the chance to observe the patterns of his speech. Does he seem obsessively detailed or unduly anxious? Does he show a flight of ideas or the disorganized thought processes that suggest a psychotic disorder? Third, try to focus his account on what you judge to be most important. Show interest and ask questions in those areas. Facilitate sparingly. Interrupt if you must, but courteously. A brief summary may help you change the topic while letting the patient know that you have heard and understood him. "As I understand it, your chest pains come frequently, last a long time, and do not necessarily stay in any one place. Now tell me about your breathing." Finally, do not let your impatience show. If you have used up the allotted time or, more likely, gone over it, explain that to the patient and arrange for a second meeting. Setting a time limit for the next appointment may be helpful. "I know we have much more to talk about. Can you come again next week? We will have a full half hour then."

Patients with Multiple Symptoms. Some patients seem to have every symptom that you mention. They have an "essentially positive review of systems." Although it is conceivable that such a patient has multiple organic illnesses, it is much more likely that he has serious emotional problems. If so, it will profit little to explore each symptom in detail. Guide the interview into a psychosocial assessment instead.

Anxious Patients. Anxiety is a frequent and natural reaction to sickness, to therapy, and to the health-care system itself. For some patients anxiety has importantly colored their reactions to life stress and may have contributed to their illnesses. Be sensitive to nonverbal and verbal clues.

For example, an anxious patient may sit tensely, fidgeting with his fingers or clothes. He may sigh frequently, lick his dry lips, sweat more than average, or actually tremble. His carotid pulsations may betray a rapid heart rate. Some anxious patients fall silent, unable to speak freely or confide. Others try to cover their feelings with words, busily avoiding their own basic problems. When you sense an underlying anxiety, encourage the patient to talk about his feelings.

Reassurance. When you are talking with such a patient, it is tempting to reassure him: "Don't worry. Everything is going to be all right." This approach is usually counterproductive. Unless you and the patient have had a chance to explore fully what he is anxious about, you may well be reassuring him about the wrong thing. Moreover, premature reassurance blocks further communication. Since admitting anxiety exposes a weakness, it requires encouragement, not a coverup. The first step to effective reassurance involves identifying and accepting the patient's feelings. This helps him feel more secure. The final steps come much later in the health-care process, after you have completed the interview, the physical examination, and perhaps some laboratory studies. Then you can interpret for the patient what is happening and deal openly with his real concerns.

Anger and Hostility. Patients have reasons to be angry: they are ill, they have suffered loss, they lack their accustomed control over their own lives, they feel relatively powerless in the health-care system. They may direct this anger toward you. It is possible that you have justly earned their hostility. Were you late for your appointment, inconsiderate, insensitive, or angry yourself? If so, recognize the fact and try to make amends. More often, however, the patient is displacing his anger onto you as a symbol of all that is wrong. Allow him to get it off his chest. Accept his feelings without getting angry in return. Beware of joining the patient in his hostility toward another part of the clinic or hospital, even when you privately harbor similar feelings. After he has calmed down, you may be able to identify specific steps that will help in the future. Rational solutions to emotional problems are not always possible, however, and patients need time to resolve their angry feelings.

The Obstreperous Inebriate. Few patients can disrupt the clinic or emergency room more quickly than acutely intoxicated persons who are angry, belligerent, and uncontrolled. Before interviewing such a patient, it is wise to alert the security force of the hospital. In approaching the patient greet him by name and title, introduce yourself, and offer a handshake. In this situation it is especially important to accept the patient, not challenge him. To do this, avoid all but the briefest eye contact and keep your posture relaxed and nonthreatening, your hands loosely open rather than clenched into fists. Do not try to make the patient lower his voice or stop cursing at you or the staff, but listen carefully and try to understand what he is saying. Since some such persons feel trapped in small rooms, it is usually best to talk with them in an open area, and you are likely to feel more comfortable there, too. In addition, an offer of food, coffee, or a cigarette may help to quiet the agitated person and bring some calm to the stormy scene.

Crying. Like anger, crying is an important clue to emotions. Rarely should it be suppressed. If the patient seems on the verge of tears, gentle confrontation or an empathic response may allow him to cry. Quiet acceptance is then appropriate. Offer a tissue; wait for recovery; perhaps make a facilitating or supportive remark: "It's good to get it out." Most of the time the patient will soon compose himself and, if properly accepted, will feel better and capable of continuing the discussion.

Depression. Masquerading as fatigue, weight loss, insomnia, or mysterious aches and pains, depression is one of the commonest problems in clinical medicine, and is commonly missed or ignored. Be alert for it, identify it, and explore its manifestations. Be sure you know how bad it is. Just as you would evaluate the severity of angina pectoris, you must evaluate the severity of depression. Both are potentially lethal. You need not fear that asking about suicide will suggest it to the patient. A sequence of questions is useful, continued as far as the patient's responses warrant.

Do you get pretty discouraged (or depressed or blue)?

How low do you feel?

What do you see for yourself in the future?

Do you ever feel that life isn't worth living? Or that you would just as soon be dead?

Have you ever thought of doing away with yourself?

How did (do) you think you would do it?

What would happen after you were dead?

Sexually Attractive or Seductive Patients. Practitioners of both sexes may occasionally find themselves attracted to their patients. If you become aware of such feelings, accept them as normal human responses but prevent them from affecting your behavior. Keep your relationship with the patient within professional bounds.

Occasionally patients may be frankly seductive or may make sexual advances. Calmly, but firmly, you should make clear that your relationship is professional, not personal. You may also wish to review your own image. Have you been overly warm with the patient? expressed your affection physically? sought his or her emotional support? Has your dress or demeanor been unconsciously seductive? Avoid this problem when you can.

Confusing Behaviors or Histories. At times you may find yourself baffled, frustrated, and confused in your interaction with the patient. His history is vague and difficult to understand; his ideas poorly related to one another; his language hard to follow. Even though you word your questions carefully, you seem unable to get clear answers. His manner of relating to you may also seem peculiar: distant, aloof, inappropriate, or bizarre. Symptoms may be described in bizarre terms: "My fingernails feel too heavy," or "My stomach knots up like a snake." These characteristics should alert you to possible mental illnesses, such as schizophrenia. With the usual nondirective techniques you may be able to get more information about the unusual qualities of the symptoms. You should also include in your interview an assessment of the patient's mental status, with special attention to mood, thought, and perceptions (see pp. 432–434).

Since drug therapy for schizophrenia and other psychotic disorders has become prevalent, many psychotic patients are functioning, with varying degrees of success, in the community. Such patients are frequently capable of telling you freely about their diagnosis, their symptoms, their hospitalizations, and their current medications. You should feel comfortable inquiring about these without embarrassment or circumlocution.

Schizophrenia is not the only cause of confusing histories. Some patients have underlying disorders of cognitive function—disorders generally classified as organic brain syndromes, such as delirium or dementia. Be particularly alert for delirium when dealing with an acutely ill or intoxicated patient, for dementia when dealing with an elderly patient. These patients may be unable to give clear histories. They are vague and inconsistent about symptoms or events and unable to report when and how things happened. They may be inattentive to your questions and hesitant in their answers. Occasionally such a patient may confabulate, that is, make up part of his history in order to fill in the gaps in his memory. When you suspect an organic brain syndrome, do not spend too much time trying to get a detailed history. You will only tire and frustrate the patient. Switch your inquiry instead to an evaluation of his mental status, checking particularly on level of consciousness, orientation, and memory (see pp. 431, 434–435). You can work the initial questions smoothly into the interview. "When was your last appointment in the clinic? . . . Let's see, then, that was about how long ago?" "Your address now is? . . . And your phone number?" Responses can all be checked against the chart (presuming, of course, that the chart is accurate).

Patients with Limited Intelligence. Patients of moderately limited intelligence can usually give adequate histories. You may, in fact, overlook their limitations and thereby make mistakes, such as omitting their dysfunction from a disability evaluation or giving instructions they cannot understand. If you suspect such a problem, pay special attention to the patient's schooling. How far did he go in school? Why did he drop out? How was he doing at the time? What kinds of courses is (was) he taking? High school seniors of normal intelligence are not usually taking simple arithmetic. If your patient is, you can make a smooth transition into a mental status examination, including simple calculations, vocabulary, information, and tests of abstract reasoning (see pp. 436–437).

When patients suffer from severe mental retardation, you will have to obtain their history from family or friends. By showing interest in the patient himself, however, and by engaging him in simple conversation, try to establish a personal relationship.

Literacy. Although it is not synonymous with intelligence, literacy should sometimes be assessed, especially before giving written instructions. Some patients who cannot read because of a language barrier, learning disorder, or poor vision will admit it on direct questioning. Others, however, will deny it. You can check, as if testing their vision, by asking them to read some words or sentences for you.

Language Barriers. Nothing will more surely convince you that a history is essential than having to do without one. When you cannot communicate with your patient because you speak different languages, take every possible step to find a translator. A few broken words and gestures are no substitute. The ideal translator is a neutral, objective person who is familiar with both languages. When family members or friends try to help, they are more likely to distort meanings and may also present problems in confidentiality to both the patient and interviewer. Many translators try to speed the process by telescoping a long communication into a few words. Try to make clear at the beginning that you need the translator to translate, not to interpret or summarize. Make your questions clear and short. You can also help the translator by outlining the goals for each segment of your history.

When available, written bilingual questionnaires are invaluable, especially for the review of systems. Before using one, however, be sure the patient can read in his own language or can get help with it.

The Hearing-Impaired and Deaf Mute. Communicating with people who have impaired hearing or are totally deaf presents many of the same problems as does communicating with a patient who speaks a different language. Here, again, written questionnaires are a great help. Although very time-consuming, handwritten questions and answers may be the only solution. If a deaf mute patient knows sign language, make every effort to find a translator who speaks, hears, and can use it. If a patient has partial hearing impairment or can read lips, face him directly, in good light. Speak slowly and in a relatively low-pitched voice. Do not let your voice trail off at the ends of sentences, avoid covering your mouth, and use gestures to reinforce your words. If the patient has a "good" ear, arrange the seating to take advantage of it; if he has a hearing aid he should, of course, wear it. Supplement any oral instructions with writing.

Blind Patients. When talking with a blind patient, be especially careful to announce yourself and explain who and what you are. Taking his hand may help to establish contact and let him know where you are. If the room is unfamiliar to the patient, orient him to it, explain what is there and whether anyone else is present. Remember to respond vocally when he speaks, since facilitative postures and gestures will not work. At the same time guard against raising your voice unnecessarily.

Fatally Ill Patients. In communicating with fatally ill or dying patients, most interviewers face problems within themselves—their own discomforts, anxieties, and desires to avoid the subject or even avoid the patients themselves. With the help of reading and discussion, you will need to work through your own feelings. As in any clinical situation, it is helpful to know what reactions the patient is likely to have. Kübler-Ross has described five stages in a patient's response to his own impending death: denial and isolation, anger, bargaining, depression or preparatory grief, and acceptance. Regardless of the stage, your approach to the patient is basically the same. Be alert to the patient's feelings and to cues that he wants to talk about them. Help him to bring them out with nondirective techniques. Make openings for him to ask questions: "I wonder if you have any concerns about the operation? . . . your illness? . . . how it will be when you go home?" Explore these concerns and provide whatever information the patient is asking for. Be wary of inappropriate reassurance. If you can explore and accept the patient's feelings, if you can answer the patient's questions, if you can assure and demonstrate your ability to stay with the patient throughout his illness, reassurance will grow within the patient himself.

Fatally ill or dying patients rarely want to talk about their illness all the time, nor do they wish to confide in everyone they meet. Give such patients opportunities to talk, and listen receptively; but if the patient prefers to keep the conversation on a lighter plane, you need not feel like a failure. Remember that illness—even a terminal one—is only one small part of personhood. A smile, a touch, an inquiry after a family member, a comment on the day's ballgame, or even some gentle kidding all recognize and reinforce other parts of the patient's individuality and help to sustain the living person. To communicate appropriately you have to get to know the patient: that is part of the helping process.

Talking with Families or Friends. Some patients are totally unable to give their own histories. Others may be unable to describe parts of them such as their behavior during a convulsion. Under these circumstances you must try to find a third person from whom to get the story. At times, although you may think you have a reasonably comprehensive knowledge of the patient, other sources may offer surprising and important information. A spouse, for example, may report significant family strains, depressive symptoms, or drinking habits that the patient has denied. When you suspect such discrepancies, look for opportunities to get additional information from persons other than the patient.

When you decide to seek information from a third person, it is usually wise to get the patient's approval. Assure him that you will keep confidential what he has already told you, or get his permission to share certain information. Data from other persons must also be held in confidence.

The basic principles of interviewing apply to your conversations with relatives or friends. Find a private place to talk. Leaning against opposite sides of a hospital corridor is not conducive to good communication. Introduce yourself, state your purpose, inquire how the person is feeling under the circumstances, and recognize and acknowledge his concerns. As you listen to his version of the history, be alert for clues as to the quality of his relationship with the patient. These may color his credibility or give you helpful ideas in planning the patient's care.

Responding to Patients' Questions. Patients' questions may seek simple factual information. More often, however, they express feelings or concerns. Try to elicit these feelings or delve further, lest you offer a misguided answer.

Patient:	What are the effects of this blood pressure medicine?
Response:	There are several effects. Why do you ask?
Patient:	(Pause) Well, I was reading up on it in a friend's book. I read it could make me impotent.

Similar caution is indicated when patients seek advice for personal problems. Should the patient quit a stressful job, for example, or move to Arizona, or have an abortion? Before responding, find out what approaches he or she has considered, what pros and cons there might be to the possible solutions. A chance to talk through the problem with you is usually much more valuable than any possible answer you could give.

Finally, when the patient is asking for specific information about his diagnosis, progress, or treatment plan, answer when you can but be careful that your responses do not conflict with those provided by others. When you are unsure of the answer, offer to find out if you can. Alternatively, you can tell the patient that he should ask Dr. X because Dr. X knows more about his case or is making that decision. Beware, however, of using this approach to avoid a difficult issue. If you carry the primary patient responsibility yourself, share your opinions and plans and the patient's prognosis with other members of the health team so that each in turn can communicate with the patient effectively.

A FINAL NOTE

This chapter is intended as a guide—to the information you need, to the ways of obtaining it, and to the methods of establishing effective relationships with your patients. Its suggestions are not intended to be iron-clad rules fettering your every move or question. In the last analysis you are a sensitive, aware human being interacting with and trying to help another.

Chapter 2
PHYSICAL EXAMINATION: APPROACH AND OVERVIEW

Most patients view a physical examination with at least some anxiety. They feel vulnerable, physically exposed, apprehensive about possible pain, and uneasy over what the clinician may find. At the same time, they often appreciate detailed concern for their problems and may even enjoy the attention they receive.

Mindful of such feelings, the skillful clinician is thorough without wasting time, systematic without being rigid, gentle yet not afraid to cause discomfort if this should be required. By listening, looking, touch, and smell, the skillful clinician examines each body part and at the same time senses the whole patient, notes the wince or worried glance, and calms, explains, and reassures.

Early in their experience, students, like patients, are apprehensive—uncertain in their ambiguous roles as student-professionals and uneasy with their newfledged competencies. This stage of anxiety is unavoidable. With study, repetitive practice, and time, however, both competence and confidence grow. As a beginning student, you will make notable gains within a few weeks; continuing progress should be a lifetime goal.

Despite inevitable insecurities as you begin to examine patients, you should take command of your own demeanor and affect. Try to look calm, organized, and competent, even when you do not exactly feel that way. If you forget a portion of your examination, as you undoubtedly will, you do not need to get flustered. Simply do that part out of sequence—smoothly. If you have already left the patient, return and ask if you can check one more thing. Avoid expressions of disgust, alarm, distaste, or other negative reactions. They have no place at the bedside, even when you come upon an ominous mass, a deep and smelly ulcer, or even a pubic louse.

As in the interview, be sensitive to the patient's feelings. The patient's facial expression or an apparently casual question such as "Is it okay?" may give you clues to previously unexpressed worries. Ascertain them when you can. Pay attention to the patient's physical comfort as well. Adjust the slant of the bed or examining table according to the patient's needs insofar as it is possible, and use pillows or blankets to position him comfortably or keep him warm. Assure as much privacy as possible by using drapes appropriately and closing doors.

As an examiner you too should be comfortable, because awkward positions may impair your perceptions. Adjust the bed to a convenient height, and ask the patient to move toward you if this will help you reach him more comfortably.

Good lighting and a quiet environment contribute importantly to what you can see and hear but may be remarkably hard to find in a hospital. Do the best you can. If a nearby patient's television is interfering with your ability to hear the sounds in your patient's chest, ask him politely to lower the volume. The usual patient cooperates readily. Remember to thank him when you are through.

As you proceed with your examination, keep the patient informed as to what you intend to do, especially when you anticipate possible embarrassment or discomfort. Patients vary considerably in their knowledge of examination procedures and hence in their need for information. Some people want to know what you are doing when you listen to the lungs or feel for a liver, while others already know or perhaps do not care. By words or gestures, be as clear as possible in your instructions. When telling patients what to do, be courteous rather than authoritarian. "I would like to examine your heart now. Would you please lie down" carries a different and better message than "I'm going to examine your heart now. Lie down on the table." Authority stems from competence and personal relationship, not from command.

Clinicians differ in how and when they report their findings to their patients. Beginning students should avoid almost all such interpretive statements since they do not yet carry the primary responsibility for the patient and may give conflicting or erroneous information. As experience and responsibility increase, however, sharing findings with the patient becomes appropriate. If you know or suspect the patient has specific concerns, it may be helpful to make a reassuring comment as you finish examining the relevant area. A steady series of reassuring comments, however, presents at least one potential problem: what to say when you find an unexpected abnormality. You may wish you had maintained judicious silence.

All students, however, should develop one habit with which they can reassure their patients and avoid unnecessary alarm. As a beginner, you may spend much more time with some procedures, such as the ophthalmoscopic examination or cardiac auscultation, than does the experienced clinician. Whenever you realize you are doing this, pause and explain: "I would like to spend a long time examining your heart because I want to listen to each of the heart sounds carefully. It does not mean that I hear anything wrong." Be forthright with the patient about your status as a student. Such openness will clarify your relationship and probably reduce anxieties on both sides.

No dogmatic answers can be given to two common questions: How complete should the examination be? What is the best sequence? The outline that follows describes a fairly comprehensive examination such as you might perform on a new adult patient. The patient's age, sex, and history, however, may suggest a specific abnormality or place him at higher than average risk for certain conditions. If so, you may select special techniques that are not part of your usual examining sequence. Techniques such as these are described in later chapters. In contrast, omissions from your usual sequence are sometimes appropriate. The asymptomatic adolescent does not usually need a rectal examination, for example, and you can better spend your time exploring portions of the history or examination that are more likely to be significant.

Despite these possible variations, you should follow a sequence of examination that is personally comfortable, then use it repetitively until you have mastered it and do not forget important details. Some students like to write a brief outline of the examination on index cards and use it unobtrusively during their first several examinations. Soon the cards become superfluous.

As you gain experience, you may modify the sequence outlined in the following pages and work out your own plan. Keep in mind a few basic principles. Try to minimize the number of times that a patient has to change positions. Minimize your own movements too, in order to increase your efficiency. Usually you can carry out most of the examination by standing at the right side of the patient's bed. Be systematic so that you will not forget items, and have all of your equipment readily at hand.

Sequence must vary in some situations. A few bed patients, for example, may be unable to sit up or stand. You can examine the head, neck, and anterior trunk of such a person as he lies supine. Then roll him onto each side to listen to his lungs, examine his back, and inspect the skin. Acute problems, such as coma, indicate a different approach from your usual procedures, as discussed in Chapter 15. And, on repeated examinations of the same person, you will probably focus primarily on the active problems—no one needs a "complete" examination every day.

You may wish to skim the following outline now to get an overview of the physical examination. Subsequent chapters deal with individual body regions or systems, each considered in isolation. After you have completed the study and practice involved in several chapters, reread this overview to see how each component of the examination fits into an integrated whole.

General Survey. Observe the patient's state of health, stature and habitus, and sexual development. Weigh him, if possible. Note his posture, motor activity, and gait; his dress, grooming, and personal hygiene; any odors of body or breath. Watch the patient's facial expressions and note his manner, affect, and reaction to the persons and things around him. Listen to his speech and note his state of awareness or level of consciousness.

The survey continues throughout the history and examination.

Vital Signs. Count the pulse and respiratory rate. Measure the blood pressure and, if indicated, the body temperature.

Skin. Observe the skin and its characteristics. Identify any lesions, noting their location, distribution, arrangement, type, and color. Inspect and palpate the hair and nails. Study the patient's hands.

The patient is sitting on the edge of the bed or examining table, unless his condition contraindicates this position. You should be standing in front of the patient, moving to either side as you need to.

Begin your assessment of the skin with the exposed areas—the hands, forearms, and face. Continue it as you examine other body regions such as the thorax, abdomen, genitalia, and limbs.

Head. Examine the hair, scalp, skull, and face.

Eyes. Check visual acuity and, if indicated, the visual fields. Note the position and alignment of the eyes. Inspect the eyebrows, irides, and pupils. Test the pupillary reactions to light and accommodation, and check the extraocular movements. With an ophthalmoscope inspect the ocular fundi.

The room should be darkened for the ophthalmoscopic examination.

Ears. Inspect the auricles, canals, and drums. Check auditory acuity. If acuity is diminished, check lateralization and compare air and bone conduction.

Nose and Sinuses. Examine the external nose, nasal mucosa, septum, and turbinates. Palpate for tenderness of the frontal and maxillary sinuses.

Mouth and Pharynx. Inspect the lips, buccal mucosa, gums, teeth, roof of the mouth, tongue, and pharynx.

Neck. Inspect and palpate the cervical nodes. Note any masses or unusual pulsations in the neck. Feel for any deviation of the trachea, and palpate the thyroid gland.

Move behind the sitting patient to feel the thyroid gland and to examine the back, posterior thorax, and lungs.

Back. Inspect and palpate the spine and muscles of the back. Check for costovertebral angle tenderness.

Posterior Thorax and Lungs. Inspect, palpate, and percuss the chest. Listen to the breath sounds, and identify any added sounds.

Breasts, Axillae, and Epitrochlear Nodes. In a woman, inspect the breasts with her arms relaxed and then elevated, then with her hands pressed on her hips. In either sex, inspect the axillae and feel for the axillary nodes. Feel for the epitrochlear nodes.

Move to the front again.

By this time you have examined the patient's hands, surveyed the back and, at least in women, made a fair estimate of the range of motion at the shoulders. Your examination of the anterior thorax will include inspection of additional musculoskeletal structures. Use these observations, together with the patient's history and the ease with which he moves throughout the examination, in deciding whether or not to continue with a full musculoskeletal examination.

If you need to do a more complete examination, it is convenient to examine the hands, arms, shoulders, neck, and jaw while the patient is still in the sitting position. Inspect and palpate the joints and check their range of motion.

Breasts. Inspect and palpate the breasts.

The patient is supine. You should stand on the right side of the patient's bed.

Anterior Thorax and Lungs. Inspect, palpate, and percuss the chest. Listen to the breath sounds and identify any added sounds.

Heart. Inspect and palpate the precordium. Assess the apical impulse. Listen in each auscultatory area, using both the bell and the diaphragm of your stethoscope. Correlate your findings with the carotid pulsations and jugular venous pulses. Identify any abnormal heart sounds or murmurs. Use special positions to bring out aortic murmurs, mitral murmurs, and the third and fourth heart sounds.

Some elevation of the patient's upper body is helpful and often necessary.

The patient should sit up, lean forward, and exhale; then roll onto his left side.

Carotid Pulsations and Jugular Venous Pulses. Inspect and palpate the carotid pulsations. Listen for carotid bruits. Identify the jugular venous pulsations, and measure the jugular venous pressure in relation to the sternal angle.

Elevate the upper body of the supine patient so as to maximize the jugular venous pulses and to visualize their highest point.

Abdomen. Inspect, auscultate, and percuss the abdomen. Palpate lightly, then deeply. Try to feel the liver, spleen, and kidneys.

The patient is supine.

Inguinal Area. Feel for the inguinal nodes, and palpate the femoral arteries.

Rectal Examination in Men. Examine the anus, rectum, and prostate. If the patient cannot stand, examine the genitalia before doing the rectal.

The patient is lying on his left side for the rectal examination.

Legs. Inspect the legs, noting any evidence of peripheral vascular, mus-

The patient is supine.

culoskeletal, or neurologic abnormalities. Palpate for edema. Check the dorsalis pedis and posterior tibial pulses. Continue a complete musculoskeletal examination, if this is indicated, by inspecting and palpating the joints and checking their range of motion.

Musculoskeletal System. Examine the range of motion of the spine, the alignment of the legs, and the feet.

The patient is standing. You should sit on a chair or stool.

Peripheral Vascular System. Inspect for varicose veins.

Genitalia and Hernias in Men. Examine the penis and scrotal contents and check for hernias.

Screening Neurologic Examination. Observe the patient's gait and his ability to walk heel-to-toe, walk on his toes, walk on his heels, hop in place, and do shallow knee bends. Check Romberg's sign.

Then assess sensory function by testing pain and vibration in the hands and feet, light touch on the limbs, and stereognosis in the hands.

The patient is sitting or supine.

Check the muscle stretch reflexes and the plantar responses.

Full Neurologic Examination. If indicated, go on to a more thorough examination, including:

Motor. Muscle tone, strength, and coordination

Sensory. Pain, temperature, light touch, position, vibration, and discrimination

Abdominal reflexes

Mental Status. Check cognitive functions, if indicated and not previously done.

Other portions of the mental status examination are usually completed during the history.

Genitalia and Rectal Examination in Women. Examine the external genitalia, vagina, and cervix. Obtain Pap smears. Palpate the uterus and the adnexa. Do a rectovaginal and rectal examination.

The patient is supine in the lithotomy position. You should be seated at first, then standing at the foot of the examining table.

Alternatively, this examination is conveniently done right after the abdominal and inguinal examinations.

When you have completed your examination, tell the patient what he should expect next and what you want him to do. If you are examining a hospitalized patient, rearrange the patient's immediate environment to suit him. If you initially found the bed rails up, it is usually advisable to put them back in this position unless you are sure he doesn't need them. Lower the bed so he can get in and out easily without risking falls.

When you record the physical examination, the sequence you use will not be exactly the same as this one. Refer to Chapter 19 for a sample of a patient's record.

Chapter 3
THE GENERAL SURVEY

Anatomy and Physiology

Much of the specific anatomy and physiology relevant to the general survey may be found in later chapters. This section deals briefly with the more general topics of body height, weight, and habitus, and will introduce the concept of sexual maturity ratings.

In all these attributes people vary importantly according to the region of the world in which they live, their socioeconomic status, nutrition, genetic makeup, early illnesses, gender, and the era in which they were born. The apparent shortening of aging Americans, for example, is partially illusory. Although people do shrink with age, their heights also vary according to the year of their birth. Young adults today on the average have grown taller than their parents, and the parents taller than the grandparents. This section cannot deal with all the variations of "normal" resulting from these many factors, but the clinician should be extremely cautious in applying the norms of one group to a person of another.

Height, Growth, and Habitus. Persons grow in height from birth to late adolescence. When the annual gain in height is measured and charted, one can readily discern an *adolescent growth spurt,* which in girls peaks at the approximate age of 12 and in boys at the approximate age of 14 years. Bone and muscle are involved in this growth spurt, with variations in degree and timing according to gender. A boy's shoulders, for example, broaden more than a girl's, while a girl's hips widen more than a boy's. These changes are summarized in the illustration on the next page.

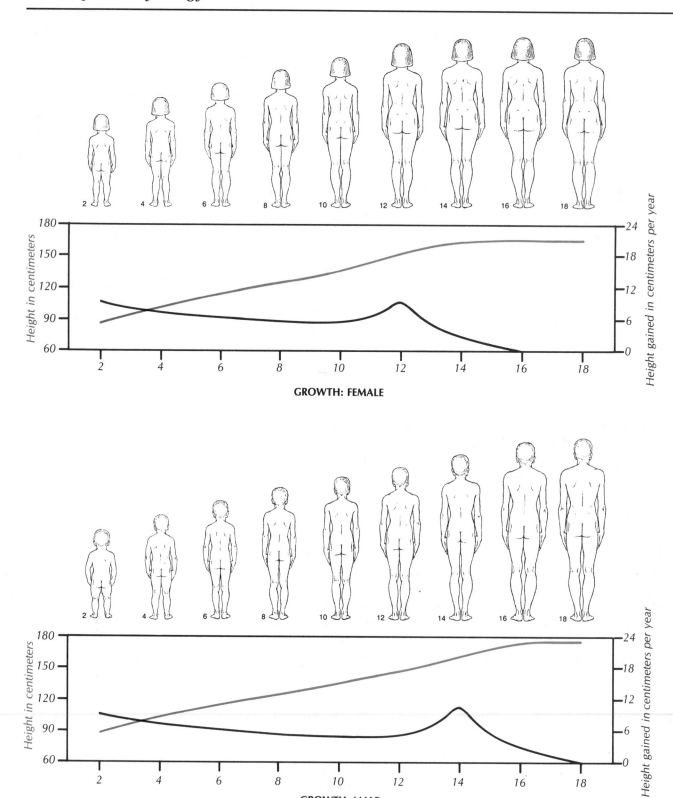

(Modified from Tanner JM: *Growing up. Scientific American* 229: 36–37, September 1973)

Toward the other end of the lifespan other changes occur. People decrease in height, and posture may become somewhat stooped as the thoracic spine becomes more convex and the knees and hips fail to extend fully. Fat tends to concentrate near the hips and lower abdomen and, together with weakening of the abdominal muscles, often produces a potbelly. The figure below illustrates some of the changes occurring in persons ranging in age from 78 to 94. These and other changes with age are further detailed in subsequent chapters.

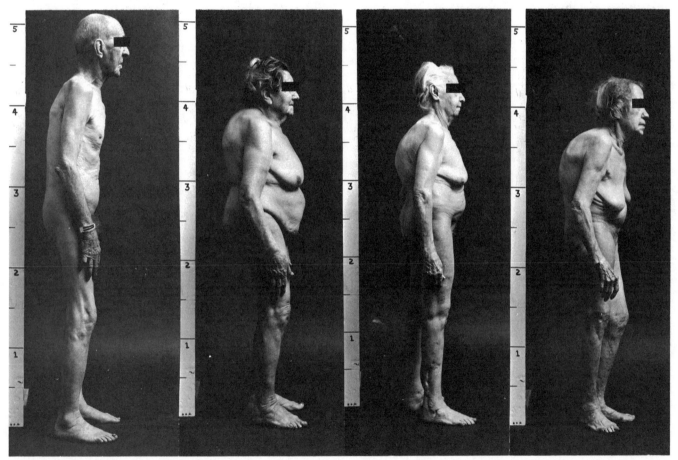

A man, age 82, and three women, ages 78, 79, and 94 respectively. (Rossman I: Clinical Geriatrics, 2nd ed, p 4. Philadelphia, J B Lippincott, 1979)

Weight. Definitions of normal weights for adults have become increasingly controversial and probably derive more from aesthetic preference and cultural attitudes than they do from scientific knowledge. People on either extreme—the very thin and the very fat—have higher mortality rates than others, and both obesity and cachexia increase the risk of specific health problems. The ranges of "normal" or "ideal" weights, however, seem to be much broader than previously believed, and their exact limits remain unclear.

Sexual Maturity Ratings. Changes in an adolescent's reproductive organs and secondary sex characteristics are closely related to the growth spurt. Later chapters describe sexual maturity ratings by which the clinician can assess sexual development: in breasts and pubic hair of girls and in genitalia and pubic hair of boys. The interrelationships between these sexual characteristics and the adolescent growth spurt give the clinician a biological yardstick with which to assess an adolescent's growth and development and with which to identify significant deviations from normal patterns. They also help the clinician to interpret for the adolescent whether growth and sexual maturation are proceeding normally and to predict what further changes may be expected.

During your initial survey of the adolescent patient, you measure only one of these variables—height. You may also make a few preliminary observations of breast and muscular development, pitch of voice, and facial hair. The full meaning of these observations, however, does not emerge until you correlate them with other data: the patient's body habitus, growth pattern over time, muscular development, sexual maturity ratings, psychosexual feelings, attitudes, and knowledge. During the assessment process, you will bring these interrelated variables together, and try to understand the patient's development and any related problems as well as you can.

Techniques of Examination

Begin your observations from the first moment you see the patient. Does the patient hear you when you call his name in the waiting room? Does he rise with ease, and how does he walk? If the patient is hospitalized when you first meet, what is he doing: sitting up and enjoying television? or lying in bed? What occupies the bedside table: a magazine? a flock of "get well" cards? a Bible or rosary? an emesis basin? or nothing at all? Each of these observations should raise one or more tentative hypotheses and guide your further assessments. Throughout the interview and examination, make note of the following:

State of Awareness and Level of Consciousness. Is the patient awake and alert? Does he seem to understand your questions and to respond appropriately and reasonably quickly, or does he lose track of the topic, ramble, become silent, or even fall asleep?

Inattentiveness, drowsiness, stupor. See Table 15-2, Abnormalities of Consciousness (p. 413).

Apparent State of Health. This judgment is an evaluative summary that should be supported by specific observations. Try to define the attributes that substantiate your conclusions. A thin, weak octogenarian with a tottering gait and a quavery voice suggests frailty, for example, while an ashen, sweaty face suggests an acute illness such as shock.

Acutely or chronically ill, frail, feeble, vigorous, robust

Signs of Distress. For example,

Cardiorespiratory Distress

Labored breathing, wheezing, cough

Pain

Facial expression, sweating, protectiveness of a painful part

Anxiety

Anxious face, fidgety movements, cold moist palms

Skin Color, together with any *lesions.* See Chapter 4 for further details.

Pallor, cyanosis, jaundice, changes in pigmentation

Stature and Habitus. If possible, measure the patient's height in stocking feet. Is he unusually short or tall? Is the build slender and lanky, muscular, or stocky? Is the body symmetrical? Note the general bodily proportions and look for any deformities.

Very short stature in Turner's syndrome and in achondroplastic, renal, and hypopituitary dwarfism; long limbs in proportion to the trunk in hypogonadism and Marfan's syndrome

Sexual Development. Are the voice, facial hair, and breast size appropriate to the patient's age and gender?

Delayed or precocious puberty, hypogonadism, virilism

Weight. Is the patient emaciated, slender, plump, obese, or somewhere in between? If obese, is the fat distributed rather evenly or does it concentrate in the trunk?

Generalized fat in simple obesity; truncal fat with relatively thin limbs in Cushing's syndrome

If possible, weigh the patient. Although narrowly construed "ideal weights" have been effectively challenged, a record of weight change over time provides valuable diagnostic data about individual patients.

Causes of weight loss include malignancy, diabetes, hyperthyroidism, chronic infection, depression, and successful dieting.

Posture, Motor Activity, and Gait. What is the patient's preferred posture?

Preference for sitting up in left-sided heart failure, and for leaning forward with arms braced in chronic obstructive pulmonary disease

Is the patient restless or quiet? How often does he move about? How fast are the movements?

Fast, frequent movements of hyperthyroidism; slumped posture and slowed activity of depression

Are there apparently involuntary motor activities, or are some bodily parts immobile?

Tremors or other involuntary movements; paralyses

Does the patient walk easily, with comfort, self-confidence, and good balance, or is there a limp, discomfort on walking, fear of falling, loss of balance, or abnormality in motor pattern?

See Table 15-5, Abnormalities of Gait and Posture (pp. 418–419).

Dress, Grooming, and Personal Hygiene. How is the patient dressed? Is clothing appropriate to the temperature and weather? Is it clean, properly buttoned, and zipped? How does it compare with clothing worn by people of comparable age and social group?

Dress may reveal the cold intolerance of hypothyroidism, the embarrassment of a skin rash, or personal preferences in lifestyle.

Glance at the patient's shoes. Have holes been cut in them? Are the laces tied? Or is the patient wearing slippers?

Cut-out holes or slippers may indicate gout, bunions, or other painful foot conditions. Untied laces or slippers also suggest edema.

Is the patient wearing any unusual jewelry?

Copper bracelets are sometimes worn for arthritis.

Note the patient's hair and fingernails, together with any use of cosmetics.

Nail polish and hair coloring that has "grown out" suggest loss of interest in personal appearance and may even help in estimating its duration.

Do the patient's personal hygiene and grooming seem appropriate to his age, lifestyle, occupation, and socioeconomic group? There are, of course, wide variations in norms.

Unkempt appearance may be seen in depression and chronic organic brain disease, but this appearance must be compared with the patient's probable norm.

Odors of Body or Breath. Although odors may give important diagnostic clues, avoid one common mistake: never assume that alcohol on a patient's breath explains his mental or neurological findings. Alcoholics may have other serious and potentially correctable problems such as hypoglycemia or a subdural hematoma; and an alcoholic breath does not necessarily mean alcoholism.

Breath odors of alcohol, acetone (diabetes), pulmonary infections, uremia, or liver failure

Facial Expression. Observe facial expression at rest, during conversation about specific topics, during the physical examination, and in interaction with others.

Anxiety, depression, embarrassment, anger, apathy; the stare of hyperthyroidism; the immobile face of parkinsonism

Manner, Affect, and Relationship to Persons and Things. Note the patient's manner toward you and toward others such as family members, friends, or staff. Watch the patient's face and gestures and listen to his words and voice for clues to affect and feelings.

Uncooperativeness, hostility, anger, resentment, depression, tearfulness, distrustfulness, suspiciousness, elation, relief, confidence, resignation, withdrawal, seductiveness

Speech. Listen for the pace of speech, its pitch, clarity, and spontaneity.

Fast speech of hyperthyroidism; slow, thick, hoarse voice of myxedema; lack of spontaneity in depression; dysphasia; dysarthria

Vital Signs. Note the pulse, blood pressure, respiratory rate, and temperature. You may choose to make these measurements at the beginning of the examination or integrate them with your cardiovascular and thoracic assessments. If you do them now, count the radial pulse. Then, with your fingers still on the patient's wrist, count the respiratory rate without the patient's realizing it. (A person may breathe differently when he becomes conscious of his own respirations.) Check the blood pressure; if it is high, repeat your measurement later in the examination.

See Table 7-15, Abnormalities of the Arterial Pulse (p. 209). See Table 6-1, Abnormalities in Rate and Rhythm of Breathing (p. 149).

Although measurement of *temperature* may be omitted in many ambulatory visits, take it if symptoms or signs suggest a possible abnormality. Oral thermometers are more convenient and more acceptable to patients than rectal ones, but oral glass thermometers should not be used when patients are unconscious, restless, or unable to close their mouths.

Hyperpyrexia refers to extreme elevation in body temperature, above 41.1° C (106° F). *Fever* or *pyrexia* refers to an elevated temperature, while *hypothermia* refers to an abnormally low temperature, below 35° C (95° F) rectally. Causes of fever include infections, trauma (such as surgery or crushing injury),

To take an *oral temperature* with a glass thermometer, shake the thermometer down to below 35.5° C (96° F), insert it under the patient's tongue, instruct him to close his lips, and wait 3 to 5 minutes. Then, read the thermometer, reinsert it for a minute, and read it again. If the temperature is still rising, repeat this procedure until the reading remains stable. It may take as long as 8 minutes to obtain an accurate oral temperature.

To take a *rectal temperature* select a rectal thermometer (with a stubby tip), lubricate it, and insert it about 3 cm to 4 cm (one and one half inches) into the anal canal, in a direction pointing toward the umbilicus. Remove and read it after 3 minutes.

Electric thermometers with disposable probe covers are available for both rectal and oral temperatures. They shorten the time required to record an accurate temperature to about 10 seconds.

Whether an oral temperature is taken with a glass or an electric thermometer, drinking hot or cold liquids may alter it artifactually. Wait 10 to 15 minutes before measurement.

The average oral temperature, usually quoted at 37°C (98.6° F), fluctuates considerably and must be interpreted accordingly. In the early morning hours it may be as low as 35.8° C (96.4° F), in the late afternoon or evening as high as 37.3° C (99.1° F). Rectal temperatures average 0.4° to 0.5° C (0.7° to 0.9° F) higher than oral readings, but this difference varies considerably.

malignancies, infarctions, blood disorders (such as acute hemolytic anemia), and immune disorders (such as drug fevers and collagen diseases). The chief cause of hypothermia is exposure to cold, but some acute illnesses may also produce it. Elderly people are especially susceptible to hypothermia and are less likely to develop fever.

Chapter 4

THE SKIN

Anatomy and Physiology

The skin is composed of three layers: the epidermis, the dermis, and the subcutaneous tissues.

The most superficial layer, the *epidermis*, is thin, devoid of blood vessels, and itself divided into two layers: an outer horny layer of dead keratinized cells, and an inner cellular layer where both melanin and keratin are formed.

The epidermis depends on the underlying *dermis* for its nutrition. The dermis is well supplied with blood. It contains connective tissue, the sebaceous glands, and some of the hair follicles. It merges below with the *subcutaneous tissues* which contain fat, the sweat glands, and the remainder of the hair follicles.

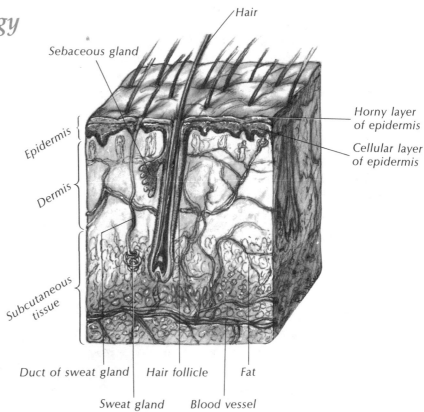

Hair, nails, and sebaceous and sweat glands are considered appendages of the skin. Adults have two types of hair: vellus and terminal. Vellus hair is short, fine, inconspicuous, and unpigmented, while terminal hair in contrast is coarser, thicker, more conspicuous, and usually pigmented. Scalp hair and eyebrows are examples of terminal hair.

Sebaceous glands secrete a protective fatty substance which gains access to the skin surface through the hair follicles. These glands are present on all skin surfaces except for the palms and soles. Sweat glands are of two types: eccrine and apocrine. The eccrine glands are widely distributed, open directly onto the skin surface, and by their sweat production help to control body temperature. In contrast, the apocrine glands are found chiefly in the axillary and genital regions, usually open into hair follicles, and are stimulated by emotional stress. Bacterial decomposition of apocrine sweat is responsible for adult body odor.

CHANGES WITH AGE

During the pubertal years coarse, or terminal, hair appears in new places: the face in boys, and the axillae and pubic areas in both sexes. Hair on the trunk and limbs increases through and after puberty, more obviously in men. Apocrine glands enlarge during puberty, axillary sweating increases, and the characteristic adult body odor appears.

As people age, their skin wrinkles, becomes lax, and loses turgor. The vascularity of the dermis decreases and the skin of white persons tends to look paler and more opaque. Where skin has been long exposed to the sun it looks weatherbeaten: thickened, yellowed, and deeply furrowed. Skin on the backs of the hands and forearms appears thin, fragile, loose, and transparent, and may show whitish, depigmented patches known as pseudoscars. Well demarcated, vividly purple macules or patches, termed senile purpura, may also appear in the same areas, fading after several weeks. These purpuric spots come from blood that has leaked through poorly supported capillaries and has spread within the dermis. Dry skin (asteatosis)—a common problem—is flaky, rough, and often itchy. It is frequently shiny, especially on the legs, where a network of shallow fissures often creates a mosaic of small polygons.

Brown macules known as liver spots, or senile lentigines, frequently appear on the backs of the hands and forearms or, less commonly, on the face. Unlike the familiar freckles, they do not fade spontaneously when protected from the sun. Also common are seborrheic keratoses—pigmented, raised, warty, and often slightly greasy lesions that develop most often on the trunk but also occur on the face and hands. Actinic (or senile) keratoses, which are less common, develop on exposed surfaces, first as small reddened areas and then as raised, rough, yellow to brown lesions. From middle life on, senile seba-

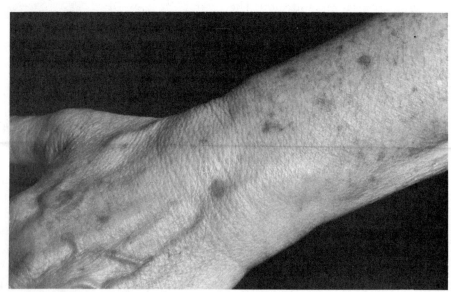

Senile lentigenes in a 58-year-old woman.

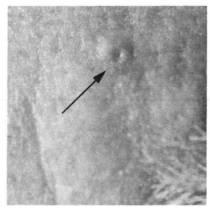

Sebaceous adenoma in a 53-year-old woman.

ceous adenomas may appear on the face, where they must be differentiated from basal cell carcinomas. Benign, yellowish, flattened papules with central depressions, they look like diminutive doughnuts and range in size from 1 mm to 3 mm or more in diameter.

Cherry angiomas are very common, first appearing fairly early in adulthood (p. 50). Most frequently found on the trunk, they have no significance.

While all these changes occur so frequently that they may be considered part of normal aging, two less common findings in older people are distinctly abnormal: squamous cell carcinoma, which sometimes develops in an actinic keratosis, and basal cell carcinoma (p. 98).

Nails lose some of their luster with age and may yellow and thicken, especially on the toes.

Hair on the scalp loses its pigment, producing the well known graying. At as early as 20 years of age a man's hairline may start to recede at the temples; hair loss at the vertex follows. Many women show loss of hair in a similar pattern, but it is less severe. Balding in this distribution is genetically determined. In both sexes the number of scalp hairs decreases in a generalized, more subtle pattern, and the diameter of each hair diminishes.

Less familiar, but probably more important clinically, is the normal hair loss elsewhere on the body: the trunk, pubic area, axillae, and limbs. These changes will be discussed, where relevant, in later chapters. Coarse facial hairs appear on the chin and upper lip of many women by the approximate age of 55, but do not increase further thereafter.

Most of the observations described here pertain to white persons and do not necessarily apply to other racial groups. For example, Native American men have relatively little facial and body hair compared to whites and should not be evaluated by white norms.

Techniques of Examination

Begin your observation of the skin with your general survey and continue it throughout the rest of your examination.

Inspect and palpate the skin. Note its:

Color. For example, brownness, cyanosis, redness, yellowness, or pallor

See Table 4-1, Variations in Skin Color (pp. 48–49).

Vascularity and evidence of *bleeding or bruising*

See Table 4-2, Vascular and Purpuric Lesions of the Skin (p. 50).

Moisture. For example, dryness, sweating, oiliness

Dryness in hypothyroidism, oiliness in acne

Temperature. Feel the skin with the backs of your fingers to assess temperature.

Texture. For example, roughness, smoothness

Roughness in hypothyroidism

Thickness

Mobility and Turgor. Lift a fold of skin and note the ease with which it is moved (mobility) and the speed with which it returns into place (turgor).

Decreased mobility in edema, scleroderma; decreased turgor in dehydration

Observe Any Lesions of the Skin.

1. First, identify their *anatomic location* and their *distribution* over the entire surface of the body. Where are the lesions? Are they generalized or localized? Do they, for example, involve only the exposed surfaces, or the intertriginous (skin fold) areas, or areas exposed to specific contacts such as wrist bands or rings?

Many skin diseases have characteristic distributions. For example, acne affects the face, upper chest, and back; psoriasis, the knees and elbows (among other areas); and Monilia infections, the intertriginous areas.

2. Then note the *grouping* or *arrangement* of the lesions. They may be linear, or clustered, or annular (in a ring), or arciform (in an arc), or they may be dermatomal (*i.e.,* covering a skin band that corresponds to a sensory nerve root; see pp. 376–377).

Vesicles in a unilateral dermatomal pattern are typical of herpes zoster.

3. Then try to identify the *type of skin lesions* (*e.g.,* macules, papules, vesicles, and the like). If possible, find representative and recent lesions that have not been traumatized by scratching or otherwise altered.

See Table 4-3, Basic Types of Skin Lesions (pp. 51–52).

4. Note the *color* of the lesions.

Inspect and palpate the fingernails and toenails. Note their color, shape, and any lesions.

See Table 4-4, Abnormalities and Variations of the Nails (p. 53).

Inspect and palpate the hair. Note its quantity, distribution, and texture.

Inspection of the mucous membranes should be correlated with your examination of the skin, but will be described in later chapters.

The differential diagnosis of skin abnormalities is beyond the scope of this book. After familiarizing yourself with the basic types of lesions, you would do well to peruse a relatively brief but well illustrated textbook of dermatology. Whenever you see a skin lesion, make a consistent habit of looking it up in such a text. The type of lesions, their location, and their distribution, together with other information from the history and the examination, should equip you well for this search and, in time, for arriving at specific dermatologic diagnoses.

Table 4-1

Table 4-1 Variations in Skin Color

COLOR	PROCESS	SELECTED CAUSES	TYPICAL LOCALIZATION
BROWN	Deposition of melanin	Genetic	Generalized
		Sunlight	Exposed area
		Pregnancy	Face, nipples, areolae, linea nigra, vulva
		Addison's disease and some pituitary tumors	Exposed areas, points of pressure and friction, nipples, genitalia, palmar creases, recent scars; often generalized
GRAYISH TAN OR BRONZE	Deposition of melanin and hemosiderin	Hemochromatosis	Exposed areas, genitalia and scars; often generalized
BLUE (CYANOSIS)	Increased amount of reduced hemoglobin secondary to hypoxia. This may be either—		
	Peripheral, or	Anxiety or cold environment	The nails, sometimes lips
	Central (arterial)	Heart or lung disease	Lips, mouth and nails
	Abnormal hemoglobin	Congenital or acquired methemoglobinemia; sulfhemoglobinemia	Lips, mouth, and nails
REDDISH BLUE	Combination of increase in total amount of hemoglobin, increase in reduced hemoglobin, and capillary stasis	Polycythemia	Face, conjunctivas, mouth, hands and feet
RED	Increased visibility of normal oxyhemoglobin because of—		
	Dilatation or increased numbers of superficial blood vessels or increased blood flow	Fever, blushing, alcohol intake, local inflammation	Face and upper chest or local area of inflammation
	Decreased oxygen use in the skin	Cold exposure	The cold area (e.g., ears)

Continued

Table 4-1

Table 4-1 (Cont'd)

COLOR	PROCESS	SELECTED CAUSES	TYPICAL LOCALIZATION
YELLOW JAUNDICE	Increased bilirubin levels	Liver disease, red blood cell hemolysis	First in scleras, then mucous membranes and generalized
CAROTENEMIA	Increased levels of carotenoid pigments	Increased intake of carotene-containing vegetables and fruits; myxedema, hypopituitarism, diabetes	Palms, soles, face; does not involve scleras or mucous membranes
CHRONIC UREMIA	Retention of urinary chromogens, superimposed on the pallor of anemia	Chronic renal disease	Most evident in exposed areas, may be generalized; does not involve scleras or mucous membranes
DECREASED COLOR	Decreased melanin		
	Congenital inability to form melanin	Albinism	Generalized lack of pigment in skin, hair, eyes
	Acquired loss of melanin	Vitiligo	Patchy, symmetrical, often involving the exposed areas
		Tinea versicolor (a common fungus infection)	Chest, upper back, and neck
	Decreased visibility of oxyhemoglobin		
	Decreased blood flow in superficial vessels	Syncope, shock, some normal variations	Most evident in face, conjunctivas, mouth, nails
	Decreased amount of oxyhemoglobin	Anemia	Most evident in face, conjunctivas, mouth, nails
	Edema (Edema of the skin masks the colors of melanin and hemoglobin and prevents the appearance of jaundice.)	Nephrotic syndrome	The edematous areas

Table 4-2

Table 4-2 Vascular and Purpuric Lesions of the Skin

	VASCULAR			PURPURIC	
	CHERRY ANGIOMA	**SPIDER ANGIOMA**	**VENOUS STAR**	**PETECHIA**	**ECCHYMOSIS**
COLOR	Bright or ruby red; may become brownish with age	Fiery red	Bluish	Deep red or reddish purple	Purple or purplish blue, fading to green, yellow, and brown with time
SIZE	1–3 mm	Very small up to 2 cm	Variable, from very small to several inches	Usually 1–3 mm	Variable, larger than petechiae
SHAPE	Round, sometimes raised, may be surrounded by a pale halo	Central body, sometimes raised, surrounded by erythema and radiating legs	Variable. May resemble a spider or be linear, irregular, cascading	Round, flat	Round, oval, or irregular; may have a central subcutaneous flat nodule
PULSATILITY	Absent	Often demonstrable in the body of the spider, when pressure with a glass slide is applied	Absent	Absent	Absent
EFFECT OF PRESSURE	May show partial blanching, especially if pressure is applied with a pinpoint's edge	Pressure over the body causes blanching of the spider.	Pressure over center does not cause blanching.	None	None
DISTRIBUTION	Trunk, also extremities	Face, neck, arms, and upper trunk, almost never below the waist	Most often on the legs, near veins; also anterior chest	Variable	Variable
SIGNIFICANCE	None; increase in size and numbers with aging	Liver disease, pregnancy, vitamin B deficiency, occurs in some normal people	Often accompanies increased pressure in the superficial veins, as in varicose veins	Blood extravasated outside the vessels; may suggest increased bleeding tendency or emboli to skin	Blood extravasated outside the vessels; often secondary to trauma; also seen in bleeding disorders

Table 4-3

Table 4-3 Basic Types of Skin Lesions

PRIMARY LESIONS (*May Arise from Previously Normal Skin*)

CIRCUMSCRIBED, FLAT, NONPALPABLE CHANGES IN SKIN COLOR

Macule—Small, up to 1 cm.* Example: freckle, petechia

Patch—Larger than 1 cm. Example: vitiligo

PALPABLE ELEVATED SOLID MASSES

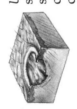

Papule—Up to 0.5 cm. Example: an elevated nevus

Plaque—A flat, elevated surface larger than 0.5 cm, often formed by the coalescence of papules

Nodule—0.5 cm to 1–2 cm; often deeper and firmer than a papule

Tumor—Larger than 1–2 cm.

Wheal—A slightly irregular, relatively transient, superficial area of localized skin edema. Example: mosquito bite, hive

CIRCUMSCRIBED SUPERFICIAL ELEVATIONS OF THE SKIN FORMED BY FREE FLUID IN A CAVITY WITHIN THE SKIN LAYERS

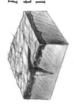

Vesicle—Up to 0.5 cm; filled with serous fluid. Example: herpes simplex

Bulla—Greater than 0.5 cm; filled with serous fluid. Example: 2nd degree burn

Pustule—Filled with pus. Examples: acne, impetigo

SECONDARY LESIONS (*Result from Changes in Primary Lesions*)

LOSS OF SKIN SURFACE

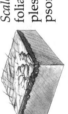

Erosion—Loss of the superficial epidermis; surface is moist but does not bleed. Example: moist area after the rupture of a vesicle, as in chickenpox

Ulcer—A deeper loss of skin surface; may bleed and scar. Examples: stasis ulcer of venous insufficiency, syphilitic chancre

Fissure—A linear crack in the skin. Example: athlete's foot

MATERIAL ON THE SKIN SURFACE

Crust—The dried residue of serum, pus, or blood. Example: impetigo

Scale—A thin flake of exfoliated epidermis. Examples: dandruff, dry skin, psoriasis

*Authorities vary somewhat in their definitions of skin lesions by size. Dimensions given in this table should be considered approximate, not rigid.

Continued

Table 4-3

Table 4-3 (Cont'd)

SECONDARY LESIONS *(Result from Changes in Primary Lesions)*

MISCELLANEOUS

Lichenification—Thickening and roughening of the skin with increased visibility of the normal skin furrows. Example: atopic dermatitis

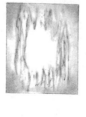

Scar—Replacement of destroyed tissue by fibrous tissue

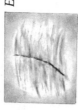

Atrophy—Thinning of the skin with loss of the normal skin furrows; the skin looks shinier and more translucent than normal. Example: arterial insufficiency

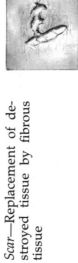

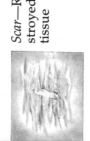

Keloid—A hypertrophied scar

Excoriation—A scratch mark

Table 4-4

Table 4-4 Abnormalities and Variations of the Nails

CLUBBING OF THE NAILS
NORMAL

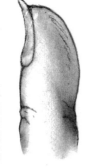

Normal angle 160°

The angle between the normal finger nail and nail base is about 160°. When palpated the nail base feels firm.

EARLY CLUBBING

Straightened angle (180°)

Springy, floating

In early clubbing the angle between nail and nail base straightens out. The nail base gives a springy or floating sensation when palpated. You can simulate this by squeezing your middle finger from each side between your thumb and ring finger of the same hand, just behind the nail. Then palpate the nail base with the index finger of the opposite hand.

LATE CLUBBING

Angle greater than 180°

Swollen, springy, floating

In late clubbing the base of the nail becomes visibly swollen and the angle between nail and nail base exceeds 180°.

Clubbing has many causes, including hypoxia and lung cancer.

CURVED NAILS

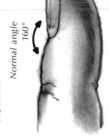

Curved nail

Normal angle

Curved nails, a variant of normal, should not be confused with clubbing. Here, although the nails show a convex curve as they may in clubbing, the normal angle between nail and nail base is preserved.

SPOON NAILS (KOILONYCHIA)

Spoon nails are characterized by concave curves. Spoon nails are sometimes seen in iron deficiency anemia, although they are not specific for this disorder.

BEAU'S LINES

Beau's lines are transverse depressions in the nails associated with acute severe illness. Appearing some weeks later, they grow out with the nail gradually over several months.

PARONYCHIA

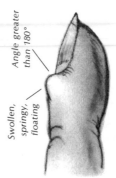

The term paronychia refers to inflammation of the skin around the nail. It is characterized by swelling and sometimes redness and tenderness.

SPLINTER HEMORRHAGES

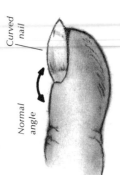

Splinter hemorrhages are red or brown linear streaks in the nail bed, parallel to the long axis of the fingers. Although traditionally associated with subacute bacterial endocarditis and trichinosis, they are nonspecific, often occurring with minor trauma or without apparent cause. They have been described in from 10% to 20% of hospitalized adults.

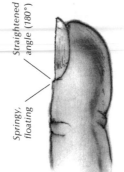

Chapter 5
THE HEAD AND NECK

Anatomy and Physiology

THE HEAD

Regions of the head take their names from the underlying bones (*e.g.,* frontal area, occipital area). Familiarity with the anatomy of the skull is helpful, therefore, in localizing and describing physical findings. Shown also in this diagram are the two salivary glands that can be examined clinically: the parotid gland, which when enlarged is sometimes visible and palpable superficial to and behind the mandible, and the submaxillary gland, which is located deep to the mandible. The openings of the parotid and submaxillary glands are visible within the oral cavity.

The superficial temporal artery passes upward just in front of the ear, where it is readily palpable. In many normal people, especially thin and elderly ones, its tortuous course can be traced across the forehead.

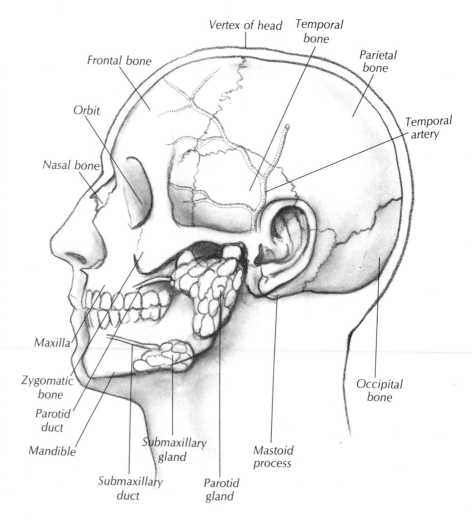

THE EYE

Gross Anatomy. Review the external anatomy of the eye, identifying the diagrammed structures.

Note that the upper eyelid normally covers a portion of the iris but does not usually overlap the pupil. The white sclera may be somewhat buff-colored peripherally.

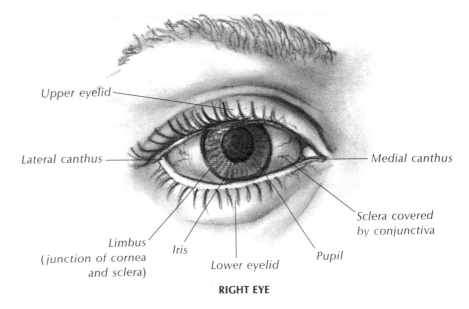

Upper eyelid

Lateral canthus

Medial canthus

Sclera covered by conjunctiva

Limbus (junction of cornea and sclera)

Iris

Lower eyelid

Pupil

RIGHT EYE

Except for the cornea, the parts of the eyeball visible anteriorly are covered by the conjunctiva. At the margin of the cornea (limbus), the conjunctiva merges with the corneal epithelium. A portion of the conjunctiva with its vessels lies loosely on the surface of the sclera and is called the bulbar conjunctiva. Above and below, it forms a deep recess and then folds forward to join the tissues of the eyelids (palpebral conjunctiva). The eyelids themselves are given form and consistency by thin strips of connective tissue known as the tarsal plates. Within each tarsal plate lies a row of parallel meibomian glands which open near the posterior margin of the lid. By secreting sebaceous material they lubricate the lids. The levator palpebrae muscle, which raises the upper eyelid, has a dual innervation: from the oculomotor nerve (3rd cranial nerve) and from the sympathetic system.

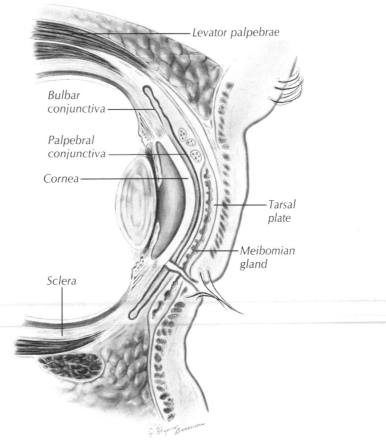

Levator palpebrae

Bulbar conjunctiva

Palpebral conjunctiva

Cornea

Tarsal plate

Meibomian gland

Sclera

SAGITTAL SECTION OF ANTERIOR EYE

The conjunctiva and cornea are lubricated by secretions from the lacrimal gland and conjunctiva. Tears drain out through the puncta at the lid margins, into the lacrimal ducts and sac, and on into the nose through the nasolacrimal duct. The puncta are the only portions of the lacrimal apparatus normally visible without special maneuvers.

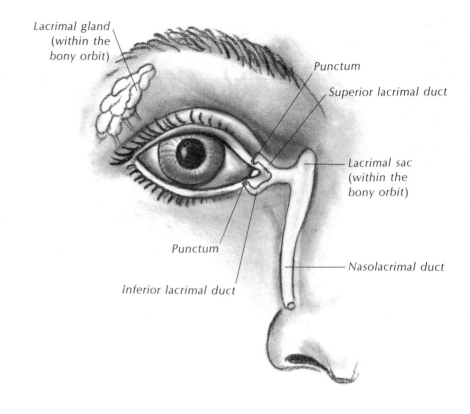

The eyeball itself is a spherical structure designed to focus a controlled amount of light on the neurosensory elements within the retina. Muscles within the iris control pupillary size. Muscles of the ciliary body control the thickness of the lens, enabling the normal eye to focus in turn on objects both near and far away. At the posterior pole of the eye the retinal surface shows a slight depression—the fovea centralis—which marks the point of central vision. The retina immediately around it is called the macula. The optic nerve with its retinal vessels joins the eye somewhat medial to this point. It is visible ophthalmoscopically as the optic disc. That portion of the eye posterior to the lens is termed the fundus of the eye. It includes most of the structures normally inspected with the ophthalmoscope: retina, choroid, fovea, macula, optic disc, and retinal vessels. The most anterior parts of the retina and the ciliary body are visible with the ophthalmoscope only by use of special techniques.

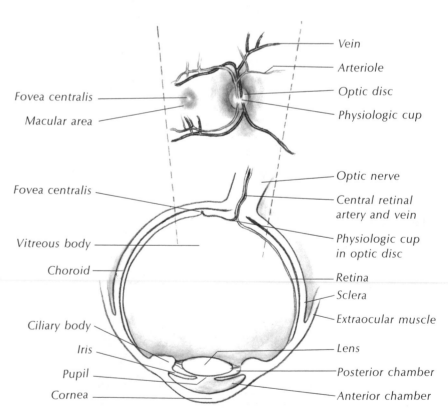

CROSS SECTION OF THE RIGHT EYE FROM ABOVE SHOWING A PORTION OF THE FUNDUS COMMONLY SEEN WITH THE OPHTHALMOSCOPE

A clear liquid called *aqueous humor* fills the anterior and posterior chambers of the eye. Aqueous humor is produced by the ciliary body, circulates from the posterior chamber through the pupil into the anterior chamber, and then drains out through the canal of Schlemm. Pressure within the eye depends primarily upon this circulatory system.

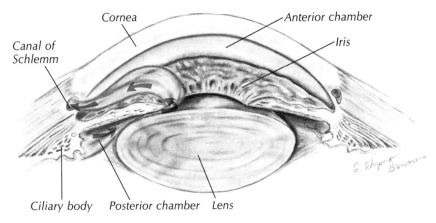

CIRCULATION OF AQUEOUS HUMOR

Visual Pathways. For a clear visual image, reflected light from an object must pass through the cornea, aqueous humor, lens, and vitreous, and be focused on the retina. Images so formed are upside down and reversed right to left. An object in the upper temporal visual field, therefore, strikes the lower nasal quadrant of the retina.

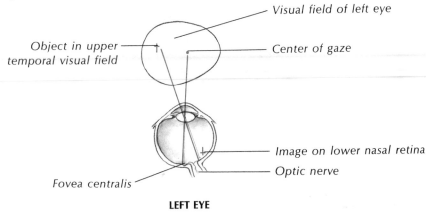

LEFT EYE

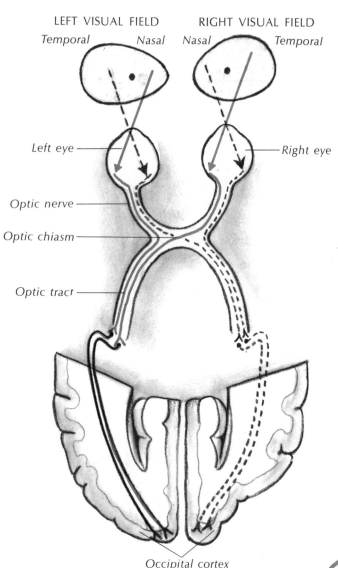

LEFT VISUAL FIELD   RIGHT VISUAL FIELD

Temporal   *Nasal*   *Nasal*   *Temporal*

Left eye

Right eye

Optic nerve

Optic chiasm

Optic tract

Occipital cortex

In response to this light stimulus, nerve impulses are conducted through the retina, optic nerve, and optic tract, and thence to the visual cortex of the occipital lobes. The spatial arrangements of nerve fibers in the retina are preserved in the optic nerves: temporal fibers run laterally in the nerve; nasal fibers run medially. At the optic chiasm, however, the nasal or medial fibers cross over so that the left optic tract contains fibers only from the left half of each retina and the right optic tract contains fibers only from the right half.

Visual Reflexes. By the sequence of events just described, light rays produce conscious vision. Light also stimulates reflex action of two kinds.

The Light Reflex. A light beam shining onto the retina causes reflex pupillary constriction of that eye (*direct light reflex*) and also of the opposite eye (*consensual light reflex*). The initial sensory pathways are similar to those described above: retina, optic nerve, and optic tract. The pathways diverge, however, in the midbrain, and through a series of synapses impulses are transmitted through the oculomotor nerve (3rd cranial nerve) and thence to the constrictor muscles of the iris on each side.

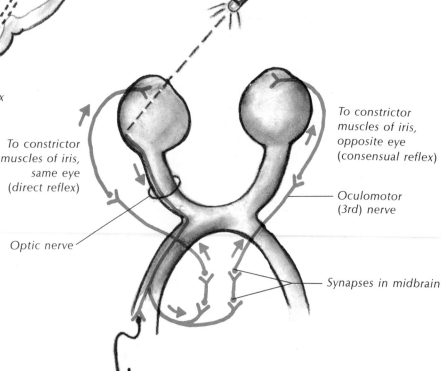

To constrictor muscles of iris, same eye (direct reflex)

Optic nerve

To constrictor muscles of iris, opposite eye (consensual reflex)

Oculomotor (3rd) nerve

Synapses in midbrain

To occipital cortex

Accommodation. Accommodation is the process by which a clear visual image is maintained as the gaze is shifted from a distant to a near point. There are three components of the accommodation reaction: convergence of the eyes, pupillary constriction, and thickening of the lens through contraction of the ciliary muscles. Only the first two are visible to the examiner.

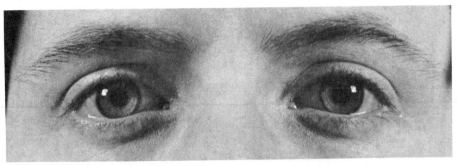

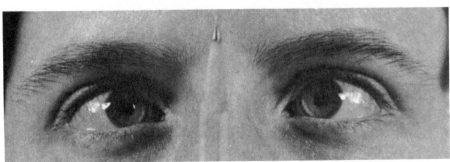

Sensory pathways for accommodation are similar to those involving conscious vision. Nerve impulses then pass from the occipital cortex to the frontal cortex, thence to the midbrain and the oculomotor nerve.

Autonomic Nerve Supply to the Eyes. Fibers traveling in the oculomotor nerve and producing pupillary constriction as described above are part of the parasympathetic nervous system. The iris is also supplied by sympathetic fibers. When these are stimulated, pupillary dilatation and also some elevation of the eyelid result. The sympathetic fibers travel through the sympathetic trunk and ganglia in the neck, then follow a nerve plexus around the carotid artery and its branches into the orbit.

Extraocular Movements. The movement of each eye is controlled by the coordinated action of six muscles, the four rectus and two oblique muscles. The function of each muscle, together with that of the nerve that supplies it, may be tested by asking the patient to move his eye in the direction predominantly controlled by that muscle. There are six such directions, known as the *cardinal fields of gaze.* These are shown in the next diagram. When the patient looks down and to the right, for example, the right inferior rectus (3rd cranial nerve) is principally responsible for moving the right eye while the left superior oblique (4th cranial nerve) is principally responsible for moving the left. If one of these muscles is paralyzed, deviation of the eyes from their normal conjugate, or parallel, positions will be most obvious in this direction of gaze.

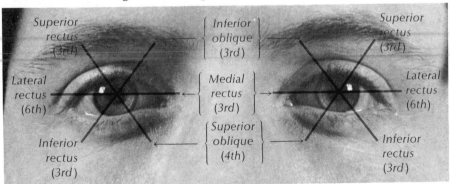

These muscles are correctly diagrammed for the intact person but differ from the individual muscle functions described in many textbooks of anatomy and physiology. Purpose explains the difference. The clinician is trying to detect which muscle is weak or paralyzed in a living person, while the basic scientist is analyzing the function of each muscle, acting alone.

THE EAR

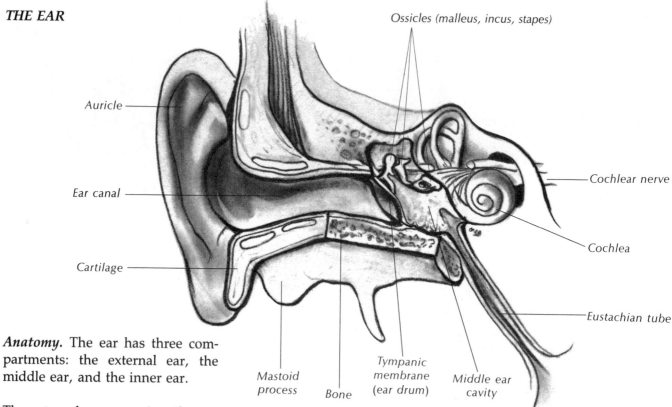

Anatomy. The ear has three compartments: the external ear, the middle ear, and the inner ear.

The external ear comprises the auricle and ear canal. The auricle consists chiefly of cartilage covered by skin and has a firm, elastic consistency. The mastoid process, a bony prominence which is not part of the external ear, can be located just posterior to the lobule. It is the point of insertion for the sternomastoid muscle.

Behind the tragus of the ear opens the somewhat curving ear canal. Its outer portion is surrounded by cartilage, its inner portion by bone. The skin lining the bony portion is exquisitely sensitive, a point always to remember while examining the patient.

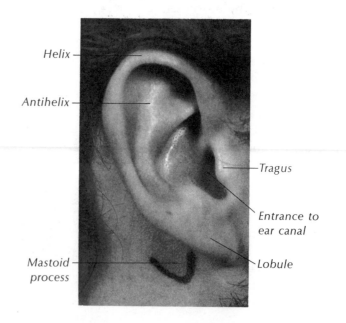

At the end of the ear canal lies the tympanic membrane or eardrum, marking the lateral limits of the middle ear. The middle ear is an air-filled cavity across which sound is transmitted by way of three tiny bones, the ossicles. It is connected by the eustachian tube to the nasopharynx and is also contiguous with some air-filled cells in the adjacent mastoid portion of the temporal bone.

Inspection of the eardrum gives significant information about the condition of the middle ear; hence, knowledge of its landmarks is important. The eardrum may be visualized as an oblique membrane pulled inward at its center by one of the ossicles, the malleus. The short process of the malleus protrudes into the eardrum above the handle. Most of the eardrum is rather taut—the pars tensa—and gives a characteristic reflection known as the cone of light. Superiorly the pars flaccida is less tensely stretched.

Much of the middle ear and all of the inner ear are inaccessible to direct examination. Some inferences concerning their condition can be made, however, by testing auditory function.

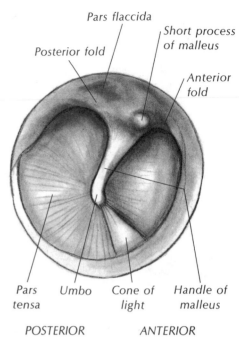

RIGHT EAR DRUM

Pathways of Hearing. Vibrations of sound pass through the air of the external ear and are transmitted through the eardrum and ossicles of the middle ear into the cochlea or inner ear.

Here nerve impulses are initiated and sent to the brain by way of the cochlear nerve (a portion of the 8th cranial nerve). This pathway is the usual one in normal hearing. An alternate pathway used for testing purposes bypasses the external and middle ear by setting the bone of the skull into vibration and thereby stimulating the inner ear directly.

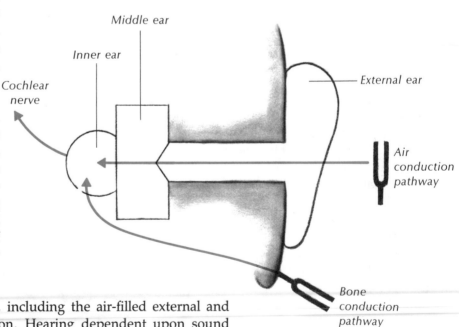

Hearing over the usual pathways, including the air-filled external and middle ear, is called air conduction. Hearing dependent upon sound transmitted through bone to the inner ear is called bone conduction. In the normal person, the usual pathway (*i.e.,* air conduction) is the more sensitive.

Equilibrium. The inner ear has an additional important function in controlling balance. A discussion of this, however, is beyond the scope of this book.

THE NOSE AND PARANASAL SINUSES

Review the terms used to describe the external anatomy of the nose.

Approximately the upper third of the nose is supported by bone, the lower two thirds by cartilage. Air enters the nasal cavity by way of the anterior naris on either side, then passes into a widened area known as the vestibule, and on through the slitlike nasal passage to the nasopharynx. The medial wall of each nasal cavity is formed by the nasal septum which, like the external nose, is supported by both bone and cartilage. It is covered by a mucous membrane well supplied with blood.

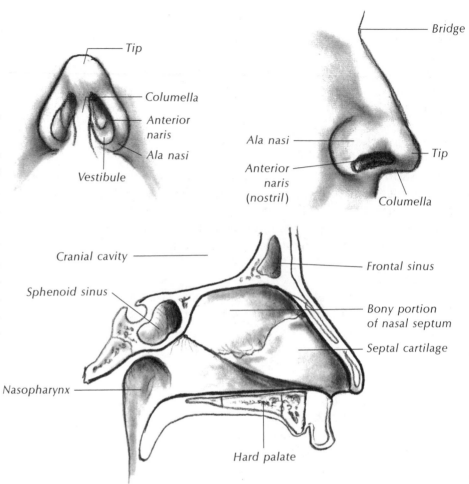

MEDIAL WALL—RIGHT NASAL CAVITY
(Mucous membrane removed to show the structure of the nasal septum)

Laterally the anatomy is more complex. Curving bony structures, the turbinates, covered by a highly vascular mucous membrane, protrude into the nasal cavity. Below each turbinate is a groove, or meatus, each named according to the turbinate above it. Into the inferior meatus drains the nasolacrimal duct; into the middle meatus drain most of the paranasal sinuses. Their openings however, are not usually visible.

The additional surface area provided by the turbinates, and the mucosa covering them, aid the nasal cavities in their principal functions: cleansing, humidification, and temperature control of inspired air.

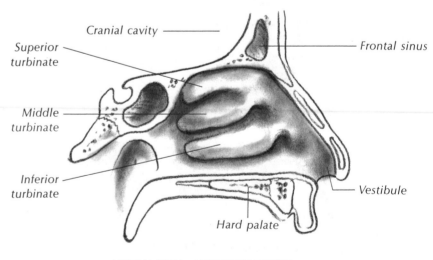

LATERAL WALL—LEFT NASAL CAVITY

Inspection of the nasal cavity through the anterior naris is usually limited to the vestibule, the anterior portion of the septum, and the lower and middle turbinates. Examination by means of a nasopharyngeal mirror is required for detection of posterior abnormalities. It is beyond the scope of this book.

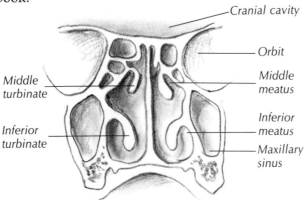

Cranial cavity

Orbit

Middle meatus

Inferior meatus

Maxillary sinus

Middle turbinate

Inferior turbinate

CROSS SECTION OF NASAL CAVITY—ANTERIOR VIEW

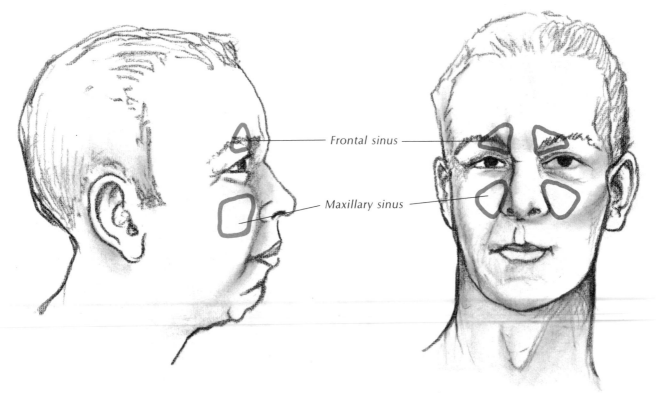

Frontal sinus

Maxillary sinus

The paranasal sinuses are air-filled cavities within the bones of the skull. Like the nasal cavities into which they drain, they are lined by mucous membrane. Their locations are diagrammed above. Only the frontal and maxillary sinuses are readily accessible to clinical examination.

THE MOUTH AND THE PHARYNX

Structures in the mouth and pharynx are illustrated below.

The dorsum of the tongue is covered by papillae, giving it a roughened surface. A thin white coating is frequent and normal. Often just visible toward the back of the tongue are the large vallate papillae. These should not be confused with tumor nodules.

Above and behind the tongue rises an arch formed by the anterior and posterior pillars, soft palate, and uvula. The tonsils can be seen in the fossae, or cavities, between the anterior and posterior pillars. The posterior pharynx may normally show small blood vessels and patches of lymphoid tissue on its surface.

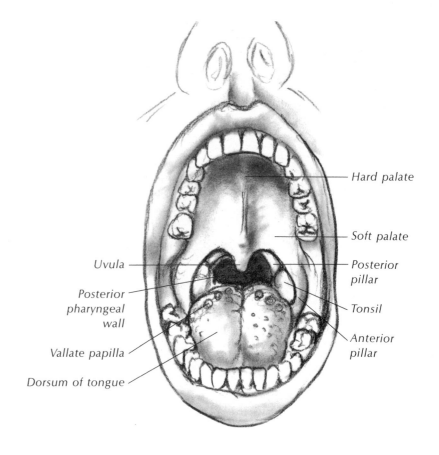

The undersurface of the tongue is smooth. At its base can be seen Wharton's ducts—ducts of the submaxillary glands—and their openings. The parotid duct (Stensen's duct) opens onto the buccal mucosa near the upper 2nd molar, where its location is frequently marked by a small papilla.

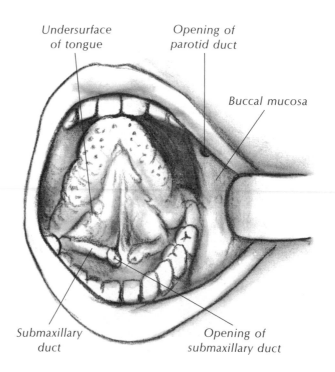

A full complement of 32 adult teeth
(16 in each jaw) is identified here.

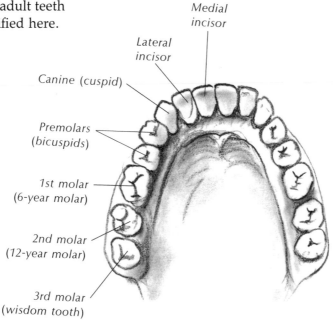

*Medial
incisor*

*Lateral
incisor*

Canine (cuspid)

*Premolars
(bicuspids)*

*1st molar
(6-year molar)*

*2nd molar
(12-year molar)*

*3rd molar
(wisdom tooth)*

THE NECK

For descriptive purposes each side
of the neck is divided into two tri-
angles by the sternomastoid muscle. The anterior triangle is bounded
above by the mandible, laterally by
the sternomastoid, and medially by
the midline of the body. The posterior triangle extends from the
sternomastoid to the trapezius and
is bounded below by the clavicle. A
portion of the omohyoid muscle
crosses its lower portion and can be
mistaken by the uninitiated for a
lymph node or mass.

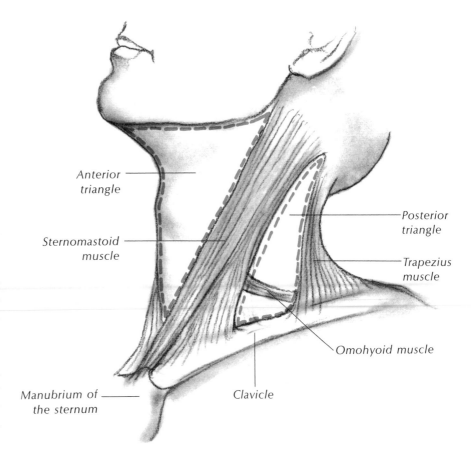

*Anterior
triangle*

*Sternomastoid
muscle*

*Posterior
triangle*

*Trapezius
muscle*

Omohyoid muscle

*Manubrium of
the sternum*

Clavicle

From above down identify the following midline structures: (1) the mobile hyoid bone just below the mandible, (2) the thyroid cartilage, readily identified by the notch on its superior edge, (3) the cricoid cartilage, (4) the tracheal rings, and (5) the soft thyroid isthmus which lies across the trachea below the cricoid. The lateral lobes of the thyroid curve posteriorly around the sides of the trachea and the esophagus. They are partially covered by the sternomastoid muscles and are not usually palpable.

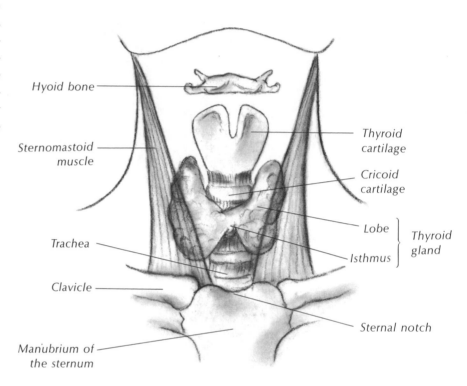

Deep to the sternomastoids run the great vessels of the neck: the carotid artery and internal jugular vein. The external jugular vein passes diagonally over the surface of the sternomastoid.

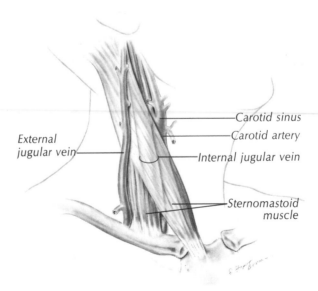

The lymph nodes of the head and neck have been classified in a variety of ways. One system of classification is shown here, together with the directions of lymphatic drainage. The deep cervical chain is largely obscured by the overlying sternomastoid muscle, but at its two extremes the tonsillar node and the supraclavicular nodes may be palpable. Note that the tonsillar, submaxillary, and submental nodes drain portions of the mouth and throat as well as the more superficial tissues of the face. Knowledge of the lymphatic system is important to a sound clinical habit: whenever a malignant or inflammatory lesion is observed, look for involvement of the regional lymph nodes that drain it; whenever a node is enlarged or tender, look for a source in the area that it drains.

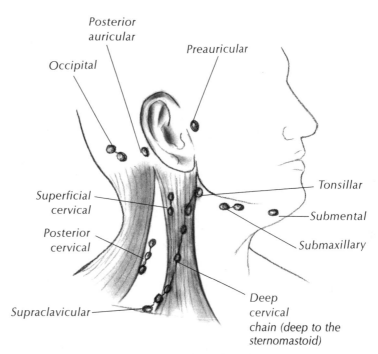

LYMPH NODES OF THE HEAD AND NECK

From abdomen, breast, thorax, and arm

⟵—— *External lymphatic drainage*

⟵--- *Internal lymphatic drainage (e.g., from mouth and throat)*

LYMPHATIC DRAINAGE OF THE HEAD AND NECK

CHANGES WITH AGE

Several changes in the head and neck accompany adolescence. In boys the voice begins to deepen and the thyroid cartilage enlarges perceptibly during the adolescent growth spurt. Facial hair appears on the upper lip, then on the cheeks and the lower lip, and finally on the chin. The facial contours of both boys and girls change subtly as children turn into young adults. Lengthening of the eyeballs in their anteroposterior diameter may cause or accentuate myopia, or nearsightedness. The comedones (blackheads) and pustules of acne appear on the face so commonly that they are almost considered an adolescent norm. Lymphoid tissues, which grow rapidly in late childhood (see p. 447), are still relatively prominent in adolescents, and cervical lymph nodes are readily palpable in most teenagers. The frequency of palpable cervical nodes gradually diminishes with age and, according to one study, falls below 50% some time between the ages of 50 and 60.

The eyes, ears, and mouth bear the brunt of old age. Visual acuity remains fairly constant between the ages of 20 and 50, then diminishes gradually until about age 70, more rapidly after that. Nevertheless most elderly people retain good to adequate vision—20/20 to 20/70 as measured by standard charts. Near vision, however, begins to blur noticeably for virtually everyone. From childhood on, the lens gradually loses its elasticity and the eye grows progressively less able to focus on nearby objects. This loss of accommodative power, called presbyopia, usually becomes noticeable in one's 40s.

While aging alters function of the eyes it also alters structure. In some elderly people the fat that surrounds and cushions the eye within the bony orbit atrophies, allowing the eyeball to recede somewhat in the orbit. The skin of the eyelids becomes wrinkled, occasionally hanging in loose folds. Fat may push the fascia of the eyelids forward, creating soft bulges especially in the lower lids and the inner third of the upper ones (p. 97). Combinations of a weakened levator palpebrae, relaxation of the skin, and increased weight of the upper eyelid may cause a senile ptosis. More important, the lower lid may fall outward away from the eyeball or turn inward onto it, resulting in ectropion and entropion respectively (p. 97). Because their eyes produce fewer lacrimal secretions, aging patients may complain of dryness of the eyes. Simple inspection, however, must usually be supplemented by special testing to make this assessment.

Corneal arcus, or arcus senilis, is common in elderly persons and in them has no clinical significance (p. 100). The corneas lose some of their luster. The pupils decrease in size with age, making ophthalmoscopic examination more difficult. They may become slightly irregular but should continue to respond to light and accommodation—normally or perhaps a little less briskly. Except for possible impairment in upward gaze, extraocular movements should remain intact.

Lenses thicken and yellow with age, impairing the passage of light to the retinas, and elderly people need more light to read and do fine work. When the lens of an elderly person is examined with a flashlight, it frequently looks gray, as if it were opaque, when in fact it permits good visual acuity and looks clear on ophthalmoscopic examination. Do not depend on your flashlight alone, therefore, to make a diagnosis of cataract—a true opacity of the lens (p. 100). Cataracts do become relatively common, however, affecting 1 out of 10 people in their 60s and 1 out of 3 in their 80s. Because the lens continues to grow over the years, it may push the iris forward, narrowing the angle between iris and cornea and increasing the risk of narrow-angle glaucoma (p. 75).

Ophthalmoscopic examination reveals fundi that have lost their youthful shine and light reflections. The arterioles look narrowed, paler, straighter, and less brilliant (see Table 5-14). Drusen (colloid bodies) may be seen (p. 108). On a somewhat more anterior plane you may be able to see some vitreous floaters—degenerative changes that may cause annoying specks or webs in the field of vision. You may also find evidence of other more serious conditions that occur more often in elderly people than in younger ones: senile macular degeneration, glaucoma, retinal hemorrhages, or possibly retinal detachment.

Acuity of hearing, like that of vision, usually diminishes with age. Early losses, which start in young adulthood, involve primarily the high-pitched sounds beyond the range of human speech and have relatively little functional significance. Gradually, however, loss continues and begins to encroach on sounds in the middle and lower ranges. When a person fails to catch the upper tones of words while hearing the lower ones, words sound distorted and conversation is difficult to understand, especially in noisy environments. Hearing loss associated with aging, known as presbycusis, becomes increasingly evident after the approximate age of 50.

The sense of smell may diminish with age and so may the sense of taste, especially for sweetness. The oral mucosa tends to be pale and dry in elderly people, and salivary secretions are diminished. Teeth may be worn down or abraded (p. 121) or may have been lost to dental caries or other conditions. Periodontal disease is the chief cause of tooth loss in most adults (p. 120). If a person has no teeth the lower portion of his face looks small and sunken, with accentuated "purse-string" wrinkles radiating out from the mouth. Overclosure of the mouth may lead to maceration of the skin at the corners—angular stomatitis (p. 117). The bony ridges of the jaws that once surrounded the tooth sockets are gradually resorbed, especially in the lower jaw.

Techniques of Examination

THE HEAD

Because abnormalities covered by the hair are so easily missed, ask the patient if he has noticed anything wrong with his scalp or hair.

Inspect and palpate:

The Hair. Note its quantity, distribution, pattern of loss if any, and texture. Identify nits (the eggs of lice) if present, differentiating them from dandruff.

Fine hair in hyperthyroidism; coarse hair in hypothyroidism. Tiny white ovoid nits adherent to hairs; loose white flakes of dandruff

The Scalp. Part the hair in several places and look for scaliness, lumps, or other lesions.

Redness and scaling in dandruff (seborrhea), psoriasis

The Skull. Observe the general size and contour of the skull. Note any deformities, lumps, or tenderness.

Enlarged skull in hydrocephalus, Paget's disease

The Face. Note the patient's facial expression and contours. Observe for asymmetry, involuntary movements, edema, and masses.

See Table 5-1, Selected Facies (p. 95).

The Skin. Observe the skin, noting its color, pigmentation, texture, thickness, hair distribution, and any lesions.

Acne in many adolescents

Hirsutism (excessive facial hair) in some women

THE EYES

Testing Vision

Visual Acuity is a test of central vision. If possible use a Snellen eye chart and light it well. Position the patient 20 feet from the chart. If he uses glasses other than reading glasses, he should wear them. Ask him to cover one eye with a card (so that he will not peek between his fingers) and to read the smallest line of print possible. Coax him to try a smaller line if he can. If the patient cannot read the largest letter, position him closer to the chart. Determine the smallest line of print from which he is able to identify more than half the letters. Record the visual acuity designated at the side of this line, together with the use of glasses, if any. Visual acuity is expressed as a fraction (*e.g.,* 20/30), in which the numerator indicates the distance of the patient from the chart, the denominator the distance at which a normal eye can read the line of letters.

Vision of 20/200 means that the patient can read at 20 feet only very large letters, which a person with normal vision could read at 200 feet. The larger the denominator, the worse the vision. "20/40 corrected" means the patient could read the 40 line with glasses (a correction).

Testing near vision with a handheld card is especially useful with middle-aged and older people. Handheld cards also enable you to test visual acuity at the bedside. When the card is held at about 13 inches from the

Presbyopia refers to the impaired near vision found in middle-aged and older people.

patient's eyes, the letters are equivalent in size to those on the larger 20-foot charts. You may, however, let the patient choose his own distance. If the patient has reading glasses, he should wear them.

Both kinds of charts are available with numbers or with *E*s that face in different directions for people who cannot read letters.

If you have no charts, screen visual acuity with any available print. If the patient cannot read even the largest letters, test his ability to count your upraised fingers and distinguish light (such as your flashlight) from dark.

Visual Fields by Confrontation is a rough clinical test of peripheral vision. This procedure is usually omitted in a routine examination but should be included whenever a neurologic problem is suspected. Because it is a rather crude method, it should be supplemented, if indicated, by special techniques such as perimetry or a tangent screen.

Poor peripheral vision can cause functional impairment even when visual acuity is normal.

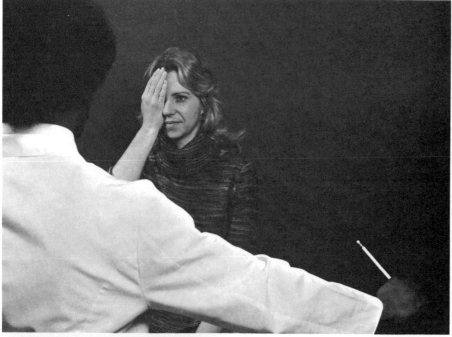

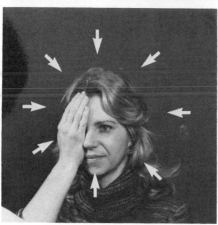

Ask the patient to cover one eye, without pressing on it, and to look at your eye directly opposite. Position yourself so that your face is directly in front and on the level with his, about 2 feet away. Close your other eye so that your own visual field is roughly superimposable on that of the patient. Bring a pencil or other small test object from the periphery into his field of vision from several directions as shown.

See Table 5-2, Visual Field Defects Produced by Selected Lesions in the Visual Pathways (p. 96).

The test object should be equidistant between you and the patient except in the temporal field. Because a normal person, even when looking straight ahead, can detect a moving object almost 90° to the side, you must test his temporal field of vision by first placing the test object somewhat behind him, a location that is unavoidably well within your visual field. Moving slowly enough to give him time to respond, ask him to indicate when the object appears. Compare his field against your own.

Repeat with the other eye.

Position and Alignment of the Eyes. Survey the eyes for their position and alignment with each other. If you note unusually prominent eyes, especially on one side, inspect them from above. Stand behind the seated patient, draw his upper lids gently upward, and note the relationship of the corneas to the lower lids.

Exophthalmos refers to an abnormal protrusion of the eyeball. Bilateral exophthalmos suggests Graves' disease. Unilateral involvement suggests a tumor or inflammatory lesion of the orbit but may also be seen in Graves' disease.

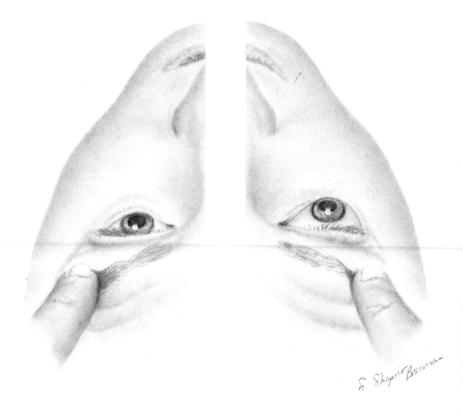

Eyebrows. Inspect the eyebrows, noting their quantity, distribution, and any scaliness of the underlying skin.

Scaliness in seborrhea; loss of lateral 3rd in myxedema and in normal aging

Eyelids. Note the position of the lids in relationship to the eyeballs. Inspect for:

See Table 5-3, Abnormalities of the Eyelids (p. 97).

Edema

Color (*e.g.,* redness)

See Table 5-4, Lumps and Swellings in and Around the Eyes (p. 98).

Lesions

Condition and direction of the eyelashes

Adequacy with which the eyelids close. Look for this especially when the eyes are unusually prominent, when there is facial paralysis, or when the patient is unconscious.

Failure of the eyelids to close exposes the corneas to serious damage.

Lacrimal Apparatus. Inspect the region of the lacrimal gland. If you suspect enlargement of the lacrimal glands because of either the patient's history or your observation, elevate the temporal aspect of the upper lid and ask the patient to look down and to the opposite side. Observe for a swollen lacrimal gland protruding between the upper lid and eyeball. In many normal people a small portion of the lacrimal gland can be brought into view by this maneuver.

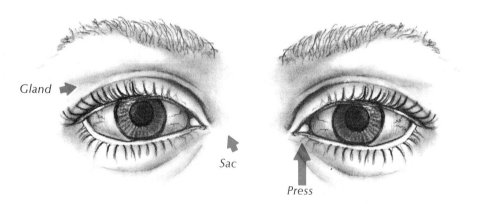

Gland

Sac

Press

Inspect the area of the lacrimal sac for swelling. If tearing is excessive, check for nasolacrimal duct obstruction by pressing on the medial aspect of the lower eyelid just inside the orbital rim. Watch for regurgitation of fluid out of the lacrimal duct openings (puncta). Palpate the area for tenderness, but press only gently on an acutely inflamed lacrimal sac.

Regurgitation of fluid from the puncta suggests an obstructed nasolacrimal duct.

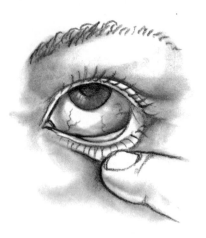

Conjunctivas and Scleras. Ask the patient to look up as you depress both lower lids with your thumbs, exposing the scleras and conjunctivas. Inspect the scleras and palpebral conjunctivas for color, and note the blood vessels against the white scleral background. Look for any nodules or swelling.

Yellow scleras of jaundice

Pale palpebral conjunctivas of anemia

Increased number and size of visible blood vessels in inflammation and other conditions. See Table 5-5, Red Eyes (p. 99).

Special Technique for Inspection of the Upper Palpebral Conjunctiva. Adequate examination of the eye in search of a foreign body requires eversion of the upper eyelid. To do this:

1. Instruct the patient to look down.
2. Get the patient to relax his eyes—by reassurance and by gentle, assured, and deliberate movements.
3. Raise the upper eyelid slightly so that the eyelashes protrude, then grasp the upper eyelashes and pull them gently down and forward.
4. Place a small stick such as an applicator or tongue blade at least 1 cm above the lid margin (and therefore at the upper border of the tarsal plate). Push down on the upper eyelid, thus everting it or turning it "inside out." Do not press on the eyeball itself.

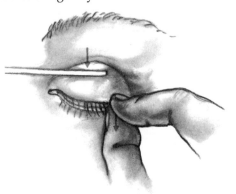

5. Secure the upper lashes against the eyebrow with your fingers and inspect the palpebral conjunctiva.
6. After your inspection, grasp the upper eyelashes and pull them gently forward. Ask the patient to look up. The eyelid will return to its normal position.

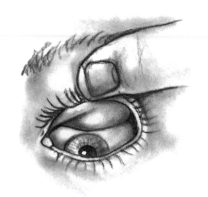

Cornea and Lens. With oblique lighting inspect the cornea of each eye for opacities and note any opacities in the lens that may be visible through the pupil.

See Table 5-6, Opacities of the Cornea and Lens (p. 100).

Iris. At the same time inspect the iris. Its markings should be clearly defined. Now look for a crescentic shadow on the side away from your light. Since the iris normally forms a relatively open angle with the cornea, oblique lighting casts no shadow.

In a small percentage of people the iris bows further forward, forming an unusually narrow angle with the cornea. The light then casts a crescentic shadow.

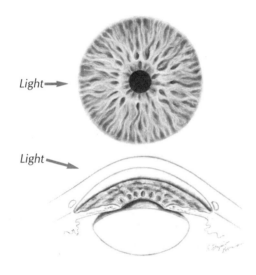 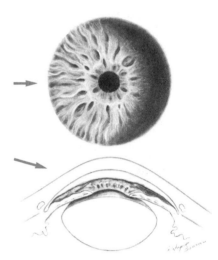

Light→

Light

In the more common kind of glaucoma—open-angle glaucoma—no shadow is cast either.

People with a narrow angle have an increased risk of acute narrow-angle (angle-closure) glaucoma—a sudden increase in intraocular pressure when drainage of aqueous humor is blocked.

Pupils. Inspect the size, shape, and equality of the pupils.

See Table 5-7, Pupillary Abnormalities (pp. 101–102).

Test the *pupillary reaction to light.* Ask the patient to look into the distance (so that accommodation will not constrict his pupils). Then shine a bright light on each pupil in turn. Inspect for:

1. The direct reaction (pupillary constriction in the same eye)
2. The consensual reaction (pupillary constriction in the opposite eye)

Always darken the room and use a bright light before deciding that a pupillary reaction is absent.

Test the *pupillary reaction to accommodation*. Ask the patient to look into the distance and then at your finger held 5 cm to 10 cm from the bridge of his nose. Note:

1. The pupillary constriction
2. Convergence of the eyes. (Convergence is also part of the extraocular muscle examination and if observed here need not be repeated.)

Extraocular Muscles. Look for weakness or imbalance of the extraocular muscles. First, shine a light onto the patient's eyes from 2 to 3 feet in front of him and ask him to look at it. You should see the light reflected symmetrically from each cornea.

Asymmetry of the corneal reflections indicates a deviation from normal ocular alignment, which may be caused by muscle weakness. If you notice asymmetry or if a patient has complained of double vision or eyestrain, do a cover test (see p. 103 and pp. 474–476). A cover test may bring out a latent muscle imbalance not otherwise seen.

Then, assess the extraocular movements. Ask the patient to follow your finger or pencil as you sweep through the six cardinal fields of gaze. Making a wide H in the air, you should lead the patient into his extreme fields of gaze: (1) to his right, (2) to his right and upward, then (3) down to the right, (4) to his left, (5) to his left and upward, and finally (6) down to his left. Move your finger or pencil at a comfortable distance from the patient. Because middle-aged or older people may have difficulty focusing on near objects, it is helpful to make this distance greater for them than for young people. Pause during upward and lateral gaze to detect nystagmus.

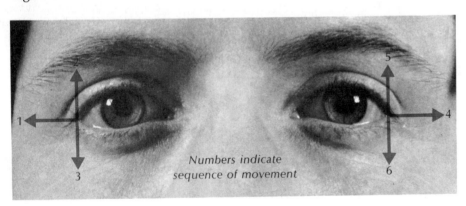

Numbers indicate sequence of movement

Inspect for:

See Table 5-8, Deviations of the Eyes (p. 103).

1. The normal conjugate, or parallel, movements of the eyes in each direction, or any deviation from normal

2. Abnormal movements of the eyes (*e.g.,* nystagmus, a rhythmic fine oscillation of the eyes). A few beats of nystagmus on extreme lateral gaze are within normal limits. If you see it, bring your finger in to within the field of binocular vision and look again.

Sustained nystagmus within the binocular field of gaze is seen in a variety of neurologic conditions. See Table 15-3, Nystagmus (pp. 414–415).

3. The relation of the upper eyelid to the globe as the eyes move from above downward. Normally, the lid overlaps the iris slightly throughout this movement. If you suspect hyperthyroidism, ask the patient to follow your finger again as you move it slowly from up to down in the midline.

Lid lag in hyperthyroidism; a rim of sclera is seen between the upper lid and iris and the lid appears to lag behind the globe.

Ask the patient to follow your finger or pencil as you move it in toward the bridge of his nose. Note convergence of the eyes. This is normally sustained to within 5 cm to 8 cm.

Poor convergence in hyperthyroidism

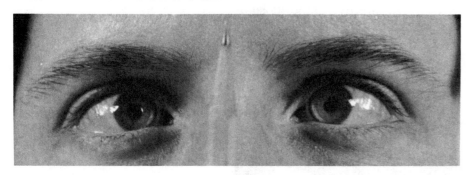

Ophthalmoscopic Examination. For most purposes you can usually perform an adequate ophthalmoscopic examination without dilating the patient's pupils. To evaluate the macula well or to investigate the cause of unexplained visual loss, however, you will need to dilate the pupils unless there is a contraindication. Use an appropriate mydriatic drug such as tropicamide (Mydriacyl).

Do not use mydriatic drops if there is any suspicion of glaucoma. Dilatation may precipitate attacks of narrow-angle glaucoma in predisposed persons.

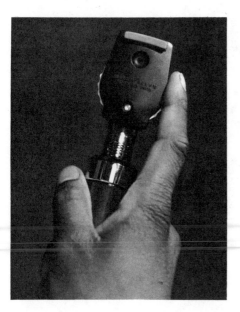

Darken the room. Switch on the ophthalmoscope light, and adjust it to the large round beam of white light.* Turn the lens disc to 0 diopters (a lens that neither converges nor diverges the light rays). Keep your index finger on the lens disc so that you can refocus the ophthalmoscope during the examination.

*Some clinicians like to use the large round beam for large pupils, the small round beam for small pupils. The other beams are rarely helpful. The slitlike beam is sometimes used to assess elevations or concavities in the retina, the green (or red-free) beam to detect small red lesions, and the grid to make measurements. Ignore the last three lights and practice with the large round white beam.

Use your *right hand* and *right eye* for the patient's *right eye;* your *left hand* and *left eye* for the patient's *left eye.*

Place the thumb of your opposite hand on the patient's eyebrow. Your thumb gives you some proprioceptive guidance as you move closer to the patient, especially when you are inexperienced; and you may use it gently to elevate the patient's upper lid if necessary. Ask the patient to look straight ahead or slightly toward the side you are examining. He should fix his gaze on a specific point on the wall. Hold the ophthalmoscope firmly braced against your face, with your eye directly behind its sight hole.

From a position about 15 inches away from the patient and about 15° lateral to his line of vision, shine the light beam on his pupil.

Note the orange glow in the pupil—the *red reflex.* Also note any opacities interrupting the red reflex.

Absence of a red reflex suggests an opacity of the lens (cataract) or possibly of the vitreous. Less commonly, a detached retina may obscure this reflex. Do not be fooled by an artificial eye, which of course has no red reflex either.

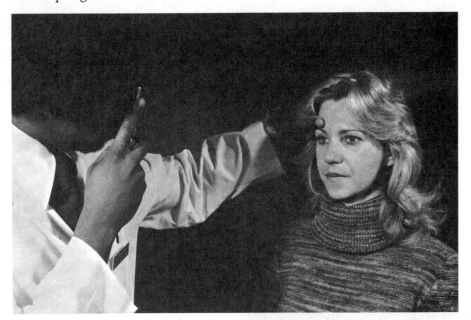

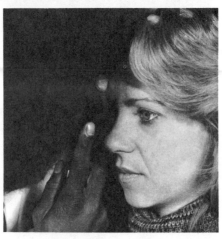

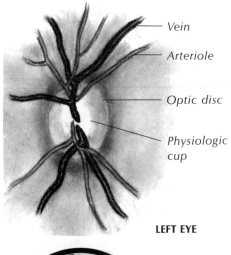

Vein

Arteriole

Optic disc

Physiologic cup

LEFT EYE

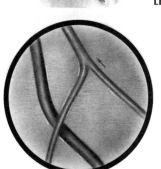

Keep your eyes relaxed, as if gazing into the distance. Try to keep both eyes open. Keeping the light beam focused on the red reflex, move in toward the pupil until your ophthalmoscope is very close to it. Your forehead should be on or very near your thumb. If you have approached horizontally on the 15° angle, you should now be seeing the retina in the vicinity of the *optic disc*—a yellowish orange to creamy pink, oval or round structure. The disc will probably fill your field of gaze. If you do not see it, follow a blood vessel centrally until you do. You can tell which way is "central" by noting the angles at which vessels branch and the progressive enlargement of vessel size as you approach the disc. Some trial and error may be necessary.

Now *bring the optic disc into sharp focus* by adjusting the lens disc. When examining a nearsighted (myopic) patient, whose eyeball is somewhat longer than normal, you will need to use a lens with a longer focus. To do this, rotate the lens disc counterclockwise to the lenses identified by the red numbers, indicating minus diopters.* When examining a farsighted patient or one whose own lens has been surgically removed, rotate the disc clockwise to the lenses of plus diopters, indicated by the black numbers. To illustrate these points:

When the lens has been surgically removed, its magnifying effect is lost. Retinal structures then look much smaller than usual, and you can see a much larger expanse of fundus.

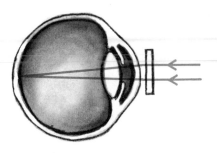

NORMAL EYE

When the patient's eye, as well as your own, is normal in size, you can usually focus clearly on the retina with a lens of 0 diopters (clear glass).

*A diopter is a unit which measures the power of a lens to converge or diverge light.

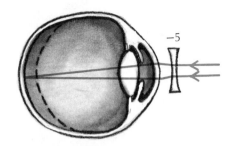

NEARSIGHTED EYE

When the patient is nearsighted, you will need a lens with a longer focus (minus diopters).

In a nearsighted (myopic) eye, retinal structures are magnified more than usual. The disc may exceed the size of your view.

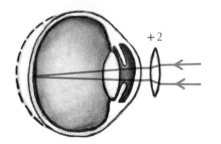

FARSIGHTED EYE

A lens with a shorter focus (*e.g.,* +1 or +2 diopters) is needed for far-sighted eyes.

In a farsighted (hyperopic) eye, retinal structures look somewhat smaller than usual.

Note:

1. The clarity of the disc outline. The nasal outline may normally be somewhat blurred.
2. The color of the disc, normally yellowish orange to creamy pink
3. The possible presence of normal white or pigmented rings or crescents around the disc
4. The size of the central physiologic cup, if present. This cup is normally yellowish white. Its horizontal diameter is usually less than half the horizontal diameter of the disc.

See Table 5-9, Normal Variations of the Optic Disc (p. 104).

See Table 5-10, Abnormalities of the Optic Disc (p. 105).

You may also see some pulsations of the veins as they cross the disc. Gentle pressure on the eye through the eyelid usually makes such pulsations evident even if you did not see them earlier. This maneuver is not, however, part of the routine examination.

The presence of venous pulsations at the disc gives some reassurance that cerebrospinal fluid pressure is normal, although exceptions occur.

Identify the *arterioles and veins*. They may be distinguished by the following features:

	ARTERIOLES	VEINS
COLOR	Light red	Dark red
SIZE	Smaller (⅔ to ⅘ the diameter of veins)	Larger
LIGHT REFLEX (or reflection)	Bright	Inconspicuous or absent

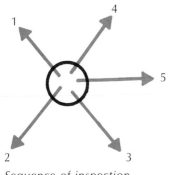

*Sequence of inspection
from disc to macula*

LEFT EYE

Follow the vessels peripherally in each of four directions, noting their relative sizes and the character of the arteriovenous crossings. Identify any lesions of the surrounding *retina* and note their size, shape, color, and distribution. As you search the retina, move your head and instrument as a unit, using the patient's pupil as an imaginary fulcrum. Until you gain experience, you may repeatedly lose your view of the retina because your light falls out of the pupil. You will improve with practice.

See Table 5-11, Retinal Arterioles and Arteriovenous Crossings: Normal and Hypertensive (p. 106).

See Table 5-12, Red Spots in the Retina (p. 107).

See Table 5-13, Light-Colored Spots in the Retina (p. 108).

See Table 5-14, Ocular Fundi (pp. 109–111).

Finally, by directing your light beam laterally or by asking the patient to look directly into the light, inspect the *macular area*. This is an avascular area somewhat larger than the disc but has no distinct margins. Except in older people the tiny bright reflection at its center—the fovea—helps to identify it. Shimmering light reflections in the macular area are common in young people.

Visualizing the macula is unfortunately difficult. Unless you use a mydriatic, the patient's pupil constricts maximally; light reflections off the cornea may further obscure your view. Moving the ophthalmoscope slightly from side to side may help you get around the reflections.

The macular area is especially important because it is responsible for central vision. Senile macular degeneration is an important cause of impaired central vision in elderly people. It takes many forms, including hemorrhages, exudates, cysts, and "holes." A common form with altered pigmentation is illustrated here.

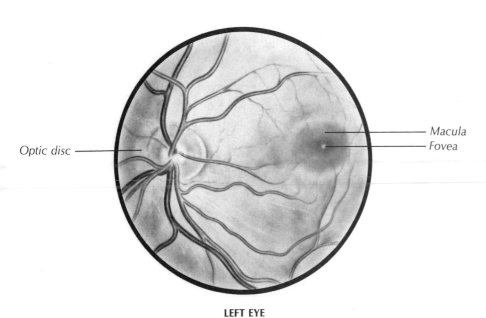

Optic disc ——

—— Macula
—— Fovea

LEFT EYE

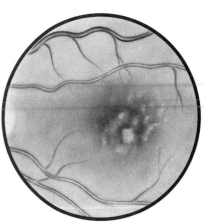

SENILE MACULAR DEGENERATION

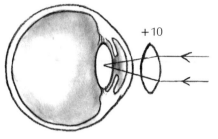

ANTERIOR STRUCTURES

If you suspect opacities in the *vitreous* or *lens,* inspect these normally transparent structures by rotating the lens disc progressively to diopters of around +10 or +12. This maneuver focuses on the anterior structures within the eyeball.

Age is the most common of the many causes of cataracts. Symptoms include impaired vision, annoying glare from bright lights, and distortion in vision.

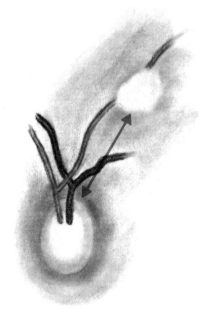

A Note on Measurement Within the Eye. Lesions of the retina can be located in relationship to the optic disc and are measured in terms of "disc diameters" and diopters. For example, "a lesion about ⅔ of a disc diameter in size located at 1 o'clock, almost 2 disc diameters from the disc" describes the abnormality shown on the left.

The elevated optic disc of papilledema can be measured by noting the differences in diopters of the two lenses used to focus clearly on the disc and on the uninvolved retina.

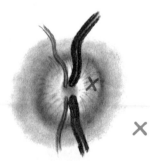

Clear focus here at +2 diopters

Clear focus here at −1 diopter

$+2 - (-1) = +3,$ therefore a disc elevation of 3 diopters

For Interest. On ophthalmoscopic examination, the normal retina is magnified about 15 times, the normal iris about 4 times. The optic disc actually measures about 1.5 mm. At the retina, 3 diopters of elevation = 1 mm.

THE EARS

The Auricle. Inspect the auricle and surrounding tissues for deformities, lumps, or skin lesions.

If ear pain, discharge, or inflammation is present, move the auricle up and down, then press on the tragus, and press firmly just behind the ear.

See Table 5-15, Nodules in and Around the Ears (p. 113).

Movement of the auricle and tragus is painful in acute otitis externa, but not in otitis media.

Tenderness behind the ear may be present in otitis media.

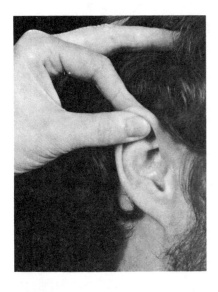

Ear Canal and Drum. The patient's head should be tipped slightly to the opposite side. Grasp the auricle firmly but gently, pulling it upward, back, and slightly out.

Insert into the canal, slightly down and forward, the largest *speculum* that the canal will accommodate. Two possible grips are illustrated below. The first feels firm and natural. The second, because your hand is lightly braced against the patient's head, is especially helpful for active patients such as children.

Nontender nodular swellings covered by normal skin deep in the ear canals suggest osteomas. These are nonmalignant overgrowths, which may obscure the drum.

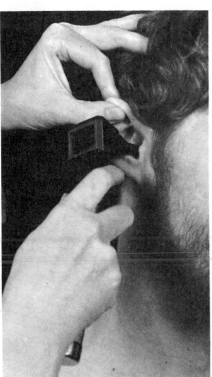
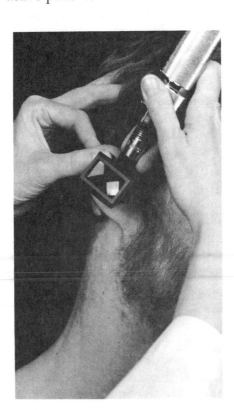

Identify wax, discharge, or foreign bodies in the ear canal. Note any redness or swelling of the canal.

Soggy pallor or redness, swelling, narrowing, and pain may be found in acute otitis externa.

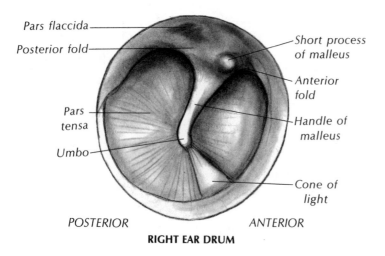

RIGHT EAR DRUM

POSTERIOR   ANTERIOR

Pars flaccida
Posterior fold
Pars tensa
Umbo
Short process of malleus
Anterior fold
Handle of malleus
Cone of light

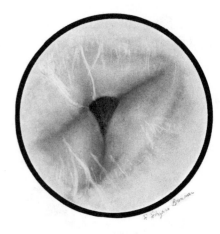

EAR CANAL IN OTITIS EXTERNA

Inspect the drum, identifying the landmarks: the pars tensa with its cone of light, the umbo, the handle and short process of the malleus, the anterior and posterior folds, and the pars flaccida.

See Table 5-16, Abnormalities of the Eardrum (p. 114).

Gently move the speculum so that you can see the entire drum, including the periphery. Note the color, thickness, and luster of the drum, and the position of the light reflex and handle of the malleus. Look for any perforations.

Fluid in the middle ear may be detected through the ear drum when a fluid level or air bubbles are identified. In most cases pneumatic otoscopy is required (see p. 481).

Auditory Acuity. To estimate hearing, test one ear at a time. Ask the patient to occlude one ear with his finger or, better still, occlude it for him. When auditory acuity on the two sides is quite different, simple occlusion of the better ear is inadequate. Under these circumstances move your finger rapidly, but gently, in the patient's ear canal. The noise so produced will help to prevent the occluded ear from doing the work of the ear you wish to test. Then, standing 1 or 2 feet away, exhale fully (so as to minimize the intensity of your voice) and whisper softly toward the unoccluded ear. Choose numbers with two equally accented syllables, such as "nine-four," and "five-two." If necessary, increase the intensity of your voice to a medium whisper, a loud whisper, then a soft, medium, and loud voice. To make sure the patient does not read your lips, cover your mouth or obstruct his vision.

If hearing loss is present, distinguish between sensorineural deafness and conduction deafness by two maneuvers, both of which require tuning forks. Use a tuning fork of 512 or 1024 Hz. These frequencies fall within the range of human speech (300 Hz–3000 Hz)—the functionally most important range. Forks with lower pitches may cause you to overestimate bone conduction and may also be felt as vibration in addition to being heard. Set the fork into *light* vibration by stroking it between thumb and index finger or by tapping it on your knuckles.

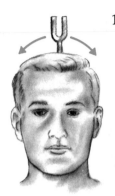

1. *Test for lateralization (Weber Test).* Place the base of the lightly vibrating tuning fork firmly on the top of the patient's head or in the middle of his forehead. Ask where he hears it: on one or both sides. Normally the sound is perceived in the midline or equally in both ears. Sometimes the normal patient perceives the sound only vaguely. If he hears nothing, press the fork more firmly on his head.

In conduction hearing loss, sound is heard in, or lateralized to, the impaired ear. In unilateral sensorineural hearing loss, sound is heard in the good ear.

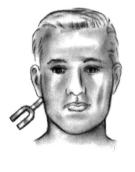

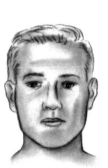

2. *Compare air (AC) and bone conduction (BC) (Rinne Test).* Place the base of a lightly vibrating tuning fork on the mastoid process until the patient can no longer hear the sound. Then quickly place the vibrating fork near the ear canal, with one side toward the ear as shown. Ascertain whether he can hear it. Normally the sound can be heard longer through air than through bone (AC > BC).

In conduction hearing loss, sound is heard longer through bone. In sensorineural hearing loss, sound is heard longer through air (the normal pattern). For explanations, see Table 5-17, Patterns of Hearing Loss (p. 115).

THE NOSE AND SINUSES

Inspect the Nose. Look for deformity, asymmetry, and inflammation.

Gently insert a nasal speculum through the nostril into the vestibule.

Two types of techniques may be used.

1. A *nasal speculum,* used with a head mirror or (by most who are not ENT specialists) a penlight. For this technique, grasp the speculum with your left hand, as shown, and insert the blades about 1 cm into the vestibule, stabilizing the instrument by placing your left finger on the patient's ala nasi. Open the blades wide in an anteroposterior direction, avoiding the sensitive septum. Do not switch examining hands for the opposite naris.

2. An *otoscope*, preferably equipped with a short, wide nasal speculum. This technique gives a narrower field of vision but has the advantages of good light and magnification. Again take care to avoid the nasal septum.

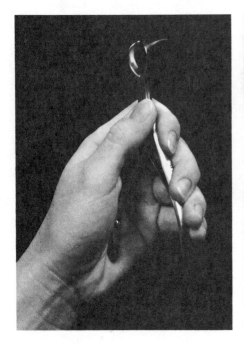
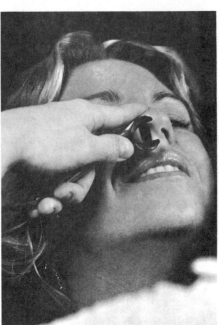

By either technique, inspect the lower portions of the nose, then the upper portions. When using a nasal speculum and head mirror, tip the patient's head back to see the upper parts as illustrated below. When using an otoscope you can move your own head and instrument to see the patient's upper nasal cavity.

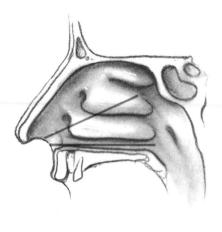

VIEW WITH HEAD ERECT

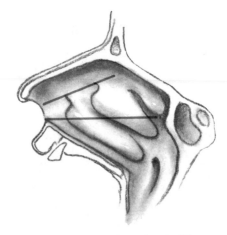

VIEW WITH HEAD TILTED BACK

Inspect:

1. The nasal mucosa, including its color (normally somewhat redder than the oral mucosa), and look for swelling, exudate, and bleeding.
2. The nasal septum, including evidence of bleeding, perforation, or deviation.
3. The inferior and middle turbinates and the middle meatus between them for color, swelling, exudate, and polyps.

See Table 5-18, Common Abnormalities of the Nose (p. 116).

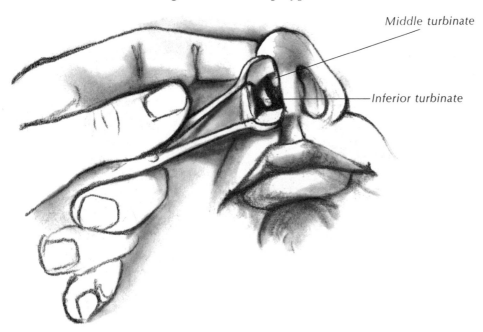

Middle turbinate

Inferior turbinate

Palpate the Sinuses. Palpate for *frontal sinus tenderness* by pressing up from deep under the bony brow on each side. Avoid pressure on the eyes.

Tenderness in acute frontal sinusitis

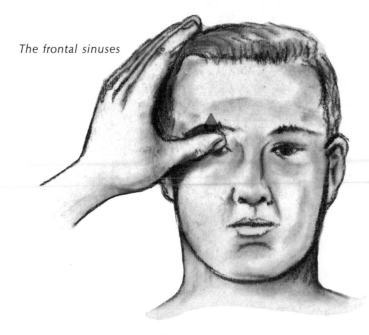

The frontal sinuses

Then press up on each *maxillary sinus.*

Tenderness in acute maxillary sinusitis

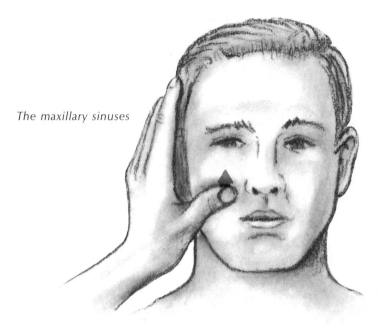

The maxillary sinuses

Transillumination of the Sinuses. Although transillumination is not part of a routine examination, it is often helpful when sinus tenderness or other symptoms suggest sinusitis. The room should be thoroughly darkened. Using a strong, narrow light source, place the light snugly deep under each brow, close to the nose. Shield the light with your hand. Look for a dim red glow as light is transmitted through the air-filled frontal sinus to the forehead.

Absence of glow on one or both sides suggests a thickened mucosa or secretions in the frontal sinus, but it may also result from developmental absence of one or both sinuses.

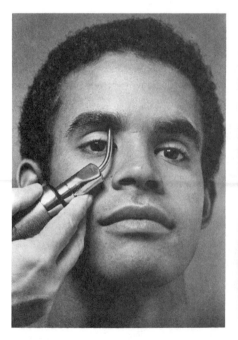 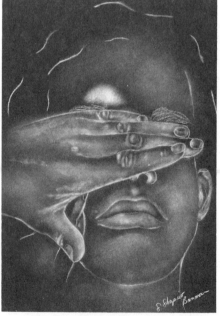

TRANSILLUMINATION OF FRONTAL SINUS

Then ask the patient to open his mouth wide and tilt his head back a little. (An upper denture should first be removed.) Shine the light downward from just below the inner aspect of each eye. Look through the open mouth at the hard palate. A reddish glow indicates a normal air-filled maxillary sinus.

Absence of a glow suggests thickened mucosa or secretions in the maxillary sinus. See page 485 for an alternative method of transilluminating the maxillary sinuses.

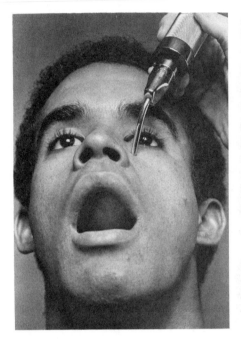 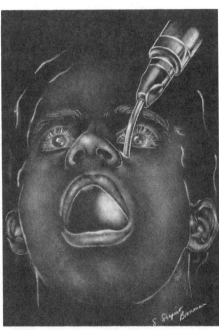

TRANSILLUMINATION OF MAXILLARY SINUS

THE MOUTH AND THE PHARYNX

If the patient wears dentures, offer him a paper towel and ask him to remove them so that you can see the mucosa underneath. If suspicious ulcers or nodules are observed, put on a glove or finger cot and palpate the lesion, noting especially any thickening or infiltration of the tissues that might suggest malignancy.

Bright red edematous mucosa underneath a denture suggests denture sore mouth. There may be ulcers or papillary granulation tissue.

Inspect:

The Lips. Look for color, moisture, lumps, ulcers, or cracking.

Cyanosis, pallor. See Table 5-19, Abnormalities of the Lips (pp. 117–118).

The Buccal Mucosa. Ask the patient to open his mouth. With a good light and the help of a tongue blade inspect the buccal mucosa for color, pigmentation, ulcers, and nodules. Patchy pigmentation is normal in black people.

See Table 5-20, Abnormalities of the Buccal Mucosa and Hard Palate (p. 119).

The Gums and Teeth. Look for:

1. Inflammation, swelling, bleeding, retraction, or discoloration of the gums
2. Loose, missing, or carious teeth and any abnormalities in the position or shape of the teeth

See Table 5-21, Abnormalities of the Gums and Teeth (pp. 120–121).

The Roof of the Mouth. Inspect the color and architecture of the hard palate.

The Tongue. Inspect the dorsum of the tongue, its color and papillae. Note any abnormal smoothness.

See Table 5-22, Abnormalities of the Tongue (p. 122).

Ask the patient to put out his tongue and inspect it for symmetry—a test of the 12th (hypoglossal) cranial nerve. Note its size.

Asymmetrical protrusion in a 12th nerve lesion and in cancer of the tongue; enlargement in myxedema, acromegaly, and amyloidosis.

Inspect the sides and the under surface of the tongue together with the floor of the mouth. These are the areas where malignancies are most likely to develop. Note any white or reddened areas, nodules, or ulcerations. Since cancer of the tongue is more common in men over age 50, especially in those who use tobacco and drink alcohol, a further maneuver is indicated in this group. Explain to the patient what you plan to do and put on gloves. Ask him to protrude his tongue. With your right hand grasp the tip of the tongue with a square of gauze and gently pull it to the patient's left. Inspect the side of the tongue, then palpate it with your gloved left hand, feeling for any induration. Reverse the procedure for the other side.

Cancer of the tongue is the second most common cancer of the mouth, second only to cancer of the lip. Any persistent nodule or ulcer, either red or white, must be suspect. Induration of the lesion further increases the possibility of malignancy. Cancer occurs most frequently on the side of the tongue, and next most often at its base.

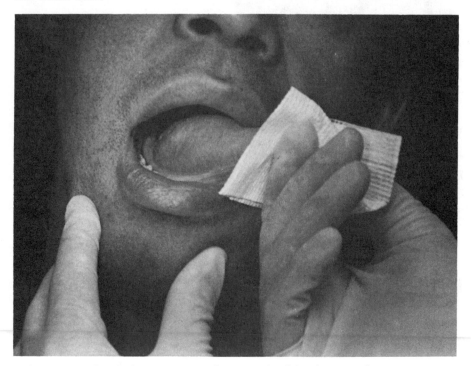

Palpate any other lesions you may have noticed in the mouth.

The Pharynx. Again ask the patient to open his mouth, this time without protruding his tongue. Press a tongue blade firmly down upon the midpoint of the arched tongue—far enough back to get good visualization of the pharynx but not so far that you cause gagging. Simultaneously ask him to say "ah" or to yawn. Note the rise of the soft palate—a test of the 10th cranial (vagus) nerve.

See Table 5-23, Abnormalities of the Pharynx (p. 123).

Inspect the soft palate, anterior and posterior pillars, uvula, tonsils, and posterior pharynx. Note their color and symmetry and any evidence of exudate, edema or ulceration, or tonsillar enlargement. If possible, palpate any suspicious area for induration or tenderness. Tonsils have crypts, or deep infoldings of squamous epithelium. Whitish spots of normal exfoliating epithelium may sometimes be seen in these crypts.

Break or discard your tongue blade after use.

THE NECK

Inspect the Neck. Note symmetry, masses, and scars. Look for enlargement of the parotid or submaxillary glands, and note any visible lymph nodes.

Lymph Nodes. Palpate the lymph nodes. Using the pads of your index and middle fingers, move the skin over the underlying tissues in each area, rather than moving your fingers over the skin. The patient should be relaxed, with his neck flexed slightly forward and, if needed, slightly toward the side of the examination.

Feel in sequence for the following nodes:

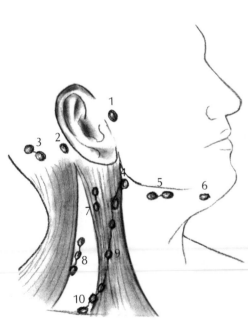

1. Pre-auricular—in front of the ear
2. Posterior auricular—superficial to the mastoid process
3. Occipital—at the base of the skull posteriorly
4. Tonsillar—at the angle of the mandible
5. Submaxillary—halfway between the angle and the tip of the mandible
6. Submental—in the midline behind the tip of the mandible
7. Superficial cervical—superficial to the sternomastoid
8. Posterior cervical chain—along the anterior edge of the trapezius
9. Deep cervical chain—deep to the sternomastoid and often inaccessible to examination. Hook your thumb and fingers around either side of the sternomastoid muscle to find them.
10. Supraclavicular—deep in the angle formed by the clavicle and the sternomastoid

White patches of exudate associated with redness and swelling, however, suggest acute exudative pharyngitis.

A scar of past thyroid surgery may give the clue to unsuspected hypothyroidism.

Enlargement of a supraclavicular node, especially on the left, suggests possible metastasis from a thoracic or abdominal malignancy.

Note their size, shape, delimitation (discrete or matted together), mobility, consistency, and any tenderness. Small, mobile, discrete, nontender nodes are frequently found in normal persons. Detection of enlarged or tender nodes, if unexplained, calls for reexamination of the regions they drain.

Tender nodes suggest inflammation; hard or fixed nodes suggest malignancy.

Trachea and Thyroid. Identify the thyroid and cricoid cartilages and the trachea below them. (The hyoid bone, high in the neck, should not be mistaken for a stony hard tumor.)

Inspect the trachea for any deviation from its usual midline position. Then feel for any deviation. Place your finger along one side of the trachea and note the space between it and the sternomastoid. Compare it with the other side. The spaces should be symmetrical.

Masses in the neck or mediastinum may push the trachea to one side. Tracheal deviation may also signify important problems in the thorax, such as atelectasis or a large pneumothorax (see p. 156).

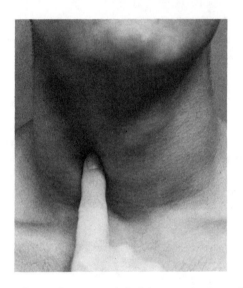

Give the patient a glass of water. Ask him to sip it and then to extend his neck slightly and swallow. Inspect the neck for any visible thyroid tissue, noting its contour and symmetry.

Thyroid tissue rises with swallowing. An enlarged thyroid gland is called a goiter.

Palpate the thyroid, noting its size, shape, symmetry, tenderness, and the presence of any nodules. There are two approaches:

1. *Palpation from in Front.* The patient's neck should be slightly extended, but not enough to tighten the sternomastoid muscles. With the pads of your index and middle fingers, feel below the cricoid cartilage for the thyroid isthmus. Ask the patient to swallow. Feel for the soft fleshy thyroid isthmus rising upward under your fingers.

   Then move your fingers laterally and deep to the anterior border of the sternomastoid. Feel for each lateral lobe before and while the patient swallows.

The larynx, trachea, and thyroid rise with swallowing; other structures such as lymph nodes do not.

Next, ask the patient to flex his neck slightly forward and to his right. Place your right thumb on the lower portion of his thyroid cartilage and displace it to the patient's right. Hook the tips of the index and middle fingers of your left hand behind the sternomastoid muscle while feeling in front of this muscle with your thumb. Your palpating fingers should be positioned below the level of the thyroid cartilage. Feel for the lateral lobe as the patient swallows. Reverse the procedure for the other the side.

See Table 5-24, Thyroid Enlargement and Nodules (p. 124).

You can sometimes feel an enlarged lobe or nodule between your thumb and fingers.

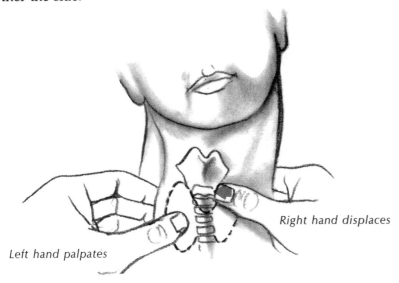

Right hand displaces

Left hand palpates

2. *Palpation from Behind.* From behind the patient you can place your fingers more naturally on the anterior surface of the thyroid and can often feel it better. Again, the patient's neck should be slightly extended. Rest your thumbs on the nape of the patient's neck, find the cricoid cartilage, and feel below it for the thyroid isthmus.

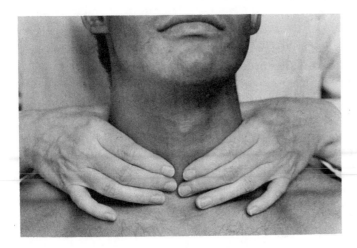

Ask the patient to swallow. Then move your fingers a little to each side and feel for the lateral lobes as the patient swallows again.

Now ask the patient to flex his neck slightly forward and to the right. Displace the thyroid cartilage to the right with the fingers of your left hand. Palpate with your right hand, placing your thumb deep to and behind the sternomastoid and your index and middle fingers in front of it. Ask the patient to swallow.

When a lobe is enlarged, you may be able to grasp it between your thumb and fingers.

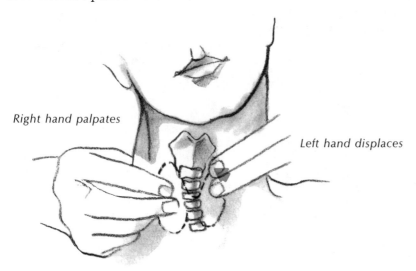

Right hand palpates

Left hand displaces

Reverse the procedure to examine the other side.

Occasionally palpation of the thyroid gland, including the lateral lobes, is more satisfactory with the patient's neck somewhat extended. In a person with a short, stocky neck the thyroid may rise from its usual low position behind the manubrium with this maneuver.

If the thyroid gland is enlarged, listen over the lateral lobes with the diaphragm of a stethoscope for a bruit (a sound similar to a cardiac murmur but of noncardiac origin).

A localized systolic bruit may occur in hyperthyroidism and is to be distinguished from a carotid artery bruit or jugular venous hum.

NOTE: The ability to see or palpate a thyroid gland varies considerably not only with thyroid size but also with the patient's habitus. In a thin person, the isthmus is usually but not always palpable. It may be impossible to find in a stocky neck. Although normal lateral lobes are sometimes palpable, they more often are not.

The Carotid Arteries and Jugular Veins. You will probably wish to defer detailed examination of the great vessels of the neck until the patient lies down for the cardiovascular examination. Jugular venous distention, however, may be visible in the sitting position and should not be overlooked. You should also be alert to unusually prominent arterial pulsations. See Chapter 9 for further discussion.

Table 5-1

Table 5-1 Selected Facies

ACROMEGALY

The increased growth hormone of acromegaly produces enlargement of both bone and soft tissues. The head is elongated, with bony prominence of the forehead, nose, and lower jaw. Soft tissues of the nose, lips, and ears also enlarge. The facial features appear generally coarsened.

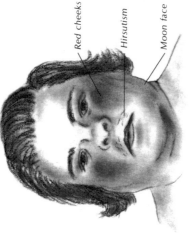

Brow prominent

Soft tissues of nose, ears, lips enlarged

Jaw prominent

MYXEDEMA

The patient with severe hypothyroidism, or myxedema, presents with a dull puffy facies. The edema, often especially pronounced around the eyes, does not pit with pressure. The hair and eyebrows are dry, coarse, and thinned. The skin is dry.

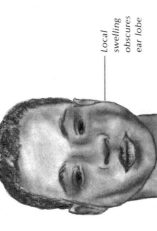

Hair dry, coarse, sparse

Lateral eyebrows thin

Periorbital edema

Puffy dull face with dry skin

NEPHROTIC SYNDROME

The face is edematous and often pale. Swelling usually appears first around the eyes. The eyes may become slitlike when edema is severe.

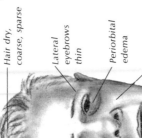
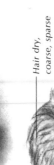

Periorbital edema

Puffy pale face

Lips may be swollen

CUSHING'S SYNDROME

The increased adrenal hormone production of Cushing's syndrome produces a round or "moon" face with red cheeks. Excessive hair growth may be present in the mustache and sideburn areas and on the chin.

Red cheeks

Hirsutism

Moon face

PAROTID GLAND ENLARGEMENT

Chronic bilateral asymptomatic parotid gland enlargement may be associated with obesity, diabetes, cirrhosis and other conditions. Note the swellings anterior to the ear lobes and above the angles of the jaw. Gradual unilateral enlargement suggests neoplasm. Acute enlargement is seen in mumps.

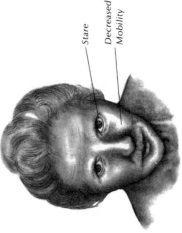
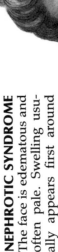

Local swelling obscures ear lobe

PARKINSON'S DISEASE

Decreased facial mobility blunts expression. A mask-like face may result, with decreased blinking and a characteristic stare. Since the neck and upper trunk tend to flex forward, the patient seems to peer upward toward the observer. Facial skin becomes oily, and drooling may occur.

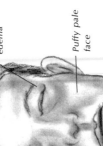

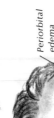

Stare

Decreased Mobility

Table 5-2 Visual Field Defects Produced by Selected Lesions in the Visual Pathways

VISUAL PATHWAYS

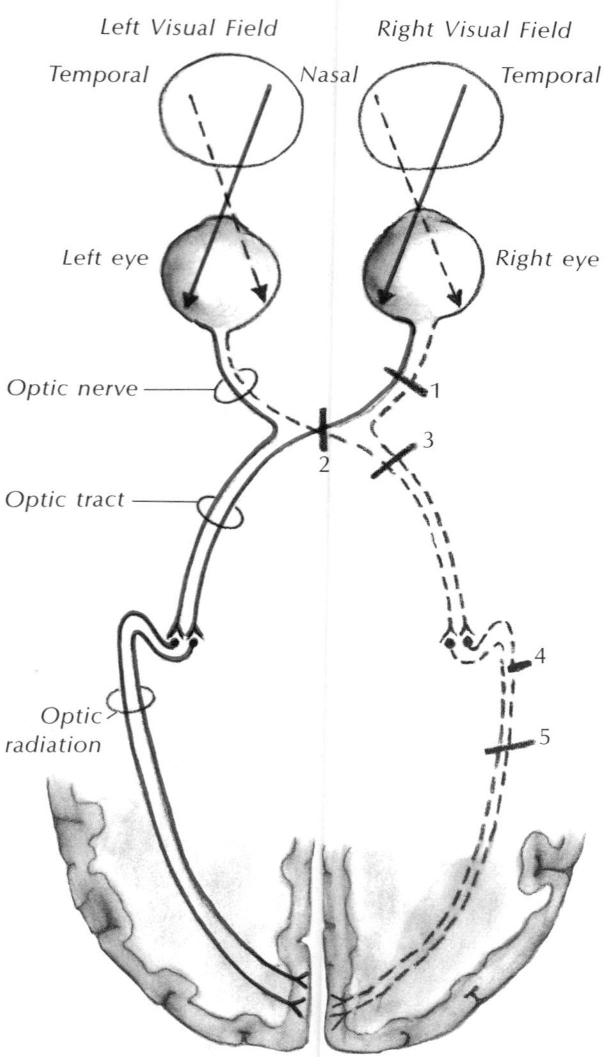

VISUAL FIELDS

BLACKENED FIELD INDICATES AREA OF NO VISION

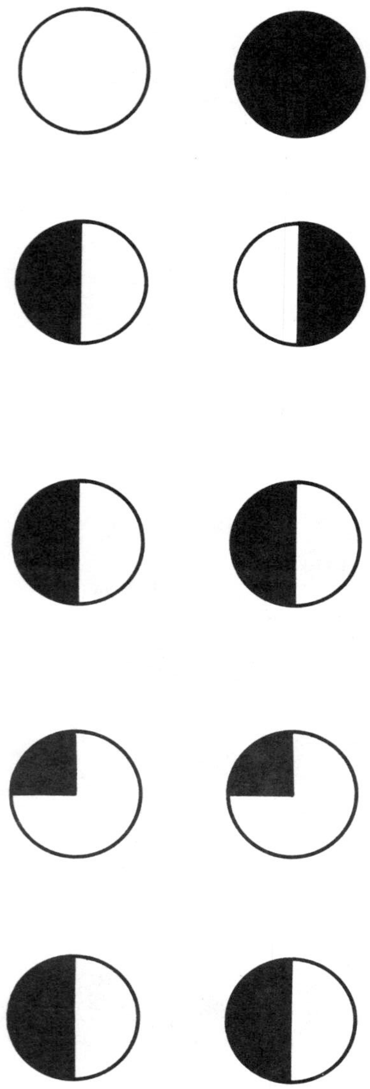

BLIND RIGHT EYE (*right optic nerve*)
A lesion of the optic nerve, and of course of the eye itself, produces unilateral blindness.

BITEMPORAL HEMIANOPSIA (*optic chiasm*)
A lesion at the optic chiasm may involve only those fibers that are crossing over to the opposite side. Since these fibers originate in the nasal half of each retina, visual loss involves the temporal half of each field.

LEFT HOMONYMOUS HEMIANOPSIA (*right optic tract*)
A lesion of the optic tract interrupts fibers originating on the same side of both eyes. Visual loss in the eyes is therefore similar (homonymous) and involves half of each field (hemianopsia).

HOMONYMOUS LEFT UPPER QUADRANTIC DEFECT (*optic radiation, partial*)
A partial lesion of the optic radiation may involve only a portion of the nerve fibers, producing, for example, a homonymous quadrantic defect.

LEFT HOMONYMOUS HEMIANOPSIA (*right optic radiation*)
A complete interruption of fibers in the optic radiation produces a visual defect similar to that produced by a lesion of the optic tract.

Table 5-3

Table 5-3 *Abnormalities of the Eyelids*

PTOSIS

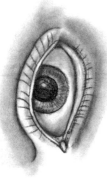

Ptosis refers to drooping of the upper eyelid. Causes include (1) muscular weakness, as in myasthenia gravis, (2) damage to the oculomotor nerve, which controls voluntary elevation of the eyelid, and (3) interference with the sympathetic nerves, which maintain smooth muscle tone of the lid (Horner's syndrome). A weakened muscle, relaxed tissues, and the weight of herniated fat may cause senile ptosis.

RETRACTION OR SPASM OF THE UPPER EYELID AND EXOPHTHALMOS

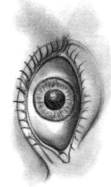

A retracted upper lid is identified by the rim of sclera between lid and iris. The eye has a stare, which is often accentuated by decreased blinking. Look for the associated lid lag when the eye moves slowly from upward to downward gaze. These signs suggest hyperthyroidism. They may simulate or accentuate exophthalmos—an actual forward protrusion of the eyeball (see p. 72).

ECTROPION

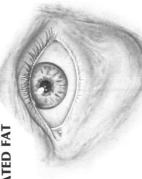

In ectropion the margin of the lid is turned outward, exposing the palpebral conjunctiva. When the punctum of the lower lid turns outward, the eye no longer drains satisfactorily and tearing occurs. Ectropion is more common in the elderly.

ENTROPION

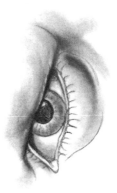

Entropion, also more common in the elderly, is an inward turning of the lid margin. The lower lashes, which are often invisible because they are turned inward, irritate the conjunctiva and lower cornea. Asking the patient to squeeze his lids together and then open them helps to demonstrate the problem when it is not obvious.

PERIORBITAL EDEMA

Since the skin of the eyelids is loosely attached to underlying tissues, edema tends to accumulate here more easily than elsewhere. Causes are many. Consider allergies, local inflammation, myxedema, fluid-retaining states such as the nephrotic syndrome, and finally, of course, recent crying.

HERNIATED FAT

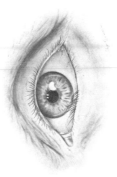

Puffy eyelids can be caused by fat as well as fluid. Fat pushes weakened fascia in the eyelids forward, producing bulges that involve the lower lids, the inner third of the upper ones, or both. Although these bulges appear more often in elderly people, they may also affect younger ones.

Table 5-4

Table 5-4 Lumps and Swellings In and Around the Eyes

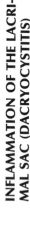

PINGUECULA

A yellowish triangular nodule in the bulbar conjunctiva on either side of the iris, a pinguecula is harmless. Pingueculae appear almost uniformly with aging, first on the nasal and then on the temporal side.

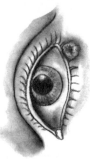

STY (ACUTE HORDEOLUM)

A painful, tender, red infection around a hair follicle of the eyelashes, a sty looks like a pimple or boil pointing on the lid margin.

CHALAZION

A chalazion is a chronic inflammatory lesion involving a meibomian gland. A beady nodule in an otherwise normal lid, it is usually painless. Occasionally a chalazion becomes acutely inflamed but, unlike a sty, usually points inside the lid rather than on the lid margin.

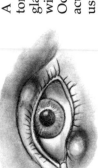

XANTHELASMA

Slightly raised, yellowish, well-circumscribed plaques in the skin, xanthelasmas appear along the nasal portions of one or both eyelids. They may accompany lipid disorders (e.g., hypercholesterolemia), but may also occur in normal persons.

BASAL CELL CARCINOMA

A slowly progressive skin cancer, a basal cell carcinoma near the eye usually involves the lower lid. It appears as a papule with a pearly border and a depressed or ulcerated center.

INFLAMMATION OF THE LACRIMAL SAC (DACRYOCYSTITIS)

A swelling between the lower eyelid and nose suggests inflammation of the lacrimal sac. It may be acute' or chronic. An *acute* inflammation is painful, red, and tender and may have a surrounding cellulitis. *Chronic* inflammation is associated with obstruction of the nasolacrimal duct. Tearing is prominent and pressure on the sac produces regurgitation of material through the puncta of the eyelids.

ENLARGEMENT OF THE LACRIMAL GLAND

An enlarged lacrimal gland may displace the eyeball downward, nasally, and forward. A swelling is sometimes visible above the lateral third of the upper lid, giving the lid margin an S-shaped curve. Look for the enlarged gland between the elevated upper lid and the eyeball. Causes of lacrimal gland enlargement include inflammation and tumors.

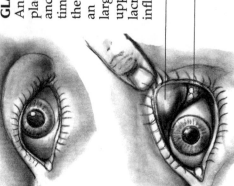

Tarsal plate and conjunctiva

Lacrimal gland

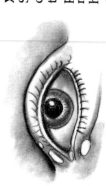

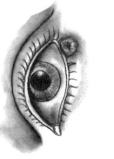

Table 5-5

Table 5-5 Red Eyes

	CONJUNCTIVAL INJECTION	CILIARY INJECTION	ACUTE GLAUCOMA	SUBCONJUNCTIVAL HEMORRHAGE	BLEPHARITIS
APPEARANCE					
PROCESS	Dilatation of the conjunctival vessels	Dilatation of branches of the anterior ciliary artery which supply the iris and related structures	Dilatation of branches of the anterior ciliary artery; may also show some conjunctival vessel dilatation	Blood outside the vessels between the conjunctiva and sclera	Inflammation of the eyelids
LOCATION OF REDNESS	Peripheral vessels of the conjunctiva, fading toward the iris	Central deeper vessels around the iris	Central deeper vessels around the iris; may also be peripheral	A homogeneous red patch, usually in an exposed part of the bulbar conjunctiva	Lid margins
APPEARANCE OF VESSELS	Irregularly branched	May radiate regularly or appear as a diffuse flush around the iris	Radiating regularly around the iris; peripherally may be irregularly branching	Vessels themselves not visible	Conjunctival and ciliary vessels normal unless there is associated disease
COLOR	Vessels bright red	Vessels more violet or rose-colored	Vessels around iris violet or rose-colored	Patch is bright red, fading with time to yellow	Lid margins red, may have yellowish scales
MOVABILITY	Conjunctival vessels can be moved against the globe by pressure on the lower lid.	Dilated vessels are deeper; cannot be moved by lid pressure.	Dilated vessels around the iris are deep; cannot be moved by lid pressure.	Not movable	Not relevant
PUPIL SIZE AND SHAPE	Normal	Normal or small and irregular	Dilated, often oval, seen through a steamy cornea	Normal	Normal
VISUAL ACUITY	Not affected	Decreased	Decreased	Not affected	Not affected
SIGNIFICANCE	Superficial conjunctival condition, as from irritation, infection, allergy, vasodilators	Disorder of cornea or inner eye. Requires prompt evaluation	Sudden increase in intraocular pressure because of blocked drainage from the anterior chamber. An ocular emergency	Often none. May result from trauma, sudden increase in venous pressure (e.g., cough), bleeding disorder	Often associated with seborrhea, staphylococcal infections

Table 5-6

Table 5-6 Opacities of the Cornea and Lens

CATARACTS

A cataract is an opacity of the lens and therefore can be viewed only through the pupil and on a deeper plane than corneal opacities. Cataracts may be classified in many ways—for example, by their causes, which are many, or by their locations within the lens. The most common cause of cataract is age—senile cataract. Two forms are illustrated, both with the pupils widely dilated so that only a narrow rim of iris shows.

CROSS SECTION OF LENS

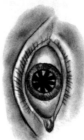

Capsule

Cortical cataract

Cortex

Nuclear cataract

NUCLEAR CATARACT

A nuclear cataract forms a central gray opacity, viewed here against a black background as you might see it with a flashlight. Through the ophthalmoscope it would appear black against the red reflex.

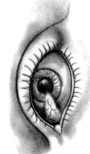

PERIPHERAL CORTICAL CATARACT A peripheral cortical cataract produces spokelike shadows that point inward—gray against black as seen with a flashlight, or black against red with an ophthalmoscope.

CORNEAL ARCUS

A corneal arcus is a thin grayish white arc or circle not quite at the edge of the cornea. It accompanies normal aging but may also be seen in younger people, especially blacks. In young people a corneal arcus suggests the possibility of hyperlipoproteinemia but does not prove it. Some surveys have revealed no relationship. An arcus does not interfere with vision.

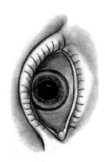

CORNEAL SCAR

A corneal scar is a superficial grayish white opacity in the cornea, secondary to an old injury, for example, or to inflammation. Size and shape are variable. It should not be confused with the opaque lens of a cataract, visible on a deeper plane and only through the pupil.

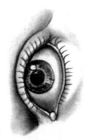

PTERYGIUM

Not a true corneal opacity, a pterygium is a triangular thickening of the bulbar conjunctiva that grows slowly across the cornea, usually from the nasal side. Reddening may occur intermittently. A pterygium may interfere with vision as it encroaches upon the pupil.

Table 5-7

Table 5-7 Pupillary Abnormalities

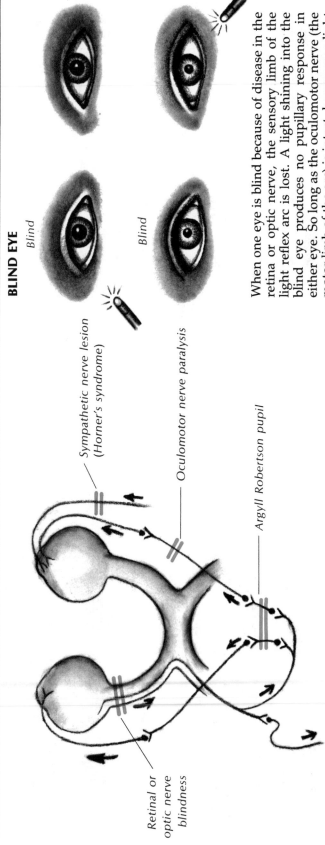

Retinal or optic nerve blindness

Sympathetic nerve lesion (Horner's syndrome)

Oculomotor nerve paralysis

Argyll Robertson pupil

To occipital cortex

BLIND EYE

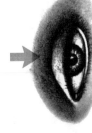

Blind

Blind

When one eye is blind because of disease in the retina or optic nerve, the sensory limb of the light reflex arc is lost. A light shining into the blind eye produces no pupillary response in either eye. So long as the oculomotor nerve (the motor limb of the arc) is intact, however, a light directed into the sound eye produces normal responses in both eyes (normal direct and consensual reactions).

HORNER'S SYNDROME

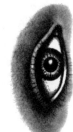

This pupil is small, regular, and unilateral. It is associated with ptosis of the eyelid and often with loss of sweating on the forehead of the involved side. Because of the ptosis, the eye may look small. Horner's syndrome is caused by interruption of the sympathetic nerve supply, most often in the neck. The pupil reacts to light and accommodation.

OCULOMOTOR NERVE PARALYSIS

A dilated pupil that reacts neither to light nor to accommodation results from injury to the oculomotor nerve. Ptosis and deviation of the eye laterally and downward may be associated.

Continued

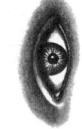
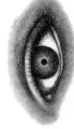
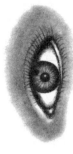

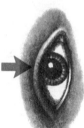
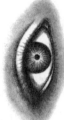
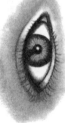

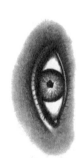
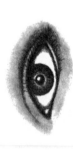
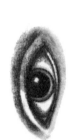

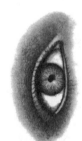
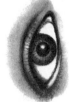
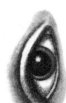

Table 5-7

Table 5-7 (Cont'd)

ARGYLL ROBERTSON PUPIL

Argyll Robertson pupils are small, irregular, and bilateral. They react to accommodation but not to light. They are often, but not necessarily, related to central nervous system syphilis (tabes dorsalis).

ADIE'S PUPIL (TONIC PUPIL)

This is a large, quite regular pupil usually confined to one side. The involved pupil reacts *very* slowly to light and accommodation. The disorder is benign and may be accompanied by diminished muscle stretch reflexes.

ANISOCORIA

Anisocoria is a descriptive, not a diagnostic, term and refers simply to inequality of the pupils. It is seen most often in dim light. Although slight pupillary inequality with normal pupillary reactions is a common normal variation, anisocoria should always be evaluated carefully.

IRIDECTOMY

Complete   *Peripheral*

A common cause of pupillary irregularity in the elderly is iridectomy, a surgical incision in the iris.

DILATED FIXED PUPILS

Bilaterally dilated and fixed pupils result from anticholinergic agents (*e.g.*, atropine, mushrooms) and from glutethimide (Doriden) poisoning. Additional causes that should be considered in the comatose patient are severe brain damage and profound hypoxia.

SMALL FIXED PUPILS

Bilaterally small, fixed, regular pupils result from morphine and related drugs, as well as from miotic drops given, for example, for glaucoma. In a comatose patient a pontine hemorrhage should also be considered.

Table 5-8

Table 5-8 Deviations of the Eyes

Deviation of the eyes from their normally parallel position (often called strabismus or squint) may be classified into two general groups: (1) paralytic, in which either the extraocular muscles or one of the nerves that supplies them is paralyzed, or (2) nonparalytic.

PARALYTIC

DEVIATION DURING TESTING IN THE SIX CARDINAL FIELDS OF GAZE

Present only in the field(s) of action of the involved muscles or nerves

FURTHER OBSERVATION

Note in which fields paralysis is present. For example, in a left 6th nerve paralysis—

Forward gaze—eyes parallel

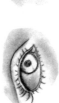

Right lateral gaze—eyes parallel

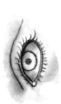

Left lateral gaze—deviation appears when the left eye does not move outward.

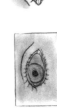

NONPARALYTIC

DEVIATION DURING TESTING IN THE SIX CARDINAL FIELDS OF GAZE

Constant in all fields

FURTHER OBSERVATION

Note whether the deviation is:

convergent—

or divergent

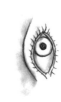

Check your findings with the *cover test*. Ask the patient to fix his gaze on a distant object.

Cover the right eye while you watch the left one.

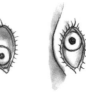

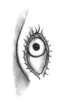

Then cover the left eye while you watch the right.

If the uncovered eye swings into place as the opposite eye is covered, it must have been deviated. Repeat the test to be sure (see also pp. 474–476).

Table 5-9

Table 5-9   Normal Variations of the Optic Disc

PHYSIOLOGIC CUPPING	RINGS AND CRESCENTS	MEDULLATED NERVE FIBERS

Labels: *Central cup*, *Temporal cup*, *Choroidal crescent*, *Scleral ring*

The physiologic cup is a small whitish depression in the optic disc from which the retinal vessels appear to emerge. Although sometimes absent, the cup is usually visible either centrally or toward the temporal side of the disc. Grayish spots are often seen at its base.	Rings or crescents are often seen around the edges of the disc. They are of two types: (1) white scleral rings or crescents, and (2) black pigmented choroidal rings or crescents.	Medullated nerve fibers are a much less common but dramatic finding. Presenting as irregular white patches with feathered margins, they obscure the disc edge and retinal vessels.

Table 5-10

Table 5-10   Abnormalities of the Optic Disc

	NORMAL	OPTIC ATROPHY	PAPILLEDEMA	GLAUCOMATOUS CUPPING
PROCESS	Tiny disc vessels give normal color to disc.	Death of optic nerve fibers leads to loss of the tiny disc vessels.	Venous stasis leads to engorgement and swelling.	Increased pressure within the eye leads to increased cupping (backward depression of the disc) and atrophy.
APPEARANCE	Color yellowish orange to creamy pink	Color white	Color pink, hyperemic	The base of the enlarged cup is pale.
	Disc vessels tiny	Disc vessels absent	Disc vessels more visible, more numerous, curve over the borders of the disc	
	Disc margins sharp (except perhaps nasally)		Disc swollen with margins blurred	
	The physiologic cup is located centrally or somewhat temporally. It may be conspicuous or absent, but its diameter from side to side is usually less than half that of the disc.		The physiologic cup is not visible.	The physiologic cup is enlarged, occupying more than half of the disc's diameter, at times extending to the edge of the disc. Retinal vessels sink in and under it, and may be displaced nasally.

Table 5-11

Table 5-11 **Retinal Arterioles and Arteriovenous Crossings: Normal and Hypertensive**

NORMAL RETINAL ARTERIOLE AND ARTERIOVENOUS (A–V) CROSSING

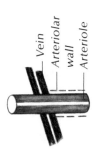

Arteriolar wall (invisible)

Column of blood

Light reflex

The normal arteriolar wall is invisible. Only the column of blood within it can usually be seen. The normal light reflex is narrow—about ¼ the diameter of the blood column.

Vein

Arteriolar wall

Arteriole

Since the arteriolar wall is transparent, a vein crossing beneath the arteriole can be seen right up to the column of blood on either side.

THE RETINAL ARTERIOLES IN HYPERTENSION

SPASM AND THICKENING OF ARTERIOLAR WALLS

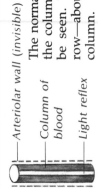

Focal narrowing

Narrowed column of blood

Narrowed light reflex

In hypertension the arterioles may show areas of focal or generalized spasm with narrowing of the column of blood. The light reflex is also narrowed. As the narrowing recurs or persists over many months or years, the arteriolar wall thickens and becomes less transparent.

SILVER WIRE AND COPPER WIRE ARTERIOLES

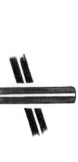

Occasionally a portion of a narrowed arteriole develops such an opaque wall that no blood is visible within it. This is a *silver wire arteriole*.

Sometimes the arterioles, especially those close to the disc, become full and somewhat tortuous and develop an increased light reflex with a bright metallic luster. Such a vessel is called a *copper wire arteriole*.

ARTERIOVENOUS CROSSINGS

Thickening of the arteriolar walls is often associated with visible changes in the arteriovenous crossings. Decreased transparency of the retina also probably contributes to the first two of the following changes.

TAPERING

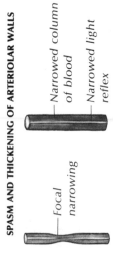

The vein appears to taper down on either side of the arteriole.

CONCEALMENT OR A–V NICKING

The vein appears to stop abruptly on either side of the arteriole.

BANKING

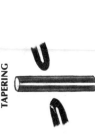

The vein is twisted on the distal side of the arteriole and forms a dark, wide knuckle.

Table 5-12

Table 5-12 Red Spots in the Retina

1. *Flame-shaped hemorrhages* are small, linear hemorrhages, often found in severe hypertension but not specific to this condition.

2. *Deep hemorrhages* are small, slightly irregular red spots often seen in diabetes. They may also be present in a number of other conditions.

3. *Microaneurysms* are tiny red spots commonly but not exclusively located in the macular area. They are characteristic of diabetic retinopathy.

4. A *preretinal hemorrhage*, located between retina and vitreous, is large and often characterized by a horizontal line separating red cells from plasma.

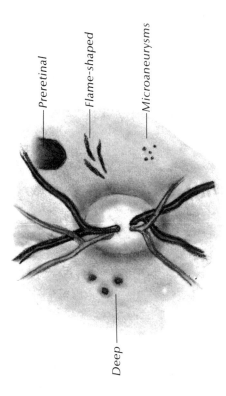

Preretinal

Flame-shaped

Microaneurysms

Deep

Table 5-13 Light-Colored Spots in the Retina

	COTTON WOOL PATCHES (Soft Exudates)	HARD EXUDATES	DRUSEN (Colloid Bodies)	HEALED CHORIORETINITIS
BORDER	Ill-defined, fuzzy	Well-defined	Defined fairly well	Well-defined, often outlined in pigment
SHAPE	Ovoid or polygonal; irregular	May be small and round or may coalesce into larger irregular spots	Round	Irregular
SIZE	Relatively large but smaller than optic disc	Small	Tiny to small	Variable—small to very large
COLOR	White or gray	Creamy or yellow, often bright	White to yellowish	White or gray with clumps of black pigment
DISTRIBUTION	No definite pattern	Often in clusters, circular or linear patterns, or stars	Haphazardly and generally distributed, may concentrate at the posterior pole	Variable
SIGNIFICANCE	Hypertension, other conditions	Diabetes, hypertension, other conditions	Concomitant of normal aging	Indicates old inflammation of many possible types

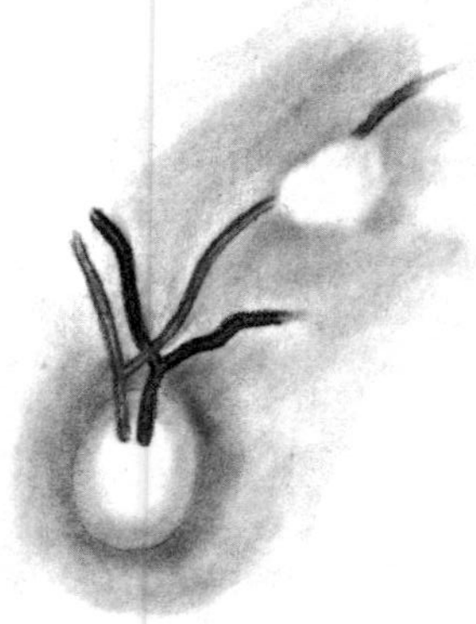

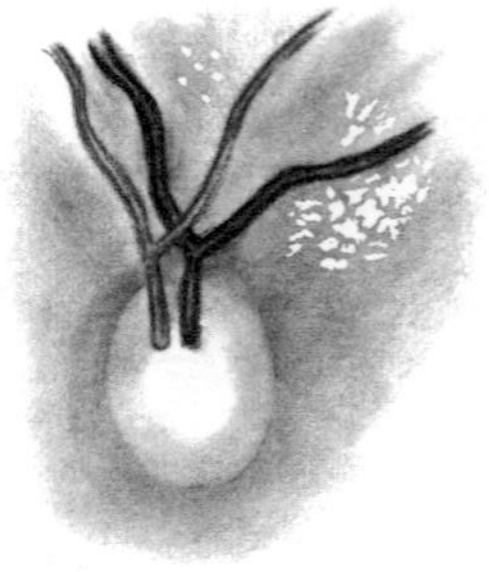

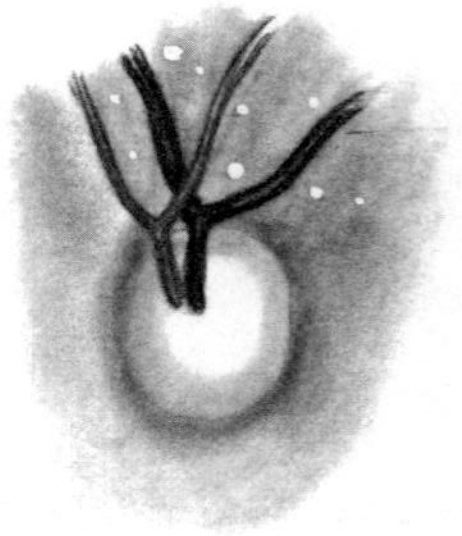

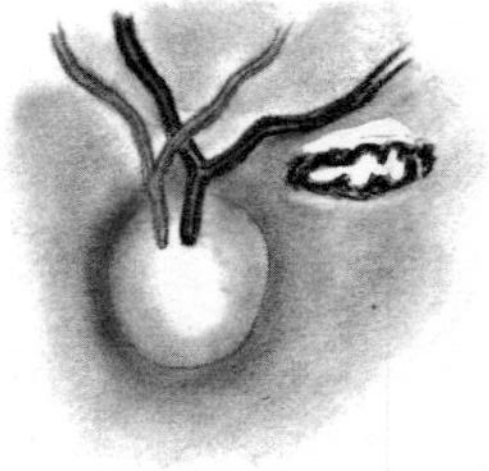

Table 5-14

Table 5-14 Ocular Fundi

To simulate an ophthalmoscopic examination, take a piece of paper and, out of its center, cut a circle approximately the size of the optic disc. Lay it on each illustration, and inspect each fundus systematically.

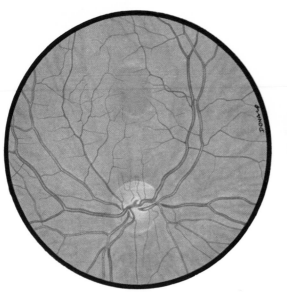 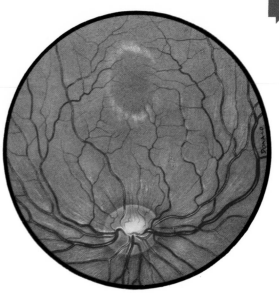

NORMAL FUNDUS OF A FAIR-SKINNED PERSON

Find and inspect the optic disc. Follow the major vessels in four directions, noting their relative sizes and the nature of the arteriovenous crossings—both normal here. Inspect the macula. The fovea is not visible in this subject. Look for any lesions in the retina. Note the striped, or tessellated, character of the fundus, especially in the lower field. This comes from normal choroidal vessels, unobscured by pigment.

NORMAL FUNDUS OF A BLACK PERSON

Again, inspect the disc, the vessels, the macula, and the retinal background. The ring around the macula is a normal light reflection. Compare the color of the fundus to that in the illustration above. It has a grayish brownish, almost purplish cast, which comes from pigment in the retina and the choroid. This pigment characteristically obscures the choroidal vessels, and no tessellation is visible. In contrast to either of the first two figures, a white person with brunette coloring has a redder fundus.

Continued

Table 5-14

Table 5-14   (Cont'd)

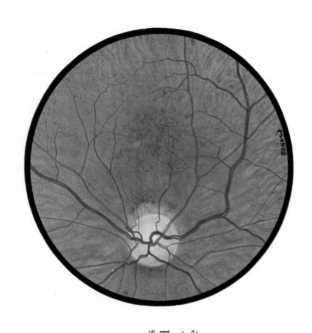

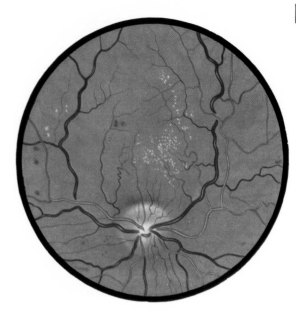

NORMAL FUNDUS OF AN AGED PERSON

Inspect the fundus as before. What differences do you observe? Two characteristics of the aging fundus can be seen in this example. The blood vessels are straighter and narrower than those in younger people, and the choroidal vessels can be easily seen. In this person the optic disc is less pink, and pigment may be seen temporal to the disc and in the macular area.

HYPERTENSIVE RETINOPATHY

Inspect the fundus as before. The nasal border of the optic disc is blurred. The light reflexes from the arterioles just above and below the disc are increased. Note the venous tapering—at the A–V crossing, about one disc diameter above the disc. Tapering and buckling can be seen at 4:30 o'clock, two disc diameters from the disc. Punctate hard exudates and a few deep hemorrhages are readily visible.

Continued

Table 5-14

Table 5-14 (Cont'd)

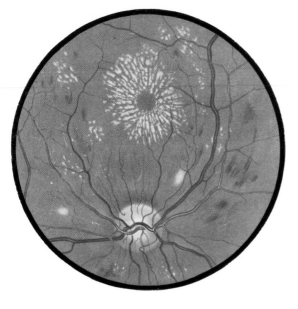 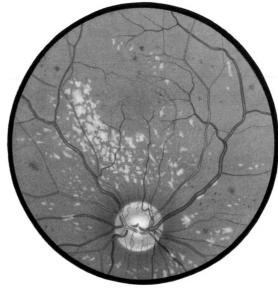

HYPERTENSIVE RETINOPATHY WITH MACULAR STAR

Punctate exudates are readily visible here. Some are scattered, while others radiate from the fovea to form a macular star. Note the two small, soft exudates about one disc diameter from the disc. A number of flame-shaped hemorrhages sweep toward 4 o'clock and 5 o'clock, and a few more may be seen toward 2 o'clock.

DIABETIC RETINOPATHY

Punctate exudates have coalesced here into homogeneous, waxy-looking patches that are typical of diabetic retinopathy. What kinds of red spots can you find? Microaneurysms are most easily visible about one disc diameter below the disc. A few deep hemorrhages can also be seen, around 2 o'clock and 3 o'clock about three disc diameters from the disc.

(Michaelson IC: Textbook of the Fundus of the Eye, 3rd ed, pp 52, 131, 141. Edinburgh, Churchill Livingstone, 1980)

Table 5-15

Table 5-15 Nodules in and Around the Ears

LYMPH NODES

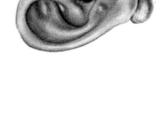

Preauricular node

Posterior auricular node

Mastoid process

Small lymph nodes just anterior to the tragus or overlying the mastoid process are quite common. Although sometimes visible, they are best detected by palpation.

SEBACEOUS CYSTS

Cyst

Punctum

Sebaceous cysts are common, especially behind the ear. They are characteristically *in* rather than beneath the skin and often show a central black dot or punctum which identifies the opening of the blocked sebaceous gland.

KELOID

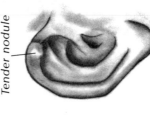

A keloid, which is a nodular, hypertrophic mass of scar tissue, may develop in an earlobe pierced for earrings. Keloids are especially common in black people.

TOPHUS

Tophi

Tophi are deposits of uric acid crystals characteristic of gout. They appear as hard nodules in the helix or antihelix. They occasionally discharge white chalky crystals.

DARWIN'S TUBERCLE

Typical location

A small elevation in the rim of the ear, a Darwin's tubercle is a harmless congenital variation from normal—the equivalent of the tip of a mammalian ear. It should not be mistaken for a tophus.

CHONDRODERMATITIS HELICIS

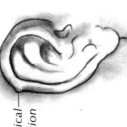

Tender nodule

This entity is characterized by a small, chronic, painful, tender nodule in the helix of the ear. It usually affects men, involving the right ear more often than the left. It may be confused with a tophus or skin cancer. Biopsy is important.

Table 5-16

Table 5-16   Abnormalities of the Eardrum

BULLOUS MYRINGITIS

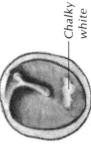

Vesicle

Vesicles form within the eardrum in infections secondary to some viruses and Mycoplasma.

SCARRING AND CALCIFIC DEPOSITS

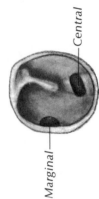

Chalky white

Past infection can leave a thickened lusterless drum or chalky white calcific deposits.

SEROUS OTITIS MEDIA

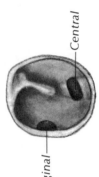

Air bubbles

Hairline air–fluid level

Fluid (amber-colored)

A viral infection or block of the eustachian tube can produce a serous otitis. Amber-colored fluid may be discerned below a hairline fluid level. Air bubbles may appear.

OLD PERFORATIONS

Central

Marginal

Perforations of the drum, as from past infection, may be either central or marginal. Search the entire edge of the drum to avoid missing the latter. Perforations are sometimes covered over by a thin, almost transparent layer of epithelium.

RETRACTED DRUM

The handle of the malleus looks shorter and more horizontal. The short process and folds stand out in sharp outline as if protruding through the membrane. The cone of light is bent, broken, or absent. Retraction of the drum results from absorption of air from the middle ear when the eustachian tube is blocked.

ACUTE PURULENT OTITIS MEDIA

Early

Hyperemic vessels

Late

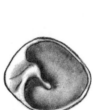

Landmarks obscured

Bulging red drum

Acute purulent otitis media begins with hyperemic vessels across the drum. Distinguish these from a few dilated vessels along the handle of the malleus which may be normal.

Later, the drum bulges outward, obscuring all landmarks. Perforation may follow.

NORMAL DRUM

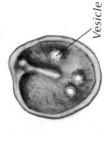

The drum is pearly gray and shows a good cone of light. The handle and short process of the malleus are readily identifiable, and the handle is at a normal angle. Compare this appearance with the abnormalities shown in the balance of the table.

Table 5-17

Table 5-17 Patterns of Hearing Loss

Hearing loss is divided into two major types: conduction and sensorineural. 1. Problems in the external or middle ear, such as otitis media or an ear canal plugged with wax, impair the normal conduction of sound to the inner ear and cause a *conduction hearing loss*. Air conduction is characteristically impaired while bone conduction remains normal. 2. Disorders of the inner ear or 8th cranial nerve, in contrast, produce a *sensorineural hearing loss*. Examples include presbycusis (the hearing loss of normal aging), drug toxicity, and pressure of a tumor on the 8th cranial nerve. In sensorineural loss both air and bone conduction are impaired but they maintain their normal relationship to each other.

Consider a patient with a unilateral hearing loss:

CONDUCTION LOSS

PROCESS

Problem in the external or middle ear

WEBER TEST

Room noise blocked

Lateralizes to the poor ear. Because the poor ear is not distracted by room noise, it can detect bone vibrations better than normal. Test this on yourself by doing a Weber test while occluding one ear with your finger. This lateralization disappears in an absolutely quiet room.

RINNE TEST

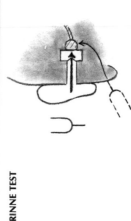

Bone conduction lasts longer than air conduction (BC > AC). Pathways of normal conduction through the external or middle ear are blocked. Vibrations through bone bypass the obstruction.

SENSORINEURAL LOSS

PROCESS

Problem in the inner ear or nerve

WEBER TEST

Lateralizes to the good ear. The inner ear or nerve is less able to receive vibrations arriving by any route, including bone. The sound is therefore heard in the better ear.

RINNE TEST

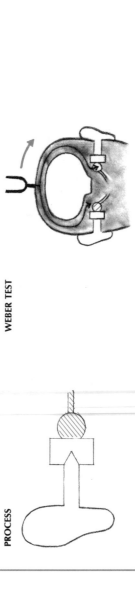

Air conduction lasts longer than bone conduction (AC > BC). The inner ear or nerve is less able to perceive vibrations arriving by either route. The normal pattern prevails.

Table 5-18

Table 5-18 Common Abnormalities of the Nose

FURUNCLE OF THE NOSE

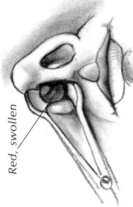

White center
Red margin

Furuncles are quite common in the nasal vestibule. The area is tender and may be red and swollen; then a typical pustule forms. Gentle examination is mandatory. Avoid manipulation since this may spread the infection.

NASAL POLYPS

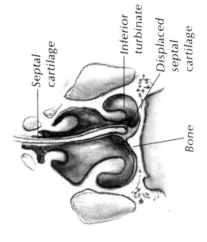

Nasal polyps may develop in patients with allergic rhinitis. They are usually found in the middle meatus, where they appear as gelatinous or soft, pale gray structures. Unlike the turbinates, for which they are sometimes mistaken, they are mobile.

ACUTE RHINITIS *(The Common Cold)*

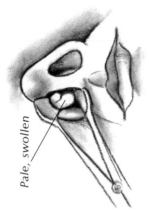

Red, swollen

The nasal mucosa is red and swollen. Nasal discharge, which is at first watery and copious, becomes thick and mucopurulent.

ALLERGIC RHINITIS

Pale, swollen

The nasal mucosa is swollen, pale, boggy, and usually gray. A dull red or bluish color may also be seen. Similar findings are seen in some patients with nonallergic vasomotor rhinitis.

SEPTAL DEVIATION

Displaced septum

Septal cartilage
Inferior turbinate
Displaced septal cartilage
Bone

Cross Section Viewed From the Front

Some degree of septal deviation is common in most adults. Illustrated here is one of the most frequent types—displacement of the septal cartilage in the anterior portion of the nose. Septal deviation may produce nasal obstruction but the turbinates often accommodate to the asymmetry. Most septal deviations are asymptomatic.

Table 5-19

Table 5-19 Abnormalities of the Lips

HERPES SIMPLEX
(Cold Sore, Fever Blister)

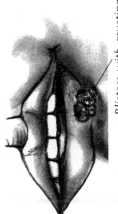

Blisters with crusting

The virus herpes simplex may produce recurrent vesicular eruptions of the lips and surrounding tissues. A small cluster of blisters develops. As these break, a crust is formed and healing ensues within 10 to 14 days.

CHANCRE

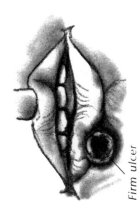

Firm ulcer

The primary lesion of syphilis may appear on the lip instead of in its more common location on the genitalia. It is a firm, buttonlike lesion which ulcerates and may become crusted. A chancre may resemble a carcinoma or a crusted cold sore. Use a glove for palpation. Dark field examination is necessary for diagnosis.

ANGULAR STOMATITIS
(Cheilosis)

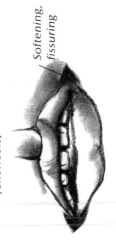

Softening, fissuring

Softening of the skin at the angles of the mouth, followed by fissuring or cracking, is called angular stomatitis or cheilosis. Although rarely secondary to riboflavin deficiency, it more commonly is caused by overclosure of the mouth, (e.g., in patients without teeth or with dentures that are too short in their vertical dimension). Saliva then wets and macerates the infolded skin, often leading to secondary infection from Monilia or bacteria. The mucous membrane remains uninvolved.

CHEILITIS

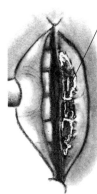

Fissures, scales and crusts

Painful fissuring with inflammation, scaling, and crust formation characterizes cheilitis. Involving chiefly the lower lip, cheilitis is often chronic. Its causes are several and may be obscure.

Continued

Table 5-19

Table 5-19 (Cont'd)

MUCOUS RETENTION CYST
(*Mucocele*)

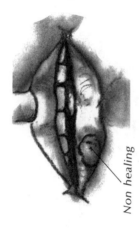

Round nodule

A round, regular, partially translucent or bluish nodule in the lip is probably a mucous retention cyst or mucocele. This is a benign lesion, having chiefly cosmetic importance. Size varies from tiny up to 1 cm to 2 cm in diameter. The cysts may also occur inside the lower lip in the buccal mucosa.

CARCINOMA OF THE LIP

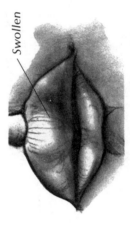

Non healing

Carcinoma of the lip usually involves the lower lip and may appear as a thickened plaque, ulcer, or warty growth. Much more frequent in men than in women, it is the most common form of oral cancer. Any sore or crusting lesion on the lip that does not heal must be considered suspicious.

PEUTZ–JEGHERS SYNDROME

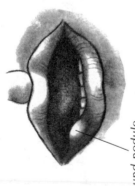

Pigmented spots

When pigmented spots on the lips are more prominent than freckling of the surrounding skin, suspect the Peutz–Jeghers syndrome. Look for abnormal pigment in the buccal mucosa to help confirm the diagnosis. Pigmented spots may also be found on the face, fingers, and hands. These findings are important because they are often associated with multiple intestinal polyps.

ANGIONEUROTIC EDEMA

Swollen

Angioneurotic edema presents as a diffuse, nonpitting, tense, subcutaneous swelling that may involve a number of structures, including the lips. It appears rather rapidly, generally disappearing in a day or two. Although usually allergic in nature and sometimes associated with hives, it does not usually itch.

Table 5-20

Table 5-20   Abnormalities of the Buccal Mucosa and Hard Palate

APHTHOUS ULCER (*Canker Sore*)

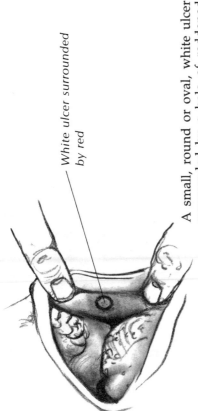

White ulcer surrounded
by red

A small, round or oval, white ulcer surrounded by a halo of reddened mucosa characterizes the common aphthous ulcer. Such ulcers are painful, may be single or multiple, and are often recurrent. Any portion of the oral mucosa may be involved.

FORDYCE SPOTS (*Granules*)

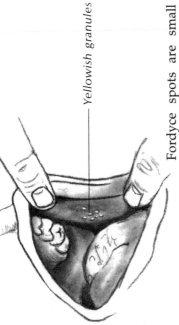

Yellowish granules

Fordyce spots are small yellowish spots visible in the buccal mucosa of most adults. They may also involve the lips. They are sebaceous glands and should not be considered an abnormality. If the patient suddenly notices and worries about them he may be reassured.

TORUS PALATINUS

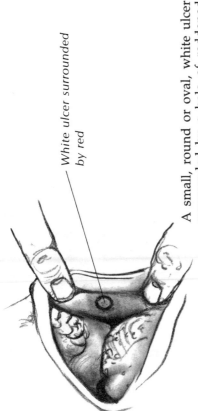

Bony

A torus palatinus is a fairly common midline bony outgrowth in the hard palate, usually developing in adulthood. Its size and lobulation vary. Although alarming at first glance, it is of no clinical consequence except perhaps in the fitting of dentures. A nodule that is not in the midline is not a torus and should suggest a tumor.

MONILIASIS (*Candidiasis, Thrush*)

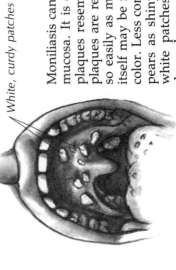

White, curdy patches

Moniliasis can involve the entire oral mucosa. It is characterized by white plaques resembling milk curds. The plaques are removable but not quite so easily as milk curds. The mucosa itself may be reddened or normal in color. Less commonly, moniliasis appears as shiny redness without the white patches. Definitive diagnosis depends on culture of the yeast.

Table 5-21

Table 5-21 Abnormalities of the Gums and Teeth

NORMAL GUMS

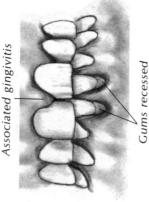

Pale red with normal stippling

Sharp interdental papilla

The gums (or gingivae) normally show a pale red stippled surface. Their margins about the teeth are sharp and the crevice between gums and teeth shallow (*e.g.*, 1 mm to 2 mm). The teeth are seated firmly in their bony sockets.

GINGIVITIS

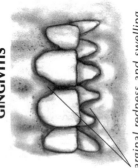

Marginal redness and swelling with bulbous interdental papillae

Redness and swelling of the margins of the gums characterize gingivitis, often the result of irritation by calculus formation. The normal stippling decreases or disappears. The gingivae between the teeth (interdental papillae) may become bulbous. The gums may bleed with light contact.

PERIODONTITIS (*Pyorrhea*)

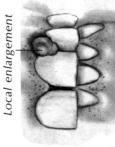

Associated gingivitis

Gums recessed

If untreated, gingivitis may progress to periodontitis, an inflammation of the deeper tissues around the teeth. This is an extremely common cause of tooth loss in adults. The crevices between the gums and teeth enlarge, and pockets containing debris and purulent material develop in these areas. The gum margins recede, exposing the necks of the teeth. The teeth may become loose.

ACUTE NECROTIZING GINGIVITIS (*Trench Mouth, Vincent's Stomatitis*)

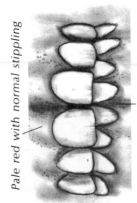

Grayish membrane over ulcerated gum margin

This is a painful gingivitis characterized by redness, swelling, and ulceration of the gingival tissues. The interdental papillae may be eroded by the ulcerative process. A grayish membrane forms over the inflamed and ulcerated gingival margins.

GINGIVAL ENLARGEMENT

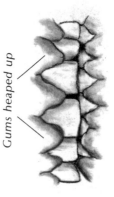

Gums heaped up

Enlargement of the gums has a variety of causes including puberty, pregnancy, Dilantin therapy, and leukemia. The gingival tissues appear heaped up and partially cover the teeth.

EPULIS

Local enlargement

Epulis is the term used to describe a localized gingival enlargement. Most are inflammatory, some are neoplastic.

Continued

Table 5-21

Table 5-21   (Cont'd)

LEAD OR BISMUTH LINE

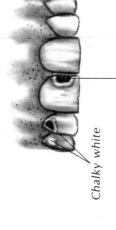

Bluish black line

In chronic lead or bismuth poisoning a bluish black line may appear on the gums about 1 mm from the gum margin. It does not appear where teeth are absent. Distinguish it from the much more common melanin pigmentation.

MELANIN PIGMENTATION

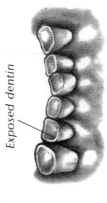

Patchy brown pigment

A brownish melanin pigmentation of the gums is frequently observed. It is normal in blacks and other dark-skinned persons and may occasionally be seen even in light-skinned persons. A similar pigment pattern may be associated with Addison's disease.

DENTAL CARIES

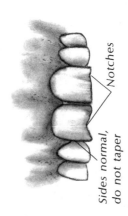

Discolored, with cavitation

Chalky white

Dental caries is first visible as a chalky white deposit in the enamel surface of the tooth. This area may then discolor to brown or black, become soft, and cavitate. Special dental techniques including x-rays are necessary for early detection.

HUTCHINSON'S TEETH

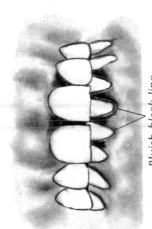

Smaller teeth, more widely spaced

Sides taper   Central notches

Hutchinson's teeth are notched on their biting surfaces, smaller than normal, and more widely spaced. Their sides taper in. The upper central incisors are most often affected; the permanent, rather than deciduous, teeth are involved. They are a sign of congenital syphilis.

ABRASION OF TEETH WITH NOTCHING

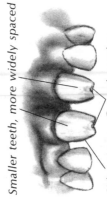

Notches

Sides normal, do not taper

The biting surface of the teeth may become abraded or notched by recurrent trauma (*e.g.*, from opening bobby pins with one's teeth, or holding nails between the teeth). Unlike Hutchinson's teeth, the sides of these teeth show their normal contours; size and spacing are unaffected.

ATTRITION OF TEETH

Exposed dentin

The teeth of many elderly people have been worn down by repetitive chewing. This flattening of the biting surfaces is called attrition. The enamel may be worn away, exposing the underlying dentin. The latter often takes on a yellow or brownish stain.

Table 5-22

Table 5-22 Abnormalities of the Tongue

SMOOTH TONGUE	HAIRY TONGUE	GEOGRAPHIC TONGUE	FISSURED TONGUE
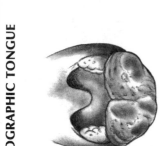	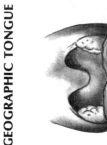	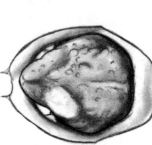	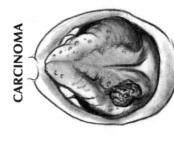

A coated tongue is normal, a smooth red tongue is not. Loss of papillae gives the tongue a red, slick appearance, often beginning at the edges. It suggests a deficiency of vitamin B$_{12}$, iron, or niacin, or may be caused by anti-cancer drugs.

The "hair" of hairy tongue consists of elongated papillae on the dorsum of the tongue and is yellowish to brown to black. Hairy tongue may follow antibiotic therapy but may also occur spontaneously. Its cause is unknown. It is harmless.

Geographic tongue is characterized by scattered red areas on the dorsum of the tongue that are denuded of their papillae and are smooth. The contrast of these areas with the normal roughened and coated surface gives a map-like pattern which changes over time. Of unknown cause, the condition is benign.

Fissures may appear in the tongue with increasing age and at times become numerous, giving rise to the alternate term "scrotal tongue." Although food debris may accumulate in the crevices and become irritating, the fissured tongue has little significance.

12TH NERVE PARALYSIS	VARICOSE VEINS OF THE TONGUE	LEUKOPLAKIA	CARCINOMA
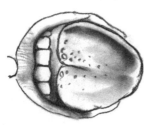	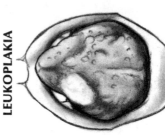	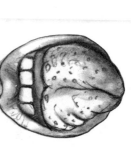	

Paralysis of the 12th cranial (hypoglossal) nerve produces atrophy and fasciculations of the involved half of the tongue. Deviation toward the paralyzed side occurs when the tongue is protruded.

Small purplish or blue black round swellings may appear under the tongue with age and have aptly been called "caviar lesions." They have no significance. As with several other tongue findings, familiarity with them pays dividends when the patient or the examiner first notices them. Reassurance is in order.

Leukoplakia is a term applied to a thickened white patch adherent to the mucous membrane. Its appearance has been likened to dried white paint. Although tongue involvement is illustrated here, leukoplakia may involve any part of the oral mucosa. Its primary significance lies in the fact that it may be premalignant.

Carcinoma of the tongue is uncommon on the dorsum of the tongue where it might be most readily noticed. Look for it at the base or edges of the tongue. Any ulcer or nodule which fails to heal in 2 or 3 weeks must be considered suspicious.

Table 5-23

Table 5-23   Abnormalities of the Pharynx

VIRAL PHARYNGITIS

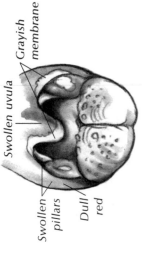

Slight
redness

Prominent
lymphoid
patches

Viral pharyngitis may present few if any signs. Mild redness, slight swelling of the pillars, and prominence of the lymphoid patches on the posterior pharyngeal wall are frequently seen.

STREPTOCOCCAL PHARYNGITIS

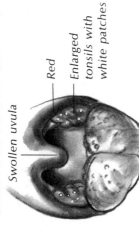

Swollen uvula

Red

Enlarged
tonsils with
white patches

Classically streptococcal infection produces redness and swelling of the tonsils, pillars, and uvula, with white or yellow patches of exudate on the tonsils. Accurate clinical diagnosis is frequently impossible, however, since streptococcal pharyngitis may occur without exudate, and some viral illnesses, including infectious mononucleosis, may produce an exudative pharyngitis.

DIPHTHERIA

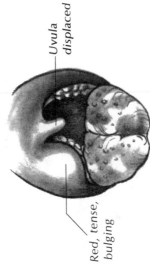

Swollen uvula

Grayish
membrane

Swollen
pillars

Dull
red

Now rare, diphtheria is included here because without prompt diagnosis and treatment it may prove fatal. The throat is dull red and swollen. A thick exudate forms on the tonsils and, unlike a streptococcal exudate, may spread over the soft palate and uvula. The throat is less painful than might be expected, the patient sick.

TONSILLAR HYPERTROPHY

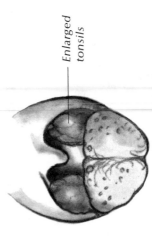

Enlarged
tonsils

The tonsils may be enlarged without being infected. They may protrude medially beyond the edges of the pillars even to the midline when the tongue is protruded. The size of the tonsils is not in itself an indicator of disease.

PARALYSIS OF THE 10ᵀᴴ CRANIAL (VAGUS) NERVE

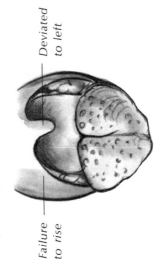

Deviated
to left

Failure
to rise

When the patient says "ah" the soft palate on the paralyzed side fails to rise. The uvula deviates to the uninvolved side.

PERITONSILLAR ABSCESS
(*Quinsy Sore Throat*)

Uvula
displaced

Red, tense,
bulging

Peritonsillar abscess occasionally complicates acute tonsillitis. Usually caused by streptococci or staphylococci, the infection spreads from tonsil to adjacent soft tissue, producing a very painful, usually unilateral, red bulge that may extend beyond the midline. Painful swallowing may cause drooling.

Table 5-24

Table 5-24 *Thyroid Enlargement and Nodules*

NORMAL THYROID GLAND

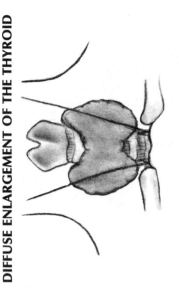

The isthmus is the only portion of the thyroid gland commonly palpable. In a short, stocky person the isthmus may lie very low, close to the sternum, and become palpable only on extension of the neck. The lobes, which curve around posteriorly, are much less frequently identifiable.

DIFFUSE ENLARGEMENT OF THE THYROID

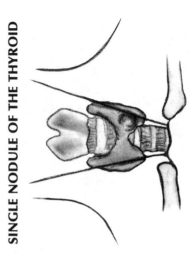

Both the isthmus and lateral lobes of a diffusely enlarged thyroid can usually be felt. The surface may feel finely lobulated but there are no discrete nodules. Such enlargement may be associated with hyperthyroidism, with endemic goiter, with Hashimoto's thyroiditis, and with some other less common conditions.

MULTINODULAR GOITER

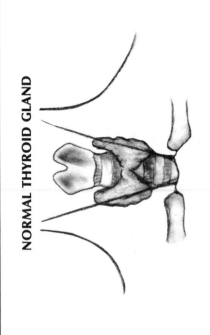

This term refers to an enlarged thyroid gland containing two or more identifiable nodules. The presence of multiple nodules suggests a metabolic rather than a malignant process, but unusual firmness and rapid enlargement of one of the nodules must raise the suspicion of neoplasm.

SINGLE NODULE OF THE THYROID

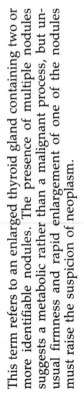

Although a clinically single nodule of the thyroid gland may be a cyst, a benign tumor, or one nodule within a multinodular gland, it always raises the question of malignancy and must be carefully evaluated. Hardness, rapid enlargement, and fixation to the surrounding tissues are especially suspicious. A single nodule can develop in any portion of the gland.

Chapter 6
THE THORAX AND LUNGS

Anatomy and Physiology

Review the *anatomy of the chest wall*, identifying the structures illustrated.

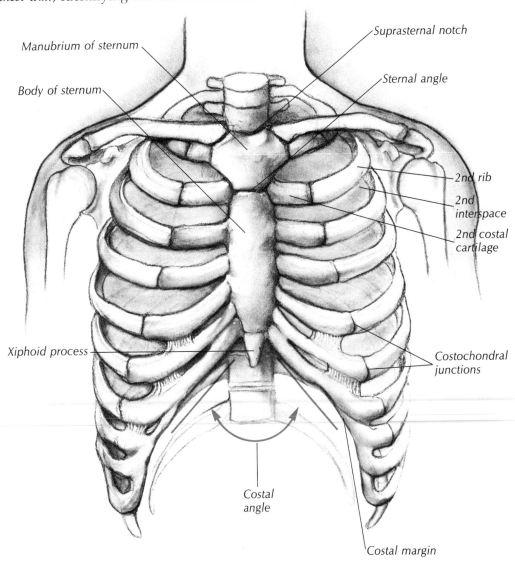

Manubrium of sternum

Body of sternum

Suprasternal notch

Sternal angle

2nd rib

2nd interspace

2nd costal cartilage

Xiphoid process

Costochondral junctions

Costal angle

Costal margin

To localize and describe a finding on the chest wall you must be able to number the ribs accurately. The sternal angle (or angle of Louis) is the best guide. To find it, first identify the suprasternal notch, then move your finger down about 5 cm or a little more to find the horizontal bony ridge that joins the manubrium to the body of the sternum. Then move your finger laterally and find the adjacent 2nd rib and costal cartilage. The interspace immediately below is the 2nd interspace. When locating ribs or interspaces lower in the anterior chest, start from the sternal angle and 2nd rib, then count downward in an oblique line several centimeters lateral to the sternal edge or costal margin. Palpation more medially may be confused by the close approximation of the costal cartilages. When counting the ribs of a woman with large breasts, you may need to displace the breast laterally or palpate a little more medially than you would otherwise.

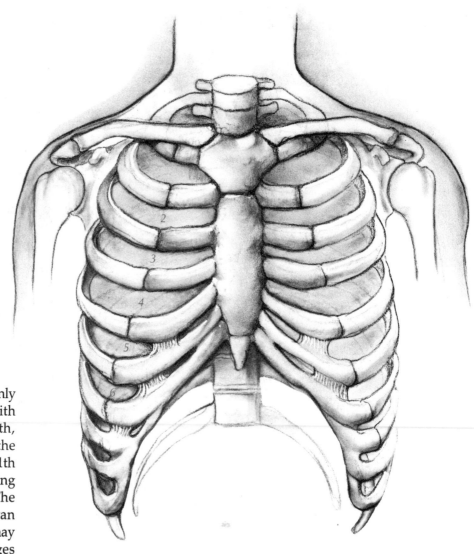

Note that the costal cartilages of only the first seven ribs articulate with the sternum. Those of the 8th, 9th, and 10th ribs articulate with the costal cartilages just above. The 11th and 12th ribs, the so-called floating ribs, have free anterior tips. The cartilaginous tip of the 11th rib can usually be felt laterally, the 12th may be felt posteriorly. Costal cartilages are not distinguishable from ribs by palpation.

Posteriorly the accurate numbering of ribs is more difficult. The inferior angle of the scapula is a helpful landmark, lying approximately at the level of the 7th rib or interspace. Findings may also be localized according to their relationship to the spinous processes. When the patient flexes his neck forward, the most prominent spinous process (the vertebra prominens) is usually that of the 7th cervical. It may, however, be the 1st thoracic. If two vertebrae appear equally prominent, they are the 7th cervical and 1st thoracic. The spinous processes below can often be felt and counted, especially when the spine is flexed. Since the processes of T4 through T12 angle obliquely downward, each overlies not its own vertebra but the body of the vertebra below. For example, the spinous process of T6 overlies the 7th thoracic vertebra and is adjacent to the 7th rib. In the lower thorax it is usually easier to identify the 12th rib, then the 11th interspace above it, and count upward from there.

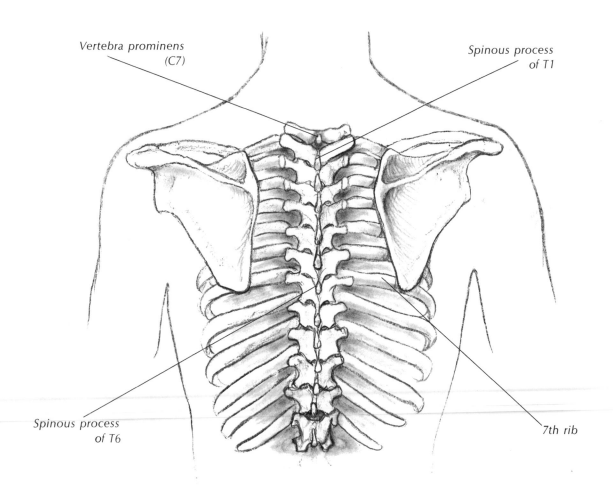

Vertebra prominens (C7)

Spinous process of T1

Spinous process of T6

7th rib

Localization of findings depends upon their relationship not only to ribs and vertebrae but also to imaginary lines drawn on the chest. Become familiar with the following:

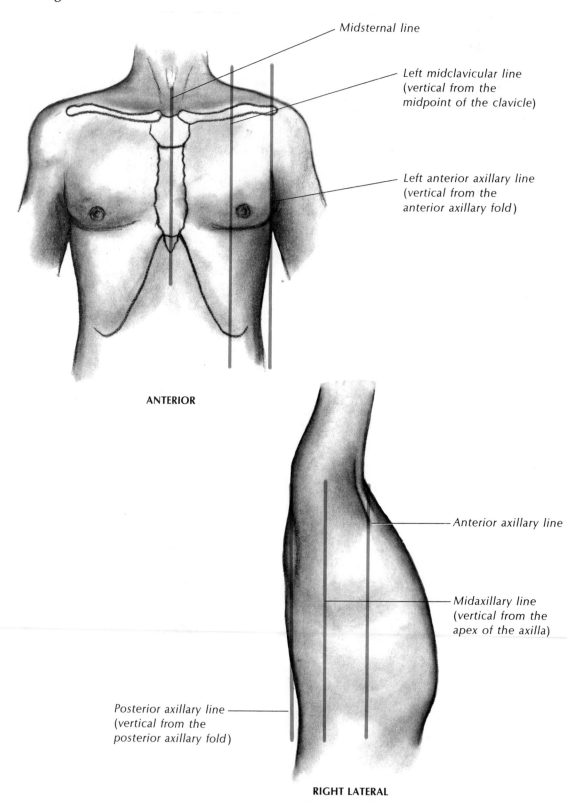

Midsternal line

Left midclavicular line (vertical from the midpoint of the clavicle)

Left anterior axillary line (vertical from the anterior axillary fold)

ANTERIOR

Anterior axillary line

Midaxillary line (vertical from the apex of the axilla)

Posterior axillary line (vertical from the posterior axillary fold)

RIGHT LATERAL

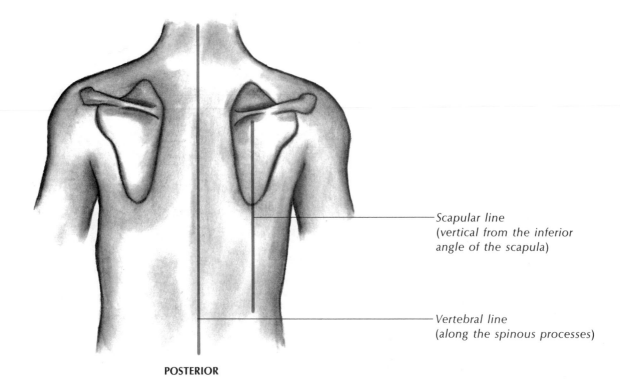

Scapular line
(vertical from the inferior
angle of the scapula)

Vertebral line
(along the spinous processes)

POSTERIOR

More general terms are also helpful: supraclavicular (above the clavicle), infraclavicular (below the clavicle), interscapular (between the scapulae), and infrascapular (below the scapula).

While examining the chest, keep in mind the probable location of the underlying lungs and their lobes. These locations can be mentally projected onto the chest wall. Key points in these surface projections include the following:

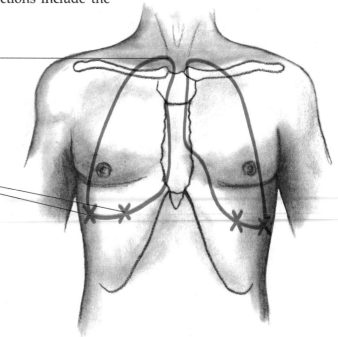

The apex of each lung rises about 2–4 cm above the inner third of the clavicle

The inferior border crosses the 6th rib at the midclavicular line, and the 8th rib at the midaxillary line

ANTERIOR

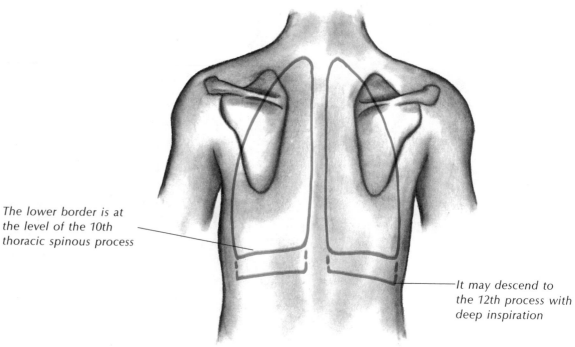

The lower border is at the level of the 10th thoracic spinous process

It may descend to the 12th process with deep inspiration

POSTERIOR

Each lung is divided approximately in half by an oblique or major fissure. Posteriorly the locations of the oblique fissures are approximated by lines drawn from the 3rd thoracic spinous process obliquely down and laterally. These lines are close to the vertebral borders of the scapulae when a person's hands are placed on top of his head. They divide upper from lower lobes.

Spinous process of T3

Left upper lobe

Right upper lobe

Oblique fissure

Left lower lobe

Right lower lobe

POSTERIOR

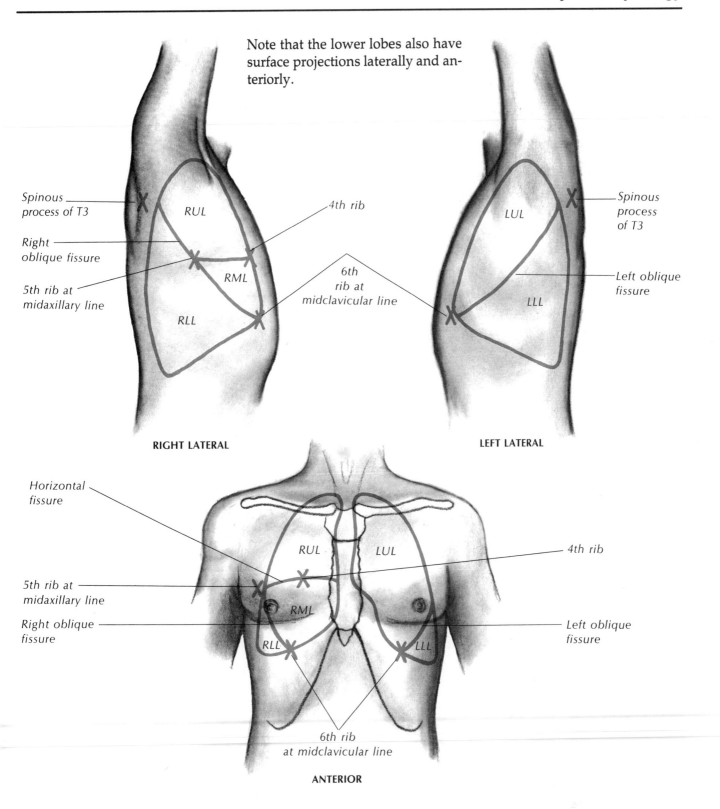

Note that the lower lobes also have surface projections laterally and anteriorly.

Spinous process of T3

Right oblique fissure

5th rib at midaxillary line

RUL

4th rib

RML

6th rib at midclavicular line

RLL

RIGHT LATERAL

LUL

Spinous process of T3

Left oblique fissure

LLL

LEFT LATERAL

Horizontal fissure

5th rib at midaxillary line

Right oblique fissure

RUL

LUL

4th rib

RML

Left oblique fissure

RLL

LLL

6th rib at midclavicular line

ANTERIOR

The right lung is further divided by the horizontal or minor fissure into the right upper and right middle lobes. This fissure runs from the right midaxillary line at the level of the 5th rib across anteriorly at the level of the 4th rib.

Although you should be mindful of the probable location of lung lobes when examining a patient's chest and when making correlations with radiologic findings, you should usually describe your physical findings in terms that are less explicit anatomically: upper, middle, and lower lung fields, for example, or the bases (lowermost portions) of the lungs. You may then infer what lobes are involved. Signs in the right upper lung field, for example, probably originate in the right upper lobe, while those at the left base almost certainly come from the left lower lobe. Signs in the right middle lung field laterally, however, could come from any of three different lobes.

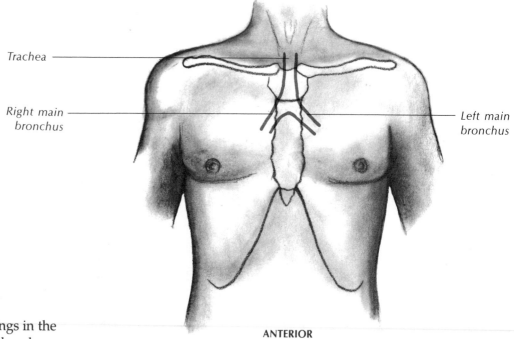

Trachea

Right main
bronchus

Left main
bronchus

ANTERIOR

Since certain physical findings in the chest are influenced by the closeness of the chest wall to the trachea and large bronchi, the location of these structures should also be familiar. Note that the trachea bifurcates at about the level of the sternal angle anteriorly and the 4th thoracic spinous process posteriorly.

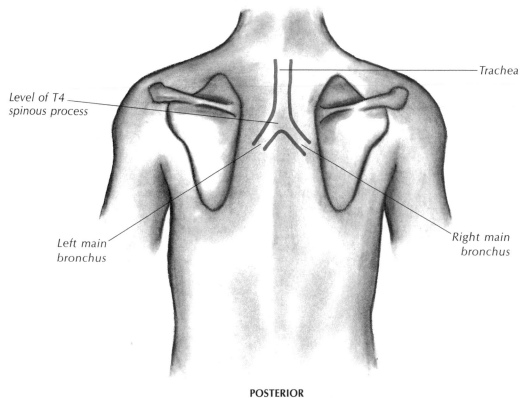

Trachea

Level of T4
spinous process

Left main
bronchus

Right main
bronchus

POSTERIOR

Breathing is largely an automatic act, controlled in the brain stem and mediated by the muscles of respiration. During inspiration the diaphragm and intercostal muscles contract, enlarging the thorax and expanding the lungs in the pleural cavities. The chest wall moves upward, anteriorly, and laterally while the diaphragm descends. As inspiratory effort stops, the lungs recoil, the diaphragm rises passively, and the chest wall relaxes into its resting position. When breathing is labored, because of exercise or disease, additional muscles come into play: the trapezii, sternomastoids, and scalenus muscles in the neck during inspiration and the abdominal muscles during expiration. Watch the muscles in your own neck in a mirror as you inhale as deeply as possible.

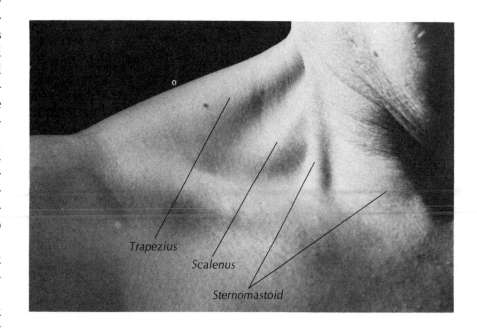

Trapezius

Scalenus

Sternomastoid

Normal breathing is quiet—barely audible near the open mouth as a faint whish. This sound has no definite pitch because it has components over a wide range of frequencies, and is called white noise. The sound of breathing originates somewhere between the pharynx and smaller bronchi, although its exact source remains under study.

Respiratory sounds are transmitted through the lungs and chest wall, where you can hear them with a stethoscope. The tissues through which they pass, however, filter out their higher-pitched components. What you hear over most of the lungs are soft, relatively low-pitched sounds that last through inspiration and fade out of your range of hearing relatively early in expiration. Such sounds have been termed *vesicular breath sounds.* Listen for them on yourself or a colleague in the lower portion of the lung—in the midaxillary line, for example, or more posteriorly. Although the expiratory component of vesicular breath sounds *seems* short to the human ear, expiration in fact continues, lasting longer than normal inspiration.

When you listen near the trachea—over the manubrium or between the scapulae, for example—your stethoscope is close enough to the source of the breath sounds so that little filtration occurs. Here the breath sounds are louder and higher in pitch. This difference is most noticeable during expiration, and you can hear relatively high-pitched breath sounds throughout expiration. These expiratory sounds last as long as the inspiratory ones or even longer. Sounds similar to these when heard at greater distances from the large airways are abnormal and are called *bronchial breath sounds.*

The characteristics of these two kinds of sounds are summarized in the table below. Note the *basic qualities for the analysis of any sound: duration, pitch, and intensity.*

BREATH SOUNDS	DURATION OF INSPIRATION AND EXPIRATION	RELATIVE PITCH OF EXPIRATION	RELATIVE INTENSITY OF EXPIRATION	NORMAL LOCATIONS
VESICULAR	Inspiratory sounds last longer than expiratory sounds.	Low	Soft	Most of the lungs, away from the trachea and large bronchi
BRONCHIAL	Expiratory sounds are equal to or longer than inspiratory sounds.	High	Loud	Near the large airways (*i.e.,* near the manubrium and between the scapulae, especially on the right)

Just as breath sounds are transmitted through the lung and chest wall to the surface, so are the sounds of the voice. You can feel them with your hand as *fremitus* or hear them through a stethoscope. As with breath sounds, the higher-pitched components of these *voice sounds* are filtered out and much attenuated as they pass through normal tissues to the surface. Normal speech is heard as a relatively low-pitched, indistinct mumble; whispered words, which lack low-pitched components, are scarcely heard at all. Abnormalities of the lungs may change both breath sounds and voice sounds and are described in Table 6-3, Alterations in Breath and Voice Sounds, (p. 151).

CHANGES WITH AGE

Throughout adult life a person's vital capacity (the maximal volume of air that can be expired after a full inspiration) declines slowly. So does the maximal rate of expiration. These functional changes (and others as well) result partly from the aging process, partly from disease. Skeletal changes associated with aging often accentuate the dorsal curve of the thoracic spine, producing kyphosis and an increased anteroposterior diameter of the chest. The resulting "barrel chest," however, does not by itself impair function.

Techniques of Examination

GENERAL APPROACH

1. The patient should be undressed to the waist and examined with good lighting.
2. Proceed in an orderly fashion:
   a. Inspection, palpation, percussion, auscultation
   b. Compare one side with the other. Variations between patients are great; to some extent at least, comparison of one side with the other allows a patient to serve as his own control.
   c. Work from above down.
3. Throughout your examination, try to visualize the underlying tissues, including the lobes of the lungs.
4. Examine the posterior thorax and lungs while the patient is still in the sitting position. His arms should be folded across his chest so that his scapulae are partly out of the way. Then ask the patient to lie down while you examine his anterior thorax and lungs.

EXAMINATION OF THE POSTERIOR CHEST

INSPECTION

Observe the *rate, rhythm,* and *effort* of breathing. A normal resting adult breathes quietly and regularly about 8 to 16 times a minute. An occasional sigh is normal.

See Table 6-1, Abnormalities in Rate and Rhythm of Breathing (p. 149).

From a midline position behind the patient note the *shape of the chest and the way in which it moves,* including:

Deformities of the thorax
Its anteroposterior diameter in proportion to its lateral diameter, normally from 1:2 to about 5:7
The slope of the ribs
Abnormal retraction of the interspaces during inspiration

See Table 6-2, Deformities of the Thorax (p. 150).

More horizontal in emphysema
Severe asthma, emphysema, tracheal or laryngeal obstruction

Abnormal bulging of the interspaces during expiration

Asthma, emphysema, massive pleural effusion

Local lag or impairment in respiratory movement

Underlying disease of lung or pleura

PALPATION

Palpation of the chest has four uses:

1. *To identify areas of tenderness.* Carefully palpate any area where pain has been reported or where lesions are evident.
2. *To assess observed abnormalities* such as masses or sinus tracts (blind, inflammatory, tubelike structures opening onto the skin)
3. *To assess further the respiratory excursion.* Place your thumbs about at the level of and parallel to the 10th ribs, your hands grasping the lateral rib cage. As you position your hands, slide them medially a bit in order to raise loose skin folds between thumbs and spine. Ask the patient to inhale deeply.

Although rare, sinus tracts usually indicate infection of the underlying pleura and lung (*e.g.*, tuberculosis, actinomycosis).

Lag or impairment of thoracic movement suggests underlying disease of the lung or pleura.

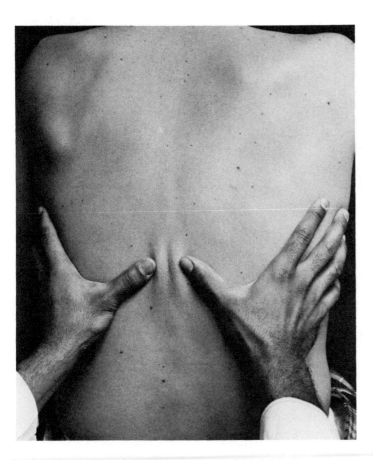

Watch the excursion of your thumbs and feel for the range and symmetry of respiratory movement.

4. *To elicit vocal or tactile fremitus.* Fremitus refers to the palpable vibrations transmitted through the bronchopulmonary system to the chest wall when the patient speaks. Ask the patient to repeat the words "ninety-nine" or "one-one-one." If fremitus is faint, ask him to speak more loudly or lower his (and especially her) voice.

Palpate and compare symmetrical areas of the lungs, using the ball of your hand (the palm of the hand at the base of the fingers). Use one hand until you become thoroughly familiar with the feel of fremitus. Some clinicians find this technique more accurate. The simultaneous use of both hands to compare sides, however, increases speed.

Fremitus is decreased or absent when the voice is decreased, the bronchus obstructed, or the pleural space occupied by fluid, air, or solid tissue. Increased fremitus is noted near the large bronchi and over consolidated lung.

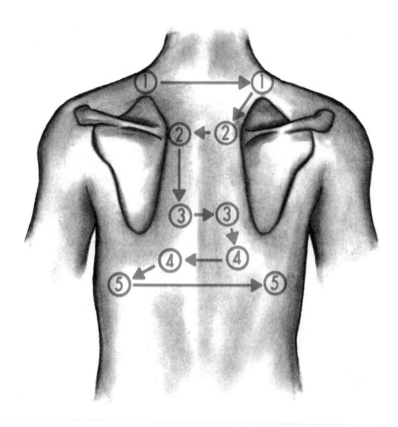

Numbers and arrows indicate sequence of examination

Identify, describe, and localize any areas of increased or decreased fremitus.

Estimate the level of the diaphragm on each side, using the ulnar side of the extended hand held parallel to the expected diaphragmatic level. Move your hand downward in progressive steps until fremitus is no longer felt. This point approximates the diaphragmatic level, which is usually slightly higher on the right.

An abnormally high level suggests pleural effusion or a high diaphragm, as from paralysis or atelectasis.

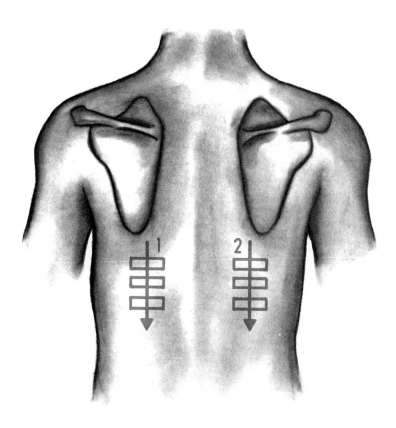

PERCUSSION

Percussion of the chest sets the chest wall and underlying tissues into motion, producing audible sounds and palpable vibrations. Percussion helps to determine whether the underlying tissues are air-filled, fluid-filled, or solid. It penetrates only about 5 cm to 7 cm into the chest, however, and will therefore not detect deep-seated lesions.

The *technique of percussion* can be practiced on any surface. The key points are:

1. Hyperextend the middle finger of your left hand (the pleximeter finger). Press its distal phalanx and joint *firmly* on the surface to be percussed. Avoid contact by any other part of the hand, since this would damp the vibrations.

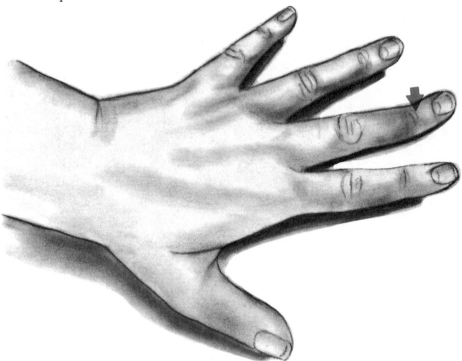

2. Position your right forearm quite close to the surface with the hand cocked upward. The right middle finger should be partially flexed, relaxed, and poised to strike.

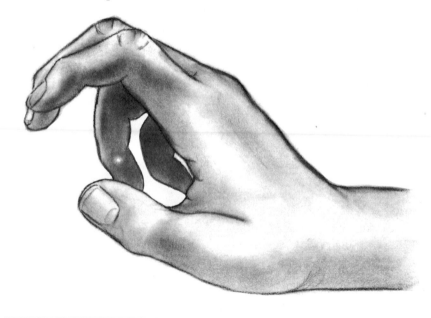

3. With a quick, sharp, but relaxed wrist motion, strike the pleximeter finger with the right middle finger (the plexor).

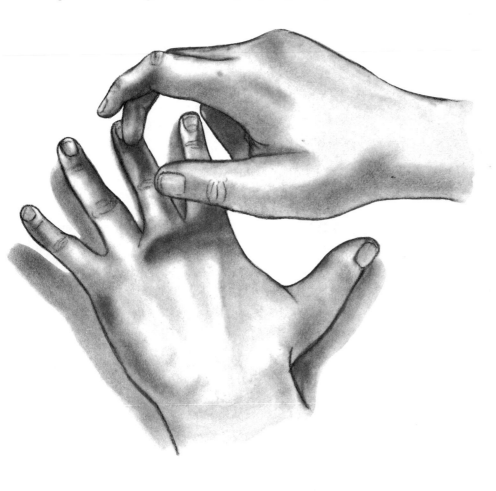

Aim at the base of the terminal phalanx or at the distal interphalangeal joint—the point overlying that portion of the pleximeter finger that is exerting maximum pressure on the surface.

Use the tip of the plexor finger, not the finger pad. The terminal phalanx should be almost at a right angle with the pleximeter. (A very short fingernail is required to avoid self-mutilation!) In percussing the lower posterior chest you can achieve the correct position more easily by standing somewhat to the side, not directly behind the patient.

4. Withdraw the plexor finger briskly to avoid damping the vibrations.

5. Strike one or two blows in one location and then move on. Keep your percussion technique uniform in comparing one part of the chest with another.

REMEMBER: The movement is at the wrist, not in the finger, elbow, or shoulder; it is a direct blow, not oblique or tangential. Use the lightest percussion that will produce a clear note.

Learn to identify five percussion notes, four of which you can reproduce on yourself. These notes can usually be distinguished by differences in their basic qualities of sound: intensity, pitch, and duration. Train your ear to detect these differences by concentrating on one quality at a time as you percuss first in one location, then in another.

	RELATIVE INTENSITY	RELATIVE PITCH	RELATIVE DURATION	EXAMPLE LOCATION
FLATNESS	Soft	High	Short	Thigh
DULLNESS	Medium	Medium	Medium	Liver
RESONANCE	Loud	Low	Long	Normal lung
HYPERRESONANCE	Very loud	Lower	Longer	Emphysematous lung
TYMPANY	Loud	*	*	Gastric air bubble or puffed-out cheek

*Distinguished mainly by its musical timbre

Percuss across the top of each shoulder to identify the approximately 5-cm band of resonance overlying each lung apex. Then, while the patient continues to keep his arms folded across his chest, percuss symmetrical areas of the lungs at about 5-cm intervals down the chest wall. Below the scapulae, percuss symmetrical areas along the sides of the chest as well as medially.

Dullness replaces resonance when fluid or solid tissue replaces air-containing lung or occupies the pleural space.

Hyperresonance is heard over the hyperinflated lung of emphysema.

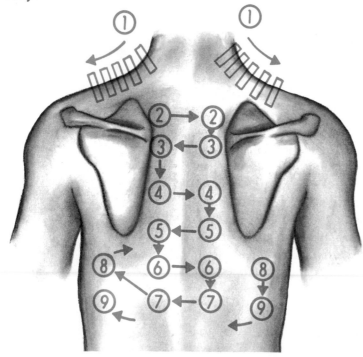

Omit the scapular areas, since the thickness of musculoskeletal structures usually precludes worthwhile percussion there.

Identify, describe, and localize any area of abnormal percussion note.

With the pleximeter finger held parallel to the expected border of diaphragmatic dullness, percuss in progressive steps downward. Identify the level of diaphragmatic dullness on each side during quiet respiration. This level is often slightly higher on the right. Check the level laterally as well as medially.

An abnormally high level suggests pleural effusion or a high diaphragm, as from paralysis or atelectasis.

A typical left pleural effusion of moderate size is represented below.

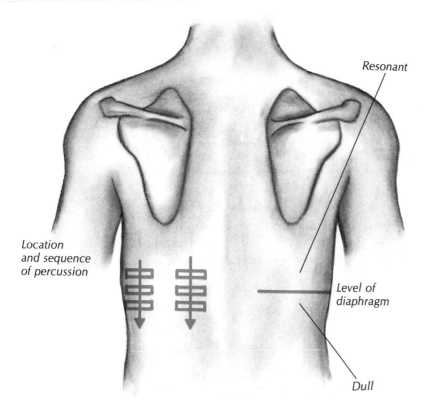

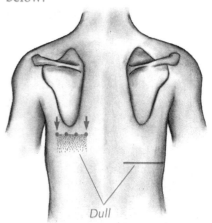

Diaphragmatic excursion may be measured by noting the distance between the levels of dullness on full expiration and full inspiration, normally around 5 cm or 6 cm.

Note that, on each of the patient's sides, you are percussing the boundary between resonant lung tussue above and dullness below. If this boundary lies at a normal level, you infer that it reflects the normal diaphragmatic boundary between lung and solid subdiaphragmatic tissue. You cannot, of course, find the diaphragm itself by percussion, or determine where it is within a dull area like that on this patient's left.

AUSCULTATION

Auscultation of the lungs is useful in estimating air flow through the tracheobronchial tree, detecting obstruction, and assessing the condition of the surrounding lungs and pleural space.

With the diaphragm of a stethoscope, listen to the patient's lungs as he breathes through his mouth somewhat more deeply than normal. Using locations similar to those recommended for percussion, compare symmetrical areas of the lungs, from above down. Listen to at least one full breath in each location. Be alert for patient discomfort secondary to hyperventilation (*e.g.*, light-headedness, faintness), and allow him to rest as needed. Listen for:

1. *The breath sounds.* Note their intensity. Breath sounds may be decreased when the patient fails to breathe deeply enough or has a very thick chest wall, as in obesity.

   Listen for the pitch, intensity, and duration of the expiratory and inspiratory sounds. In normal vesicular breathing, the expiratory sound is relatively low-pitched, soft, and shorter than the inspiratory sound. Is this kind of sound normally distributed over the patient's chest wall? Or are there bronchial breath sounds in unexpected places?

Breath sounds may be decreased when air flow is decreased (as by obstructive lung disease or muscular weakness), or when pleural fluid or air blocks the transmission of sound (as in pleural effusion or pneumothorax).

See Table 6-3, Alterations in Breath and Voice Sounds (p. 151).

2. *Any added sounds* (*i.e.,* crackles, wheezes, or rubs). Note what kinds of sounds you hear, where in the respiratory cycle you hear them, and where on the chest wall they are located.

See Table 6-4, Added Lung Sounds: Crackles, Wheezes, and Rubs (pp. 152–153).

If breath sounds are diminished, or if you suspect but cannot hear signs of obstructive breathing, ask the patient to breathe hard and fast with his mouth open. The diminished breath sounds associated with obesity may become readily audible; wheezes that were previously inaudible may appear.

Breath sounds remain decreased in emphysema. Wheezes may appear in asthma or bronchitis.

If you have discovered abnormalities in tactile fremitus, percussion, or auscultation, continue on to check *spoken and whispered voice sounds.*

See Table 6-3, Alterations in Breath and Voice Sounds (p. 151).

1. Ask the patient to say "ninety-nine" or "eee." Listen in symmetrical areas of the lungs, noting the intensity and clarity of the sounds. Normally the sounds are muffled.
2. Ask the patient to whisper "ninety-nine." Normally the whispered voice is heard only faintly and indistinctly.

See Table 6-5, Physical Signs in Selected Abnormalities of Bronchi and Lungs (pp. 154–156).

EXAMINATION OF THE ANTERIOR CHEST

The patient should be supine and comfortable, with his arms slightly abducted away from his chest.

INSPECTION

Observe the *rate, rhythm,* and *effort* of breathing. A normal resting patient can lie supine without respiratory difficulty and does not use his accessory muscles of respiration.

The sternomastoids, scaleni, and trapezii may contract visibly when breathing is labored. Patients with severe chronic obstructive lung disease may exhale through pursed lips and prefer to sit leaning forward with arms supported on knees or table.

At the same time *listen to the patient's breathing.* In the normal resting person inspiratory breath sounds are not audible at a distance of more than a few centimeters from the mouth.

In asthma and chronic bronchitis the white noise of inspiratory breath sounds increases in intensity and may be audible even across the room.

Observe the *shape of the patient's chest* and the *way in which it moves. Note:* Deformities of the thorax

See Table 6-2, Deformities of the Thorax (p. 150).

The width of the costal angle (usually less than 90° except in patients with short, heavy builds)

Wider in emphysema

Abnormal retraction of the interspaces and supraclavicular fossae during inspiration

Severe asthma, emphysema, tracheal obstruction

Abnormal bulging of the interspaces during expiration

Asthma, emphysema, massive pleural effusion

Local lag or impairment in respiratory movement

Underlying disease of lung or pleura

PALPATION

Palpation has four uses:

1. *To identify areas of tenderness*

2. *To assess any observed abnormality*

3. *To assess further the respiratory excursion.* Place your thumbs along each costal margin, your hands along the lateral rib cage. As you position your hands, slide them medially a bit to raise a loose skin fold between the thumbs. Ask the patient to inhale deeply. Watch for divergence of your thumbs as the thorax expands, and feel for the range and symmetry of respiratory movement.

Tender pectoral muscles or costal cartilages tend to corroborate, but do not prove, a musculoskeletal origin of chest pain.

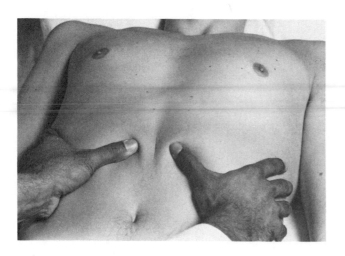

4. *To elicit vocal or tactile fremitus.* Compare symmetrical areas of the lungs, anteriorly and laterally, using the ball of your hand. When examining a woman, gently displace the breasts as necessary. Note that fremitus is usually decreased or absent over the precordium.

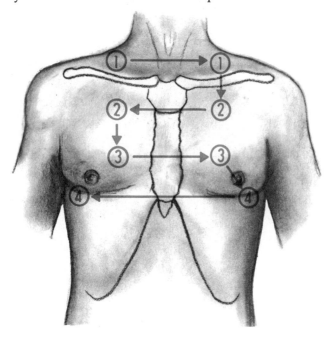

PERCUSSION

Percuss the anterior and lateral chest, again comparing symmetrical points, including the supraclavicular areas, the infraclavicular areas, and successive points down the chest wall about 5 cm apart. The heart normally produces an area of dullness to the left of the sternum from the 3rd to the 5th interspaces.

Dullness replaces resonance when fluid or solid tissue replaces air-containing lung or occupies the pleural space. Since pleural fluid usually sinks to the lowest part of the pleural space (posteriorly in a supine patient), only a very large effusion can be detected anteriorly.

The hyperresonance of emphysema may totally replace cardiac dullness.

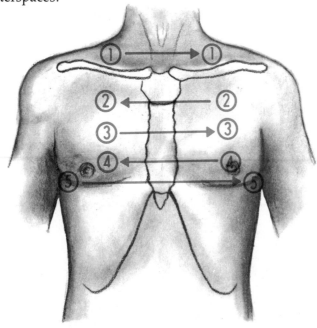

When a woman's breast interferes with percussion, gently displace it with your left hand while percussing with the right.

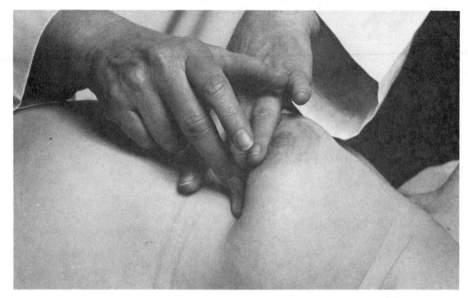

Alternatively you may ask the patient to move her breast for you.

Identify, describe, and localize any area of abnormal percussion note.

With your pleximeter finger parallel to the expected upper border of liver dullness, percuss in progressive steps downward in the right midclavicular line. Identify the upper border of liver dullness.

By a similar maneuver on the left, identify the usually tympanitic gastric air bubble.

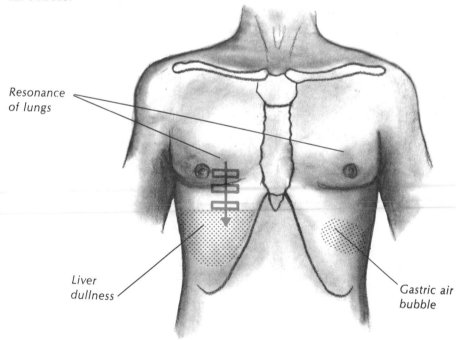

AUSCULTATION

Listen to the patient's chest, anteriorly and laterally, as he breathes through his mouth somewhat more deeply than normal. Compare symmetrical areas of the lungs, from above downward.

1. Listen to the *breath sounds*, noting their intensity and identifying any variations from normal vesicular breathing. Bronchial breathing may be heard over the large airways, especially on the right.

2. Identify any *added sounds*, time them in the respiratory cycle, and locate them on the chest wall.

See Table 6-4, Added Lung Sounds: Crackles, Wheezes, and Rubs (pp. 152–153).

If breath sounds are diminished, or if you suspect but cannot hear signs of obstructive breathing, ask the patient to breathe hard and fast with his mouth open.

If indicated, proceed to *spoken and whispered voice sounds.*

A note on examining the patient who cannot sit up. Because physical signs in the chest are often masked or distorted in the supine patient, try to get help in sitting the patient up for an examination of his posterior lung fields. If this is not possible, position the patient on each side and examine the upper lung.

CLINICAL ASSESSMENT OF PULMONARY FUNCTION

An informative but frequently overlooked way to assess the complaint of breathlessness in an ambulatory patient is to walk with him down the hall or climb one flight of stairs.

Marked generalized reduction of breath sounds in a patient with chronic bronchitis or emphysema suggests severe obstructive lung disease. A "match test" may be useful here. Hold a lighted book match 15 cm (6 inches) from the patient's lips and ask him to blow it out with his mouth open (not with lips pursed). Dentures, if any, should be removed for this test.

Inability to blow out the match indicates severe obstruction and carries a relatively poor prognosis.

Table 6-1

Table 6-1 Abnormalities in Rate and Rhythm of Breathing

When observing respiratory patterns think in terms of rate, depth, and regularity of the patient's breathing. Describe what you see in these terms. Traditional terms, such as tachypnea, are given below so that you will understand them, but simple descriptions are recommended for use.

NORMAL

Inspiration Expiration

Time

Volume of air

The respiratory rate is about 8 to 16 per minute in adults and up to 44 per minute in infants.

RAPID SHALLOW BREATHING
(Tachypnea)

Rapid shallow breathing has a number of causes, including restrictive lung disease, pleuritic chest pain, and an elevated diaphragm.

RAPID, DEEP BREATHING
(Hyperpnea, Hyperventilation)

Rapid deep breathing also has a number of causes, including exercise, anxiety, and metabolic acidosis. In the comatose patient, infarction, hypoxia, or hypoglycemia affecting the midbrain or pons should be considered. *Kussmaul breathing* is deep breathing associated with metabolic acidosis. It may be fast, normal in rate, or slow.

SLOW BREATHING
(Bradypnea)

Slow breathing may be secondary to such causes as diabetic coma, drug-induced respiratory depression, and increased intracranial pressure.

CHEYNE–STOKES BREATHING

Hyperpnea   Apnea

Respiration waxes and wanes cyclically so that periods of deep breathing alternate with periods of apnea (no breathing). Children and aging people may normally show this pattern in sleep. Other causes include heart failure, uremia, drug-induced respiratory depression, and brain damage (typically on both sides of the cerebral hemispheres or diencephalon).

ATAXIC BREATHING
(Biot's Breathing)

Ataxic breathing is characterized by unpredictable irregularity. Breaths may be shallow or deep and stop for short periods. Causes include respiratory depression and brain damage, typically at the medullary level.

SIGHING RESPIRATION

Sighs

Breathing punctuated by frequent sighs should alert you to the possibility of hyperventilation syndrome—a common cause of dyspnea and dizziness.

Occasional sighs are normal.

OBSTRUCTIVE BREATHING

Prolonged expiration

Air trapping

In obstructive lung disease expiration is prolonged because of increased airway resistance. If the patient must increase his respiratory rate, he lacks sufficient time for full expiration. His chest overexpands (air trapping) and his breathing becomes more shallow.

<Table 6-2>

Table 6-2 Deformities of the Thorax

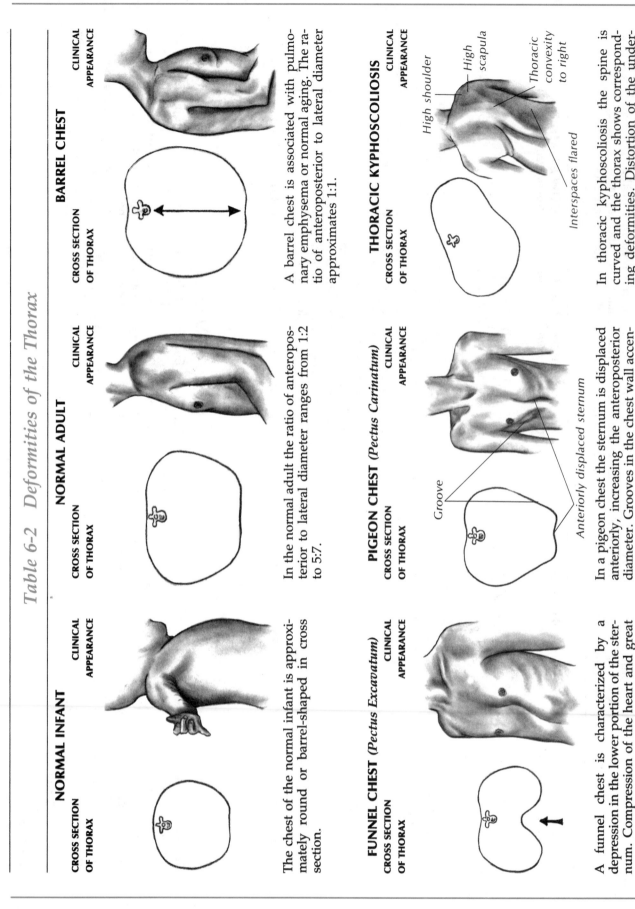

NORMAL INFANT

CROSS SECTION OF THORAX

CLINICAL APPEARANCE

The chest of the normal infant is approximately round or barrel-shaped in cross section.

FUNNEL CHEST (*Pectus Excavatum*)

CROSS SECTION OF THORAX

CLINICAL APPEARANCE

A funnel chest is characterized by a depression in the lower portion of the sternum. Compression of the heart and great vessels may cause murmurs.

NORMAL ADULT

CROSS SECTION OF THORAX

CLINICAL APPEARANCE

In the normal adult the ratio of anteroposterior to lateral diameter ranges from 1:2 to 5:7.

PIGEON CHEST (*Pectus Carinatum*)

CROSS SECTION OF THORAX

CLINICAL APPEARANCE

Groove

Anteriorly displaced sternum

In a pigeon chest the sternum is displaced anteriorly, increasing the anteroposterior diameter. Grooves in the chest wall accentuate the deformity.

BARREL CHEST

CROSS SECTION OF THORAX

CLINICAL APPEARANCE

A barrel chest is associated with pulmonary emphysema or normal aging. The ratio of anteroposterior to lateral diameter approximates 1:1.

THORACIC KYPHOSCOLIOSIS

CROSS SECTION OF THORAX

CLINICAL APPEARANCE

High shoulder

High scapula

Thoracic convexity to right

Interspaces flared

In thoracic kyphoscoliosis the spine is curved and the thorax shows corresponding deformities. Distortion of the underlying lungs may make interpretation of lung findings very difficult.

Table 6-3

Table 6-3   Alterations in Breath and Voice Sounds

When normally air-filled lung tissue becomes airless or solid, the sounds transmitted to the chest wall through an open bronchial tree undergo much less attenuation than normal. Higher-pitched components of the sounds, which are normally filtered out, come through more readily. Characteristic alterations in breath and voice sounds occur in areas overlying the abnormal tissue. These changes have been known as bronchial breath sounds, bronchophony, egophony, and whispered pectoriloquy, although some authorities recommend simple descriptions such as "increased clarity of whispered and spoken voice." Causes include the consolidation of lung tissue associated with lobar pneumonia and the compression of lung tissue produced toward the upper level of a pleural effusion.

BRONCHIAL BREATH SOUNDS
The expiratory sound is higher-pitched and louder than in vesicular breath sounds. It is equal to or lasts longer than the inspiratory component. Sounds like these are normal over the trachea and large bronchi but not in the more peripheral parts of the lung.

EGOPHONY
Altered filtration of sound may give a nasal bleating quality to voice sounds and change the patient's "ee" to what sounds like "ay."

BRONCHOPHONY
Voice sounds are louder and clearer than usual because their higher-pitched components are better transmitted through airless lung tissue.

WHISPERED PECTORILOQUY
Whispered sounds are louder and heard more clearly than normal because of enhanced transmission through airless lung tissue.

Table 6-4

Table 6-4 Added Lung Sounds: Crackles, Wheezes, and Rubs

Added sounds in the lungs are of two basic kinds: (1) discrete, non-continuous sounds, called *crackles*, and (2) continuous musical sounds of greater duration, called *wheezes*. Pleural rubs are technically categorized as crackling sounds. The terminology of lung sounds, confused for over a century, is changing, and common usages vary. Rales and crepitations, for example, are older terms for crackles, and many American clinicians like to distinguish two types: the soft, very short, and high-pitched *fine crackles* and the louder, slightly longer, and lower-pitched *coarse crackles*. Moreover, a distinction may be made between two continuous sounds: the sonorous, low-pitched *rhonchus* and the sibilant, higher-pitched *wheeze*. Presented here is a simple classification, based primarily on the work of Forgacs.

CRACKLES

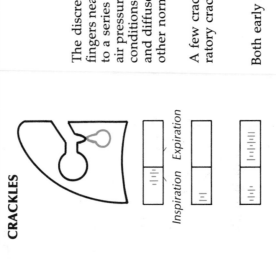

Inspiration   Expiration

The discrete, noncontinuous sounds termed crackles may be simulated by rolling a lock of hair between your fingers near your ear. Crackles that are heard relatively late in inspiration, as illustrated on the left, are attributed to a series of tiny explosions produced when previously deflated airways are reinflated during inspiration and air pressures between the two previously separated air-containing compartments are suddenly equalized. These conditions are met in pneumonia, and in the dependent portions of patients' lungs in congestive heart failure and diffuse pulmonary fibrosis. Crackles may also be present at the lung bases of elderly, bedridden, and some other normal people, and clear with deep breathing. These latter crackles have no pathological significance.

A few crackles may be heard in obstructive chronic bronchitis. In contrast to the previous group of late inspiratory crackles, these tend to occur early in inspiration and are also audible at the mouth.

Both early inspiratory and expiratory crackles have been described in bronchiectasis.

Loud gurgling and bubbling sounds during both inspiration and expiration may be produced by secretions in the trachea and large bronchi. Such sounds may be heard in pulmonary edema and in moribund or other patients who cannot cough up their secretions. It is this sound that has been called a death rattle.

WHEEZES

Wheezes are musical sounds produced by the rapid passage of air through a bronchus that is narrowed to the point of closure. The walls of the bronchus oscillate between closed and barely open positions, and generate audible sound.

Wheezes are characteristic of obstructive lung disease. They are typically expiratory but may occur in both inspiration and expiration. Although wheezes vary in pitch, no inferences can be made from the pitch as to the size of the airways involved.

A single wheeze may have a variety of musical components, each with a different pitch, all starting and stopping at the same time. Such a wheeze is called *polyphonic*.

Continued

Table 6-4

Table 6-4 (Cont'd)

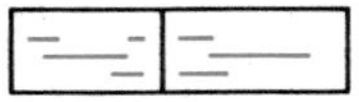

In contrast, several separate wheezes, each with its own pitch, may be heard. This diagram shows a series of such *monophonic* wheezes.

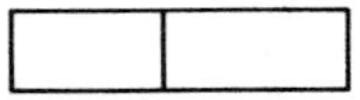

Occasionally a patient with severe obstructive lung disease worsens to the point that he is no longer able to force enough air through his narrowed bronchi to produce wheezing. The disappearance of wheezing in such a patient should signal concern and not be mistaken for improvement.

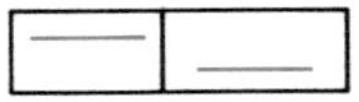

A persistent single, monophonic wheeze may indicate partial obstruction of a bronchus by tumor, scarring, or a foreign body. It may be inspiratory, expiratory, or both.

PLEURAL RUB

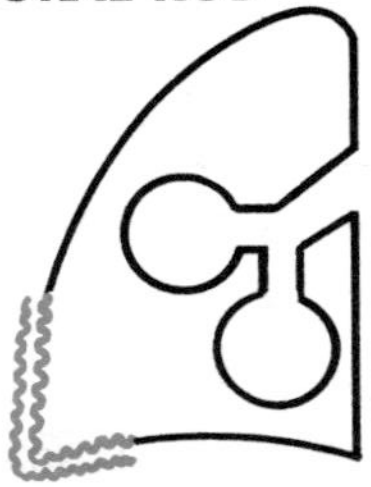

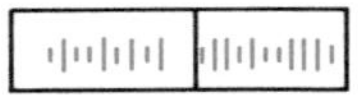

Normal pleural surfaces move smoothly and noiselessly against each other during respiration. When pleural surfaces become inflamed, however, they move jerkily as they are momentarily and repeatedly delayed by increased friction. These movements, with their associated vibrations, produce crackling sounds known as a pleural rub. The sounds tend to be loud, low-pitched, and confined to a relatively small area of the chest wall. They are often both inspiratory and expiratory but are sometimes confined to inspiration.

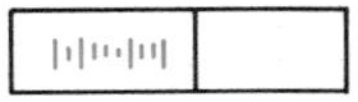

Pleural rubs resemble crackles acoustically, although they are produced by quite different pathologic processes. Rubs, especially when confined to inspiration, may therefore be difficult to distinguish from pulmonary crackles.

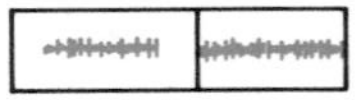

The crackling sounds of a rub may be discrete, but sometimes they are so numerous that they merge into a continuous sound.

Table 6-5

Table 6-5 Physical Signs in Selected Abnormalities of Bronchi and Lungs

CONDITION	DESCRIPTION	PERCUSSION NOTE	TACTILE FREMITUS, VOICE SOUNDS, WHISPERED VOICE SOUNDS	BREATH SOUNDS	ADDED SOUNDS
NORMAL *Bronchus* *Pleura* *Alveoli*	The tracheobronchial tree and alveoli are clear; the pleurae are thin and close together; the mobility of the chest wall is unimpaired.	Resonant	Normal	Vesicular, except perhaps for bronchial breath sounds near the large bronchi	None, except perhaps for a few transient, inspiratory crackles at the bases after recumbency or sleep
LEFT-SIDED HEART FAILURE *Swollen mucosa (sometimes)* *Deflated airway*	In left-sided heart failure, some airways in the dependent portions of the lungs are deflated abnormally during expiration. The bronchial mucosa may be swollen.	Resonant	Normal	Normal or sometimes prolonged expiration	Crackles at lung bases; sometimes wheezes
PLEURAL FLUID OR THICKENING *Pleural fluid or thickening*	Pleural fluid or fibrotic thickening muffles all sounds.	Dull to flat	Decreased to absent; however, when fluid compresses the underlying lung, bronchophony, egophony, and whispered pectoriloquy may appear.	Decreased vesicular or absent; however, when fluid compresses the lung, a bronchial quality may appear.	None unless there is underlying disease

Continued

Table 6-5

Table 6-5 (Cont'd)

CONDITION	DESCRIPTION	PERCUSSION NOTE	TACTILE FREMITUS VOICE SOUNDS, WHISPERED VOICE SOUNDS	BREATH SOUNDS	ADDED SOUNDS
PULMONARY CONSOLIDATION (e.g., LOBAR PNEUMONIA) 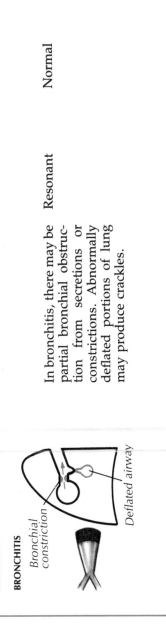 *Deflated airway* *Alveoli filled with fluid, red and white cells*	A consolidated lung is dull to percussion but, as long as the large airways are clear, fremitus, breath and voice sounds are transmitted as if they came directly from the larynx and trachea. Abnormally deflated portions of the lungs produce crackles.	Dull	Increased, with bronchophony, egophony, whispered pectoriloquy	Bronchial	Crackles
BRONCHITIS *Bronchial constriction* *Deflated airway*	In bronchitis, there may be partial bronchial obstruction from secretions or constrictions. Abnormally deflated portions of lung may produce crackles.	Resonant	Normal	Normal or prolonged expiration	Wheezes or crackles
EMPHYSEMA 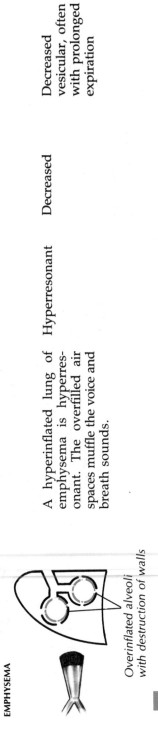 *Overinflated alveoli with destruction of walls*	A hyperinflated lung of emphysema is hyperresonant. The overfilled air spaces muffle the voice and breath sounds.	Hyperresonant	Decreased	Decreased vesicular, often with prolonged expiration	None, or signs of bronchitis

Continued

155

Table 6-5

Table 6-5 (Cont'd)

CONDITION	DESCRIPTION	PERCUSSION NOTE	TACTILE FREMITUS VOICE SOUNDS, WHISPERED VOICE SOUNDS	BREATH SOUNDS	ADDED SOUNDS
PNEUMOTHORAX 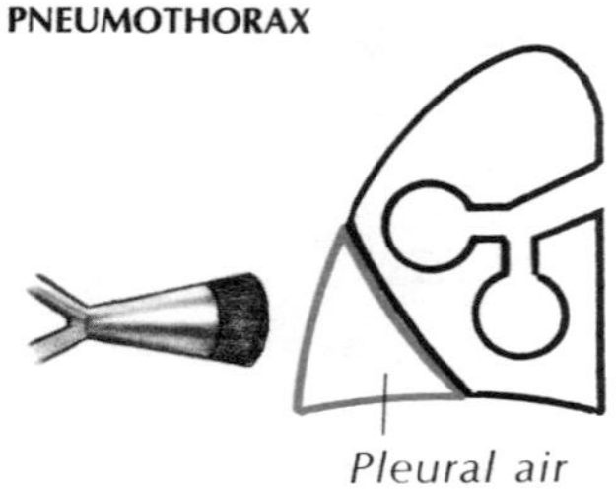 *Pleural air*	The free pleural air of pneumothorax may mimic obstructive lung disease but is usually unilateral and may shift the trachea to the opposite side. The air-filled pleural space gives a hyperresonant percussion note but muffles voice and breath sounds.	Hyperresonant	Decreased to absent	Decreased to absent	None
ATELECTASIS 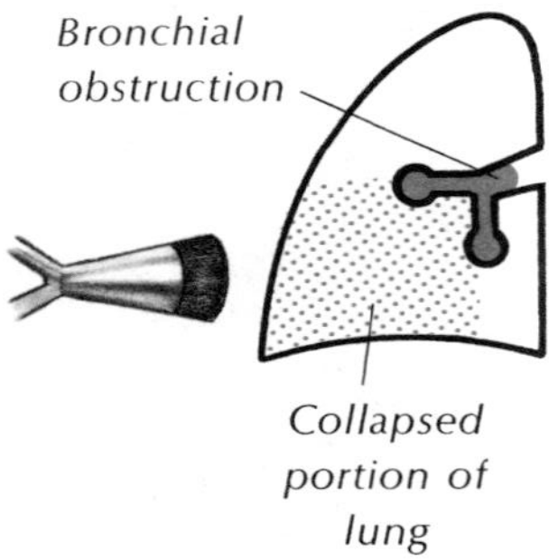 *Bronchial obstruction* *Collapsed portion of lung*	A collapsed or atelectatic lung is dull to percussion. Bronchial obstruction (shown here but not always present) prevents transmission of breath and voice sounds. The trachea may shift to the same side.	Dull	Decreased to absent	Decreased vesicular or absent	None

THE HEART, PRESSURES, AND PULSES

Anatomy and Physiology

SURFACE PROJECTIONS OF THE HEART AND GREAT VESSELS

The heart is assessed chiefly by examination through the anterior chest wall. Most of the anterior cardiac surface is made up of right ventricle. This chamber and the pulmonary artery may be visualized roughly as a wedge lying behind and to the left of the sternum.

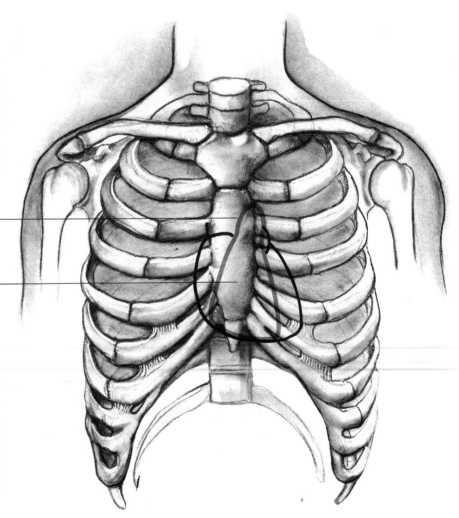

Pulmonary artery —————

Right ventricle —————

The inferior border of the right ventricle rests at a level somewhat below the junction of sternum and xiphoid process. The right ventricle narrows superiorly and meets the pulmonary artery at the level of the 3rd left costal cartilage close to the sternum.

The left ventricle, lying to the left and behind the right ventricle, makes up only a small portion of the anterior cardiac surface. It is clinically important, however, forming the left border of the heart and producing the apical impulse.* This impulse is a brief systolic beat usually found in the 5th interspace, 7 cm to 9 cm from the midsternal line.

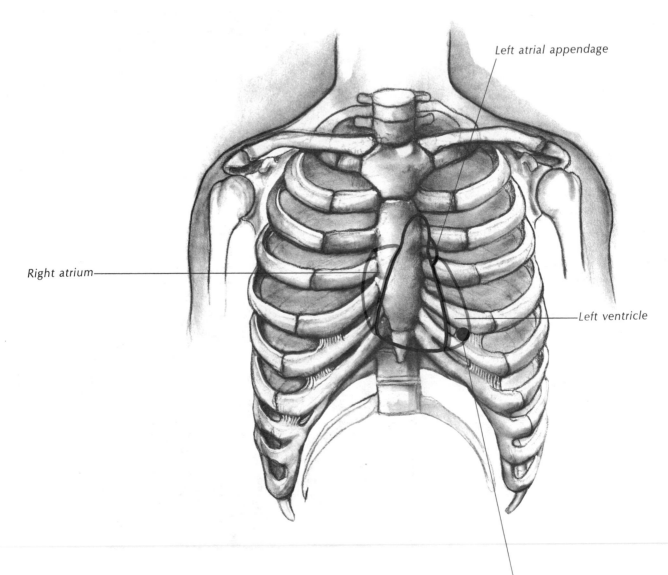

Left atrial appendage

Right atrium

Left ventricle

Apical impulse

The right border of the heart is formed by the right atrium, a chamber not usually identifiable on physical examination. The left atrium is mostly posterior and cannot be examined directly, although its small atrial appendage may make up a segment of the left cardiac border between pulmonary artery and left ventricle.

*The apical impulse is sometimes called the point of maximum impulse, or P.M.I. Since in some conditions the most prominent cardiac impulse may not be apical, this term is not recommended.

Above the heart lie the great vessels. The pulmonary artery, already mentioned, bifurcates quickly into its left and right branches. The aorta curves upward from the left ventricle to the level of the sternal angle, where it arches backward and then down. On the right the superior vena cava empties into the right atrium.

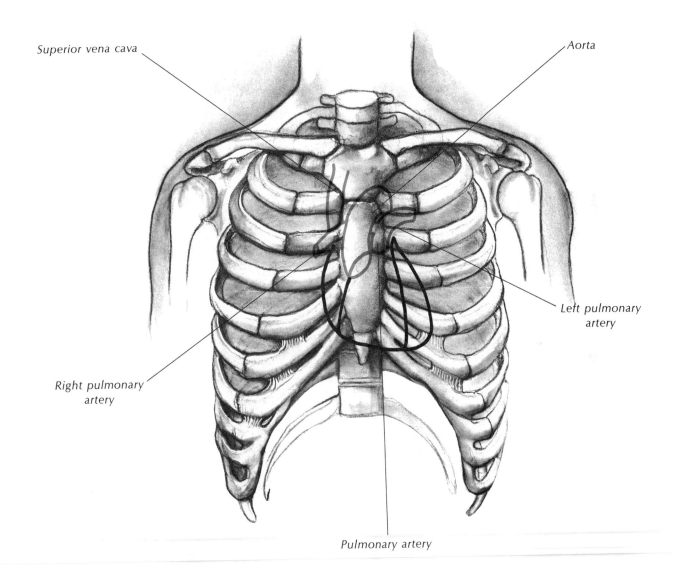

Superior vena cava

Aorta

Left pulmonary artery

Right pulmonary artery

Pulmonary artery

Although not illustrated above, the inferior vena cava also empties into the right atrium. The superior and inferior venae cavae carry venous blood from the upper and lower portions of the body respectively.

CARDIAC CHAMBERS, VALVES, AND CIRCULATION

Circulation through the heart is illustrated in the following diagram, which identifies the cardiac chambers, valves, and direction of blood flow. Because of their positions, the tricuspid and mitral valves are often called atrioventricular valves. The aortic and pulmonic valves are called semilunar valves because their leaflets have a half-moon configuration.

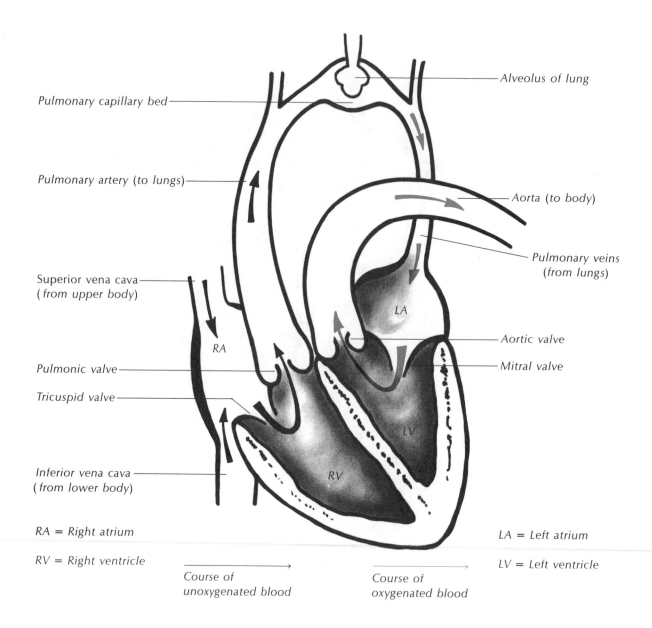

RA = Right atrium

RV = Right ventricle

LA = Left atrium

LV = Left ventricle

Course of unoxygenated blood

Course of oxygenated blood

Although this diagram shows all valves in an open position, they are not all open at the same time in the living heart. Closure of the valves is responsible for normal heart sounds. Their positions and movements must be understood in relation to events in the cardiac cycle.

EVENTS IN THE CARDIAC CYCLE

If one were to measure the pressure in the left ventricle throughout the cardiac cycle, one would find a pressure curve like the following:

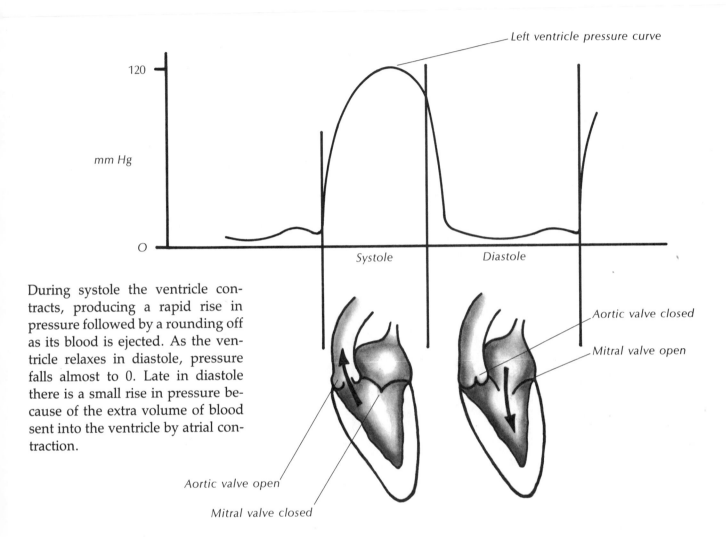

During systole the ventricle contracts, producing a rapid rise in pressure followed by a rounding off as its blood is ejected. As the ventricle relaxes in diastole, pressure falls almost to 0. Late in diastole there is a small rise in pressure because of the extra volume of blood sent into the ventricle by atrial contraction.

Note that during systole the aortic valve is open, allowing ejection of blood from the left ventricle into the aorta. The mitral valve is closed, preventing blood from regurgitating back into the left atrium. In contrast, during diastole the aortic valve is closed, preventing regurgitation of blood from the aorta back into the left ventricle. The mitral valve is open, allowing blood to flow from the left atrium into the relaxed left ventricle.

The interrelationships of the pressures in these three chambers—left atrium, left ventricle, and aorta—together with the position and movement of the valves are fundamental to the understanding of heart sounds. Events on the right side of the heart also contribute, of course, but for the sake of clarity will be discussed later.

During diastole, pressure in the blood-filled left atrium slightly exceeds that in the relaxed left ventricle, and blood flows from left atrium to left ventricle across the open mitral valve. Just before the onset of ventricular systole, atrial contraction produces a slight pressure rise in both chambers.

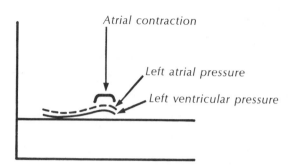

As the ventricle starts to contract, pressure within it rapidly exceeds left atrial pressure, thus shutting the mitral valve. Closure of the mitral valve produces the first heart sound (S_1).*

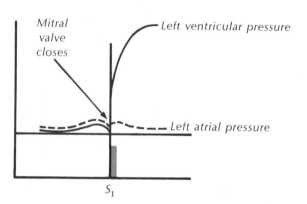

As the ventricular pressure continues to rise, it exceeds the diastolic pressure in the aorta and forces the aortic valve open. Opening of the aortic valve is not usually heard, but in some pathologic conditions is accompanied by an early systolic ejection sound (Ej).

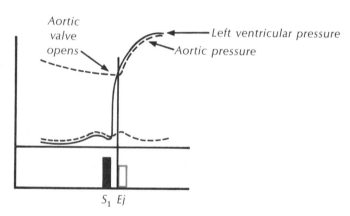

As the ventricle ejects most of its blood, its pressure begins to fall. When left ventricular pressure drops below the aortic pressure, the aortic valve shuts. Aortic valve closure causes the second heart sound (S_2).

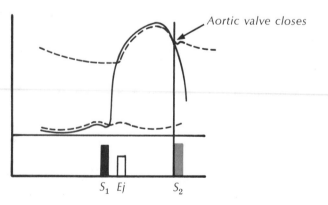

*An extensive literature deals with the exact causes of heart sounds (*e.g.*, actual closure of valve leaflets, tensing of related structures, and the impact of columns of blood). The explanations given here are oversimplified but retain clinical usefulness.

As the left ventricular pressure continues to drop during ventricular relaxation, it falls below left atrial pressure. The mitral valve opens. This is usually a silent event but may be audible as an opening snap (O.S.) in mitral stenosis.

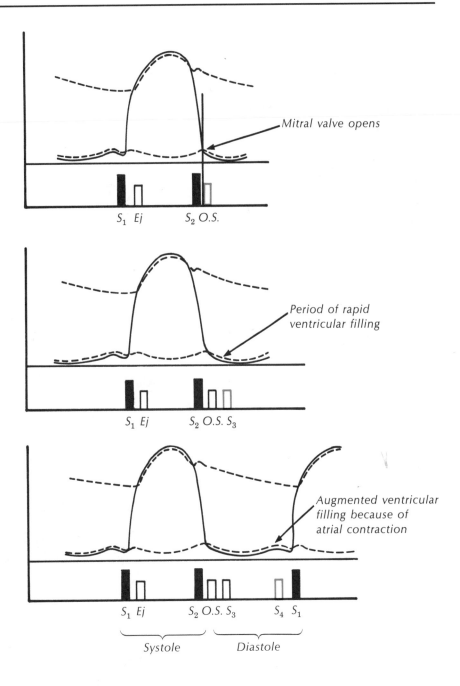

Next occurs a period of rapid ventricular filling as blood flows early in diastole from left atrium to left ventricle. In children and young adults this period may be marked by a third heart sound (S_3).

Finally, although not often heard in normal adults, a fourth heart sound (or S_4) marks atrial contraction. It immediately precedes S_1 of the next beat.

While these events are occurring on the left side of the heart, similar changes are occurring on the right, involving the right atrium, right ventricle, tricuspid valve, pulmonic valve, and pulmonary artery. Right ventricular and pulmonary arterial pressures are significantly lower than corresponding levels on the left side. Furthermore, right-sided events usually occur slightly later than those on the left. Instead of a single heart sound, therefore, you may hear two discernible components, the first from left-sided valvular closure, the second from right-sided closure. The normal second heart sound, for example, typically splits during inspiration into aortic and pulmonic components, then becomes single again during expiration.

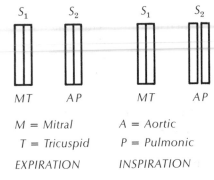

M = Mitral   A = Aortic
T = Tricuspid   P = Pulmonic
EXPIRATION   INSPIRATION

RELATION OF HEART SOUNDS TO THE CHEST WALL

Events related to the movement of heart valves and to flow across them are best heard *not over their anatomic locations* but in the following *auscultatory areas* that bear their names. These names do not imply, however, that sounds heard there come only from those valves.

Aortic area—right 2nd interspace close to the sternum

Pulmonic area—left 2nd interspace close to the sternum

these two areas together are sometimes called the "base" of the heart

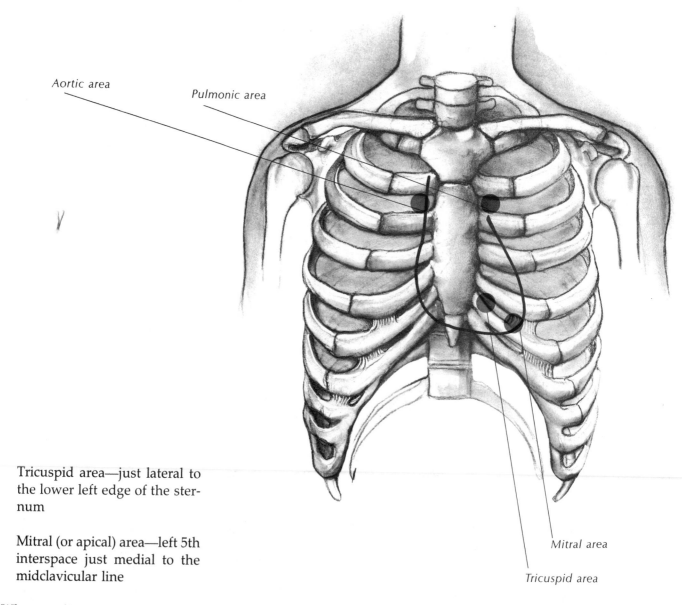

Aortic area

Pulmonic area

Mitral area

Tricuspid area

Tricuspid area—just lateral to the lower left edge of the ster-num

Mitral (or apical) area—left 5th interspace just medial to the midclavicular line

When cardiovascular structures are altered by disease, the best areas for auscultation may change accordingly.

From a knowledge of pressure changes in the cardiac cycle, one can correctly predict the relative intensities of heart sounds in these areas. S_2 is produced by closure of the two semilunar valves, the aortic and pulmonic. Aortic valve closure under the relatively high aortic pressure produces the major component of S_2. This component (A_2) is loudest in the aortic area and can be heard throughout the precordium. In the pulmonic area, one can additionally distinguish that component of S_2 produced by closure of the pulmonic valve (P_2). P_2 is softer because of the lower pressure in the pulmonary artery. It can be heard normally only in the vicinity of the left 2nd or 3rd interspace. Physiologic splitting of S_2, therefore, is usually heard only in these areas.

The first sound, S_1, is produced by the closure of the atrioventricular valves, primarily the mitral, with probably an additional soft tricuspid component. Although usually audible throughout the precordium, S_1 is loudest, as expected, in the mitral area. In the tricuspid area the tricuspid component of S_1 sometimes becomes distinguishable from the louder mitral component, and S_1 is accordingly split.

THE CONDUCTION SYSTEM

Muscular contraction of the cardiac chambers should be distinguished from the electrical conduction system that stimulates and coordinates it.

Each normal impulse is initiated in a group of cardiac cells known as the sinus node. Located in the right atrium, the sinus node acts as cardiac pacemaker and automatically discharges an impulse about 60 to 100 times a minute. This impulse travels through both atria to the atrioventricular (or AV) node, a specialized group of cells located low in the atrial septum. Here the impulse is delayed somewhat before its passage down the bundle of His and its branches and thence to the ventricular myocardium. Muscular contraction follows: first the atria, then the ventricles. The normal conduction pathway is diagrammed in simplified form at the right.

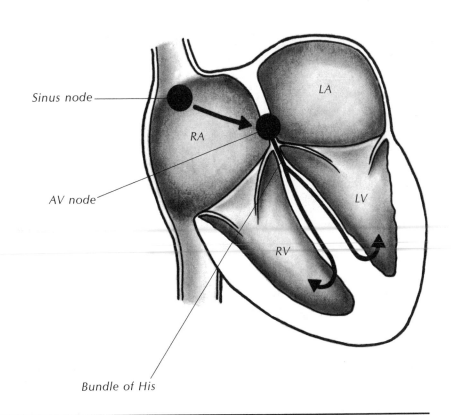

Sinus node

RA

AV node

LA

LV

RV

Bundle of His

The electrocardiogram records these events. Each normal impulse produces a series of waves:

A *small P wave* of atrial depolarization (electrical activation)

A *larger QRS complex* of ventricular depolarization. Each consists of one or more of the following:

A *Q wave*, formed whenever the initial deflection is downward

An *R wave*, the upward deflection

An *S wave*, a downward deflection following an R wave

A *T wave* of ventricular repolarization (or recovery)

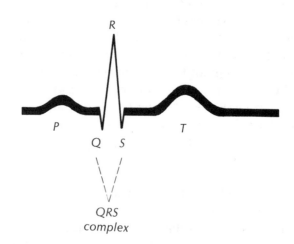

The electrical impulse slightly precedes the myocardial contraction that it stimulates. The relation of electrocardiographic waves to the cardiac cycle is shown below.

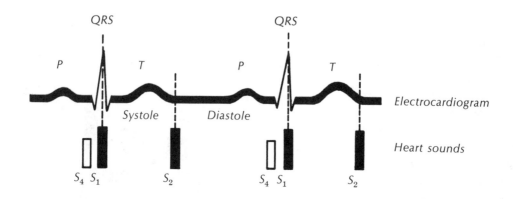

ARTERIAL PULSES AND BLOOD PRESSURE

With each contraction the left ventricle ejects a volume of blood (stroke volume) into the aorta and thence on into the arterial tree. A pressure wave moves rapidly through the arterial system where it can be felt as the *arterial pulse*. Although the pressure wave travels quickly—about ten times faster than the blood itself—a palpable delay between ventricular contraction and peripheral pulses makes the latter unsuitable for timing cardiac events. Always use the carotid arteries instead.

Blood pressure in the arterial system varies with the cardiac cycle, reaching a systolic peak and diastolic trough, the levels of which are measured by sphygmomanometry. The difference between systolic and diastolic pressures is known as the pulse pressure.

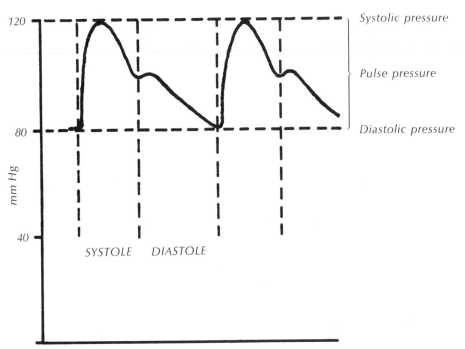

Several factors influence arterial pressure:

1. *Cardiac Output.* The pumping action of the left ventricle is of course essential to the maintenance of blood pressure. It affects chiefly the systolic pressure.
2. *Elastic Recoil of the Aorta and Large Arteries.* As the left ventricle forces blood into the aorta and large arteries, it distends their elastic walls. Recoil of the vessel walls during diastole advances the blood down the arterial tree and helps to maintain diastolic pressure. A competent aortic valve is also necessary to assure forward flow.
3. *Peripheral Resistance.* Peripheral resistance to blood flow depends primarily on the caliber of the arterioles, under control of the autonomic nervous system. It is the chief determinant of diastolic blood pressure.
4. *Volume of Blood in the Arterial System*
5. *Viscosity of the Blood*

Changes in any of these five factors alter systolic pressure, diastolic pressure, or both. Blood pressure levels fluctuate strikingly through any 24-hour period, varying, for example, with physical activity, emotional state, pain, noise, environmental temperature, the use of coffee, tobacco, and other drugs, and even with the time of day.

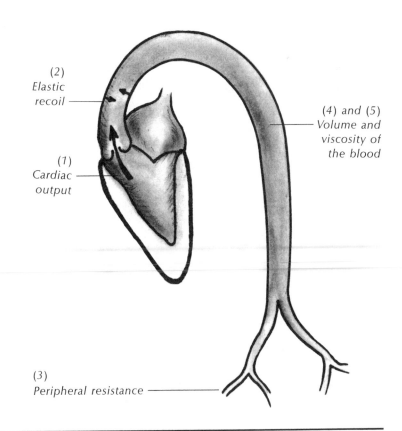

JUGULAR VENOUS PRESSURE AND PULSES

Pressure on the venous side of the circulatory system is much lower than on the arterial side. It is ultimately dependent upon left ventricular contraction, but much of this force is dissipated as the blood passes through the arterial tree and capillary bed. Other important determinants of venous pressure include (1) blood volume, and (2) the capacity of the right heart to receive blood and to eject it onward into the pulmonary arterial system. When any of these variables is altered pathologically, abnormalities in venous pressure result. For example, the venous pressure falls when left ventricular output or blood volume is significantly reduced; it rises when the right heart fails or when increased pressure in the pericardial sac impedes the return of blood to the right atrium.

In the laboratory, venous pressure is measured from a zero point in the right atrium. Since it is difficult to establish this point reliably during physical examination, a stable and reproducible landmark is substituted—the sternal angle. In most positions, whether a patient is upright or supine, the sternal angle is roughly 5 cm above the right atrium.

Although it is possible to measure venous pressure elsewhere in the venous system, the best estimate of right atrial pressure, and therefore of right heart function, is made from the internal jugular veins. If these are impossible to see, the external jugular veins can be used but they are less reliable. The level of venous pressure is determined by finding the highest point of oscillation in the internal jugular veins or, if necessary, the point above which the external jugular veins appear collapsed. The vertical distance in centimeters between either of these points and the sternal angle is recorded as the venous pressure. The zero point (*i.e.,* the sternal angle) should also be stated. A jugular venous pressure 2 cm above the sternal angle is roughly equivalent to a central venous pressure of 7 cm.

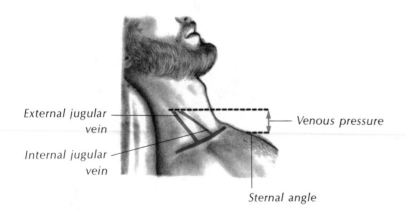

External jugular vein

Internal jugular vein

Venous pressure

Sternal angle

In order to see the venous pressure level, it may be necessary to alter the patient's position. In the illustration above, for example, consider an internal jugular venous pressure of 0—just level with the sternal angle. The venous pulsations would be visible scarcely, if at all, just above the clavicle. By lowering the head of the patient's bed you should see them more satisfactorily higher in the patient's neck. Conversely, if the patient's pressure were extremely high—up to his ear lobe, for example—you could not be sure of its top. If you sat the patient upright, however, the top of the oscillating column would probably drop into view.

Pressures more than 3 cm or 4 cm above the sternal angle are considered elevated.

The oscillations that you see in the internal jugular veins (and sometimes in the externals as well) do not arise in the venous system itself. They reflect instead changing pressures within the right atrium. Of all the visible veins, the right internal jugular has the most direct channel to the right atrium and usually, therefore, reflects these pressure changes most satisfactorily.

Careful observation reveals that the internal jugular pulse is composed of two, or sometimes three, waves. These are called *a*, *c*, and *v* waves. Their analysis gives important information about the cardiac events and pressures in the right atrium.

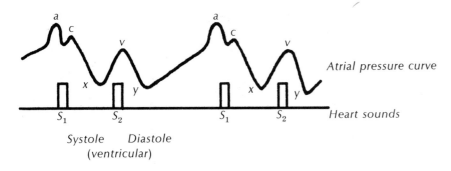

Atrial pressure curve

Heart sounds

Systole   Diastole
(ventricular)

The *a wave* represents a slight rise in atrial pressure that occurs with atrial contraction, just before ventricular systole. With the beginning of ventricular systole, the tricuspid valve closes and the atrium relaxes. The resulting fall in right atrial pressure is reflected in the jugular venous pulse as a fall in the height of the blood column—a trough known as the *x descent*. As the venous return to the right atrium continues and the chamber begins to fill, there is another rise in right atrial pressure, seen as the *v wave*. This wave begins during the latter part of ventricular systole. With the beginning of diastole and the opening of the tricuspid valve, the right atrium empties rapidly into the right ventricle. The right atrial pressure again falls, forming a second trough or *y descent*. Sometimes a *c wave* is visible. It is a reflected wave from the nearby carotid artery.

CHANGES WITH AGE

Cardiovascular findings vary importantly with age. The apical impulse, which is usually felt easily in children and young adults, may get harder to find with age as the chest deepens in its anteroposterior diameter. For the same reason, splitting of the second heart sound may be harder to hear in older people as its pulmonic component becomes less audible. A physiologic third heart sound, commonly heard in children and young adults, may persist as late as the age of 40, especially in women. After the approximate age of 40, however, an S_3 strongly suggests either ventricular failure or volume overloading of the ventricle caused by valvular heart disease such as mitral regurgitation. In contrast, an S_4 is seldom heard in young adults. It may, however, be heard in apparently healthy older people, but is also frequently associated with heart disease. (See Table 7-8, Extra Heart Sounds in Diastole, p. 199.)

At some time over the life span almost everyone has cardiovascular murmurs. These are sounds that last longer than heart sounds and are caused by turbulent blood flow or valvular vibrations. Most of these murmurs are benign in that they occur without other evidence of cardiovascular abnormality and may, therefore, be considered normal variants. The nature of these common murmurs varies importantly with age, and familiarity with their patterns helps to distinguish normal from abnormal.

Children, adolescents, and young adults frequently have soft *pulmonic systolic murmurs* (see p. 203).

Many women late in pregnancy and during lactation have a so-called mammary souffle* secondary to increased blood flow in their breasts. Although this murmur may be noted anywhere in the breasts, it is often most easily heard in the 2nd or 3rd interspace on either side of the sternum. A mammary souffle is typically both systolic and diastolic, but sometimes only the louder systolic component is audible.

Many middle-aged and older adults have *aortic systolic murmurs.* These have been heard in about a third of people near the age of 60, and in well over half of those reaching 85. Aging thickens the bases of the aortic cusps with fibrous tissue, calcification follows, and audible vibrations result. Turbulence produced by blood flow into a dilated aorta may contribute to this murmur. In most people this valvular fibrosis and calcification—known as aortic sclerosis—do not impede blood flow. In some, however, the valve cusps become progressively calcified and immobile, and true aortic stenosis, or obstruction of flow, develops. The aortic systolic murmur then loses its benignity. Differentiation between benign aortic sclerosis and the pathologic aortic stenosis may be extremely difficult.

A similar aging process affects the mitral valve, usually about a decade later than aortic sclerosis. Here degenerative changes with calcification impair the ability of the mitral valve to close normally during systole, and cause the *systolic murmur of mitral regurgitation.* Although these changes

---

*Souffle is pronounced soó-fl, not like cheese soufflé. Both words come from a French word meaning puff.

are fairly common, a murmur of mitral regurgitation cannot be considered benign.

Murmurs may originate in large blood vessels as well as in the heart. The *jugular venous hum,* which is very common in children and may still be heard through young adulthood, illustrates this point (see pp. 207–208). A second, more important example is the *cervical systolic murmur* or *bruit.* In older people systolic bruits heard in the middle or upper portions of the carotid arteries suggest, but do not prove, the possibility of partial arterial obstruction secondary to atherosclerosis. In contrast, cervical bruits in younger people are usually innocent. In children and young adults systolic murmurs (or bruits) are frequently heard just above the clavicle. One study has shown that, while cervical bruits can be heard in almost 9 out of 10 children under the age of 5, their prevalence falls steadily to about 1 out of 3 in adolescence and young adulthood and to less than 1 out of 10 in middle age. For further information on cardiovascular murmurs, see Tables 7-10 through 7-14, pages 201 to 208.

The aorta and large arteries stiffen with age as they become arteriosclerotic. As the aorta becomes less distensible, a given stroke volume causes a greater rise in systolic blood pressure; *systolic hypertension* with a *widened pulse pressure* may ensue. Peripheral arteries tend to lengthen, become tortuous, and feel harder and less resilient. These changes do not necessarily indicate atherosclerosis, however, and you can make no inferences from them as to disease in the coronary or cerebral vessels. Lengthening and tortuosity of the aorta and its branches occasionally result in kinking or buckling of the carotid artery low in the neck, especially on the right. The resulting pulsatile mass, which occurs chiefly in hypertensive women, may be mistaken for a carotid aneurysm. A tortuous aorta occasionally raises the pressure in the left-sided jugular veins by impairing their drainage in the chest.

Both systolic and diastolic blood pressures tend to rise from childhood through the approximate ages of 65 or 70, and distinctions between normal and abnormally high levels become increasingly difficult with age. On the other extreme, some elderly people develop an increased tendency toward *postural* (or *orthostatic*) *hypotension*—a sudden drop in blood pressure when they rise to a sitting or standing position. This is an important problem with multiple, often correctable causes, and should not be missed.

Techniques of Examination

THE HEART

The patient should be supine or lying with his upper body somewhat elevated. The latter position is especially helpful when the patient is orthopneic or when you are correlating cardiac signs with the jugular venous pulse. Stand at the patient's right side. When examining a woman with large breasts, you may need to displace the left breast upward or to the left. Alternatively, ask her to do this for you. The room must be quiet.

Abnormalities should be described in terms of:

1. Their timing in relation to the cardiac cycle

2. Their location (*i.e.*, the interspace and distance from the midsternal, midclavicular, or axillary lines). The midsternal line has the advantage of being the most reliable from one observer to another. When using it, hold the ruler tangential to the anterior chest, not curving around it.

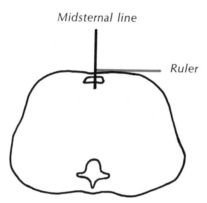

INSPECTION AND PALPATION

As you examine the patient's anterior chest, visualize the underlying cardiac chambers and great vessels: the right and left ventricles, the aorta, and the pulmonary artery. Try to detect any abnormal pulsations that they may produce. You may sometimes actually feel accentuated heart sounds, extra heart sounds, and the vibrations of loud cardiac murmurs. These last vibrations, which feel like the throat of a purring cat, are called thrills (a term that should be explained to the patient when it is used at the bedside!).

You can see and feel cardiovascular pulsations more easily when patients are thin. In contrast, a thick chest wall may obscure them, and lung tissue may intervene when age or emphysema increases the anteroposterior diameter of the chest. Keep these common variations in mind as you make your assessments.

Since inspection and palpation reinforce each other, they will be described together. Note that:

1. Tangential lighting helps you detect pulsations. Observing the chest surface tangentially is also useful, allowing you to see the pulsation "on edge."

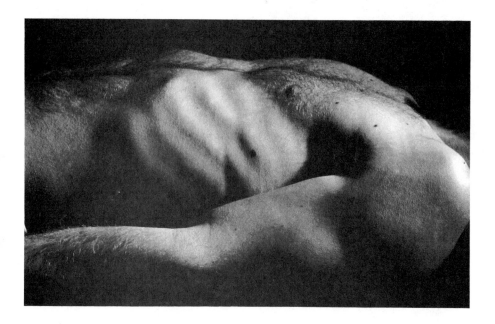

2. The "ball of the hand" (the palmar surface of the hand at the base of the fingers) is most sensitive to vibrations. It may, therefore, be especially useful in detecting thrills. The finger pads are more helpful in detecting and analyzing pulsations.

3. In order to time puzzling pulsations or thrills in relation to systole and diastole, feel the carotid pulse or listen to the heart as you palpate (see pp. 176–177 for the relationships of these events).

Proceed in an orderly fashion to examine:

1. *The Aortic Area* (2nd interspace to the right of the sternum). Observe for any pulsation or thrill or the vibration of aortic valve closure.

Pulsation of aortic aneurysm; thrill of aortic stenosis; accentuated aortic valve closure sound of hypertension

2. *The Pulmonary Area* (2nd left interspace; observe also the 3rd left interspace for events of the pulmonic valve and artery). Observe for any pulsation or thrill or the vibration of pulmonic valve closure.

Pulsation of increased pressure or flow in the pulmonary artery; thrill of pulmonic stenosis; accentuated pulmonic valve closure sound of pulmonary hypertension

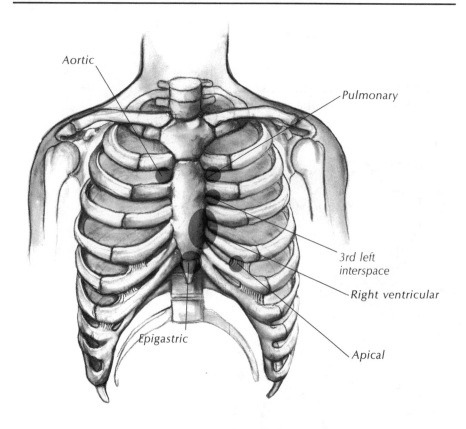

Aortic

Pulmonary

3rd left interspace

Right ventricular

Epigastric

Apical

3. *The Right Ventricular Area* (lower half of the sternum and the parasternal area, especially on the left). Observe for a diffuse lift or heave or any thrills.

Thin adults may have a brief right ventricular impulse here.

In patients with anemia, anxiety, hyperthyroidism, fever, or pregnancy, where cardiac output is increased, a brief right ventricular impulse may be felt.

A sustained systolic lift in right ventricular enlargement

Systolic thrill of ventricular septal defect

4. *The Apical or Left Ventricular Area* (the 5th intercostal space at or just medial to the midclavicular line). Inspect the chest wall in and around this area including the 4th, 5th, and 6th interspaces; try to identify the apical impulse. This is the lowest and most lateral point on the chest where you can detect a cardiac impulse. Normally the apical impulse is just medial to the midclavicular line in either the 5th or 4th interspace. You can see or feel it in at least half of adults. Asking the patient to exhale and then hold his breath out may help you find it.

The apical impulse may be displaced upward and to the left by pregnancy or a high left diaphragm. It may also be displaced by deformities of the chest wall and by heart disease. When cardiac output is increased, as in anemia, anxiety, hyperthyroidism, fever, or pregnancy, the apical impulse may have an increased amplitude.

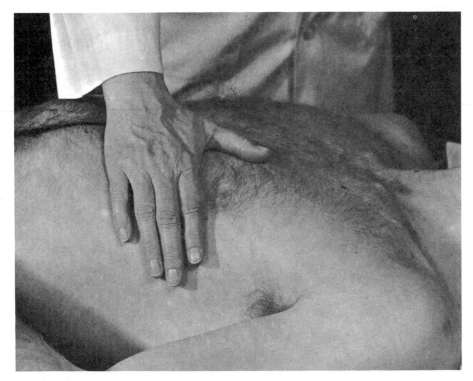

With the palm of your hand try to locate the apical impulse.

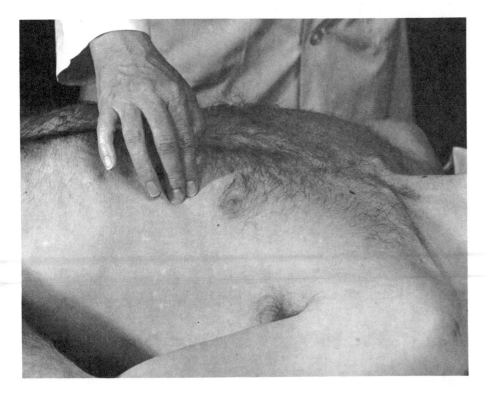

Then make finer assessments with your fingertips.

Define the location of the apical impulse by identifying the interspace(s) in which you feel it, and measure its distance in centimeters from the midsternal line. Assess the diameter of the impulse, its amplitude, force, and duration. To estimate the duration of the impulse, listen to the heart sounds while you are palpating, or watch the movement of your stethoscope as you listen at the apex. Estimate the proportion of systole occupied by the palpable pulsation. Normally the apical impulse is a light tap, felt in an area about 1 cm to 2 cm in diameter or less. It begins about at the time of the first heart sound and is sustained during the first third to half of systole.

If you cannot feel the apical impulse, ask the patient to turn onto his left side. This maneuver may shift the heart toward the chest wall and make the apical impulse more accessible. Since this position displaces the apical impulse, however, you should not use it for localization.

Look and feel carefully for any extra impulses, such as those that may coincide with S_3 or S_4. Feel for any thrills.

5. *The Epigastric Area.* Note any pulsations. The pulsation of the abdominal aorta may often be seen and felt here in a normal person. In addition, the pulsation of an enlarged right ventricle can sometimes be felt. To distinguish these two, place the palm of your hand on the epigastric area and slide your fingers up under the rib cage. The aortic pulsations thrust forward against the palmar surfaces of your fingers; the pulsations of an enlarged right ventricle thrust downward against your fingertips.

AUSCULTATION

With your stethoscope identify the first and second heart sounds (S_1 and S_2), starting at the aortic or pulmonic area. The following clues are helpful:

1. At normal and slow rates S_1 is the first of the paired heart sounds, following the longer diastolic period and preceding the shorter systole.

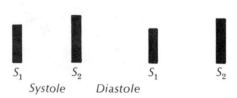

S_1 S_2 S_1 S_2

Systole   *Diastole*

2. At the base (aortic and pulmonic areas) S_2 is normally louder than S_1. This fact is especially helpful at rapid heart rates when systole and diastole may be approximately equal in length. Through a process of "inching," auscultation at the base may serve as a guide when listening in other areas of the heart. Having identified S_2 at the base, gradually move or "inch" your stethoscope down toward the apex. Concentrate on S_2 and its rhythmic recurrence in the cardiac cycle, using it as a guide to time other sounds. If you get confused, return to the base and inch back down again.

Examples of Abnormalities:

See Table 7-1, Comparison of the Apical Impulse in Normal People and in Those With Left Ventricular Enlargement (p. 191).

A rare patient has dextrocardia—a heart situated in the right chest. The cardiac impulses will then be found on the right side.

Thrills of mitral regurgitation and stenosis

Increased aortic pulsation in aneurysm of the abdominal aorta and aortic regurgitation; right ventricular pulsation in right ventricular enlargement

3. S_1 is approximately synchronous with the onset of the apical impulse.

4. S_1 just precedes the carotid impulse.

Identify the heart rate. Count the rate per minute. If the rhythm is perfectly regular and seems to be normal in rate, you may count for 15 seconds and multiply by 4. This short period of observation, however, produces errors. If there is any irregularity, if the heart rate is unusually fast, and especially if the heart rate is slow, count for at least a minute.

Identify the rhythm. Is it regular or irregular? If irregular, try to identify a pattern: (1) Do early beats appear on a basically regular rhythm? (2) Does the irregularity vary consistently with respiration? Or (3) is the rhythm totally irregular?

See Tables 7-2 to 7-4, Differentiation of Selected Heart Rates and Rhythms (pp. 192–195).

Listen in order in the following locations:

1. Aortic area (2nd right interspace close to the sternum)
2. Pulmonic area (2nd left interspace close to the sternum)
3. 3rd left interspace close to the sternum, where murmurs of both aortic and pulmonic origin may often be heard
4. Triscuspid area (lower left sternal border)
5. Mitral (apical) area (5th left interspace just medial to the midclavicular line)

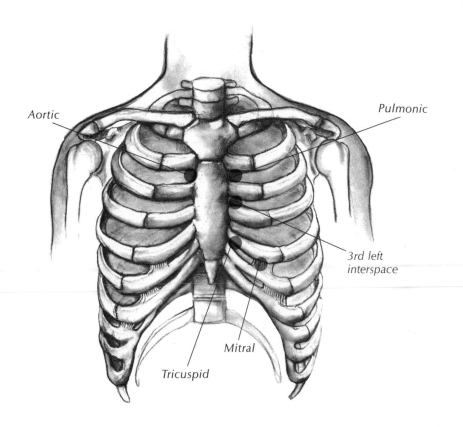

All heart sounds may be diminished in the presence of a thick chest wall or pulmonary emphysema.

Listen first with the diaphragm in all areas, then with the bell. The diaphragm is better for picking up relatively high-pitched sounds such as S_1, S_2, the murmurs of aortic and mitral regurgitation, and pericardial friction rubs. Press it firmly onto the chest. The bell is more sensitive to low-pitched sounds such as S_3, S_4, and the diastolic murmur of mitral stenosis. Apply it lightly, with just enough pressure to produce an air seal with its full rim.

Take your time at *each auscultatory area*, concentrating in turn on each of the six following points:

1. Listen carefully to the first heart sound. Note its intensity and listen for any splitting.

   See Table 7-5, Variations in the First Heart Sound (p. 196).

2. Listen to the second heart sound. Note its intensity and listen for splitting. Pay special attention to splitting in the left 2nd and 3rd interspaces, where S_2 usually splits slightly during inspiration but becomes single during expiration. When listening for splitting, ask the patient to breathe quietly, then slightly more deeply than normally but through his nose. (Mouth breathing makes louder breath sounds that obscure the heart sounds.) A thick chest wall or increased anteroposterior diameter of the chest, as with age, may make the pulmonic component of S_2 inaudible.

   See Table 7-6, Variations in the Second Heart Sound (p. 197).

3. Listen for extra sounds in systole such as ejection sounds or systolic clicks. Note their location, timing, intensity, pitch, and the effects of respiration on the sounds.

   See Table 7-7, Extra Heart Sounds in Systole (p. 198).

4. Listen for extra sounds in diastole such as S_3, S_4, or an opening snap. Note their location, timing, intensity, pitch, and the effects of respiration on the sounds.

   See Table 7-8, Extra Heart Sounds in Diastole (p. 199).

   See Table 7-9, Three Causes of an Apparently Split First Heart Sound (p. 200).

5. Listen for systolic murmurs. Murmurs are differentiated from heart sounds by their longer duration.

   See Table 7-10, Mechanisms of Heart Murmurs. (p. 201).

6. Listen for diastolic murmurs.

If systolic or diastolic murmurs are present, note the following characteristics:

Timing. For example:

> *Systolic murmurs* may be described as early, mid-, or late systolic or, when heard throughout systole, pansystolic or holosystolic.

   See Table 7-11, Midsystolic Ejection Murmurs (pp. 202–203), and Table 7-12, Pansystolic Regurgitant Murmurs (p. 204).

Diastolic murmurs are classified as early, mid- , and late diastolic. Late diastolic murmurs are sometimes also called presystolic.

See Table 7-13, Diastolic Murmurs (pp. 205–206).

Some murmurs and other cardiovascular sounds, such as pericardial friction rubs or venous hums, have *both systolic and diastolic components*. Observe and describe these sounds according to the same characteristics used for systolic and diastolic murmurs.

See Table 7-14, Differentiation of Cardiovascular Sounds with Both Systolic and Diastolic Components (pp. 207–208).

Location of maximal intensity—described in terms of interspace and relation to the sternum, the midsternal, the midclavicular, or one of the axillary lines

For example, a murmur best heard in the 2nd right interspace close to the sternum or in the 5th left interspace 10 cm from the midsternal line

Radiation or *transmission* from the point of maximal intensity. Explore the surrounding chest surface to determine where else you can hear the murmur.

Aortic murmurs often radiate to the neck or down the left sternal border to the apex; mitral murmurs may radiate to the left axilla.

Intensity

    Grade 1—very faint, heard only after the listener has "tuned in"; may not be heard in all positions

    Grade 2—quiet but heard immediately upon placing the stethoscope on the chest

    Grade 3—moderately loud

    Grade 4—loud

    Grade 5—very loud, may be heard with a stethoscope partly off the chest

    Grade 6—may be heard with the stethoscope entirely off the chest

thrills are associated

For example, you might describe a harsh, medium-pitched, grade 3, midsystolic murmur, best heard in the aortic area, with radiation to the neck vessels.

Pitch—high, medium, or low

Quality—blowing, rumbling, harsh, or musical

Variations of murmurs with respiration may also be helpful in your interpretation.

Murmurs originating in the right side of the heart tend to change more with respiration than do left-sided murmurs.

Changing the patient's position may give you further information about heart sounds and murmurs. You should make auscultation in two of these positions part of your regular cardiac examination.

1. Ask the patient to *sit up, lean forward, exhale completely, and hold his breath* in expiration.

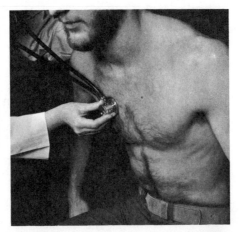

With the diaphragm of your stethoscope pressed on the chest, listen at the aortic area and down the left sternal border to the apex, pausing periodically so the patient may breathe.

This position accentuates or brings out aortic murmurs. You may easily miss the murmur of aortic regurgitation unless you use this position.

2. Ask the patient to *roll onto his left side.* Find the apical impulse. Then, using the bell of your stethoscope in light contact with the chest, listen carefully over the apical impulse.

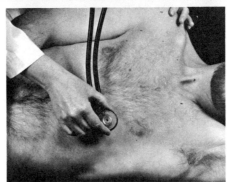

This position accentuates or brings out S_3, S_4, and mitral murmurs, especially the murmur of mitral stenosis.

Asking the patient to sit up from a lying position may also be useful. Do this when evaluating a split S_2 that fails to disappear when the patient is supine. Expiratory splitting should disappear when the patient sits up. Moreover, innocent pulmonic murmurs often disappear in the sitting position.

THE ARTERIAL PULSE

By examining arterial pulses you can count the rate of the heart, determine its rhythm, assess the amplitude and contour of the pulse wave, and sometimes detect obstructions to blood flow.

Rate and Rhythm. The radial pulse is conveniently used to assess heart rate and rhythm. With the pads of your index and middle fingers, compress the radial artery until a maximum pulsation is detected. Count the rate, and note any variations in rhythm or amplitude. Abnormalities are best evaluated by cardiac auscultation. See page 310 for further discussion of the radial pulse.

Dropped or apparently absent beats suggest premature contractions. See Table 7-15, Abnormalities of the Arterial Pulse (p. 209).

Amplitude and Contour. These are best assessed in the carotid arteries because of their proximity to the heart. The carotid arteries may also give important information about cerebral blood flow.

First inspect the neck for pulsations. Carotid pulsations may be visible just medial to the sternomastoid muscles.

A unilateral pulsatile bulge of a kinked carotid artery (see p. 171).

Then feel the carotid pulse, comparing one side with the other. Turn the patient's head slightly toward the side you are examining. The sternomastoid muscles should be relaxed. Place the tips of your index and middle fingers along the medial border of the sternomastoid in the lower half of the neck, press posteriorly, and feel the carotid pulsations. Avoid the carotid sinus, since pressure here may cause a reflex drop in pulse rate or blood pressure. Note any palpable thrills.

Decreased pulsations may be caused by decreased stroke volume or aortic stenosis, but they may also be due to local factors in the neck such as arterial narrowing or occlusion.

A thrill may radiate from the aortic valve or may originate in the carotid artery itself.

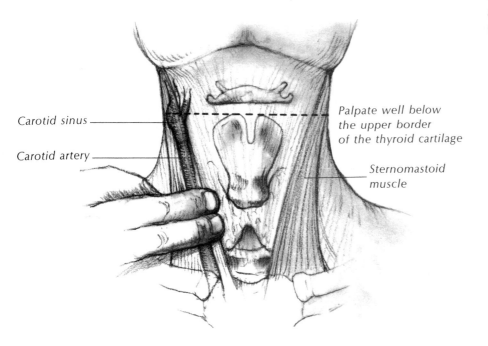

Carotid sinus

Carotid artery

Palpate well below the upper border of the thyroid cartilage

Sternomastoid muscle

Now, using the side on which you can feel the pulse more easily, carefully assess the amplitude and contour of the pulse. Simultaneously listen to the base of the heart so that you can correlate your observations with the heart sounds. Slowly increase the pressure of your fingers on the carotid until you feel a maximal pulsation, then slowly release the pressure. Try to assess:

1. The amplitude of the pulse

Small weak pulses and large bounding pulses. See Table 7-15, Abnormalities of the Arterial Pulse (p. 209).

2. The contour of the pulse wave (*i.e.*, the speed of its upstroke, the duration of its summit, and the speed of its downstroke). The normal upstroke is smooth and rapid and follows the first heart sound almost immediately. The summit is smooth, rounded, and roughly midsystolic. The downstroke is less abrupt than the upstroke.

3. Any variations in amplitude—
   a. from beat to beat

                                                              Pulsus alternans, bigeminal pulse

   b. with respiration

                                                              Paradoxical pulse

Amplitude of the pulse can be correlated with the pulse pressure as measured by sphygmomanometry. You cannot, however, estimate the blood pressure itself by palpating an artery.

If the patient is middle-aged or elderly, or if you suspect cerebrovascular disease, listen to the carotid arteries with the diaphragm of your stethoscope. Ask the patient to hold his breath so that breath sounds do not obscure a bruit.

> A bruit here suggests but does not prove narrowing of the carotid artery. It may also be secondary to radiation of a systolic murmur from the aortic area.

BLOOD PRESSURE

Choice of Sphygmomanometer. Blood pressure may be measured satisfactorily with a sphygmomanometer of either the aneroid or the mercury type. Since an aneroid instrument often becomes inaccurate with repeated use, it should be recalibrated periodically. Select a cuff with an inflatable bag of appropriate size. Proper size depends on the circumference of the limb on which the cuff is to be used. The width of the bag should be about 40% of this circumference—12 cm to 14 cm in an average adult. The length of the bag should be about 80% of this circumference (range 60% to 100%)—almost long enough to encircle the arm.

> Cuffs that are too short or narrow may give falsely high readings. Using a regular cuff on an obese arm may lead to a false diagnosis of hypertension. For an obese arm, select a cuff with a larger than standard bag.

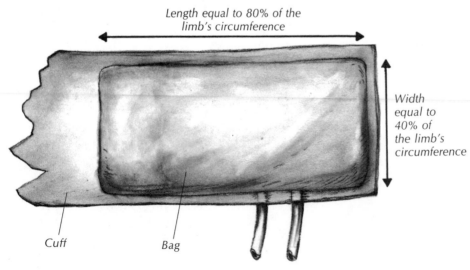

Length equal to 80% of the limb's circumference

Width equal to 40% of the limb's circumference

Cuff   *Bag*

Technique. The patient should be as comfortable and relaxed as possible, his arm free of clothing. Center the inflatable bag over the brachial artery on the inside of the arm. The lower border should be about 2.5 cm above the antecubital crease. Secure the cuff snugly. Position the patient's arm so that it is slightly flexed at the elbow. Support it yourself or rest it on a pillow, table, or other steady surface, making sure that the cuff lies at heart level. Find the brachial artery—usually just medial to the biceps tendon.

A loose cuff or a bag that balloons outside the cuff leads to falsely high readings.
If the patient supports his own arm, the sustained muscular contraction may raise his diastolic pressure as much as 10%.

If the brachial artery is much below heart level the blood pressure will appear falsely high. Conversely, if the artery is much above heart level blood pressure will appear falsely low. A 13.6 cm difference between arterial and cardiac levels produces a blood pressure error of 10 mm Hg.

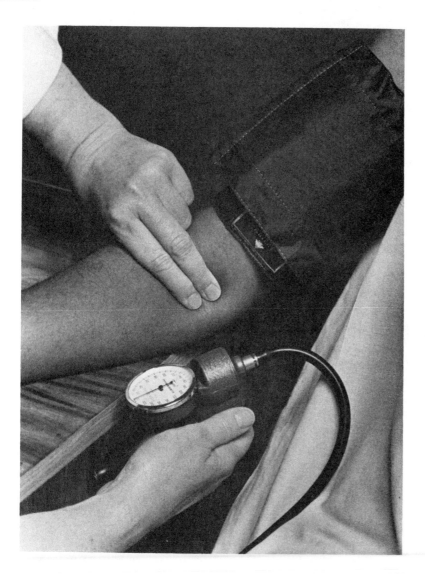

An occasional patient has an auscultatory gap—a silent interval part way between systolic and diastolic pressures. If this is not recognized, it may lead to serious underestimation of systolic or overestimation of diastolic pressure.

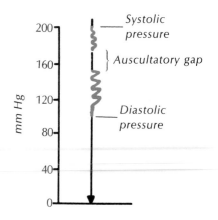

With the thumb or fingers of one hand resting on the brachial artery, rapidly inflate the cuff to about 30 mm Hg above the level at which the pulsations disappear. Deflate the cuff slowly until you again feel the pulse. This is the palpatory systolic pressure and helps you avoid being misled by an auscultatory gap. Deflate the cuff completely.

Record your findings completely (*e.g.*, 200/98 with an auscultatory gap from 170 to 150).

Now place the bell of a stethoscope lightly over the brachial artery. Since the sounds to be heard are relatively low in pitch, they can be heard better with a bell.

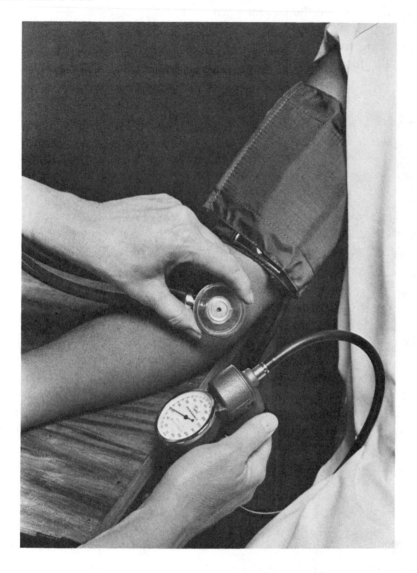

Inflate the cuff again, to about 30 mm Hg above the palpatory systolic pressure. Then deflate the cuff slowly, allowing the pressure to drop at a rate of about 3 mm Hg per second. Note the level at which you hear the sounds of at least two consecutive beats. This is the systolic pressure.

Continue to lower the pressure slowly until the sounds become muffled and then disappear. Then deflate the cuff rapidly to zero. The disappearance point, which is usually only a few mm Hg below the muffling point, marks the generally accepted diastolic pressure.

Rapid deflation will lead to underestimation of the systolic and overestimation of the diastolic pressure.

In some people the muffling point and the disappearance point are farther apart. Occasionally, as in aortic regurgitation, the sounds never disappear. If there is more than 10 mm Hg difference, record both figures (*e.g.*, 154/80/68).

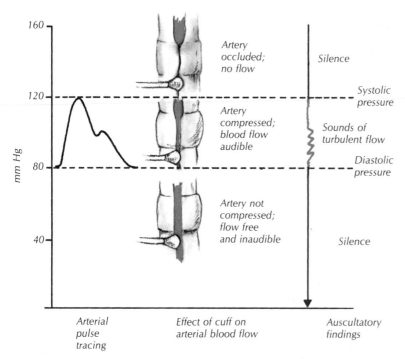

160

120

mm Hg

80

40

Artery
occluded;
no flow

Silence

Systolic
pressure

Artery
compressed;
blood flow
audible

Sounds of
turbulent flow

Diastolic
pressure

Artery not
compressed;
flow free
and inaudible

Silence

Arterial
pulse
tracing

Effect of cuff on
arterial blood flow

Auscultatory
findings

When using a mercury sphygmomanometer, keep the manometer vertical (unless you are using a tilted floor model) and make all readings at eye level with the meniscus. When using an aneroid instrument, hold the dial so that it faces you directly. Avoid slow or repetitive inflations of the cuff, because the resulting venous congestion can cause false readings. If you need to repeat your measurements, wait a minute or two after the cuff has deflated completely.

By making the sounds less audible, venous congestion may produce artifactually low systolic and high diastolic pressures.

Blood pressure should be taken in both arms at least once. You should do this too when evaluating a patient with symptoms of cerebrovascular insufficiency. Normally there may be a difference in pressure of 5 mm Hg, sometimes up to 10 mm Hg. Subsequent readings should be made on the arm with the higher pressure.

Pressure difference of over 10 mm Hg to 15 mm Hg suggests arterial compression or obstruction on the side with the lower pressure. With cerebrovascular symptoms, consider the subclavian steal syndrome.

When the patient is taking antihypertensive medications, when he has a history of fainting or postural dizziness, or when you suspect depletion of blood volume, take his blood pressure in three positions—supine, sitting, and standing (unless, of course, these positions are contraindicated). Normally, as the patient rises from the horizontal to a standing position his systolic pressure drops slightly or remains unchanged while his diastolic pressure rises slightly.

A substantial fall in systolic pressure (20 mm Hg or more), especially when accompanied by symptoms, indicates orthostatic (postural) hypotension. The diastolic pressure may also fall. Causes include drugs, depletion of blood volume, prolonged bedrest, and diseases of the peripheral autonomic nervous system.

Upper limits of normal blood pressure in adults have traditionally been set between 140/90 and 160/95. Even the lower of these two criteria would be suspiciously high, however, in a young adult. Blood pressure readings on at least three separate visits should usually be taken before making a diagnosis of hypertension.

Lower limits of normal blood pressure, sometimes estimated at 90/60 in adults, should always be interpreted in the light of past readings and the patient's present clinical state.

A pressure of 110/70 might well be normal, for example, but could also indicate significant hypotension in a patient whose past pressures have been high.

Special Problems

1. *The Apprehensive Patient.* Anxiety is a frequent cause of high blood pressure, especially on a first visit. Try to get the patient relaxed. Repeat your measurements later during the encounter and on subsequent visits before concluding that the patient has persistent hypertension.

2. *The Obese Arm.* If you have difficulty fitting the cuff to an obese arm, you may apply a standard cuff to the forearm and listen over the radial artery.

3. *Leg Pulses and Pressures.* In order to rule out coarctation of the aorta, two observations should be made at least once in every hypertensive patient:

   a. Compare the volume and timing of the radial and femoral pulses.

   b. Compare blood pressures in the arm and leg.

A diminished, delayed femoral pulse in relation to the radial pulse suggests coarctation of the aorta or occlusive aortic disease. Blood pressure lower in the legs than in the arms is confirmatory.

   To determine blood pressure in the leg, use a wide long cuff on the lower third of the thigh. Center the bag over the posterior surface, wrap it securely, and listen over the popliteal artery. If possible the patient should be prone. If he cannot lie on his abdomen, flex his leg slightly. By sphygmomanometry, systolic pressure in the legs is usually found to be substantially higher than in the brachial artery. This does not reflect a true difference in intra-arterial pressures. A systolic pressure lower in the legs than the arms is abnormal.

4. *Inaudible Blood Pressure.* Consider the following possibilities and act accordingly:

   a. Erroneous placement of your stethoscope. Search again for the brachial artery.

   b. Venous engorgement of the arm from repeated inflation of the cuff. Remove the cuff. Elevate the patient's arm over his head for one or two minutes, then reapply the cuff and try again.

   c. Shock. Try to get the systolic pressure by palpation. It may be impossible to measure the blood pressure of a patient in shock without direct arterial puncture.

5. *Arrhythmias*. Irregular rhythms produce variations in pressure and therefore unreliable measurements. Ignore the effects of an occasional premature contraction. With frequent premature contractions and in atrial fibrillation, take an average of several observations and note that your measurements are approximate.

JUGULAR VENOUS PRESSURE AND PULSES

Examination of the jugular veins and their pulsations allows quite accurate estimation of the central venous pressure, and therefore gives important information about cardiac compensation. The internal jugular pulsations, although somewhat harder to see than the external jugulars, give a more accurate reading.

Position the patient so that he is relaxed and comfortable, with his head slightly elevated on a pillow and his sternomastoid muscles relaxed. Adjust the head of the bed so as to maximize the jugular venous pulsations and make them visible above the clavicles but well below the jaw. Usually the head of the bed needs slight elevation (*e.g.*, 15° to 30° from the horizontal). When the patient's venous pressure is increased, however, an elevation to 45° or even to 90° may be required.

Use tangential (oblique) lighting and examine *both sides* of the neck. Unilateral distention, especially of an external jugular vein, may be deceptive: it can be caused by local factors in the neck.

Identify the external jugular vein on each side. Then *find the pulsations of the internal jugular vein.* Since this vein lies deep to muscle, you will not see the vein itself. Watch instead for the pulsations transmitted through the surrounding soft tissues. Look for them in the suprasternal notch, between the attachments of the sternomastoid on the sternum and clavicle, or just posterior to the sternomastoid. Distinguish these pulsations from those of the adjacent carotid artery by the following points:

INTERNAL JUGULAR PULSATIONS	CAROTID PULSATIONS
Rarely palpable	Palpable
Soft undulating quality, usually with 2 or 3 outward components (*a*, *c*, and *v* waves)	A more vigorous thrust with a single outward component
Pulsation eliminated by light pressure on the vein just above the sternal end of the clavicle	Pulsation not eliminated
Level of pulsation usually descends with inspiration	Pulsation not affected by inspiration
Pulsations vary with position	Pulsations unchanged by position

Identify the highest point at which pulsations of the internal jugular vein can be seen. With a centimeter ruler measure the vertical distance between this point and the sternal angle. A sturdy square-cornered piece of paper helps establish the horizontal and vertical relationships that underlie this measurement. A second observer at some distance from you can help establish a truly horizontal line.

Increased pressure suggests right-sided heart failure or, less commonly, constrictive pericarditis or superior vena cava obstruction. In patients with obstructive lung disease, venous pressure may appear elevated on expiration only; the veins collapse on inspiration. This finding does not indicate congestive heart failure.

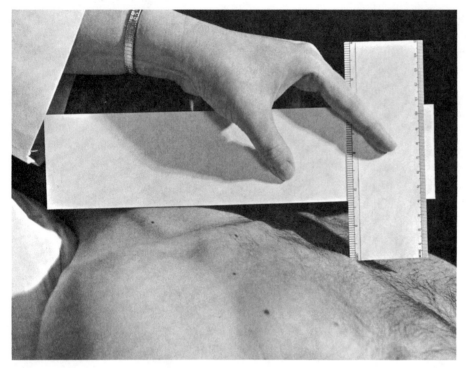

If the highest point of venous pulsation is below the sternal angle, hold the ruler at the neck rather than at the sternal angle.

If the neck veins stay flat when the patient is horizontal, depletion of blood volume may be suspected.

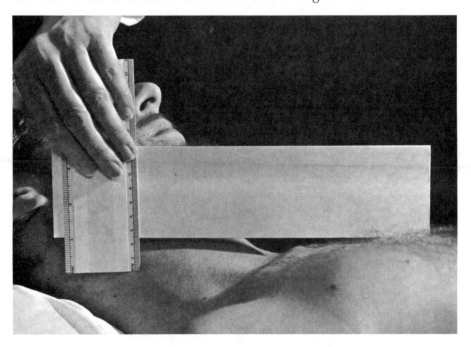

If you are unable to visualize pulsations in the internal jugular veins, look for them in the external jugulars, although they are not usually visible here. If you see none, identify *the point above which the external jugular veins appear to be collapsed*. Make this observation on each side of the neck. Measure the vertical distance of this point from the sternal angle.

Unilateral distention of the external jugular vein is usually due to local kinking or obstruction. Occasionally even bilateral distention has a local cause.

By either technique, record the distance in centimeters above or below the sternal angle, together with the angle at which the patient was lying (*e.g.,* "The internal jugular venous pulse is 6 cm above the sternal angle, with the head of the bed elevated to 45°"). Venous pressure greater than 3 cm or 4 cm above the sternal angle is considered elevated.

If congestive heart failure is suspected, whether or not the jugular venous pressure appears elevated, *check for a hepatojugular reflux.* Adjust the position of the patient so that the highest level of pulsation is readily identifiable in the lower half of the neck. Exert firm and sustained pressure with your hand over the patient's right upper quadrant for 30 to 60 seconds. Be sure the patient remains relaxed and continues to breathe easily. If a tender right upper quadrant prevents this, press on another part of the abdomen. Watch for an increase in the jugular venous pressure during this maneuver. A rise of more than 1 cm is abnormal.

A rise in jugular venous pressure with this maneuver (a positive hepatojugular reflux) suggests congestive heart failure.

Observe the amplitude and timing of the jugular venous pulsations. In order to time these pulsations, listen to the heart simultaneously. The *a* wave is approximately synchronous with S_1. The *x* descent can be seen as a systolic collapse between S_1 and S_2. The *v* wave coincides approximately with S_2. Look for absent or unusually prominent waves.

The *a* waves disappear in atrial fibrillation.

Giant *a* waves are seen in tricuspid stenosis and severe cor pulmonale.

Large *v* waves characterize tricuspid regurgitation.

Considerable practice and experience are required to master jugular venous pulsations. A beginner is probably well advised to concentrate primarily on jugular venous pressure.

A NOTE ON CARDIOVASCULAR ASSESSMENT

A good cardiovascular examination requires more than observation. You need to think about the possible meanings of your individual observations, fit them together in a logical pattern, and correlate your cardiac findings with the patient's blood pressure, arterial pulses, venous pulsations, venous pressure, and the remainder of your history and physical examination.

Evaluating the common systolic murmur illustrates this point. In examining an asymptomatic teenager, for example, you might hear a Grade 2 midsystolic murmur localized in the 2nd and 3rd left interspaces. Since this suggests a murmur of pulmonic origin, you should pay special attention to the size of the right ventricle by carefully palpating the left parasternal area. Because pulmonic stenosis and atrial septal defects can occasionally cause such murmurs, listen carefully to the splitting of the second heart sound and try to hear any ejection sounds. Listen to the murmur after the patient sits up. Look for evidence of anemia, hyperthyroidism, or pregnancy that could produce such a murmur by increasing the flow across the pulmonic valve. If all your findings are normal, your patient probably has an *innocent murmur*—one with no pathological significance.

In contrast, in examining a 60-year-old person with anginal pains, you might hear a Grade 3 harsh midsystolic murmur maximal in the right 2nd interspace and radiating to the neck vessels. You cannot feel a thrill. These findings suggest aortic stenosis, but could be related to a sclerotic valve without stenosis, to a dilated aorta, or to increased flow across a normal valve. Evaluate the apical impulse for evidence of left ventricular enlargement. Listen for the murmur of aortic regurgitation as the patient leans forward and exhales. Assess the carotid pulse contour and the blood pressure for evidence of aortic stenosis. Put all this information together and make a tentative hypothesis as to the nature of the murmur.

Table 7-1

Table 7-1 Comparison of the Apical Impulse in Normal People and in Those with Left Ventricular Enlargement

	AMPLITUDE	DURATION	LOCATION	DIAMETER
NORMAL HEART	Small amplitude, light or even absent	Less than ⅔ and usually less than half of systole	5th or sometimes the 4th interspace, 7–9 cm from the midsternal line	1–2 cm; usually occupies only one interspace
LEFT VENTRICULAR ENLARGEMENT	Larger amplitude, feels more forceful and thrusting	Usually lasts throughout systole, up to S₂	May be displaced to the left and downward	3 cm or more; occupies two or more interspaces

When the left ventricle is hypertrophied but not dilated, increased amplitude and duration of the impulse are the principal signs.

When the left ventricle is dilated as well as hypertrophied, the apical impulse is also both displaced and enlarged.

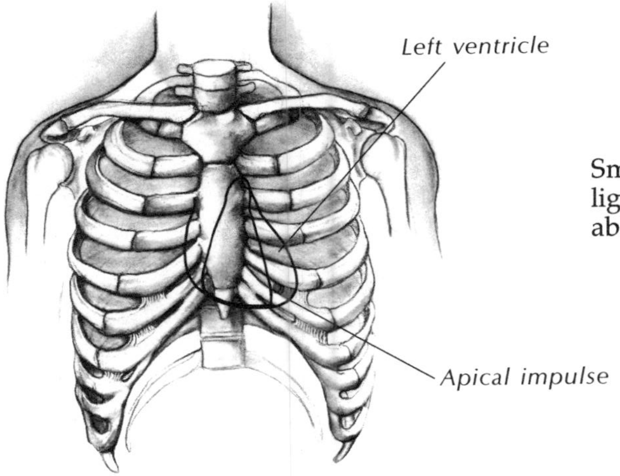

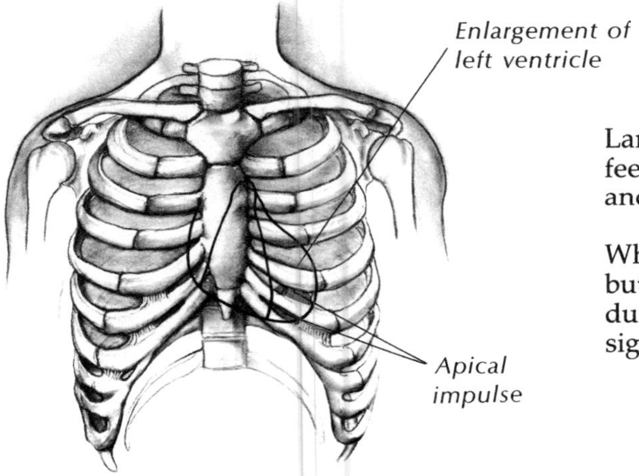

Left ventricle

Apical impulse

Enlargement of left ventricle

Apical impulse

Table 7-2

Table 7-2 Approach to the Differentiation of Selected Heart Rates and Rhythms

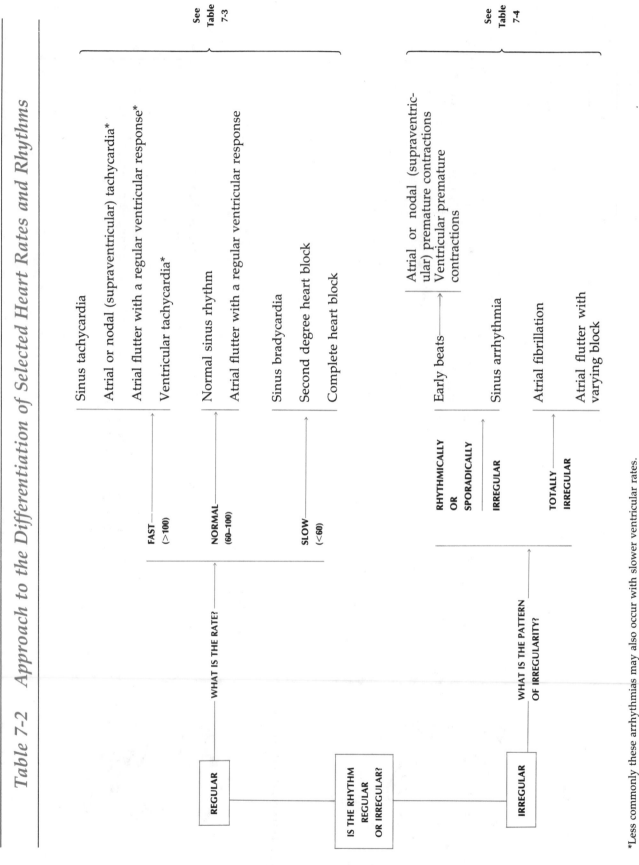

			See Table 7-3
REGULAR	WHAT IS THE RATE?	FAST (>100) →	Sinus tachycardia Atrial or nodal (supraventricular) tachycardia* Atrial flutter with a regular ventricular response* Ventricular tachycardia*
		NORMAL (60–100) →	Normal sinus rhythm Atrial flutter with a regular ventricular response
		SLOW (<60) →	Sinus bradycardia Second degree heart block Complete heart block

IS THE RHYTHM REGULAR OR IRREGULAR?

			See Table 7-4
IRREGULAR	WHAT IS THE PATTERN OF IRREGULARITY?	RHYTHMICALLY OR SPORADICALLY IRREGULAR →	Early beats → Atrial or nodal (supraventricular) premature contractions Ventricular premature contractions Sinus arrhythmia
		TOTALLY IRREGULAR →	Atrial fibrillation Atrial flutter with varying block

*Less commonly these arrhythmias may also occur with slower ventricular rates.

Table 7-3

Table 7-3 Differentiation of Selected Regular Rhythms

RHYTHMS WITH FAST VENTRICULAR RATES	DESCRIPTION	CLINICAL MANIFESTATIONS			1ST AND 2ND HEART SOUNDS
		VENTRICULAR RATE			
		USUAL RESTING RATE	RESPONSE TO EXERCISE	RESPONSE TO VAGAL STIMULATION*	
SINUS TACHYCARDIA	A fast rhythm originating normally in the sinus node and conducted over normal pathways through the heart. Causes include exercise, anxiety, fever, hyperthyroidism, and blood loss.	100–150	—	Smooth slowing	Normal
ATRIAL OR NODAL (SUPRAVENTRICULAR) TACHYCARDIA	A fast rhythm typically occurring in episodes or paroxysms. Young adults with no other evidence of heart disease are often affected. Conduction within the atria is abnormal, but the ventricles usually respond to each impulse.	160–200	—	Abrupt slowing or no change	Normal
ATRIAL FLUTTER WITH A REGULAR VENTRICULAR RESPONSE	A very fast atrial rhythm, often around 300 to 320 per minute. There is usually a partial conduction block at the AV node. In a 2:1 block, for example, every second atrial beat is followed by a ventricular response.	150–160	—	Abrupt slowing or no change	Normal
VENTRICULAR TACHYCARDIA	A fast rhythm originating in the ventricles. This is an ominous arrhythmia, usually associated with organic heart disease, and may herald ventricular fibrillation and sudden death.	150–200	—	No change	Split S_1, S_2; varying intensity of S_1

*Vagal stimulation may be produced by holding a deep breath, by the induction of gagging or retching, and by carotid sinus massage. Careful monitoring is required.

Continued

Table 7-3

Table 7-3 (Cont'd)

CLINICAL MANIFESTATIONS

		VENTRICULAR RATE		
DESCRIPTION	USUAL RESTING RATE	RESPONSE TO EXERCISE	RESPONSE TO VAGAL STIMULATION*	1ST AND 2ND HEART SOUNDS
RHYTHMS WITH NORMAL VENTRICULAR RATES				
NORMAL SINUS RHYTHM — A rhythm of normal origin and conduction through the heart. Note, however, that a regular rhythm with a normal rate is not necessarily a normal sinus rhythm.	60–100	Smooth increase	Smooth slowing	Normal
ATRIAL FLUTTER WITH A REGULAR VENTRICULAR RESPONSE — A very fast atrial rhythm, as described above, but with a greater degree of AV block, such as a 4:1 block, in which every fourth atrial impulse is followed by a ventricular response.	60–100	Abrupt increase or no change	Abrupt slowing or no change	Normal
RHYTHMS WITH SLOW VENTRICULAR RATES				
SINUS BRADYCARDIA — A slow rhythm with normal sinus origin and normal conduction. A very common rhythm, it may indicate excellent physical fitness. Other causes include hypothyroidism, hypothermia, acute myocardial infarction, the sick sinus syndrome, and drugs such as digitalis and propranolol.	50–60, may be down to 40	Smooth increase	—	Normal
SECOND DEGREE HEART BLOCK — A slow rhythm produced by impaired conduction through the AV node or the bundle of His. Some of the atrial impulses fail to get through to the ventricles. Causes include heart disease and drugs such as digitalis.	35–60	Smooth increase	—	Normal S_1, S_2; atrial sounds may also be heard
COMPLETE HEART BLOCK — A very slow rhythm produced by a complete block of conduction through the AV node, the bundle of His, or its branches. Ventricular beats originate in the ventricles themselves. The most common cause is an acute myocardial infarction.	25–45, may be up to 60	No change	—	Varying S_1

*Vagal stimulation may be produced by holding a deep breath, by the induction of gagging or retching, and by carotid sinus massage. Careful monitoring is required.

Table 7-4

Table 7-4   Differentiation of Selected Irregular Rhythms

TYPE OF RHYTHM	DIAGRAMMATIC REPRESENTATION	RHYTHM	HEART SOUNDS
ATRIAL OR NODAL (SUPRAVENTRICULAR) PREMATURE CONTRACTIONS	QRS, P, T, Aberrant P wave, Normal QRS and T, S_1 S_2, Early beat, Pause	A beat of atrial or nodal origin comes earlier than the expected normal beat. A pause follows and the rhythm resumes.	S_1 may differ in intensity from normal beats, S_2 may be decreased, but both sounds are otherwise similar to normal beats.
VENTRICULAR PREMATURE CONTRACTIONS	No P wave, Aberrant QRS and T, S_1 S_2, Early beat with split sounds, Pause	A beat of ventricular origin comes earlier than the expected normal beat. A pause follows and the rhythm resumes.	S_1 may differ in intensity from the normal beats, S_2 may be decreased, but both sounds are likely to be split.
SINUS ARRHYTHMIA	S_1 S_2 S_1 S_2 S_1 S_2 S_1 S_2 S_1 S_2 S_1 S_2, INSPIRATION, EXPIRATION	The heart varies cyclically, usually speeding up with inspiration and slowing down with expiration.	Normal, although S_1 may vary with the heart rate.
ATRIAL FIBRILLATION AND ATRIAL FLUTTER WITH VARYING AV BLOCK	No P waves, Fibrillation waves, S_1 S_2 S_1 S_2 S_1 S_2 S_2 S_1 S_2 S_1 S_2	The ventricular rhythm is totally irregular, although short runs may seem regular.	S_1 varies in intensity.

Table 7-5

Table 7-5 Variations in the First Heart Sound

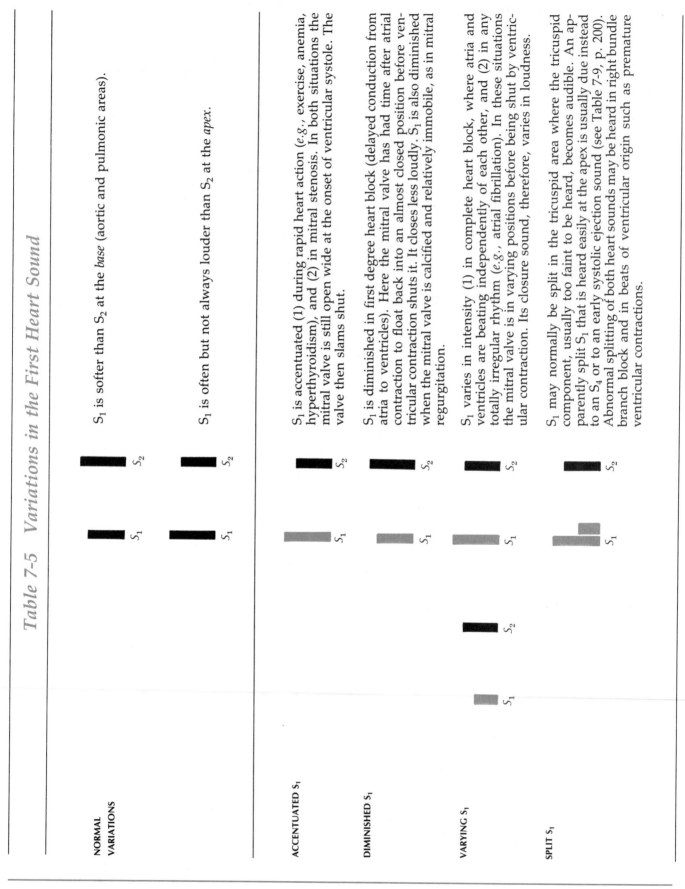

NORMAL VARIATIONS

S_1 is softer than S_2 at the *base* (aortic and pulmonic areas).

S_1 is often but not always louder than S_2 at the *apex*.

ACCENTUATED S_1

S_1 is accentuated (1) during rapid heart action (*e.g.*, exercise, anemia, hyperthyroidism), and (2) in mitral stenosis. In both situations the mitral valve is still open wide at the onset of ventricular systole. The valve then slams shut.

DIMINISHED S_1

S_1 is diminished in first degree heart block (delayed conduction from atria to ventricles). Here the mitral valve has had time after atrial contraction to float back into an almost closed position before ventricular contraction shuts it. It closes less loudly. S_1 is also diminished when the mitral valve is calcified and relatively immobile, as in mitral regurgitation.

VARYING S_1

S_1 varies in intensity (1) in complete heart block, where atria and ventricles are beating independently of each other, and (2) in any totally irregular rhythm (*e.g.*, atrial fibrillation). In these situations the mitral valve is in varying positions before being shut by ventricular contraction. Its closure sound, therefore, varies in loudness.

SPLIT S_1

S_1 may normally be split in the tricuspid area where the tricuspid component, usually too faint to be heard, becomes audible. An apparently split S_1 that is heard easily at the apex is usually due instead to an S_4 or to an early systolic ejection sound (see Table 7-9, p. 200). Abnormal splitting of both heart sounds may be heard in right bundle branch block and in beats of ventricular origin such as premature ventricular contractions.

Table 7-6

Table 7-6 Variations in the Second Heart Sound

	EXPIRATION	INSPIRATION	
PHYSIOLOGICAL SPLITTING	S_1 S_2	S_1 — A_2 P_2 S_2	*Physiological splitting* of the second heart sound can usually be detected in the pulmonic area. The pulmonic component of S_2 is usually too faint to be heard at the apex or aortic area where S_2 is single and derived from aortic valve closure alone. Normal splitting is accentuated by inspiration and usually disappears on expiration. In some patients, however, especially younger ones, S_2 may not become completely single on expiration. It may do so when the patient sits up.
PATHOLOGICAL SPLITTING (*All of these suggest heart disease.*)	S_1 S_2	S_1 S_2	*Wide splitting* of S_2 refers to an increase in the usual splitting and can be heard throughout the respiratory cycle. Wide splitting can be caused by delayed closure of the pulmonic valve (*e.g.*, by pulmonic stenosis or right bundle branch block). As illustrated here, right bundle branch block also causes splitting of S_1 into its mitral and tricuspid components. Wide splitting can also be caused by early closure of the aortic valve, as in mitral regurgitation.
	S_1 S_2	S_1 S_2	*Fixed splitting* refers to wide splitting that does not vary with respiration. It occurs in atrial septal defect and right ventricular failure.
	S_1 P_2 A_2 S_2	S_1 S_2	*Paradoxical* or *reversed splitting* refers to splitting that appears on expiration and disappears on inspiration. Closure of the aortic valve is abnormally delayed so that A_2 follows P_2 in expiration. Normal inspiratory delay of P_2 makes the split disappear. The most common cause of paradoxical splitting is left bundle branch block.

INCREASED INTENSITY OF S_2 IN THE AORTIC AREA (where S_2 is composed entirely of the aortic closure sound) occurs in arterial hypertension and aortic valve syphilis.

DECREASED INTENSITY OF S_2 IN THE AORTIC AREA is heard in aortic stenosis.

INCREASED INTENSITY OF THE PULMONIC COMPONENT OF S_2. When P_2 is equal to or louder than the aortic component, or when splitting of S_2 can be heard at the apex, pulmonary hypertension can be suspected.

DECREASED INTENSITY OF THE PULMONIC COMPONENT OF S_2 is heard in pulmonic stenosis.

Table 7-7

Table 7-7 Extra Heart Sounds in Systole

Extra heart sounds in systole are of two kinds: (1) early ejection sounds, and (2) clicks, most commonly heard in mid- and late systole.

EARLY SYSTOLIC EJECTION SOUNDS

$S_1 \quad E_j \qquad S_2$

Early systolic ejection sounds occur shortly after the first heart sound, coincident with the opening of the aortic and pulmonic valves. They are relatively high in pitch and have a clicking quality.

An *aortic ejection sound* is heard at both base and apex and may be louder at the apex. It does not usually vary with respiration. An aortic ejection sound may accompany a dilated aorta or aortic valve disease.

A *pulmonic ejection sound* is best heard in the 2nd and 3rd left interspaces. When the first heart sound, usually relatively soft in this area, appears to be loud, you may instead be hearing a pulmonic ejection sound. Decreased intensity of the sound during inspiration gives another clue. Causes include dilatation of the pulmonary artery, pulmonary hypertension, and pulmonary stenosis.

MID- AND LATE SYSTOLIC CLICKS

$S_1 \qquad \qquad S_2$

Mid- to late systolic clicks are usually related to mitral valve prolapse—an abnormal ballooning of part of the mitral valve. This is a common cardiac abnormality affecting about 5% of young adults. The click is usually single, but more than one are sometimes heard. The click is often followed by a systolic murmur (see p. 204). Findings often vary from time to time: a click only, a click and murmur, or only a late systolic murmur.

Table 7-8

Table 7-8   Extra Heart Sounds in Diastole

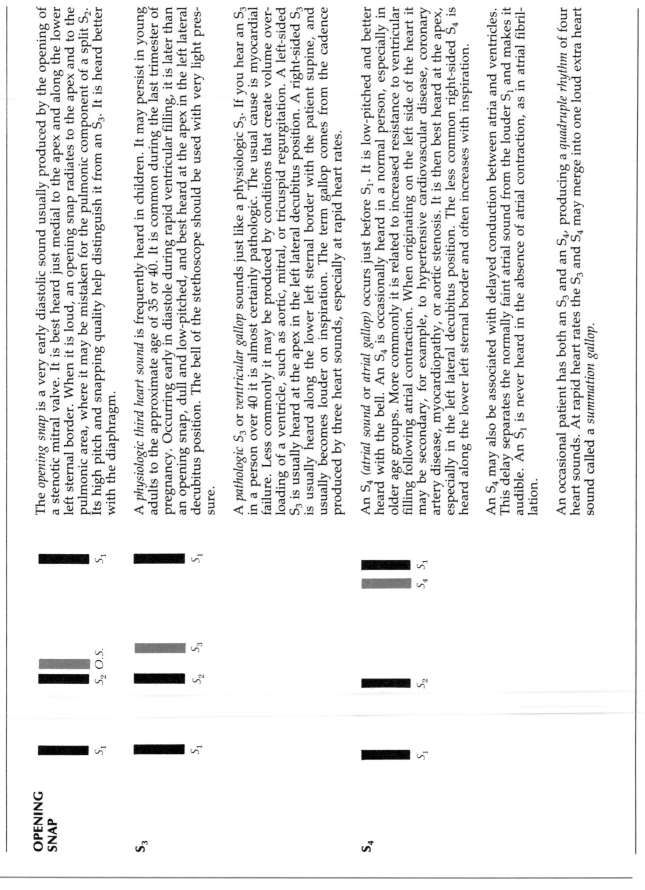

OPENING SNAP

The *opening snap* is a very early diastolic sound usually produced by the opening of a stenotic mitral valve. It is best heard just medial to the apex and along the lower left sternal border. When it is loud, an opening snap radiates to the apex and to the pulmonic area, where it may be mistaken for the pulmonic component of a split S_2. Its high pitch and snapping quality help distinguish it from an S_3. It is heard better with the diaphragm.

S_3

A *physiologic third heart sound* is frequently heard in children. It may persist in young adults to the approximate age of 35 or 40. It is common during the last trimester of pregnancy. Occurring early in diastole during rapid ventricular filling, it is later than an opening snap, dull and low-pitched, and best heard at the apex in the left lateral decubitus position. The bell of the stethoscope should be used with very light pressure.

A *pathologic* S_3 or *ventricular gallop* sounds just like a physiologic S_3. If you hear an S_3 in a person over 40 it is almost certainly pathologic. The usual cause is myocardial failure. Less commonly it may be produced by conditions that create volume overloading of a ventricle, such as aortic, mitral, or tricuspid regurgitation. A left-sided S_3 is usually heard at the apex in the left lateral decubitus position. A right-sided S_3 is usually heard along the lower left sternal border with the patient supine, and usually becomes louder on inspiration. The term gallop comes from the cadence produced by three heart sounds, especially at rapid heart rates.

S_4

An S_4 *(atrial sound or atrial gallop)* occurs just before S_1. It is low-pitched and better heard with the bell. An S_4 is occasionally heard in a normal person, especially in older age groups. More commonly it is related to increased resistance to ventricular filling following atrial contraction. When originating on the left side of the heart it may be secondary, for example, to hypertensive cardiovascular disease, coronary artery disease, myocardiopathy, or aortic stenosis. It is then best heard at the apex, especially in the left lateral decubitus position. The less common right-sided S_4 is heard along the lower left sternal border and often increases with inspiration.

An S_4 may also be associated with delayed conduction between atria and ventricles. This delay separates the normally faint atrial sound from the louder S_1 and makes it audible. An S_1 is never heard in the absence of atrial contraction, as in atrial fibrillation.

An occasional patient has both an S_3 and an S_4, producing a *quadruple rhythm* of four heart sounds. At rapid heart rates the S_3 and S_4 may merge into one loud extra heart sound called a *summation gallop*.

Table 7-9 Three Causes of an Apparently Split First Heart Sound

When you hear an apparently double first heart sound, there are three possibilities:

	S_4	SPLIT S_1	EJECTION SOUND
	S_4 S_1 S_2	S_1 S_2	S_1 Ej S_2
PITCH	An S_4 is relatively low-pitched; therefore, the split is better heard with the bell.	Both components of a split S_1 are relatively high-pitched; therefore, the split is better heard with the diaphragm.	An ejection sound is relatively high-pitched; therefore the split is better heard with the diaphragm.
LOCATION	Usually the apex, although an S_4 originating in the right ventricle may be best heard along the lower sternal border	The tricuspid area, since the tricuspid component of S_1 is soft and does not radiate widely	An aortic ejection sound is usually heard in the aortic area and at the apex. A pulmonic ejection sound is usually best heard in the 2nd or 3rd left interspace.
PALPABLE SPLIT	Sometimes a palpable extra impulse at the apex	No	No

Table 7-10

Table 7-10   Mechanisms of Heart Murmurs

Heart murmurs are of longer duration than heart sounds. They originate within the heart itself or in its great vessels and are usually caused by one of the following mechanisms:

1. Flow across a partial obstruction (*e.g.*, aortic stenosis)

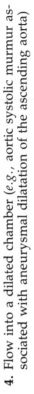

2. Flow across a valvular or intravascular irregularity without obstruction (*e.g.*, a bicuspid aortic valve without true stenosis)

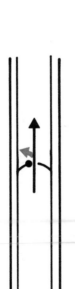

3. Increased flow through normal structures (*e.g.*, aortic systolic murmur associated with anemia)

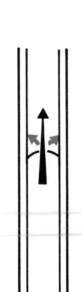

4. Flow into a dilated chamber (*e.g.*, aortic systolic murmur associated with aneurysmal dilatation of the ascending aorta)

5. Backward or regurgitant flow across an incompetent valve or defect (*e.g.*, mitral regurgitation)

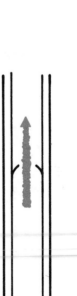

6. Shunting of blood out of a high pressure chamber or artery through an abnormal passage (*e.g.*, ventricular septal defect, patent ductus arteriosus)

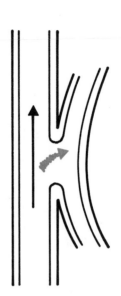

Table 7-11 Midsystolic Ejection Murmurs

Midsystolic ejection murmurs constitute the most common kind of heart murmur. They may be (1) *organic* (i.e., secondary to structural cardiovascular abnormality); (2) *functional* (i.e., secondary to a physiologic alteration with or without heart disease); or (3) *innocent* (i.e., not associated with any functional or structural abnormality). Systolic ejection murmurs are relatively easy to identify but often hard to interpret. The entire cardiovascular examination, in fact a thorough evaluation of the whole patient, is frequently necessary.

Midsystolic ejection murmurs are associated with forward flow through the semilunar valves or outflow tracts. Constriction, structural irregularity, an increased rate of flow, or flow into a dilated great vessel produces the systolic noise. The murmur has a crescendo–decrescendo (or diamond-shaped) pattern and is usually separated from the first and second heart sounds.

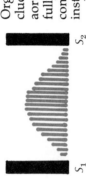

Organic causes of midsystolic ejection murmurs include aortic and pulmonic stenosis (i.e., failure of the aortic and pulmonic valves, respectively, to open as fully as they should during systole). Occasionally the constriction of flow occurs above or below the valve instead of in the valve itself. The murmurs of aortic and pulmonic valvular stenosis are contrasted below. Other causes of these murmurs are discussed on the next page.

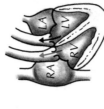

	AORTIC STENOSIS	**PULMONIC STENOSIS**
LOCATION	Aortic area	Pulmonic area and 3rd left interspace
RADIATION	Into the neck, down the left sternal border, and sometimes to the apex. Note that an apical ejection murmur, despite its location, often originates in the aortic valve.	Toward the left shoulder and upward toward the neck vessels, especially on the left
INTENSITY	Variable. If loud, a thrill may be felt in the aortic area and neck.	Variable. If loud, a thrill may be felt in the pulmonic area.
PITCH	Medium	Medium
QUALITY	Often harsh	Often harsh
ASSOCIATED SIGNS MAY INCLUDE	1. A diminished S_2 2. An early aortic ejection sound, a left-sided S_4 3. A thrusting sustained apical impulse of left ventricular hypertrophy 4. A slowly rising carotid pulse contour 5. A narrow pulse pressure	1. A widely split S_2 and diminished to absent P_2. (If P_2 is absent, there can be no splitting.) 2. An early pulmonic ejection sound, a right-sided S_4 3. A sustained parasternal lift of right ventricular hypertrophy

Continued

Table 7-11

Table 7-11 (Cont'd)

OTHER CAUSES OF AORTIC SYSTOLIC MURMURS	OTHER CAUSES OF PULMONIC SYSTOLIC MURMURS
Structural abnormality of the aortic valve without true stenosis may cause a midsystolic or early systolic ejection murmur indistinguishable from mild aortic stenosis. Two common examples are a *congenitally bicuspid but nonstenotic aortic valve* and the *sclerotic aortic valve associated with aging*. The lack of associated signs may help to make these diagnoses, but prolonged followup is often necessary.	*Increased blood flow* across the pulmonic valve may produce a murmur that sounds like that of pulmonic stenosis. It is this mechanism, not flow through the defect, that produces the systolic murmur of *atrial septal defect*. Wide splitting of S$_2$ may accompany both atrial septal defect and pulmonic stenosis.
Flow into an aorta dilated by syphilitic aortitis or by atherosclerosis may also cause this kind of systolic murmur.	Increased blood flow from causes such as anemia or hyperthyroidism can also cause a pulmonic flow murmur.
Functional murmurs associated with increased blood flow across the aortic valve must also be considered in the differential diagnosis. Anemia and hyperthyroidism, for example, may cause such murmurs. If so, the murmur will disappear when the underlying condition is corrected. Aortic regurgitation increases left ventricular volume and, thus, augments systolic flow across the aortic valve. By this mechanism aortic regurgitation may produce an early or midsystolic murmur (in addition to its own diastolic murmur) in the absence of true valvular stenosis.	Distinguishing the pulmonic murmurs of organic heart disease from the much more common *innocent murmurs* of children and young adults is a frequent and important problem. Innocent murmurs are usually (but not always) soft, grade 1 or 2, short, midsystolic, and best heard in the left 2nd and 3rd interspaces. Splitting of the second sound is normal, no ejection sound is heard, and palpation of the right ventricle is normal. There should be no diastolic murmurs. The character of an innocent murmur frequently changes with change in position, phase of respiration, and heart rate. Chest x-ray, electrocardiogram, and occasionally other tests may be needed to make sure of this diagnosis.

Table 7-12

Table 7-12 Pansystolic Regurgitant Murmurs

Pansystolic regurgitant murmurs are heard when blood flows from a chamber of high pressure to one of lower pressure through a valve or other structure that should be closed. Regurgitation (also called incompetence or insufficiency) means there is a leak. Causes of pansystolic murmurs include mitral regurgitation (LV → LA), tricuspid regurgitation (RV → RA), and ventricular septal defect (LV → RV). The murmur begins immediately with the first heart sound and continues up to the second heart sound.

Three types of pansystolic murmurs are contrasted below.

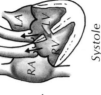

	MITRAL REGURGITATION 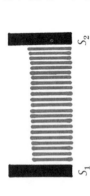 *Systole*	TRICUSPID REGURGITATION 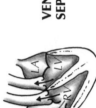 *Systole*	VENTRICULAR SEPTAL DEFECT *Systole*
LOCATION	Mitral (apical) area	Lower left sternal border	Left sternal border in the 3rd, 4th, and 5th interspaces
RADIATION	Into the left axilla	May radiate to the right of the sternum and to the left midclavicular line but not into the axilla	May radiate over the precordium but not into the axilla
INTENSITY	Variable, often loud; may be associated with an apical thrill; does not increase with inspiration	Variable; increases with inspiration	Often very loud and accompanied by a thrill
PITCH	High	High	High
QUALITY	Blowing	Blowing	Often harsh
ASSOCIATED SIGNS MAY INCLUDE	Decreased S_1 An S_3 A thrusting sustained apical impulse displaced downward and to the left (left ventricular hypertrophy and dilatation)	A left parasternal lift of right ventricular hypertrophy Systolic pulsations in the jugular venous pulse and sometimes in the liver	Signs vary with severity of defect and with associated lesions

Another form of mitral regurgitation occurs with a *prolapsed mitral valve.* Here the murmur is late systolic and often follows a mid- or late systolic click. Although the mitral valve is competent early in systole, a portion of it balloons into the left atrium later in ventricular contraction, allowing some regurgitation of blood.

Table 7-13

Table 7-13 Diastolic Murmurs

Unlike systolic murmurs, diastolic murmurs are almost always indicative of heart disease. Two general types may be distinguished:

(1) the diastolic rumble originating in the atrioventricular valves, and (2) the early diastolic murmurs of semilunar valve incompetence.

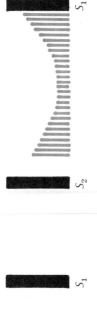

S_1 S_2 S_1

Diastolic rumbling murmurs are caused by (1) flow across distorted or stenotic mitral or tricuspid valves, or (2) increased blood flow across normal mitral or tricuspid valves. Because these valves open only after the aortic and pulmonic valves close, a short period of silence separates S_2 from the beginning of diastolic rumbles. These murmurs are low in pitch, rumbling in quality, and heard best with the bell of the stethoscope in light skin contact. They tend to be loudest in the two phases of diastole when ventricular filling is most rapid: early in diastole immediately after valvular opening, and again during atrial contraction (presystole).

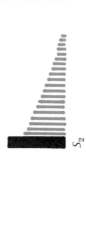

S_1 S_2 S_1

Semilunar valve incompetence may result either from valvular deformity or from dilatation of the valvular ring. In either case blood regurgitates from the great vessel back into the ventricle. Murmurs of aortic regurgitation, together with most murmurs of pulmonic regurgitation, start immediately after the second sound and then diminish in intensity. They may be described, therefore, as *decrescendo diastolic murmurs* or immediate diastolic murmurs. In contrast to the rumbling atrioventricular valve murmurs, they are high-pitched and blowing. They are best heard with the diaphragm pressed firmly on the chest.

The most common examples of these two types of diastolic murmurs are those of mitral stenosis and aortic regurgitation. They are contrasted on the next page.

Continued

Table 7-13   (Cont'd)

MITRAL STENOSIS

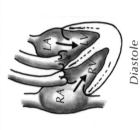

Diastole

AORTIC REGURGITATION

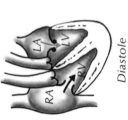

Diastole

	MITRAL STENOSIS	AORTIC REGURGITATION
LOCATION	Mitral (apical) area	Aortic area
RADIATION	Very little	Down the left sternal border, sometimes as far as the apex; also may radiate down the right sternal border
INTENSITY	Variable; may be brought out or accentuated in the left lateral decubitus position and by exercise	Variable, often faint; may be brought out by asking the patient to sit leaning forward with his breath exhaled
PITCH	Low (heard better with a bell)	High (heard better with a diaphragm)
QUALITY	Rumbling	Blowing
ASSOCIATED SIGNS MAY INCLUDE	Increased S_1 in the mitral area Opening snap Increased P_2 and left parasternal lift of right ventricular hypertrophy if pulmonary hypertension has developed	Aortic systolic murmur from increased flow. Since a relatively large volume of blood regurgitates back into the left ventricle with each diastole, it adds importantly to the volume of blood ejected across the aortic valve in the next systole. A low rumbling apical diastolic murmur resembling the murmur of mitral stenosis. This is called an *Austin Flint* murmur and is caused by a regurgitant stream of blood that impinges on the anterior leaflet of the mitral valve during diastole. S_3 A thrusting apical impulse displaced downward and laterally (left ventricular enlargement) Wide pulse pressure, large bounding pulses

Table 7-14

Table 7-14   Differentiation of Cardiovascular Sounds with Both Systolic and Diastolic Components

Some cardiovascular sounds are not confined to one portion of the cardiac cycle. Three examples are (1) a pericardial friction rub, produced by inflammation of the pericardial sac; (2) patent ductus arteriosus, a congenital abnormality in which an open channel persists between aorta and pulmonary artery; and (3) a venous hum, a benign sound produced by turbulence of blood in the jugular veins (common in children). Their characteristics are contrasted below. The term "continuous murmur" is defined as one that begins in systole and continues through the second sound into all or part of diastole. It need not continue through diastole. The murmur of patent ductus arteriosus, therefore, may be classified as continuous.

	PERICARDIAL FRICTION RUB	PATENT DUCTUS ARTERIOSUS	VENOUS HUM
	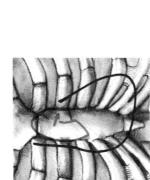	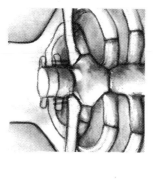	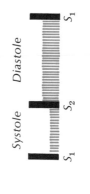
	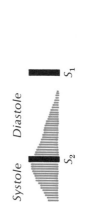		
TIMING	May have three short components, each associated with cardiac movement: (1) atrial systole, (2) ventricular systole, and (3) ventricular diastole. Usually the first two components are present; all three make diagnosis easy; only one (which is usually the systolic) invites confusion with a murmur.	Continuous murmur in both systole and diastole often with a silent interval late in diastole. Is loudest in late systole, obscures S_2, and fades in diastole	Continuous murmur without a silent interval. Loudest in diastole

Ventricular systole   *Ventricular diastole*   *Atrial systole*

S_1 S_2 S_1

Systole *Diastole*

S_1 S_2 S_1

Systole *Diastole*

S_1 S_2 S_1

Continued

Table 7-14

Table 7-14 (Cont'd)

	PERICARDIAL FRICTION RUB	PATENT DUCTUS ARTERIOSUS	VENOUS HUM
LOCATION	Variable but usually best heard in the 3rd interspace to the left of the sternum	Left 2nd interspace	Above the medial $\frac{1}{3}$ of the clavicles, especially on the right
RADIATION	Little	Toward the left clavicle	1st and 2nd interspaces
INTENSITY	Variable. May increase when the patient leans forward and exhales	Usually loud, sometimes associated with a thrill	Soft to moderate. Can be obliterated by pressure on the jugular veins
QUALITY	Scratchy, sounds close to the ear	Harsh, machinerylike	Humming, roaring
PITCH	High (heard better with a diaphragm)	Medium	Low (heard better with a bell)

Table 7-15

Table 7-15   Abnormalities of the Arterial Pulse

NORMAL	*mm Hg*	The pulse pressure is about 30–40 mm Hg. The pulse contour is smooth and rounded. (The notch on the descending slope of the pulse wave is not palpable.)
SMALL, WEAK PULSES		The pulse pressure is diminished. The pulse contour may show a slowed upstroke and prolonged peak. Causes include (1) decreased stroke volume as in heart failure or shock; and (2) mechanical obstruction to left ventricular output as in aortic stenosis.
LARGE, BOUNDING PULSES		The pulse pressure is increased. The pulse contour frequently shows a rapid rise, brief peak, and rapid fall. Causes include (1) hyperkinetic states (*e.g.*, anxiety, exercise, fever, anemia, hyperthyroidism); (2) abnormally rapid runoff of blood as in aortic regurgitation, patent ductus arteriosus; and (3) increased aortic rigidity as in aging and atherosclerosis.
BISFERIENS PULSE		A double systolic peak characterizes a bisferiens pulse. Causes include pure aortic regurgitation, combined aortic stenosis and regurgitation, and idiopathic hypertrophic subaortic stenosis.
PULSUS ALTERNANS		To make this observation the rhythm must be regular. The pulse alternates in amplitude from beat to beat. When the variation is slight, it can be detected only by sphygmomanometry: lower the cuff pressure slowly toward the systolic level; note alternating loud and soft sounds or a sudden doubling of the rate as the cuff pressure declines. Pulsus alternans is evidence of left-sided heart failure.
BIGEMINAL PULSE	*Premature contractions*	This is really a disorder of rhythm that may masquerade as pulsus alternans. Do not confuse the two. A bigeminal rhythm is usually produced by a normal beat alternating with a premature contraction. The stroke volume of the latter is diminished and the pulse varies in its amplitude, alternating between strong and weak. The rhythm here is irregular.
PARADOXICAL PULSE	*Expiration ← → Inspiration*	The pulse diminishes perceptibly in amplitude on inspiration. This is frequently detectable only by sphygmomanometry. As the patient breathes quietly, lower the cuff pressure slowly toward the systolic level. Note the pressure reading when the first sounds can be heard. Drop the cuff pressure very slowly until sounds can be heard throughout the respiratory cycle. Again note the pressure reading. If the readings are 10 mm Hg or more apart, a paradoxical pulse is present. A paradoxical pulse, an exaggeration of the normal response to respiration, is found in severe obstructive lung disease and constrictive pericardial disease.

THE BREASTS AND AXILLAE

Anatomy and Physiology

The female breast lies between the 2nd and 6th ribs, between the sternal edge and midaxillary line. About two thirds of it is superficial to the pectoralis major, about one third to the serratus anterior. The nipple is located centrally, where it is surrounded by the areola. Sebaceous glands on the areola present as small round elevations.

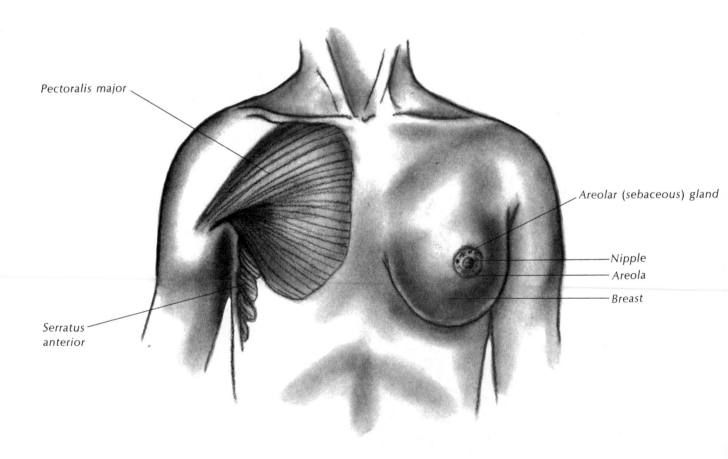

Pectoralis major

Serratus anterior

Areolar (sebaceous) gland

Nipple

Areola

Breast

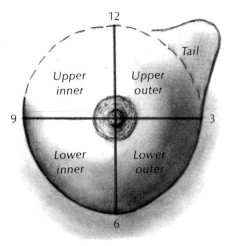

LEFT BREAST

For purposes of description, the breast may be divided into four quadrants by horizontal and vertical lines crossing at the nipple. In addition a tail of breast tissue frequently extends toward or into the axilla. An alternative method of localizing findings visualizes the breast as the face of a clock. A lesion may be located by the "time," (*e.g.*, 4 o'clock) and by the distance in centimeters from the nipple.

Breast tissue has three principal components. (1) The *glandular tissue* is organized into 12 to 20 lobes, each of which terminates in a duct that opens on the surface of the nipple. (2) This glandular tissue is supported by *fibrous tissue*, including suspensory ligaments that are connected both to the skin and to fascia underlying the breast. (3) *Fat* surrounds the breast and predominates both superficially and peripherally. The proportions of these components vary with age, the general state of nutrition, pregnancy, and other factors.

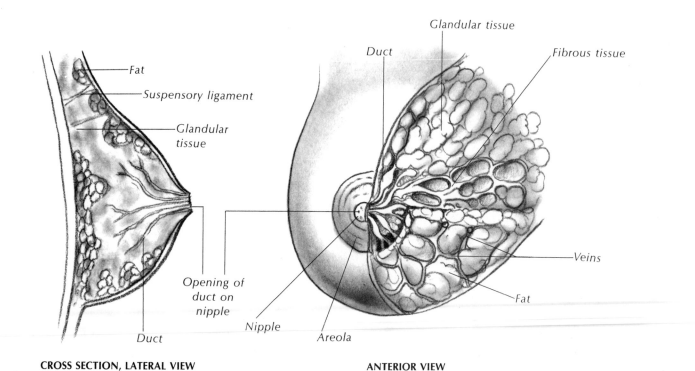

CROSS SECTION, LATERAL VIEW

ANTERIOR VIEW

The male breast consists chiefly of a small nipple and areola. These overlie a thin disc of undeveloped breast tissue that is not usually distinguishable clinically from the surrounding tissues.

CHANGES WITH AGE

Development of a woman's breasts begins during puberty. The preadolescent breast consists of a small elevated nipple with no elevation of underlying breast tissue. Between the ages of 8 and 13 years (average around 11 years) secondary sex characteristics become apparent. Breast buds appear, and further enlargement of breasts and areolae follows. The five stages of breast development as defined by Tanner's sex maturity ratings (SMR) are shown below.

Sex Maturity Ratings in Girls: Breasts

STAGE 1
Preadolescent. Elevation of nipple only

STAGE 2

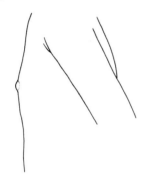

Breast bud stage. Elevation of breast and nipple as a small mound; enlargement of areolar diameter

STAGE 3

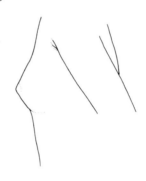

Further enlargement and elevation of breast and areola, with no separation of their contours

STAGE 4

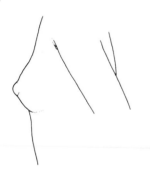

Projection of areola and nipple to form a secondary mound above the level of breast

STAGE 5

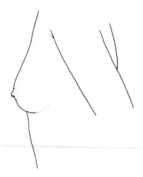

Mature stage; projection of nipple only. Areola has receded to general contour of the breast (although in some normal individuals the areola continues to form a secondary mound)

(Illustrations through the courtesy of W.A. Daniel, Jr, Division of Adolescent Medicine, University of Alabama, Birmingham)

Concomitantly, pubic hair appears and spreads, as illustrated on page 275. These two developmental changes—in breasts and pubic hair—are useful in assessing growth and maturation, although they do not necessarily proceed synchronously in any given person. The sequence from SMR 2 to SMR 5 takes about 3 years on the average, with a range of 1.5 to 6 years. Axillary hair usually appears about 2 years after pubic hair.

Menarche ordinarily occurs when a girl is in breast stage 3 or 4. By the time of menarche a girl has characteristically reached the peak of her adolescent growth spurt. Although she may continue to grow somewhat, her rate of growth has begun to taper off. The relationships of menarche to breast development and to the growth spurt are useful in counselling a girl who is worried that she may grow too tall or that her menarche is too late. The usual sequence of these changes is summarized in the diagram below.

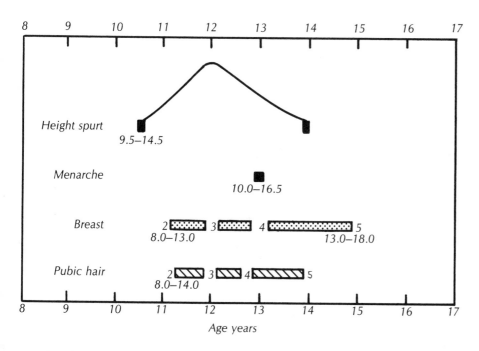

Numbers below the bars indicate the ranges in age within which certain changes occur. (Redrawn from Marshall WA, Tanner JM: Variations in the pattern of pubertal changes in boys. Arch Dis Child 45:22, 1970)

Tanner's figures are based on studies of white English girls. An American survey indicates that black girls tend to be more advanced in their secondary sex characteristics than whites of the same age. Black girls, too, develop axillary hair earlier than their white counterparts, sometimes before their pubic hair appears. These differences, together with the relatively fine, sparse pubic hair described in Oriental women, illustrate the caution required in applying group norms.

Breasts vary normally in several ways. In about 1 out of 12 girls, breasts develop at different rates, and considerable asymmetry may result. This is usually a temporary phenomenon, and unless the difference is unusually marked, reassurance is indicated. In many girls and women breasts become somewhat tender, slightly enlarged, and more nodular during the premenstrual period.

Pregnancy brings further changes. Starting in the second month the breasts enlarge and become somewhat nodular as glandular and ductal tissue increases. The nipples enlarge and become darker and more erectile. Later the areolae also darken and the venous pattern over the breasts becomes accentuated. Colostrum, a thick, yellowish fluid, can often be expressed from the nipple by gentle massage after the 16th week of gestation.

The breasts of an aging woman tend to diminish in size as glandular tissue atrophies and fat decreases. They may get flabby and hang lower on the chest, as shown on page 37. The ducts surrounding the nipple may become more easily palpable as firm stringy strands. Axillary hair diminishes.

Although adult male breasts are usually small, approximately 2 out of 3 adolescent boys develop temporary breast enlargement, or gynecomastia, on one or both sides. Usually this is a slight change consisting only of a firm plaque of breast tissue deep to the areola. Occasionally, however, more obvious enlargement develops and may cause considerable embarrassment (see p. 227). Pubertal gynecomastia usually resolves spontaneously.

LYMPHATICS

Since the lymphatics of much of the breast drain toward the axilla, an understanding of the axillary lymph nodes will help you in assessing the breasts. Of these, the central axillary nodes are most frequently palpable. They are located high in the axilla, close to the ribs and serratus anterior. Into them drain channels from three other groups of lymph nodes:

1. The pectoral (or anterior) group of nodes is located along the lower border of the pectoralis major inside the anterior axillary fold. These nodes drain the anterior chest wall and most of the breast.

2. The subscapular (or posterior) group is located along the lateral border of the scapula and is felt deep in the posterior axillary fold. These nodes drain the posterior chest wall and a portion of the arm.

3. The lateral group is felt along the upper humerus. These nodes drain most of the arm.

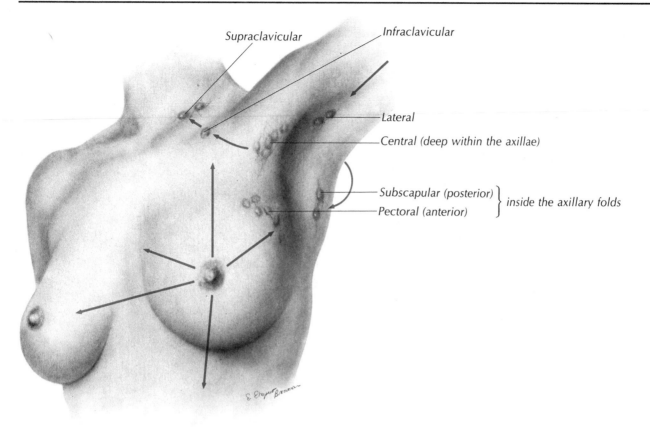

Supraclavicular

Infraclavicular

Lateral

Central (deep within the axillae)

Subscapular (posterior)
Pectoral (anterior) } *inside the axillary folds*

Arrows indicate direction of lymph flow

Lymph drains from the central axillary nodes to the infraclavicular and supraclavicular nodes.

Note that the lymphatics of the breast do not all drain into the axilla. Depending upon the location of a lesion in the breast, spread may occur directly to the infraclavicular nodes, into deep channels within the chest or abdomen, and even to the opposite breast.

Techniques of Examination

THE FEMALE BREAST

GENERAL APPROACH

Many student examiners, especially men, initially find it embarrassing to examine a woman's breasts. These feelings are normal. Women patients, too, may be embarrassed or dislike the exposure involved. With practice you can learn to do a competent examination yet remain sensitive to the patient's feelings.

Tell the patient that you are going to examine her breasts. This may be a good time to ask if she has noted any lumps or other problems or whether she does monthly self-examinations. An adequate inspection requires full exposure of the chest, but later in the examination you may find it helpful to cover one breast while you are palpating the other. Gentleness, courtesy, and a matter-of-fact approach all help the patient to relax.

If the patient is unfamiliar with self-examination, you have a good opportunity to explain what you are doing and help her to repeat maneuvers after you. Some adolescent girls, however, are hesitant to touch their own bodies or are too embarrassed to examine themselves. Adapt your approach to the patient's comfort and psychological readiness.

INSPECTION

With the patient in the sitting position, disrobed to the waist and with her arms at her sides—

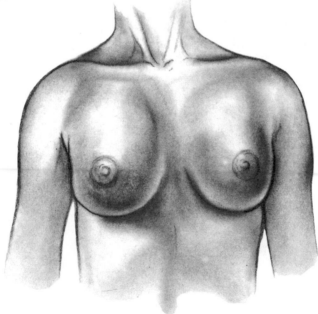

ARMS AT SIDE

Inspect the breasts. Note:

1. Their size and symmetry. Some difference in size is common and usually normal.

2. Their contour, with special reference to masses, dimpling, or flattening

See Table 8-1, Visible Signs of Breast Cancer (p. 224).

3. The appearance of the skin, including

   a. Color

   Redness in infection or inflammatory carcinoma

   b. Thickening or edema

   Edema or increased venous prominence in carcinoma

   c. Venous pattern

Inspect the nipples. Note:

See Table 8-2, Abnormalities of Nipple and Areola (p. 225).

1. Their size and shape. Simple inversion of long standing is common and usually normal

2. The direction in which they point

3. Rashes or ulcerations

4. Discharge

When examining an adolescent girl, assess her breast development according to Tanner's sex maturity ratings (SMR) described on page 212. Because an adolescent girl is often concerned about her breasts, it may be helpful to tell her that she is developing normally (if she is) and, using the diagrams, to review with her the usual developmental sequence. You will rate pubic hair development separately, later in the examination.

Breast development before the age of 8 may be considered *precocious.* If no breast development is seen by age 13, or if more than 5 years have elapsed between the beginning of breast development and menarche, puberty may be considered *delayed.*

In order to bring out dimpling or retraction that may otherwise be over-looked, ask the patient (1) to raise her arms over her head, and (2) to press her hands against her hips. Again inspect the breast contour carefully.

Dimpling or retraction of the breasts suggests an underlying cancer.

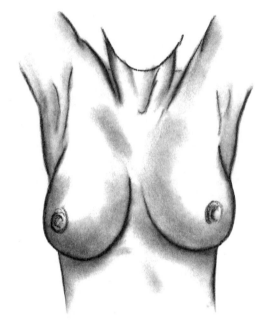

ARMS OVER HEAD

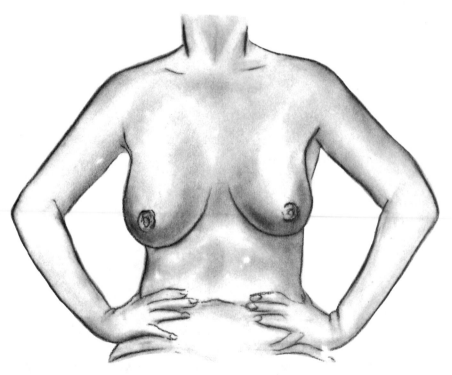

HANDS PRESSED AGAINST HIPS

Occasionally, other maneuvers may be useful:

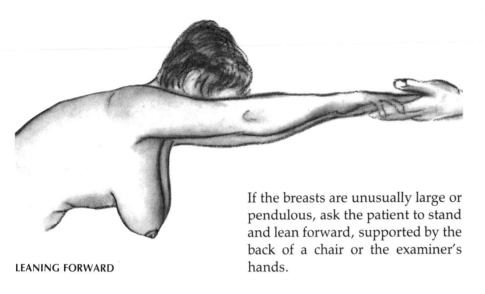

LEANING FORWARD

If the breasts are unusually large or pendulous, ask the patient to stand and lean forward, supported by the back of a chair or the examiner's hands.

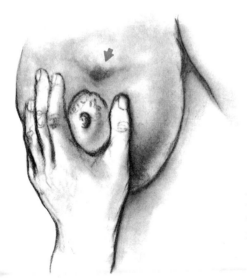

If you suspect a mass, gently move or compress the breast and watch for dimpling.

PALPATION

Ask the patient to lie down. Unless the breasts are small, place a small pillow under the patient's shoulder on the side you are examining and ask her to rest her arm over her head. These maneuvers help to spread the breast more evenly across the chest and make it easier to find nodules.

Use the pads of your three fingers in a rotary motion to compress the breast tissue gently against the chest wall. Proceed systematically, examining the entire breast including the periphery, tail, and areola.

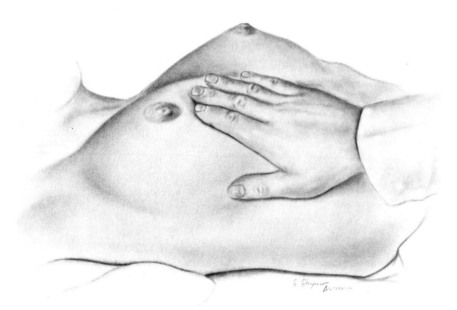

A uniform pattern of examination, as in the following diagram, helps to assure a complete assessment.

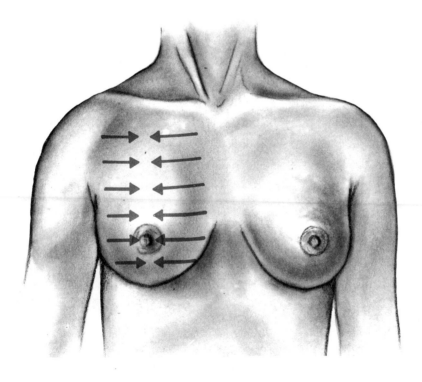

Note:

The consistency or elasticity of the tissues. Normal variations include the firm elasticity of the young breast, the lobular feel of glandular tissue, and the somewhat stringy or granular feel of the older breast. Premenstrual fullness, nodularity, and tenderness are common. Especially in large breasts a firm transverse ridge of compressed tissue may be present along the lower edge of the breast. This is the normal inframammary ridge and should not be confused with a tumor.

Induration

Tenderness

Nodules

If present, describe the following:

1. Their location, by quadrant or the clock method, with centimeters from the nipple
2. The size in centimeters
3. Shape, (*e.g.*, round or discoid, regular or irregular)
4. Consistency (*e.g.*, soft, firm, or hard)
5. Delimitation in relationship to surrounding tissues (*e.g.*, well circumscribed or not)
6. Mobility, with special reference to the skin and underlying tissues
7. Tenderness

See Table 8-3, Differentiation of Common Breast Nodules (p. 226).
Hard, poorly circumscribed nodules, fixed to the skin or underlying tissues, strongly suggest cancer.

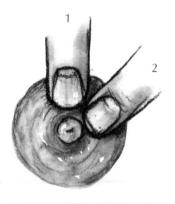

Palpate each nipple, noting it elasticity. Compress it between your thumb and index finger. Inspect for discharge. If there is a history or physical evidence of nipple discharge, try to determine its origin by compressing the areola with your index finger placed in radial positions around the nipple. Watch for discharge appearing through one of the duct openings on the nipple's surface.

Loss of elasticity in cancer.
Bloody discharge of intraductal papilloma

The tactile stimulation of examination may produce temporary erection of the nipple and wrinkling or puckering of the areola. These normal phenomena should not be confused with signs of cancer.

Inversion, flattening, or retraction of the nipple, and edema of the areola suggest cancer.

THE MALE BREAST

Examination of the male breast may be brief but should not be omitted.

See Table 8-4, Abnormalities of the Male Breast (p. 227).

Inspect the nipple and areola for nodules, swelling, or ulceration.

Palpate the areola for nodules. If the breast appears enlarged, distinguish between the soft fatty enlargement that may accompany obesity and the firm disc of glandular enlargement.

A firm disc of glandular enlargement in a male is called gynecomastia.

THE AXILLAE

Although the axillae may be examined with the patient lying down, a sitting position is preferable.

INSPECTION

Inspect the skin of each axilla, noting evidence of:

Rash

Deodorant and other rashes

Infection

Sweat gland infections (hidradenitis suppurativa)

Unusual pigmentation

Deeply pigmented, velvety axillary skin suggests the rare acanthosis nigricans, one form of which is associated with internal malignancy.

PALPATION

To examine the patient's left axilla, ask him to relax with his left arm down. Help him by supporting his left wrist or hand with your left hand. Cup together the fingers of your right hand and reach as high as you can toward the apex of his axilla. Bringing your fingers down over the surface of the ribs and serratus anterior, try to feel the central nodes by compressing them against the chest wall. Of the axillary nodes, the central nodes are most often palpable. One or two soft, small, nontender nodes may be normal.

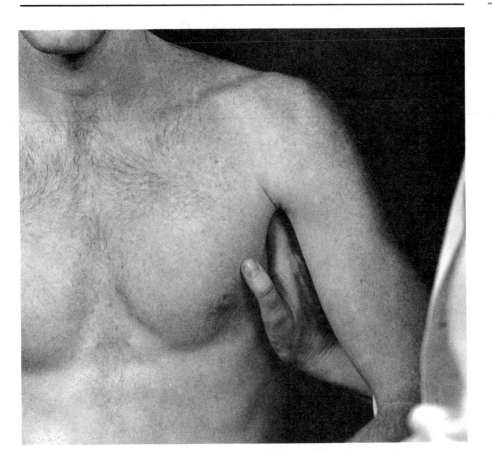

Feel inside the anterior and posterior axillary folds and against the humerus for the pectoral, subscapular, and lateral axillary nodes respectively. The subscapular and lateral nodes may be more easily identified by standing behind the patient. If you detect enlarged or tender nodes, feel for infraclavicular nodes and reexamine the supraclavicular nodes.

Now, using your left hand, reverse the procedure to examine the right axilla.

Axillary metastases of breast cancer; lymphadenitis from infection of hand or arm.

Table 8-1

Table 8-1 Visible Signs of Breast Cancer

RETRACTION SIGNS

A breast cancer frequently causes fibrosis, or scar tissue formation. Contraction of this fibrotic tissue produces *retraction signs*, including dimpling of the skin, alteration in breast contours, and flattening or deviation of the nipple.

Dimpling

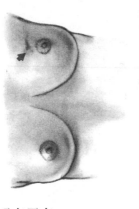

Flattening of nipple

SKIN DIMPLING

Dimpling of the skin suggests an underlying malignancy. Look for this sign at rest, during special positioning, and on moving or compressing the breasts.

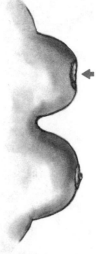

ABNORMAL CONTOURS

ARMS OVER HEAD

Alterations in contour are identified by careful inspection of the normally convex surfaces of the breasts and by comparison of one breast with the other. Changing the patient's position (*e.g.*, by elevation of her arms) also helps.

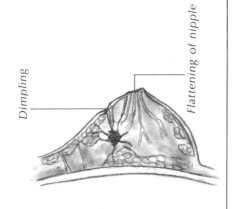

LEANING FORWARD

Here an abnormal contour and nipple retraction appear when the patient leans forward.

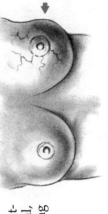

In Addition, Vascular Signs may be Noted. These Include:

EDEMA OF THE SKIN

Edema of the skin is produced by lymphatic blockade. This is manifested by thickened skin with enlarged pores—the so-called pig skin or orange peel (peau d'orange) appearance.

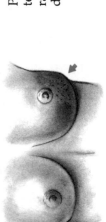

VENOUS PROMINENCE

Prominence of the venous pattern, especially when unilateral, raises suspicion of underlying disease.

Table 8-2

Table 8-2   Abnormalities of Nipple and Areola

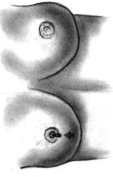
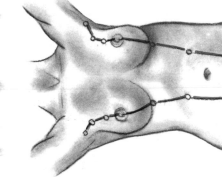

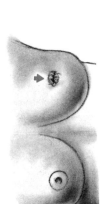
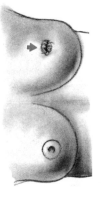

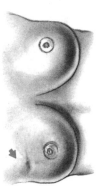

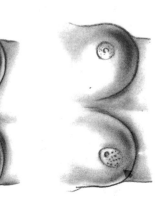

NIPPLE INVERSION

Simple nipple inversion is a common variant of normal and is usually of long standing. It may be unilateral or bilateral. The nipple can usually be pulled out of the sulcus in which it lies. Flattening, broadening, and true retraction are absent. The recent development of inversion in a previously erect nipple, however, is highly suggestive of malignancy.

NIPPLE FLATTENING OR RETRACTION

The fibrosis associated with a cancer behind the nipple pulls the nipple inward and may broaden and flatten it.

NIPPLE DEVIATION OR POINTING

The fibrosis associated with cancer may deviate the axis in which the nipple points. The nipple deviates toward the cancer.

EDEMA OF NIPPLE AND AREOLA

The pig skin or orange peel appearance produced by lymphatic blockade often affects the areola first. It strongly suggests cancer.

PAGET'S DISEASE

A form of breast cancer, Paget's disease progresses slowly from a smooth redness to rough thickening to erosion or ulceration of the nipple and areola. In any dermatitis of nipple and areola, cancer must be suspected.

NIPPLE DISCHARGE

There are many causes of nipple discharge, most of them nonmalignant. Note the color of the discharge and if possible identify its source.

SUPERNUMERARY BREASTS

One or more extra breasts may be located along the "milk line," most commonly in the axillae or below the normal breasts. A supernumerary breast usually consists of a small nipple and areola and may be mistaken for a mole. Less commonly glandular tissue is present.

Table 8-3 Differentiation of Common Breast Nodules

Despite the classic differences listed below, definitive diagnosis usually depends on aspiration of cysts or surgical biopsy. Differentiation is most difficult in cases where it is most desirable—the early small nodule.

Pathology	CYSTIC DISEASE *Single or Multiple Cysts*	ADENOFIBROMA *A Benign Neoplasm*	CANCER *A Malignant Neoplasm*
FINDINGS BY PALPATION (The illustrations do not imply visibility to inspection.)	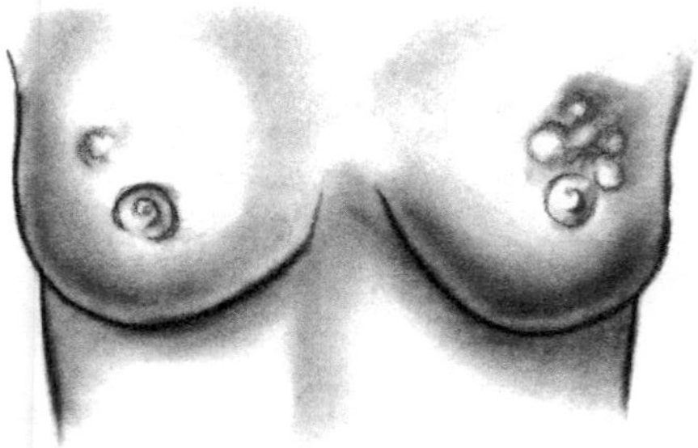	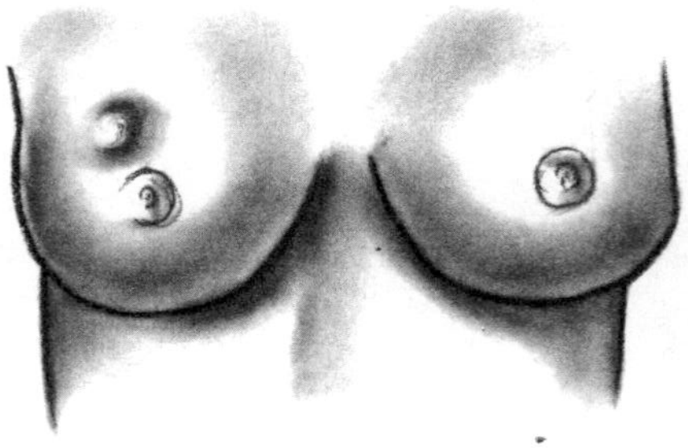	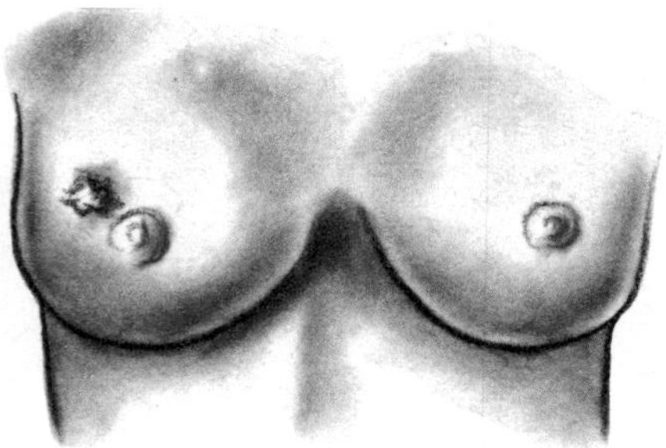
USUAL AGE	30–55, regresses after menopause	Puberty and young adulthood, up to 55	30–80, most common in middle-aged and elderly
NUMBER	Single or multiple	Usually single, may be multiple	Usually single, although may coexist with other nodular lesions
SHAPE	Round	Round, discoid, or lobular	Irregular or stellate
CONSISTENCY	Soft to firm, usually elastic	May be soft, usually firm	Firm or hard
DELIMITATION	Well delineated	Well delineated	Not clearly delineated from surrounding tissues
MOBILITY	Mobile	Very mobile	May be fixed to skin or underlying tissues
TENDERNESS	Often tender	Usually nontender	Usually nontender
RETRACTION SIGNS	Absent	Absent	Often present

Table 8-4

Table 8-4 Abnormalities of the Male Breast

GYNECOMASTIA

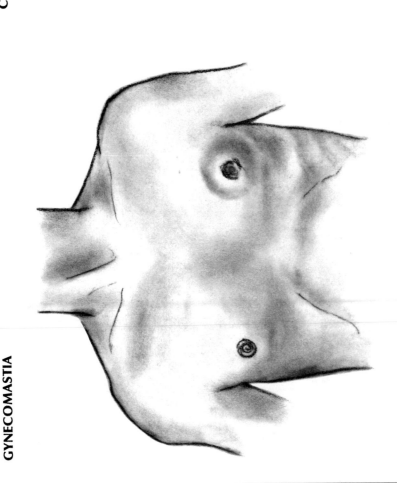

A smooth, firm, mobile, often tender disc of breast tissue centrally located behind the areola suggests gynecomastia. It may be unilateral or bilateral. Temporary gynecomastia frequently accompanies normal puberty. There are many additional causes. Among them are cirrhosis of the liver and medications such as estrogens, digitalis, spironolactone, and phenothiazines.

CANCER

A hard, irregular nodule in the areola of a man's breast suggests cancer. It is usually eccentrically placed. Frequently fixed to both nipple and underlying tissue, it tends to distort the nipple and areola.

Check the axillae for evidence of metastases.

Chapter 9
THE ABDOMEN

Anatomy and Physiology

Review the anatomy of the abdominal wall, identifying the illustrated landmarks. The rectus abdominis muscles can be identified by asking the patient to raise his head from a supine position.

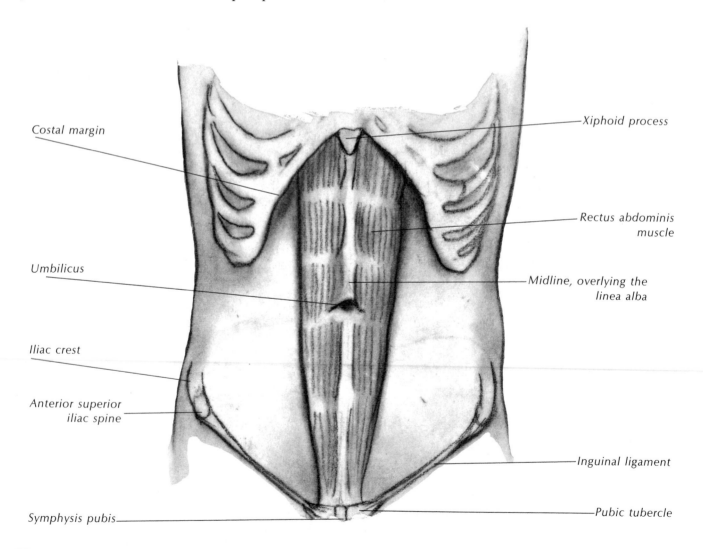

Costal margin

Xiphoid process

Rectus abdominis muscle

Umbilicus

Midline, overlying the linea alba

Iliac crest

Anterior superior iliac spine

Inguinal ligament

Symphysis pubis

Pubic tubercle

For descriptive purposes the abdomen is generally divided into four quadrants by imaginary lines crossing at the umbilicus: right upper, right lower, left upper, and left lower quadrants. Another system divides the abdomen into nine sections. Terms for three of them are commonly used: epigastric, umbilical, and hypogastric or suprapubic.

Sometimes the examiner can feel several normal structures within the abdomen. Although the liver often lies entirely up under the rib cage, its edge may sometimes be felt just below the right costal margin, especially on deep inspiration. The lower pole of the right kidney can occasionally be detected here too, especially in thin women with well relaxed abdominal walls. In some people the right kidney lies closer to the anterior abdominal wall than anatomy texts have indicated, and its lower pole may be hard to differentiate from the liver. Portions of stool-filled colon are frequently noted as tubular structures deep in the abdomen. Become thoroughly familiar with their contours and do not mistake them for tumors. Another normal structure that in thin people occasionally masquerades as a tumor—an ominous stony hard one—is the sacral promontory. Through a thin, well relaxed abdominal wall you may feel it deep in the abdomen below the umbilicus. Other misleading "tumors" include a distended bladder and a pregnant uterus. The pulsating abdominal aorta is frequently seen and usually felt in the upper abdomen, while the pulsations of the iliac arteries are sometimes palpable in the lower quadrants.

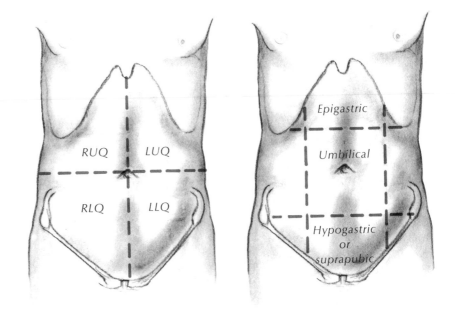

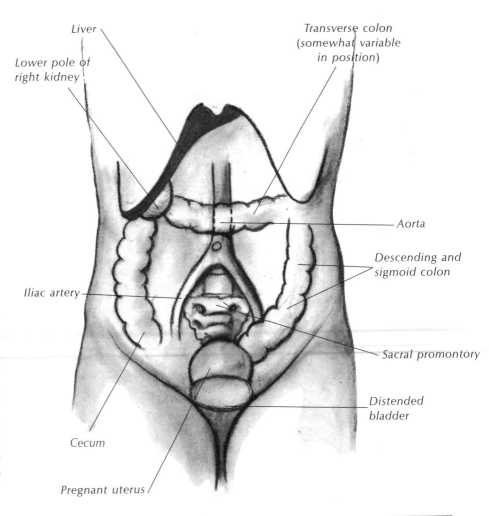

The abdomen extends up under the rib cage to the dome of the diaphragm. When organs are confined to this region they are examined chiefly by percussion. They include the liver, spleen, and stomach, as shown in the figure below at the left. The duodenum and pancreas lie deep in the upper abdomen while the gall bladder lies deep to the liver in the right upper quadrant. These three organs are not normally palpable.

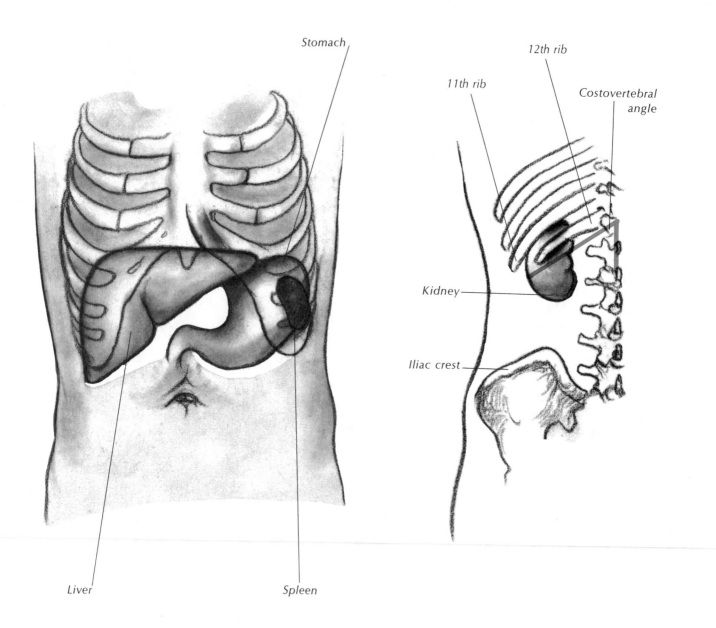

The kidneys are posterior organs, protected above by the ribs and below by the heavy back muscles. The costovertebral angles, formed by rib cage and vertebral column, are clinically useful landmarks. (See the figure above at the right.)

CHANGES WITH AGE

During the middle and later years fat tends to accumulate in the lower abdomen and near the hips, even when total body weight is stable. This accumulation, together with weakening of the abdominal muscles, often produces a potbelly. An occasional person, noting this change with concern or alarm, may interpret it as fluid or evidence of disease.

Techniques of Examination

GENERAL APPROACH

Essential conditions for a good abdominal examination include (1) good light, (2) a relaxed patient, and (3) full exposure of the abdomen from above the xiphoid process to the symphysis pubis. The groins should be visible although the genitalia should be kept draped. To encourage relaxation:

1. The patient should *not* have a full bladder.

2. Make him comfortable in a supine position with a pillow for his head, perhaps also under his knees. You can ascertain whether or not he is relaxed flat on the table by trying to insert your hand underneath his low back.

An occasional patient arches his back and thus thrusts his abdomen forward, tightening his muscles.

3. He should keep his arms at his sides or folded across the chest. Although patients commonly put their arms over their heads, this move should be discouraged because it stretches and tightens the abdominal wall and makes palpation difficult.

4. Have warm hands, a warm stethoscope, and short fingernails. Rubbing your hands together or running hot water over them may help to warm them. Anxious examiners, unfortunately, often have cold hands. This problem decreases over time.

5. Approach slowly and avoid quick, unexpected movements.

6. Distract the patient if necessary with conversation or questions.

7. If the patient is very frightened or very ticklish, begin palpation with his own hand beneath yours. In a few moments you can slip your hand under his to palpate directly.

8. Ask the patient to point to any areas of pain, and examine tender areas last.

9. Monitor your examination by watching the patient's face.

Make a habit of visualizing each organ in the region you are examining. From the patient's right side proceed in an orderly fashion: inspection, auscultation, percussion, palpation.

INSPECTION

Starting from your usual standing position at the right side of the bed, inspect the abdomen. When looking at the contour of the abdomen and watching for peristalsis, it is helpful to sit or bend down so that you can view the abdomen tangentially.

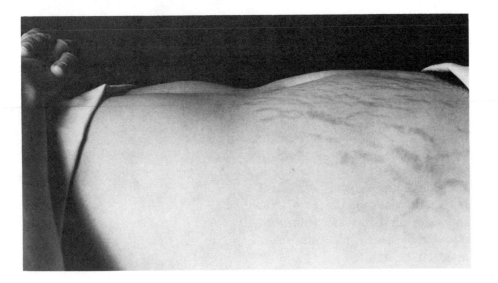

Note:

1. *The skin*, including:

   Scars. Describe their location.

   Striae. Old silver striae or stretch marks, as illustrated above, are normal.

   Dilated veins. A fine venous network may normally be present.

   Rashes and lesions

2. *The umbilicus*—its contour, location, signs of inflammation or hernia

3. *Contour of the abdomen.* Is it flat, rounded, protuberant, or scaphoid (markedly concave or hollowed)? Are there any local bulges? Include in this survey the inguinal and femoral areas. The techniques of examining for inguinal and femoral hernias are described in Chapter 10.

4. *Symmetry*

5. *Enlarged organs.* As the patient breathes, watch for an enlarged liver or spleen to descend below the rib cage.

6. *Masses*

Pink purple striae of Cushing's syndrome

Dilated veins of inferior vena cava obstruction

See Table 9-1, Abdominal Hernias and Bulges (p. 250).

See Table 9-2, Protuberant Abdomens (p. 251).

Suprapubic bulge of distended bladder or pregnant uterus

Asymmetry of an enlarged organ or mass

Lower abdominal mass of an ovarian tumor

7. *Peristalsis.* Observe for several minutes if you suspect intestinal obstruction. Peristalsis may normally be visible in very thin people.

Increased peristaltic waves of intestinal obstruction

8. *Pulsations.* The normal aortic pulsation is frequently visible in the epigastrium.

Increased pulsation of aortic aneurysm or of increased pulse pressure

AUSCULTATION

Auscultation of the abdomen is useful in assessing bowel motility and abdominal complaints, in searching for renal artery stenosis as a cause of hypertension, and in exploring for other vascular obstructions. You should practice the technique until you become thoroughly familiar with normal variations and can listen intelligently when you need to. In most other situations, however, auscultation may safely be omitted.

Listen to the abdomen before percussing and feeling it, because the latter maneuvers may alter the frequency of bowel sounds. Place the diaphragm of your stethoscope gently on the abdomen.

Listen for *bowel sounds* and note their frequency and character. Normal sounds consist of clicks and gurgles, the frequency of which has been estimated at from 5 to 34 per minute. Occasionally you may hear borborygmi—loud prolonged gurgles of hyperperistalsis—the familiar "stomach growling." Since bowel sounds are widely transmitted through the abdomen, listening in one spot, such as the right lower quadrant, is generally enough.

Bowel sounds may be altered in diarrhea, intestinal obstruction, paralytic ileus, and peritonitis. See Table 9-3, Sounds in the Abdomen (p. 252).

If the patient has high blood pressure, listen in the epigastrium and in each upper quadrant for *bruits*—vascular sounds resembling heart murmurs. Later in the examination, when the patient sits up, listen also in the costovertebral angles. For unexplained reasons some normal people, especially young adults, have epigastric bruits.

In a hypertensive patient an epigastric bruit, especially if it radiates laterally, suggests but does not prove renal artery stenosis.

If you suspect arterial insufficiency in the legs, listen for bruits over the aorta, the iliac arteries, and the femoral arteries.

Partial arterial obstruction creates turbulent blood flow and may thus cause bruits. See Table 9-3, Sounds in the Abdomen (p. 252).

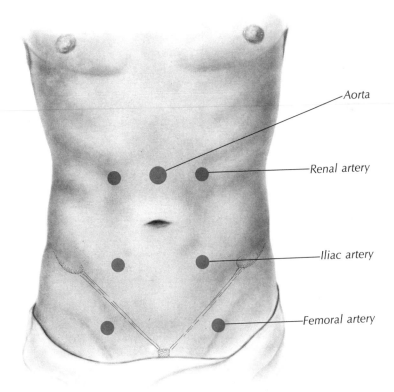

Aorta

Renal artery

Iliac artery

Femoral artery

If you suspect a liver tumor, gonococcal infection around the liver, or splenic infarction, listen over the liver and spleen for *friction rubs*.

See Table 9-3, Sounds in the Abdomen (p. 252).

PERCUSSION

Percussion is useful for orientation to the abdomen, for measuring the liver and sometimes the spleen, and for identifying ascitic fluid, solid or fluid-filled masses, and air in the stomach and bowel. Although percussion for all these purposes is described in this section, some practitioners prefer to alternate percussion with palpation as they examine liver, spleen, and other areas of the abdomen. Either approach is satisfactory.

For General Orientation. Percuss the abdomen lightly in all four quadrants to assess the general proportions and distribution of tympany and dullness. Tympany usually predominates. Check for the suprapubic dullness of a distended bladder.

See Table 9-2, Protuberant Abdomens (p. 251).

The Liver. In the right midclavicular line, starting at a level below the umbilicus (in an area of tympany, not dullness), lightly percuss upward toward the liver. Ascertain the lower border of liver dullness in the midclavicular line.

Next, identify the upper border of liver dullness in the midclavicular line. Lightly percuss from lung resonance down toward liver dullness. Now measure in centimeters the vertical span, or height, of liver dullness. If the liver appears enlarged, you may wish to outline the boundaries of liver dullness in other locations also—for example, the midsternal line and the right anterior axillary line.

The span of liver dullness is increased when the liver is enlarged.

CAUTION
Dullness of a right pleural effusion or consolidated lung, if adjacent to liver dullness, may falsely increase the estimated liver size.

CAUTION
Gas in the colon may produce tympany in the right upper quadrant, obscure liver dullness, and falsely decrease the estimated liver size.

Liver dullness may be decreased or absent when free air is present below the diaphragm, as from a perforated hollow viscus.

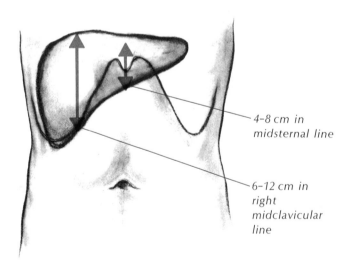

4–8 cm in midsternal line

6–12 cm in right midclavicular line

Normal liver heights are shown above. They are generally greater in men than in women, in tall people than in short. Although percussion is probably the most accurate clinical method for estimating liver size, it provides only a gross estimate. Furthermore, each border of liver dullness is sometimes obscured.

Ask the patient to take a deep breath and hold it. Again percuss the lower border of liver dullness in the midclavicular line, always percussing from tympany to dullness. Estimate its descent. This maneuver will help guide subsequent palpation.

The Stomach. Identify the tympany of the gastric air bubble, in the area of the left lower anterior rib cage. Its size is variable.

Increase in the size of the gastric air bubble, together with upper abdominal distention, suggests gastric dilatation.

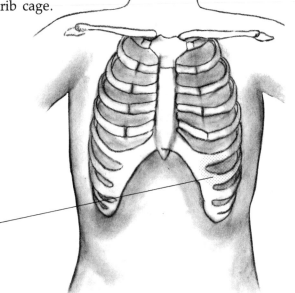

Tympany of gastric air bubble

The Spleen. Identify if possible the small oval area of splenic dullness near the left 10th rib just posterior to the midaxillary line (as illustrated on page 238). To do so percuss in several directions from resonance or tympany toward the anticipated area of dullness so that you can outline its edges. You cannot, of course, distinguish between the dullness of the posterior flank and dullness of the spleen. The dullness of a normal spleen is often obscured by gastric or colonic air. Moreover, a full stomach or feces-filled colon may simulate the dullness of splenic enlargement.

A large dull area suggests splenic enlargement.

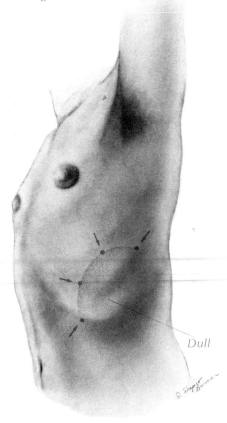

Dull

As another method of identifying splenic enlargement, percuss the lowest interspace in the left anterior axillary line. This area is usually tympanitic. Ask the patient to take a deep breath. When spleen size is normal, the percussion note usually remains tympanitic.

A change in percussion note from tympany to dullness on inspiration suggests splenic enlargement. This is a positive splenic percussion sign.

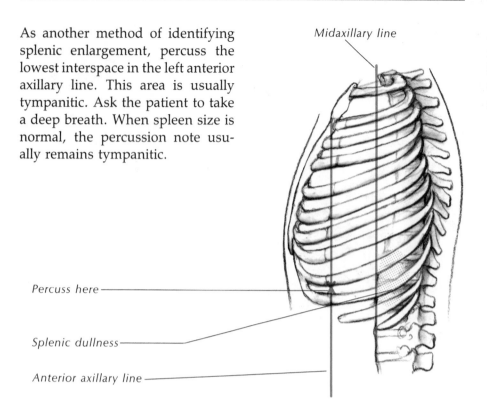

Midaxillary line

Percuss here

Splenic dullness

Anterior axillary line

LIGHT PALPATION

Light palpation is especially helpful in identifying muscular resistance, abdominal tenderness, and some superficial organs and masses. Its gentleness helps also to reassure and relax the patient.

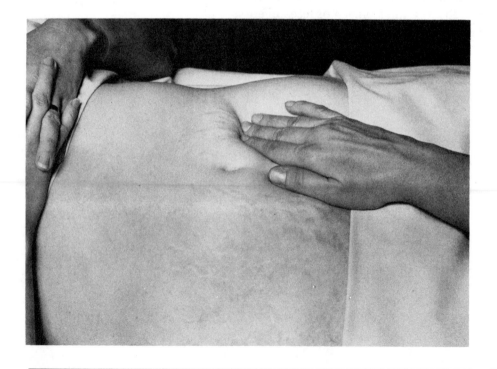

Keeping your hand and forearm on a horizontal plane, use the pads of your fingertips, with fingers together, in a light, gentle, dipping motion. Avoid short quick jabs. Moving smoothly, feel in all quadrants. Identify any organs or masses, any area of tenderness or increased resistance. If resistance is present, try to determine whether it is voluntary resistance or involuntary spasm: (1) Try all the maneuvers to relax the patient (p. 232). (2) Feel for the relaxation of the rectus muscles that normally accompanies expiration. If the rigidity remains unaltered by all these maneuvers, it is probably involuntary.

Involuntary rigidity or spasm of the abdominal muscles indicates peritoneal inflammation.

DEEP PALPATION

Deeper palpation is usually required to delineate abdominal organs and masses.

Again using the palmar surfaces of the fingers, feel in all four quadrants.

Identify any masses and note their location, size, shape, consistency, tenderness, pulsations, and mobility (*e.g.*, with respiration or with the examining hand).

Identify any tender areas. If greater than normal tenderness is present, check for rebound tenderness by firmly and slowly pressing in, then quickly withdrawing your fingers. Rebound tenderness is elicited when pain is noted during withdrawal.

See Table 9-4, Tender Abdomens (pp. 253–254).

Rebound tenderness suggests peritoneal inflammation.

When deep palpation is difficult—because of obesity, for example, or muscular resistance—use two hands, one on top of the other. Exert pressure with the outside hand while concentrating on feeling with the inside hand.

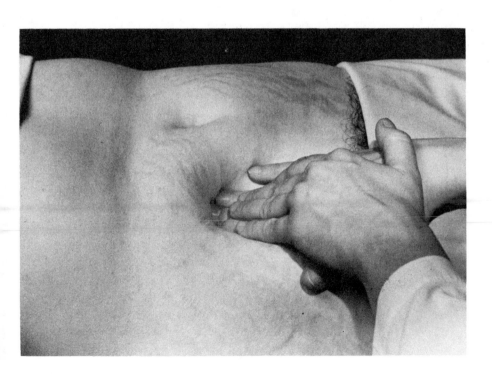

PALPATING THE LIVER, SPLEEN, KIDNEYS, AND AORTA

The Liver. Place your left hand behind the patient, parallel to and supporting his right 11th and 12th ribs. Remind the patient to relax on your hand if necessary. By pressing your left hand forward, the patient's liver is more easily felt in front.

Place your right hand on the patient's right abdomen lateral to the rectus muscle, with your fingertips well below the lower border of liver dullness. Some examiners like to point their fingers up toward the patient's head, others prefer a more oblique position. In either case, press gently in and up.

A greatly enlarged liver is sometimes missed because the examiner started too high in the abdomen and never felt its lower edge.

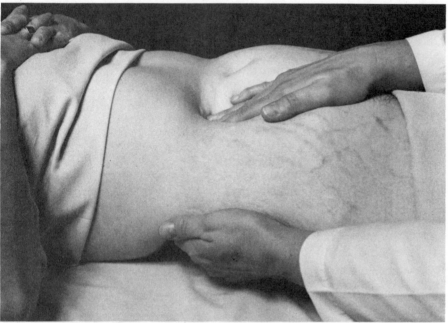

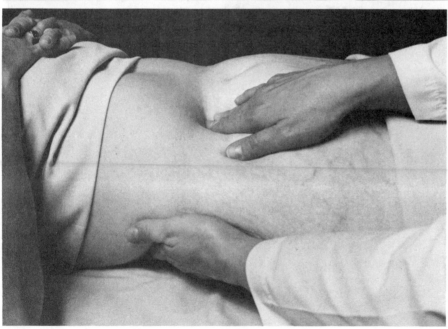

Ask the patient to take a deep breath. Try to feel the liver edge as it comes down to meet your fingertips. When palpable, a normal liver edge presents a firm, sharp, regular ridge with a smooth surface, although sometimes only a sense of increased resistance can be perceived. If unsuccessful, exert more pressure inward and repeat. Readjust the position of your right hand closer to the right costal margin and repeat.

Toward the peak of inspiration it may be helpful to release the pressure of your right hand slightly and let it ride up and over the descending liver edge. It is primarily the descending liver and not your hand, however, that moves in this maneuver.

See Table 9-5, Liver Enlargement: Apparent and Real (pp. 255–256).

If palpable, trace the liver edge both medially and laterally by repeating your maneuvers. The edge may extend over into the left upper quadrant. Describe the contour and surface of the liver and note any tenderness.

The liver may also be felt by the "hooking technique." Stand to the right of the patient and face his feet. Place both hands, side by side, on his right abdomen below the border of liver dullness. Press in with your fingers and up toward the costal margin. Ask him to take a deep breath.

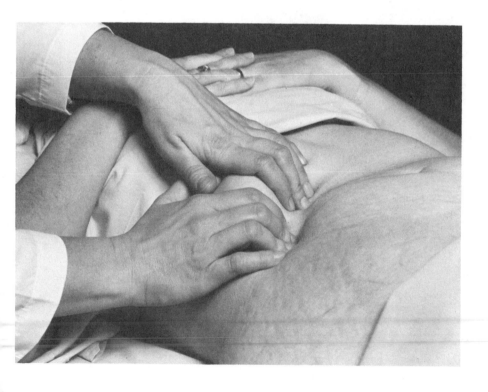

Some people, especially women, breathe primarily with their chests rather than with their diaphragms. It may be helpful to train such a patient to "breathe with the abdomen," thus bringing the liver, as well as the spleen and kidneys, into a palpable position during inspiration.

To check for liver tenderness when the organ is not palpable, place your left hand flat on the lower right rib cage, then strike your hand with the ulnar surface of your right fist. Ask the patient to compare the sensation with that produced by a similar maneuver on the left side.

Tenderness suggests inflammation, as in hepatitis.

The Spleen. With your left hand, reach over and around the patient to support and press forward his lower left rib cage. With your right hand below the left costal margin, press in toward the spleen. Begin palpation low enough to be sure that you are below a possibly enlarged spleen. Furthermore, if your hand is too close to the costal margin it is not sufficiently mobile to reach up under the rib cage. Ask the patient to take a deep breath. Try to feel the tip or edge of the spleen as it comes down to meet your fingertips.

See Table 9-6, Steps in Splenic Enlargement (p. 257). A greatly enlarged spleen is sometimes missed because the examiner started too high in the abdomen and never felt its lower edge.

If the spleen of an adult is palpable, it is probably considerably larger than normal.

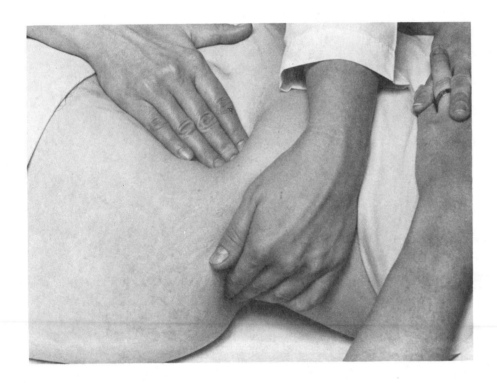

Repeat with the patient lying on his right side and his legs somewhat flexed at hips and knees. In this position, gravity may bring the spleen forward and to the right into a palpable location.

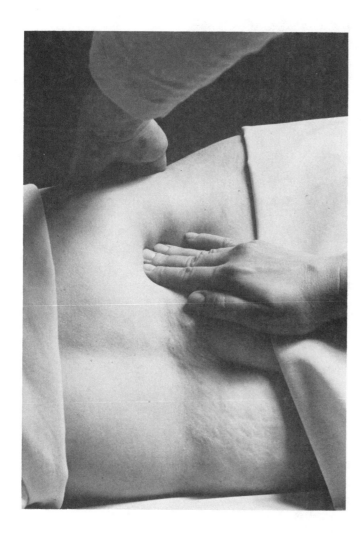

The Right Kidney. Place your left hand behind and supporting the patient's right loin, between rib cage and iliac crest. Place your right hand below the right costal margin with your fingertips pointing to the left.

Press your hands firmly together. Because of the usual posterior location of the kidneys, palpation should be deeper than when searching for the liver. As the patient takes a deep breath, try to feel the lower pole of the right kidney come down between your fingers.

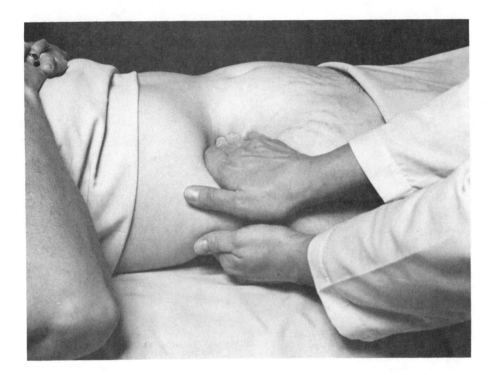

As another method of feeling the right kidney, try to "capture" it. Place your hands as before. At the peak of inspiration, press your fingers together quickly, exerting slightly more pressure above than below. Ask the patient to breathe out and then to stop breathing briefly. Slowly release the pressure of your fingers. If you have captured the kidney between your hands, you can feel it as it slips between your fingers back up into place. The patient can usually feel a capture and release, although the maneuver does not normally hurt.

If the kidney is palpable describe its size, contour, and tenderness. A right kidney, especially when located anteriorly, may be difficult to distinguish from a palpable liver. The edge of the liver tends to be sharper and to extend further medially and laterally. It cannot be captured. The lower pole of the kidney is more rounded than the usual liver edge.

Causes of kidney enlargement include hydronephrosis, neoplasm, and polycystic disease.

The Left Kidney. Use the same maneuvers. From the patient's right side, support his left loin with your left hand while your right hand palpates his anterior abdominal wall. The capture technique is more easily done from the patient's left: place your right hand behind the patient, your left in front. A normal left kidney is rarely palpable.

An enlarged left kidney may be difficult to distinguish from an enlarged spleen. A palpable notch on the medial edge of the organ favors a spleen. See Table 9-6, Steps in Splenic Enlargement (p. 257).

Although *kidney tenderness* is usually searched for posteriorly during examination of the back, thus saving the patient needless exertion, the technique will be mentioned here. Place the palm of your left hand over each costovertebral angle in turn. Strike it with the ulnar surface of your right fist. Normally the patient should perceive a jar or thud, but not pain.

Costovertebral angle tenderness suggests kidney infection.

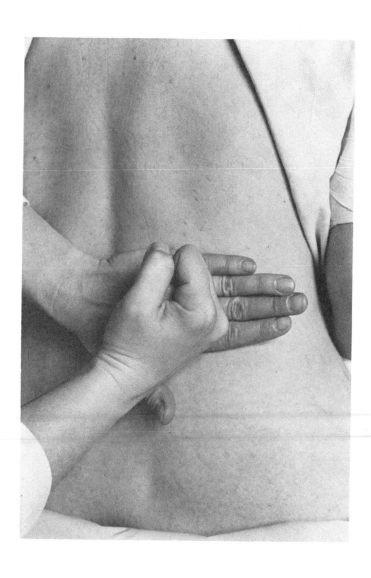

The Aorta. Press firmly deep into the upper abdomen, slightly to the left of the midline. Identify the aortic pulsation. If the pulsation is prominent, try to assess the width of the aorta and the direction of its pulsations. If the abdominal wall is relatively thick, as illustrated, press your hands deeply in the upper abdomen, one on either side of the aorta. When the abdominal wall is thin you can use one hand, the thumb on one side of the aorta and the fingers on the other side.

A prominent pulsation with lateral expansion suggests an aortic aneurysm. A normal aorta or an aorta covered by a mass transmits the pulsation forward without lateral expansion.

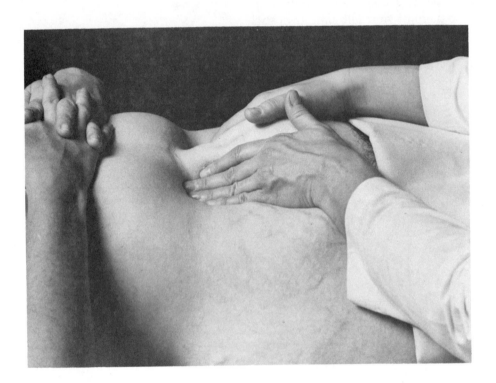

SPECIAL MANEUVERS

To Assess Possible Ascites. A protuberant abdomen with bulging flanks suggests the possibility of ascitic fluid. Since ascitic fluid characteristically sinks with gravity, percussion gives a dull note in dependent areas of the abdomen, while gas-filled loops of bowel float to the top. Look for such a pattern by percussing outward in several directions from the central area of tympany. Map the border between tympany and dullness.

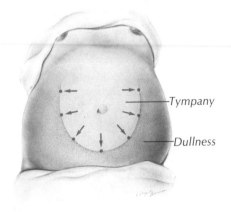

Tympany

Dullness

Two further maneuvers help to confirm the presence of ascites, although both signs may be misleading.

1. *Test for shifting dullness.* After mapping the borders of tympany and dullness, ask the patient to turn onto his side. Percuss and mark the borders again. In a person without ascites the borders between tympany and dullness usually stay relatively constant.

In ascites, dullness shifts to the more dependent side, while tympany shifts to the top.

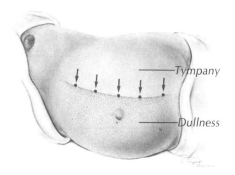

2. *Test for a fluid wave.* Ask the patient or an assistant to press the edges of his hands firmly down the midline of the abdomen. This pressure helps to stop the transmission of a wave through fat. While you tap one flank sharply with your fingertips, feel on the opposite flank for an impulse transmitted through the fluid. Unfortunately, this sign is often negative until ascites is obvious, and it is sometimes positive in people without ascites.

An easily palpable impulse suggests ascites.

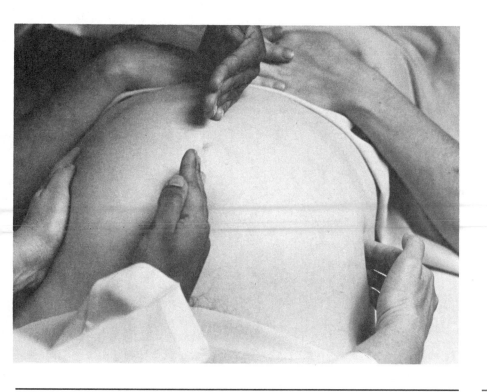

To Assess Possible Appendicitis. When the history suggests appendicitis, evaluate the patient carefully.

1. Ask the patient to point to where the pain began and where it is now.

   1. The patient with appendicitis classically points to the umbilicus, then to the right lower quadrant.

2. Search carefully for an area of local tenderness.

   2. Localized tenderness anywhere in the right lower quadrant, even in the right flank, may indicate appendicitis.

3. Feel for muscular rigidity.

   3. Early voluntary guarding may be replaced by involuntary muscular rigidity.

4. Perform a rectal examination (and also a pelvic examination in women). This maneuver may be helpful in identifying an inflamed appendix atypically located within the pelvic cavity, and also helps to identify other causes of abdominal pain. A rectal examination, however, may not discriminate well between a normal and an inflamed appendix. (These maneuvers are most conveniently done at the end of your physical assessment.)

   4. Right-sided rectal tenderness may be caused by inflamed adnexa or an inflamed seminal vesicle, for example, as well as by an inflamed appendix.

Some additional maneuvers are sometimes helpful.

5. Check the tender area for rebound tenderness. (If other signs are typically positive, you can save the patient unnecessary pain by omitting this test.)

   5. Rebound tenderness suggests peritoneal inflammation, as from appendicitis.

6. Check for Rovsing's sign and for referred rebound tenderness. Press deeply and evenly in the *left* lower quadrant. Then quickly withdraw your fingers.

   6. Pain in the *right* lower quadrant during left-sided pressure suggests appendicitis (a positive Rovsing's sign). So does right lower quadrant pain on quick withdrawal (referred rebound tenderness).

7. Look for a psoas sign. Place your hand just above the patient's right knee and ask him to flex his leg against it. Alternatively, ask him to turn on to his left side; then extend his right leg at the hip.

   7. Increased abdominal pain on either maneuver constitutes a positive psoas sign, suggesting irritation of the psoas muscle by an inflamed appendix.

8. Look for an obturator sign. Flex the patient's right thigh at the hip, with his knee bent, and rotate the leg internally at the hip.

8. Right hypogastric pain constitutes a positive obturator sign, suggesting irritation of the obturator muscle.

9. Look for cutaneous hyperesthesia. At a series of points down the abdominal wall gently pick up a fold of skin between your thumb and index finger, without pinching it. This maneuver should not normally be painful.

9. Localized pain with this maneuver, in all or part of the right lower quadrant, may accompany appendicitis.

To Distinguish an Abdominal Mass from a Mass in the Abdominal Wall.
An occasional mass is in the abdominal wall rather than inside the abdominal cavity. Ask the patient to tighten his muscles by raising his head and shoulders or by straining. Feel for the mass again.

A mass in the abdominal wall remains palpable; an intra-abdominal mass is obscured by muscular tension.

Table 9-1

Table 9-1   Abdominal Hernias and Bulges

Abdominal hernias are almost always made more evident when the patient stands or when he raises his head and shoulders from a supine position.

UMBILICAL HERNIA

In young children an umbilical hernia is centrally located. In adults it is usually partially above the umbilicus.

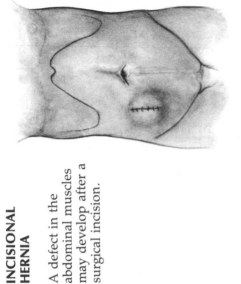

INFANT

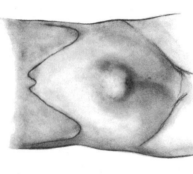

ADULT

INCISIONAL HERNIA

A defect in the abdominal muscles may develop after a surgical incision.

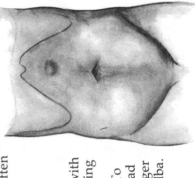

DIASTASIS RECTI

Not a true hernia, a diastasis recti is a separation of the two rectus abdominis muscles often caused by pregnancy or obesity. The increased intra-abdominal pressure produced when the patient raises his head and shoulders causes a midline ridgelike bulge. It is of no clinical consequence.

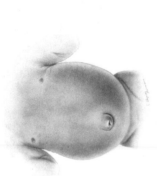

Palpable separation

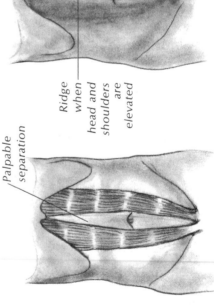

Ridge when head and shoulders are elevated

HERNIA OF THE LINEA ALBA

This is a small, often tender, midline nodule usually located in the epigastrium and best discovered with the patient standing up. Its pain may mimic an ulcer. To find it, run the pad of your index finger down the linea alba.

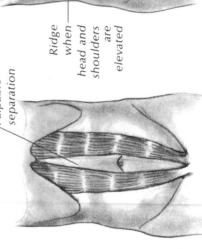

Table 9-2

Table 9-2 Protuberant Abdomens

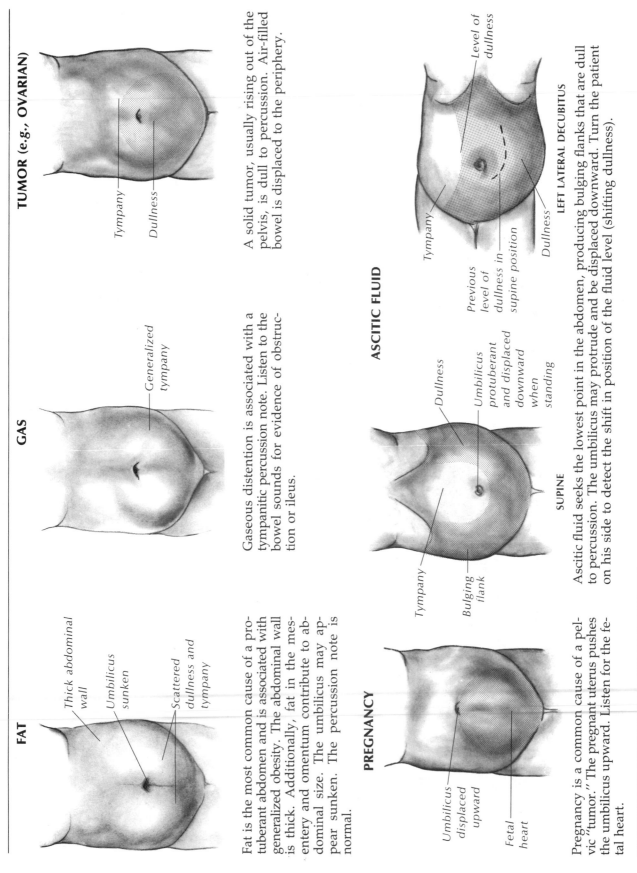

FAT

Thick abdominal wall

Umbilicus sunken

Scattered dullness and tympany

Fat is the most common cause of a protuberant abdomen and is associated with generalized obesity. The abdominal wall is thick. Additionally, fat in the mesentery and omentum contribute to abdominal size. The umbilicus may appear sunken. The percussion note is normal.

GAS

Generalized tympany

Gaseous distention is associated with a tympanitic percussion note. Listen to the bowel sounds for evidence of obstruction or ileus.

TUMOR (e.g., OVARIAN)

Tympany

Dullness

A solid tumor, usually rising out of the pelvis, is dull to percussion. Air-filled bowel is displaced to the periphery.

PREGNANCY

Umbilicus displaced upward

Fetal heart

Pregnancy is a common cause of a pelvic "tumor." The pregnant uterus pushes the umbilicus upward. Listen for the fetal heart.

ASCITIC FLUID

Dullness

Umbilicus protuberant and displaced downward when standing

Tympany

Bulging flank

SUPINE

Level of dullness

Tympany

Previous level of dullness in supine position

Dullness

LEFT LATERAL DECUBITUS

Ascitic fluid seeks the lowest point in the abdomen, producing bulging flanks that are dull to percussion. The umbilicus may protrude and be displaced downward. Turn the patient on his side to detect the shift in position of the fluid level (shifting dullness).

Table 9-3

Table 9-3 Sounds in the Abdomen

BOWEL SOUNDS

Bowel sounds may be:

1. Increased, as from diarrhea or early intestinal obstruction.
2. Decreased, then absent, as in paralytic ileus and peritonitis. Before deciding that bowel sounds are absent, sit down and listen where shown for two minutes or even longer.

High-pitched tinkling sounds suggest intestinal fluid and air under tension in a dilated bowel. Rushes of high-pitched sounds coinciding with an abdominal cramp indicate intestinal obstruction.

SYSTOLIC BRUITS

Renal artery

Aorta

Iliac artery

Systolic bruits are vascular sounds resembling cardiac murmurs. They suggest partial arterial obstruction or turbulent flow, as in an aneurysm. Do not be misled by a cardiac murmur radiating to the abdomen.

VENOUS HUM

Epigastric and umbilical

A venous hum is rare. It is a soft humming noise with both systolic and diastolic components. It indicates increased collateral circulation between portal and systemic venous systems, as in hepatic cirrhosis.

FRICTION RUBS

Hepatic

Splenic

Friction rubs are rare. They are grating sounds with respiratory variation. They indicate inflammation of the peritoneal surface of an organ as from a liver tumor, gonococcal perihepatitis, or splenic infarct. When a systolic bruit accompanies a hepatic friction rub, suspect carcinoma of the liver.

Table 9-4

Table 9-4   Tender Abdomens

ABDOMINAL WALL TENDERNESS

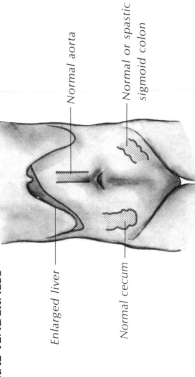

Superficial lesions

Muscle

Deep lesions

Occasionally tenderness originates from the abdominal wall, not within the abdominal cavity. Distinguish these two sources by asking the patient to raise his head and shoulders or to strain down. Tenderness of a superficial lesion persists on light palpation; tenderness of a deeper lesion decreases because of muscle guarding.

VISCERAL TENDERNESS

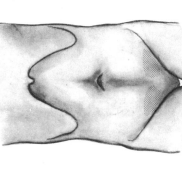

Normal aorta

Normal or spastic sigmoid colon

Enlarged liver

Normal cecum

The structures shown may be tender to deep palpation. Usually the discomfort is dull and there is no muscular rigidity or rebound tenderness. When normal structures are tender, a reassuring explanation to the patient may prove quite helpful.

TENDERNESS FROM DISEASE IN THE CHEST AND PELVIS

ACUTE PLEURISY

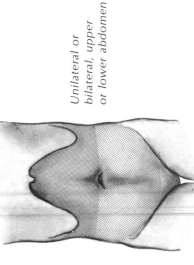

Unilateral or bilateral, upper or lower abdomen

Abdominal pain and tenderness may be secondary to acute inflammation of the pleurae. When unilateral it may mimic the findings of acute cholecystitis or even acute appendicitis. Rebound tenderness and rigidity are less common, and chest signs are usually present.

Continued

ACUTE SALPINGITIS

Frequently bilateral, the tenderness of acute salpingitis is usually maximal just above the inguinal ligaments. Rebound tenderness and rigidity may be present. On pelvic examination, motion of the uterus causes pain.

Table 9-4

Table 9-4 (Cont'd)

TENDERNESS OF PERITONEAL INFLAMMATION

Tenderness associated with peritoneal inflammation is usually more severe than visceral tenderness. Muscular rigidity and rebound tenderness are frequently but not necessarily present. Examples follow:

ACUTE CHOLECYSTITIS

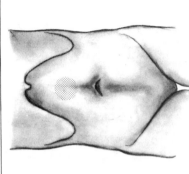

Signs are maximal in the right upper quadrant. Press your left thumb just under the right costal margin and ask the patient to take a deep breath. A sharp increase in tenderness with a sudden stop in inspiratory effort constitutes a positive Murphy's sign of acute cholecystitis.

ACUTE APPENDICITIS

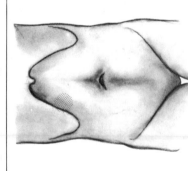

Just below the middle of a line joining the umbilicus and the anterior superior iliac spine

Right rectal tenderness

Right lower quadrant signs are typical of acute appendicitis but may be absent early in the course. The typical area of tenderness is illustrated. Explore other portions of the right lower quadrant also, as well as the right flank.

ACUTE PANCREATITIS

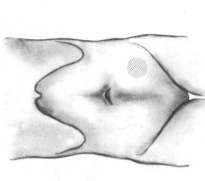

In acute pancreatitis epigastric tenderness and rebound are usually present but the abdominal wall may be soft.

ACUTE DIVERTICULITIS

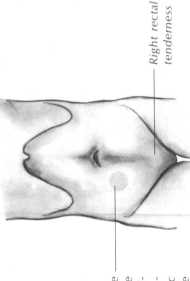

Acute diverticulitis resembles a left-sided appendicitis.

Table 9-5

Table 9-5   Liver Enlargement: Apparent and Real

Estimates of liver size should be based upon full evaluation by both percussion and palpation. A palpable liver edge does not necessarily indicate hepatomegaly.

DOWNWARD DISPLACEMENT OF THE LIVER BY A LOW DIAPHRAGM

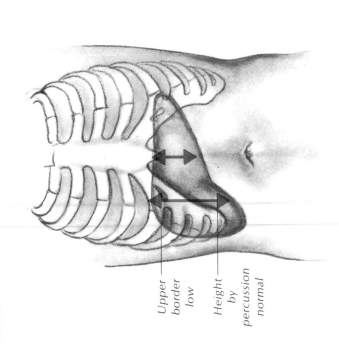

Upper border low

Height by percussion normal

This is a common finding (*e.g.*, in emphysema) where the diaphragm is low. The liver edge may be readily palpable well below the costal margin. Percussion, however, reveals a low upper edge also, and the total span or height is normal.

NORMAL VARIATIONS IN LIVER SHAPE

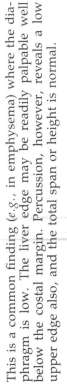

Elongated right lobe

In some persons, especially those with a lanky build, the liver tends to be somewhat elongated so that its right lobe is easily palpable as it projects downward toward the iliac crest. Such an elongation represents a variation in shape, not an increase in liver volume or size. This variant illustrates the basic limitations of assessing liver size. We can only estimate the upper and lower borders of an organ that has three dimensions and differing shapes. Some error is unavoidable.

Continued

Table 9-5

Table 9-5 (Cont'd)

SMOOTH NONTENDER LIVER

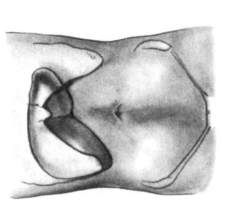

Cirrhosis may produce an enlarged liver with a firm nontender edge. The liver is not always enlarged in this condition, however, and many other diseases may produce similar findings.

SMOOTH TENDER LIVER

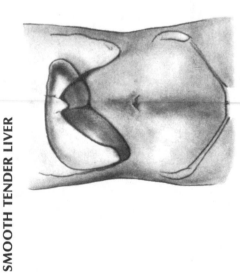

An enlarged liver with a smooth tender edge suggests inflammation, as in hepatitis, or venous congestion, as in right-sided heart failure.

IRREGULAR LIVER

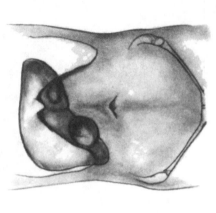

An enlarged liver that is firm or hard and that presents an irregular edge or surface suggests malignancy. There may be a single or multiple nodules. The liver may or may not be tender.

Table 9-6

Table 9-6   Steps in Splenic Enlargement

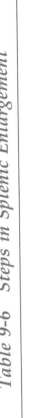

1. Normal splenic dullness (10th rib posterior to the midaxillary line). This may enlarge.

2. The first sign of splenomegaly may be a change from normal tympany to splenic dullness as an enlarged spleen descends toward the costal margin on deep inspiration. For this sign, percuss in the lowest interspace in the anterior axillary line.

3. The spleen tip then becomes palpable on inspiration below the left costal margin.

4. A markedly enlarged spleen descends into the left lower quadrant. A notch can frequently be felt along its medial border and may be helpful in distinguishing this organ from an enlarged left kidney.

5. A massively enlarged spleen may extend across the midline.

Chapter 10
MALE GENITALIA AND HERNIAS

Anatomy and Physiology

Review the anatomy of the male genitalia.

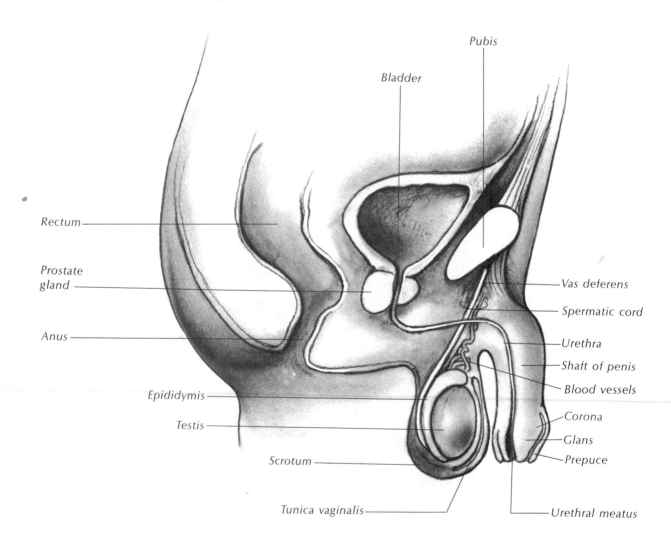

The shaft of the penis is formed by three columns of vascular erectile tissue bound together by fibrous tissue. At the end of the penis is the cone-shaped glans with its expanded base, or corona. Unless the person has been circumcised, the glans is covered by a loose, hoodlike fold of skin called the prepuce, or foreskin. The urethra is located ventrally in the shaft of the penis, within one of the vascular columns, and urethral abnormalities may sometimes be felt here. The urethra opens into the vertical, slitlike urethral meatus, located somewhat ventrally at the tip of the glans.

The scrotum is a loose, wrinkled pouch divided into two compartments, each of which contains a testicle. The testes are ovoid, somewhat rubbery structures, about 4.5 cm long in the adult, with a range from 3.5 cm to 5.5 cm. The left usually lies somewhat lower than the right. On the posterolateral surface of each testis is the softer, comma-shaped epididymis. It is most prominent along the superior margin of the testis. (The epididymis may be located anteriorly in 6% to 7% of males.) Surrounding the testis, except posteriorly, is the tunica vaginalis, a serous membrane enclosing a potential cavity.

The vas deferens, a cordlike structure, begins at the tail of the epididymis, ascends within the scrotal sac, and passes through the external inguinal ring on its way to the abdomen and pelvis. Behind the bladder it is joined by the duct from the seminal vesicle and enters the urethra within the prostate gland. Sperm thus pass from the testis and the epididymis through the vas deferens into the urethra. In its course through the scrotum the vas is closely associated with blood vessels, nerves, and muscle fibers, with which it makes up the spermatic cord.

Lymphatics from the penile and scrotal surfaces drain into the inguinal nodes. When you find an inflammatory or possibly malignant lesion on these surfaces, assess the inguinal nodes especially carefully for enlargement or tenderness. The lymphatics of the testes, however, drain into the abdomen, where enlarged nodes are clinically undetectable. See page 308 for further discussion of the inguinal nodes.

Since hernias are relatively common, it is important to understand the anatomy of the groin. The basic landmarks are the anterior superior iliac spine, the pubic tubercle, and the inguinal ligament which runs between them. Find these on yourself or a colleague.

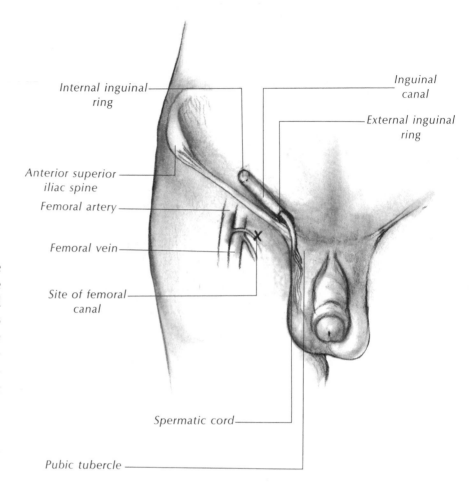

Internal inguinal ring

Inguinal canal

External inguinal ring

Anterior superior iliac spine

Femoral artery

Femoral vein

Site of femoral canal

Spermatic cord

Pubic tubercle

The inguinal canal, which lies above and approximately parallel to the inguinal ligament, forms a tunnel for the vas deferens as it passes through the abdominal muscles. The exterior opening of the tunnel—the external inguinal ring—is a triangular slitlike structure palpable just above and lateral to the pubic tubercle. The internal opening of the canal—or internal inguinal ring—is about 1 cm above the midpoint of the inguinal ligament. Neither canal nor internal ring is palpable through the abdominal wall. When loops of bowel force their way through weak areas of the inguinal canal they produce inguinal hernias, as illustrated on page 271.

Another potential route for a herniating mass is the femoral canal. This lies below the inguinal ligament. Although you cannot see it, you can estimate its location by placing your right index finger, from below, on the right femoral artery. Your middle finger will then overlie the femoral vein; your ring finger, the femoral canal. Femoral hernias protrude here.

CHANGES WITH AGE

Important anatomic changes in the male genitalia accompany puberty and help to define its progress. A noticeable increase in the size of the testes constitutes the first reliable sign and usually begins between the ages of 9.5 years and 13.5 years. Next, pubic hair appears and the penis begins to grow. The complete change from preadolescent to adult form requires about 3 years, with a range from less than 2 years to almost 5 years.

Sex Maturity Ratings in Boys

In assigning SMRs in boys, observe each of the three characteristics separately because they may develop at different rates. Record two separate ratings: pubic hair and genital. If the penis and testes differ in their stages, average the two into a single figure for the genital rating.

| | PUBIC HAIR | GENITAL | |
		PENIS	TESTES AND SCROTUM
STAGE 1	Preadolescent—no pubic hair except for the fine body hair (vellus hair) similar to that on the abdomen	Preadolescent—same size and proportions as in childhood	Preadolescent—same size and proportions as in childhood
STAGE 2	Sparse growth of long, slightly pigmented, downy hair, straight or only slightly curled, chiefly at the base of the penis	Slight or no enlargement	Testes larger; scrotum larger, somewhat reddened, and altered in texture
STAGE 3	Darker, coarser, curlier hair spreading sparsely over the pubic symphysis	Larger, especially in length	Further enlarged
STAGE 4	Coarse and curly hair, as in the adult; area covered greater than in stage 3 but not as great as in the adult and not yet including the thighs	Further enlarged in length and breadth, with development of the glans	Further enlarged; scrotal skin darkened
STAGE 5	Hair adult in quantity and quality, spread to the medial surfaces of the thighs but not up over the abdomen	Adult in size and shape	Adult in size and shape

(Illustrations through the courtesy of W.A. Daniel, Jr, Division of Adolescent Medicine, University of Alabama, Birmingham)

By observing the pubic hair and the development of the penis, testes, and scrotum, you can assess sexual development according to the five stages described by Tanner. These are outlined and illustrated above.

In about 80% of men, pubic hair spreads further up the abdomen in a triangular pattern pointing toward the umbilicus. Because this kind of spread, known as stage 6, is not completed until the mid-20s or later, however, it is not considered a pubertal change.

An average developmental sequence is diagrammed below. Note the rather wide age ranges for the start and completion of pubertal changes. Some normal boys may have completed their genital development while others of the same age have not yet begun. Boys often begin to experience ejaculation as they approach SMR 3, and sometimes mistake nocturnal emissions for the discharge of venereal disease. Discussion and explanation are indicated.

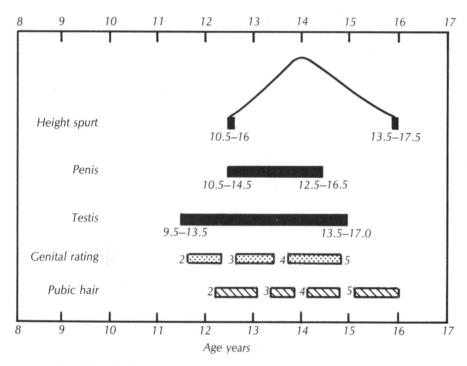

Numbers below the bars indicate the ranges in age within which certain changes occur. (Redrawn from Marshall WA, Tanner JM: Variations in the pattern of pubertal changes in boys. Arch Dis Child 45:22, 1970)

In elderly patients pubic hair may decrease and become gray. The penis decreases in size and the testicles hang lower in the scrotum. Although the testes often decrease in size with protracted, debilitating illnesses, they do not necessarily decrease with aging *per se.*

Techniques of Examination

GENERAL APPROACH

Many students—especially women but also men—feel anxious about examining a man's genitalia. "How will the patient react?" "Will he have an erection?" "Will he let me examine him?" These feelings are normal, and it is often helpful to talk them through with your instructor or another experienced clinician. In fact, a male patient, regardless of who examines him, does occasionally have an erection, though not very often, and is probably more embarrassed about it than you are. You should explain to him that this is a normal response, finish your examination, and proceed on with an unruffled demeanor. Occasionally, too, a man may refuse to be examined by a woman just as a woman sometimes refuses to allow a man to do a pelvic examination. Your own comfort with the procedures will minimize these difficulties, but you should respect the patient's wishes and rights. A male colleague can check a male patient, just as a female colleague can examine a woman, if the patient wants it that way.

A good genital examination can be done with the patient either standing or supine. To check for hernias or varicoceles, however, the patient should stand, and you should sit comfortably on a chair or stool. A gown conveniently covers the patient's chest and abdomen. If you suspect an infectious process, wear gloves. Expose the genitalia and groins.

ASSESSMENT OF SEXUAL DEVELOPMENT

Assess sexual maturation by noting the size and shape of the penis and testes, the color and texture of the scrotal skin, and the character and distribution of the pubic hair.

Make two separate sex maturity ratings according to Tanner's stages: one for pubic hair, the other for genital development. If a boy's testes have increased in size to 2.5 cm or more, or if his pubic hair has reached stage 2, you can tell him that his sexual development has started. You may also use Tanner's diagrams to show your patient how he is developing, to review the wide range of normals for his age, and to answer any questions he may have.

If no testicular increase has occurred by 13.5 years of age and if pubic hair has not reached stage 2, *puberty* may be considered *delayed*, although it is not necessarily abnormal. Delay is also suggested if the boy has not reached stage 3 within 4 years of reaching stage 2. *Puberty* may be considered *precocious* if it starts before age 9 or 9.5 years.

THE PENIS

INSPECTION

Inspect the penis, including:

See Table 10-1, Abnormalities of the Penis (p. 268).

1. The skin

2. The prepuce or foreskin. If present, retract it or ask the patient to retract it. This step is essential for the detection of many chancres and carcinomas. A cheesy, whitish material called smegma may normally accumulate under the foreskin.

Phimosis is a tight prepuce that cannot be retracted over the glans. Paraphimosis is a tight prepuce that, once retracted, gets caught behind the glans and cannot be returned. Edema ensues.

3. The glans

Look for any ulcers, scars, nodules, or signs of inflammation.

Balanitis (inflammation of the glans); balanoposthitis (inflammation of the glans and prepuce)

Check the skin around the base of the penis for excoriations or inflammation. Look for nits or lice at the bases of the pubic hairs.

Pubic or genital excoriations suggest the possibility of lice (crabs) or sometimes scabies.

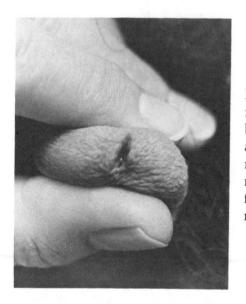

Note the location of the urethral meatus. Compress the glans gently between your index finger above and your thumb below. This maneuver should open the urethral meatus and allow you to inspect it for discharge. Normally there is none.

The discharge of gonococcal urethritis tends to be profuse and yellow, while that of nongonococcal urethritis tends to be scanty and white or clear. Definitive diagnosis, however, requires a Gram stain and culture.

If the patient has reported a discharge but you do not see any, ask him to strip, or milk, the shaft of the penis from its base to the glans. Alternatively, do it yourself. This maneuver may bring some discharge out of the urethral meatus for appropriate examination. Have a glass slide and culture materials ready.

PALPATION

Palpate any abnormality of the penis, noting any tenderness or induration. Palpate the shaft of the penis between your thumb and first two fingers, noting any induration. Palpation of the shaft may be omitted in a young asymptomatic male patient.

If you retracted the foreskin, replace it before proceeding on to the scrotum.

Induration along the ventral surface of the penis suggests a urethral stricture or possibly a carcinoma. Tenderness of such an indurated area suggests periurethral inflammation secondary to a urethral stricture.

THE SCROTUM

INSPECTION

Inspect the contour of the scrotum, noting any lumps or swelling. Inspect the scrotal skin, noting any nodules, ulcers, excoriations, or signs of inflammation. Lift up the scrotum so that you can see its posterior surface as well.

Tender, painful scrotal swellings occur in acute epididymitis, acute orchitis, torsion of the spermatic cord, and strangulated hernia. See Table 10-2, Abnormalities in the Scrotum (pp. 269–270).

PALPATION

Between your thumb and first two fingers palpate each testis and epididymis.

If one or possibly both testicles are not palpable, consider cryptorchidism (undescended testicles). The scrotum on the involved side is poorly developed. Try to find the testicle within the scrotum or within the inguinal canal (see also p. 497).

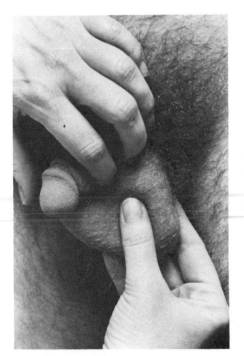

Note their size, shape, consistency, and tenderness; feel for any nodules. Pressure on the testis normally produces a deep visceral pain.

Identify each spermatic cord with its vas deferens, and palpate it between your thumb and fingers along its course from epididymis to superficial inguinal ring.

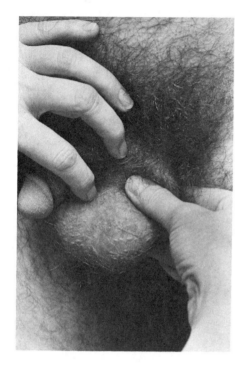

Note any nodules or swellings.

Any swelling in the scrotum other than the testicles should be evaluated by transillumination. After darkening the room, shine the beam of a strong flashlight from behind the scrotum through the mass. Look for transmission of the light as a red glow.

Swellings containing serous fluid transilluminate (*i.e.*, light up with a red glow); those containing blood or tissue do not.

HERNIAS

INSPECTION

Inspect the inguinal and femoral areas carefully for bulges. While you continue your observation, ask the patient to strain down.

A bulge that appears on straining suggests a hernia.

PALPATION

Using in turn your right hand for the patient's right side and your left hand for the patient's left side, invaginate loose scrotal skin with your index finger. Start at a point low enough to ensure full mobility of your finger. This may be the bottom of the scrotal sac. Follow the spermatic cord upward to the triangular slitlike opening of the external inguinal ring. This is just above and lateral to the pubic tubercle. If the ring is somewhat enlarged, it may admit your index finger. If possible, gently follow the inguinal canal laterally in its oblique course. With your finger located either at the external ring or within the canal, ask the patient to strain down or cough. Note any palpable herniating mass as it touches your finger.

See Table 10-3, Course and Presentation of Hernias in the Groin (p. 271).

See Table 10-4, Differentiation of Hernias in the Groin (p. 272).

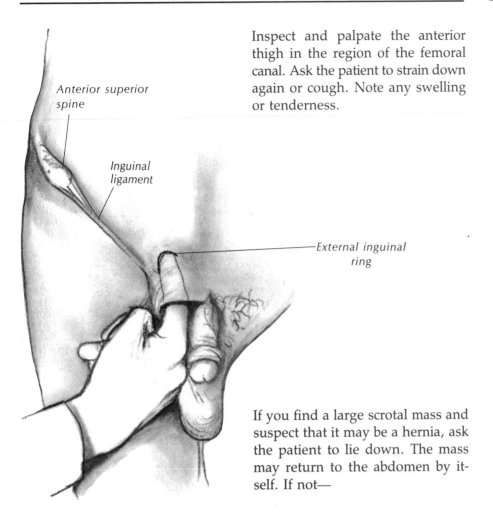

Anterior superior spine

Inguinal ligament

External inguinal ring

Inspect and palpate the anterior thigh in the region of the femoral canal. Ask the patient to strain down again or cough. Note any swelling or tenderness.

If you find a large scrotal mass and suspect that it may be a hernia, ask the patient to lie down. The mass may return to the abdomen by itself. If not—

1. Can you get your fingers above the mass in the scrotum?

2. Listen to the mass with a stethoscope for bowel sounds.

If you can, suspect a hydrocele.

Bowel sounds may be heard over a hernia, but not over a hydrocele.

If the findings suggest a hernia, gently try to reduce it (return it to the abdominal cavity) by sustained pressure with your fingers. Do not attempt this maneuver if the mass is tender or the patient reports nausea and vomiting.

History may be helpful here. The patient can usually tell you what happens to his swelling on lying down and may demonstrate how he reduces it himself. Remember to ask him.

A hernia is *incarcerated* when its contents cannot be returned to the abdominal cavity. A hernia is *strangulated* when the blood supply to the entrapped contents is compromised. Suspect strangulation in the presence of tenderness, nausea, and vomiting.

Table 10-1

Table 10-1 Abnormalities of the Penis

HYPOSPADIAS

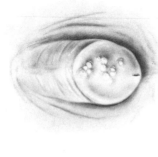

SYPHILITIC CHANCRE

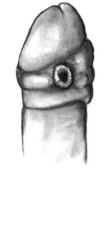

GENITAL HERPES

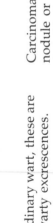

Hypospadias is a congenital displacement of the urethral meatus to the inferior surface of the penis. A groove extends from the actual urethral meatus to its normal location on the tip of the glans.

A syphilitic chancre presents as an oval or round, dark red, painless erosion or ulcer with an indurated base. It feels like a button just beneath the skin. Nontender enlarged inguinal lymph nodes are usually associated.

A cluster of small vesicles, followed by shallow, painful, nonindurated ulcers on red bases, suggests a herpes simplex infection. The lesions may occur anywhere on the penis. Recurrent infections usually have fewer lesions than the first one.

VENEREAL WART
(Condyloma acuminatum)

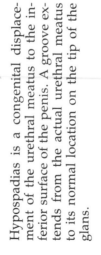

CARCINOMA OF THE PENIS

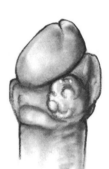

PEYRONIE'S DISEASE

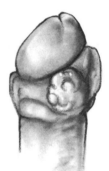

A variant of the ordinary wart, these are rapidly growing warty excrescences.

Carcinoma may present as an indurated nodule or ulcer that is usually nontender. Limited almost completely to men who are not circumcised in childhood, it may be masked by the prepuce. Any persistent penile sore must be considered suspicious.

In Peyronie's disease the patient has palpable nontender hard plaques just beneath the skin, usually along the dorsum of the penis. He complains of crooked, painful erections.

Table 10-2

Table 10-2 Abnormalities in the Scrotum

HYDROCELE

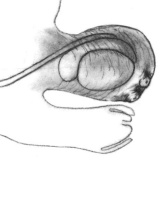

Fingers can get above mass

A hydrocele is a nontender, fluid-filled mass that occupies the space within the tunica vaginalis. The examining fingers can get above the mass within the scrotum. The mass transilluminates.

SCROTAL HERNIA

Fingers cannot get above mass

A hernia located within the scrotum is usually an indirect inguinal hernia. Since it comes through the external inguinal ring, the examining fingers cannot get above it in the scrotum.

TUMOR OF THE TESTIS

EARLY

A tumor of the testis usually presents as a painless nodule. It does not transilluminate. Any nodule within the testis must raise the suspicion of malignancy.

LATE

As a testicular neoplasm grows and spreads, it may seem to replace the entire organ. The testicle characteristically feels heavier than normal.

SPERMATOCELE OR CYST OF THE EPIDIDYMIS

A painless, movable cystic mass just above the testis, a spermatocele or cyst of the epididymis transilluminates.

VARICOCELE

A varicocele consists of varicose veins of the spermatic cord, usually occurring on the left. It feels like a soft "bag of worms." It is separate from the testis and epididymis and slowly collapses when the scrotum is elevated in the supine position.

TUBERCULOUS EPIDIDYMITIS

The chronic inflammation of tuberculosis produces a firm enlargement of the epididymis, sometimes tender, with thickening or beading of the vas deferens.

SEBACEOUS CYSTS

These are firm, yellowish, nontender, cutaneous cysts up to about 1 cm in diameter. They are common and frequently multiple.

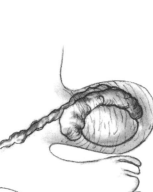
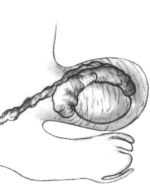
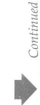

Continued

Table 10-2

Table 10-2 (Cont'd)

ACUTE ORCHITIS

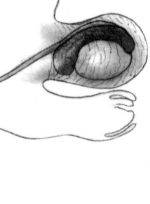

An acutely inflamed testis is painful, tender, and swollen. The testis may be difficult to distinguish from the epididymis. The scrotum may be reddened. Look for evidence of post-pubertal mumps or other less common infectious causes.

SMALL TESTIS

Adult testes are considered small when they are less than 3.5 cm long. Small firm testes (usually less than 2 cm long) suggest Klinefelter's syndrome. Small soft testes suggest atrophy, associated with several conditions (*e.g.,* cirrhosis, myotonia dystrophica, administration of estrogens, and hypopituitarism). Atrophy may also follow orchitis (*e.g.,* from mumps).

ACUTE EPIDIDYMITIS

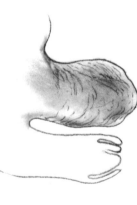

An acutely inflamed epididymis is tender and swollen and may be difficult to distinguish from the testis. The scrotum may be reddened, and the vas deferens may also be inflamed. Epididymitis occurs chiefly in adults. Coexisting urinary tract infection or prostatitis supports the diagnosis.

EMPTY SCROTAL HALF

The testis and epididymis may be absent. Check the inguinal canal and upper scrotum for an undescended testicle.

TORSION OF THE SPERMATIC CORD

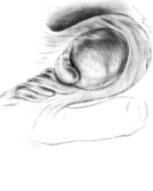

Torsion, or twisting, of the testicle on its spermatic cord produces an acutely painful, tender, and swollen organ that is retracted upward in the scrotum. The scrotum becomes red and edematous. There is no associated urinary infection. Torsion, most common in adolescents, is a surgical emergency because of obstructed circulation.

SCROTAL EDEMA

The scrotal skin may become taut with pitting edema. Scrotal edema is usually associated with generalized edema (*e.g.,* cardiac or nephrotic).

Table 10-3

Table 10-3   Course and Presentation of Hernias in the Groin

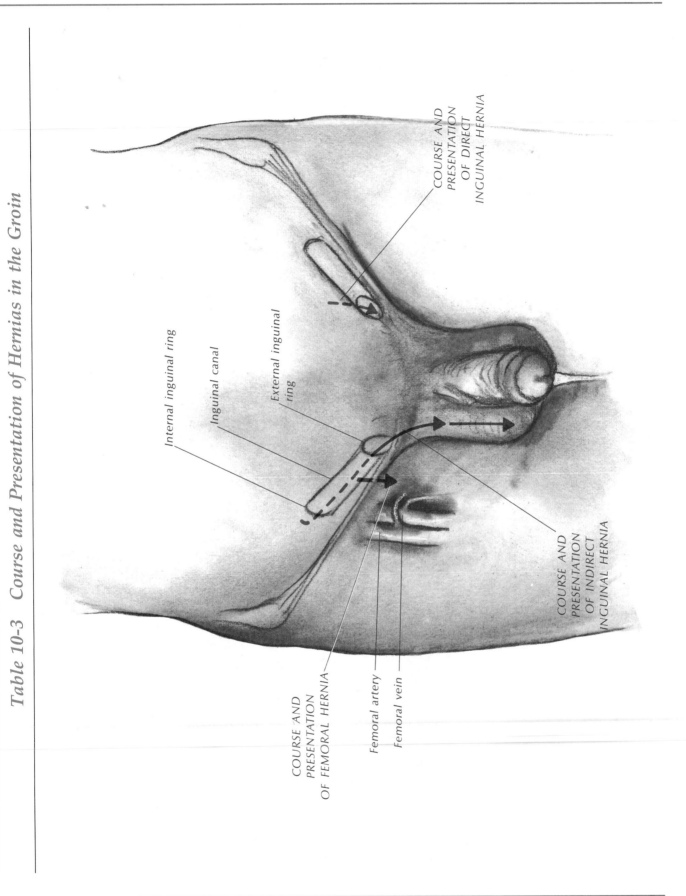

COURSE AND PRESENTATION OF DIRECT INGUINAL HERNIA

Internal inguinal ring

Inguinal canal

External inguinal ring

COURSE AND PRESENTATION OF FEMORAL HERNIA

Femoral artery

Femoral vein

COURSE AND PRESENTATION OF INDIRECT INGUINAL HERNIA

Table 10-4

Table 10-4 Differentiation of Hernias in the Groin

Differentiation between these hernias is not always clinically possible. Understanding their features, however, improves your observation.

FEATURES	INGUINAL		FEMORAL
	INDIRECT	**DIRECT**	
FREQUENCY	Most common, all ages, both sexes	Less common	Least common
AGE AND SEX	Often in children, may be in adults	Usually men over age 40, rare in women	More common in women than in men
POINT OF ORIGIN	Above inguinal ligament, near its midpoint (the internal inguinal ring)	Above inguinal ligament, close to the pubic tubercle (near the external inguinal ring)	Below the inguinal ligament, appears more lateral than an inguinal hernia and may be hard to differentiate from lymph nodes
COURSE	Often into the scrotum	Rarely into the scrotum	Never into the scrotum
(With the examining finger in the inguinal canal during straining or cough)	Hernia comes down the inguinal canal and touches the fingertip.	Hernia bulges anteriorly and pushes the side of the finger forward.	The inguinal canal is empty.

Chapter 11
FEMALE GENITALIA

Anatomy and Physiology

Review the anatomy of the external female genitalia, or vulva, including the mons pubis, a hair-covered fat pad overlying the symphysis pubis; the labia majora, rounded folds of adipose tissue; the labia minora, thinner pinkish red folds that extend anteriorly to form the prepuce; and the clitoris. The vestibule refers to the boat-shaped fossa between the labia minora. In its posterior portion lies the vaginal opening or introitus, which in virgins may be hidden by the hymen. The term perineum, as commonly used clinically, refers to the tissues between the introitus and anus.

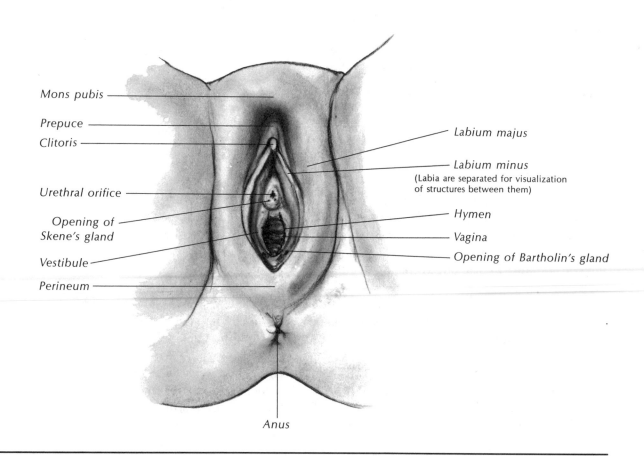

Mons pubis

Prepuce

Clitoris

Urethral orifice

Opening of Skene's gland

Vestibule

Perineum

Labium majus

Labium minus
(Labia are separated for visualization of structures between them)

Hymen

Vagina

Opening of Bartholin's gland

Anus

The urethral orifice opens into the vestibule between the clitoris and vagina. Just posterior to it on either side can sometimes be discerned the openings of the paraurethral or Skene's glands. The openings of Bartholin's glands are located posteriorly, on either side of the vaginal opening, but are not usually visible. Bartholin's glands themselves are situated more deeply.

The vagina is a hollow tube extending between urethra and rectum upward and back. It terminates in the cup-shaped fornix. At almost right angles to it sits the uterus, a flattened, pear-shaped, fibromuscular structure. Its cervix protrudes into the vagina, dividing the fornix into anterior, posterior, and lateral fornices. A round or slitlike depression, the external os of the cervix, marks the opening into the endocervical canal and uterine cavity.

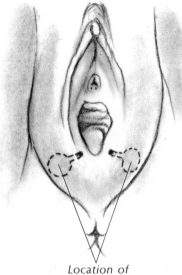

Location of
Bartholin's gland

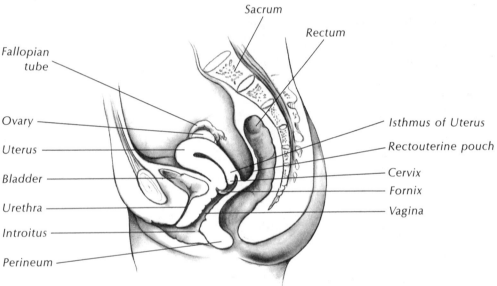

CROSS SECTION, SIDE VIEW

The upper part of the uterus is called the body or fundus; the area between the body and cervix is the isthmus. From each side of the fundus extends a fallopian tube. The fringed, funnel-shaped end of each tube curves toward the ovary. Each ovary is an almond-shaped structure, varying considerably in size but averaging about 3.5 × 2 × 1.5 cm.

Both ovaries and tubes are supported by peritoneal folds called ligaments. Neither these ligaments nor the tubes, however, are normally palpable. The term adnexa refers to the ovaries, tubes, and supporting tissues.

As in the male (see p. 297) the peritoneal surface becomes accessible to the examining finger just anterior to the rectum—beyond the posterior fornix of the vagina in the rectouterine pouch (also called the pouch of Douglas or cul-de-sac).

Lymph from the vulva and the lower third of the vagina drains to the inguinal nodes, but that from the internal genitalia, including the upper third of the vagina, flows into pelvic and abdominal lymph nodes which are not palpable clinically. Lymph from the middle third of the vagina can go in either direction. When you see a lesion of the vulva or the lower two thirds of the vagina, examine the inguinal nodes especially carefully for enlargement or tenderness.

CHANGES WITH AGE

During the pubertal years the vulva and internal genitalia grow and change to their adult proportions. Assessment of sexual maturity in girls, as classified by Tanner, depends not on internal examination, however, but on the growth of pubic hair and the development of breasts. Tanner's stages, or sex maturity ratings, as they relate to pubic hair are shown below; those relating to breasts are shown on page 212.

Sex Maturity Ratings in Girls: Pubic Hair

STAGE 1 Preadolescent—no pubic hair except for the fine body hair (vellus hair) similar to that on the abdomen

STAGE 2

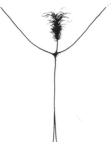

STAGE 3

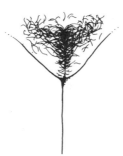

Sparse growth of long, slightly pigmented, downy hair, straight or only slightly curled, chiefly along the labia

Darker, coarser, curlier hair, spreading sparsely over the pubic symphysis

STAGE 4

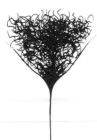

STAGE 5

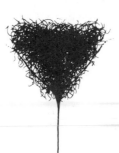

Coarse and curly hair as in adults; area covered greater than in stage 3 but not as great as in the adult and not yet including the thighs

Hair adult in quantity and quality, spread on the medial surfaces of the thighs but not up over the abdomen

---

(Illustrations through the courtesy of W.A. Daniel, Jr, Division of Adolescent Medicine, University of Alabama, Birmingham)

A girl's first sign of puberty is usually the appearance of breast buds. Sometimes, however, pubic hair appears first. On the average these changes start at around 11 years of age, with a range from 8 to 13 years for breast buds, 8 to 14 years for pubic hair. The transformation from preadolescent to adult form takes about 3 years, with a range of 1.5 to 6 years. Menarche tends to occur during breast stage 3 or 4, at ages ranging from 10 to 16.5 years. These figures are summarized in the diagram below.

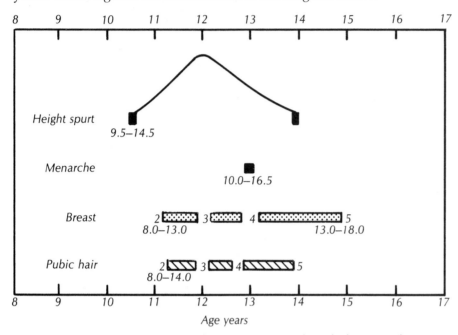

Numbers below the bars indicate the ranges in age within which certain changes occur. (Redrawn from Marshall WA, Tanner JM: Variations in the pattern of pubertal changes in boys. Arch Dis Child 45:22, 1970)

As in boys, there is a wide range of normal. Some girls may have completed the development of their secondary sex characteristics while others of the same age have not yet begun.

In 10% or more of women pubic hair spreads further up the abdomen in a triangular pattern, pointing toward the umbilicus. This spread can be classified as stage 6 but, because it is usually not completed until the mid-20s or later, it is not considered a pubertal change.

Just before menarche there is a physiologic increase in vaginal secretion—a normal change that sometimes worries a girl or her mother. As menses become established, increased secretions, or leukorrhea, coincide with ovulation. They also accompany sexual arousal. These normal kinds of discharges must be differentiated from those of infectious processes.

Ovarian function usually starts to diminish during a woman's 40s, and menstrual periods cease on the average between ages 48 and 51, with a range from about age 40 to age 55. Pubic hair becomes sparse as well as gray. With the decline of estrogenic stimulus the labia and clitoris become smaller. The vagina narrows and shortens and its mucosa becomes thin, pale, and dry. The uterus and ovaries diminish in size.

Techniques of Examination

GENERAL APPROACH

Most students feel anxious, embarrassed, or uncomfortable when first examining the genitalia of another person. These feelings are normal, and it may be useful to talk them through with your instructor or another experienced clinician. At the same time, patients bring to the examination their own concerns. Some women have had painful, embarrassing, or even demeaning experiences during previous examinations while others, especially adolescents, may be facing with apprehension their first examination. A patient's reactions and behavior give you important clues to these feelings and to her attitudes toward sexuality. If she adducts her thighs, pulls away, or expresses negative feelings during the examination, you can gently confront her as you would during the interview. "I notice you are having some trouble relaxing . . . or seem disgusted . . . . Is it just being here or is it the same way at home . . . or during intercourse . . . ?" Behavior that seems to present an annoying obstacle to your examination may become the key to understanding your patient's problem.

Getting the patient to relax is essential for an adequate pelvic examination. Sensitivity to her feelings may help here. In addition,

1) Ask the patient to empty her bladder before the examination.
2) Drape her appropriately. Some patients are more comfortable when drapes cover their thighs and knees. Others prefer to watch both the practitioner and the examination itself and object to drapes that obscure their view. A girl or woman may wish to use a mirror to see her own genitalia during the examination. Ask the patient which method she prefers.
3) The patient's arms should be at her sides or folded across her chest—not over her head, since this last position tends to tighten the abdominal muscles.
4) Explain in advance each step of the examination and tell the patient what she may feel. Avoid any sudden or unexpected movements. When beginning palpation or using a speculum, it may be helpful to make initial contact not on the genitalia themselves but on the upper inner thigh.
5) Have warm hands and a warm speculum.
6) Monitor your examination when possible by watching the patient's face. Depressing the center of the drape onto the patient's abdomen allows you to maintain eye contact while you are seated.
7) Finally, of course, be as gentle as possible.

Wear a glove on the hand you use for internal examination or, if you suspect an infectious process, on both hands. During the bimanual examination, an ungloved abdominal hand makes palpation easier.

Equipment. You should have within reach a good light, a vaginal speculum of appropriate size, and materials for bacteriologic cultures and Papanicolaou smears. Specula are made of metal or plastic and come in two basic shapes. Graves specula are usually best for sexually active women. They are available in small, medium, and large sizes. The narrow-bladed Pedersen speculum is useful for a patient with a relatively small introitus, such as a virgin or an elderly woman, and is often more comfortable for other patients as well.

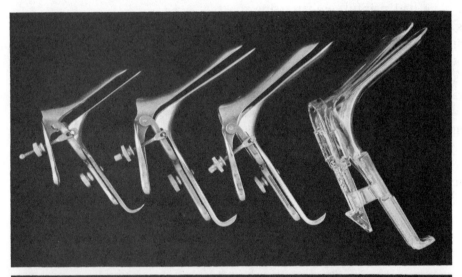

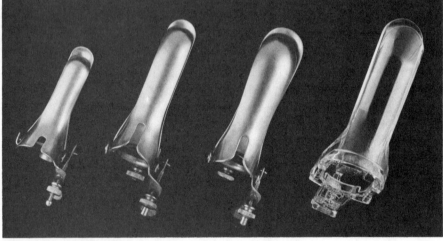

Specula, from left to right: small metal Pedersen, medium metal Pedersen, medium metal Graves, and large plastic Pedersen

Before using a speculum become thoroughly familiar with how to open and close its blades, lock the blades in an open position, and release them again. Although the instructions in this chapter refer to a metal speculum, you can easily adapt them to a plastic one by handling the speculum before using it. Plastic specula typically make a loud click when locked or released. Forewarning the patient about this click helps to avoid unnecessary surprise.

Male examiners are customarily attended by female assistants. Female examiners may or may not prefer to work alone but should be similarly attended if the patient is emotionally disturbed.

Position. Drape the patient appropriately, then assist her into the lithotomy position. Help her to place first one heel, then the other, into the stirrups. She may be more comfortable with shoes on than with bare feet. Then ask her to move toward the end of the examining table until her buttocks extend slightly beyond the edge. Her thighs should be flexed and abducted. A pillow should support her head.

EXTERNAL EXAMINATION

Assess the Sexual Maturity of an Adolescent Patient. If an adolescent girl is not sexually active and if there is no reason to suspect a problem in the genital area, you will probably choose not to do a pelvic examination. You can then assess pubic hair in conjunction with your abdominal examination rather than placing her in a lithotomy position. In any case, note the character and distribution of pubic hair and rate it according to Tanner's stages described on page 275. See page 212 for staging of breast development.

If neither pubic hair nor breast development is seen by age 13, *puberty* may be considered *delayed*.

Inspect the Patient's External Genitalia. Seat yourself comfortably and inspect the mons pubis, labia, and perineum. With your gloved hand, separate the labia and inspect:

Excoriations or itchy, small, red maculopapules suggest pediculosis pubis (lice or crabs). Look for nits or lice at the bases of the pubic hairs.

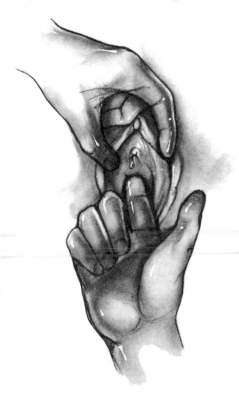

The labia minora

The clitoris

Enlarged clitoris in masculinizing conditions

The urethral orifice

The vaginal opening or introitus

See Table 11-1, Lesions of the Vulva (p. 286).
Syphilitic chancre, sebaceous cyst

Note any inflammation, ulceration, discharge, swelling, or nodules. If there are any lesions, palpate them.

If urethritis or inflammation of Skene's glands (*e.g.*, from gonorrhea) is suspected, insert your index finger into the vagina and milk the urethra gently from inside outward. Note any discharge from or about the urethral orifice. If present, culture it.

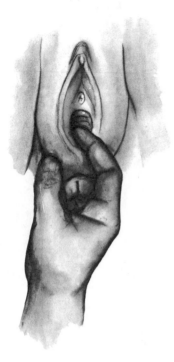

If there is a history or appearance of labial swelling, check Bartholin's glands. Insert your index finger into the vagina near the posterior end of the introitus. Place your thumb outside the posterior part of the labium majus. On each side in turn palpate between your finger and thumb for swelling or tenderness. Note any discharge exuding from the duct opening of the gland. If present, culture it.

Assess the Support of the Vaginal Outlet. With the labia separated by your middle and index finger, ask the patient to strain down. Note any bulging of the vaginal walls.

See Table 11-2, Bulges and Swellings of Vulva and Vagina (p. 287).

Cystocele and rectocele

INTERNAL EXAMINATION

Insert the Speculum. Select a speculum of appropriate size and shape, and lubricate and warm it with warm water. (Other lubricants may interfere with cytological or other studies but may be used if no such tests are planned.) By having your speculum ready during assessment of the vaginal outlet, you can ease speculum insertion and increase your efficiency by proceeding to this next maneuver while the patient is still straining down.

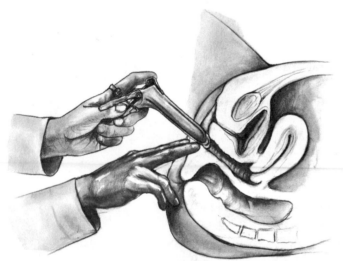

Place two fingers just inside or at the introitus and gently press down on the perineal body. With your other hand introduce the closed speculum past your fingers at a 45° angle downward. The blades should be held obliquely and the pressure exerted toward the posterior vaginal wall in order to avoid the more sensitive anterior wall and urethra. Be careful not to pull on the pubic hair nor to pinch the labia with the speculum.

After the speculum has entered the vagina, remove your fingers from the introitus. Rotate the blades of the speculum into a horizontal position, maintaining the pressure posteriorly.

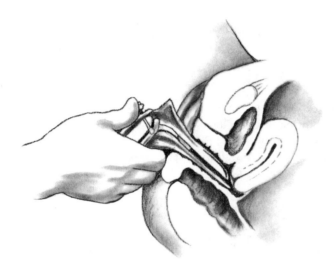

Inspect the Cervix. Open the blades after full insertion and maneuver the speculum so that the cervix comes into full view.

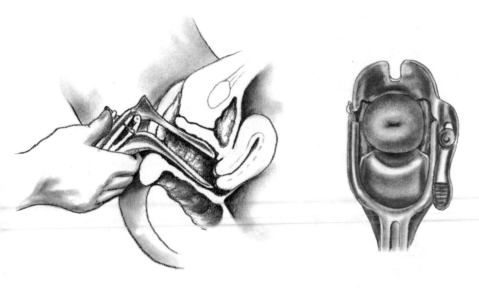

When the uterus is retroverted, the cervix points more anteriorly than diagrammed. Position the speculum more anteriorly (*i.e.*, more horizontally) in order to bring the cervix into view.

Inspect the cervix and its os. Note the color of the cervix, its position, any ulcerations, nodules, masses, bleeding, or discharge.

Secure the speculum with the blades open by tightening the thumb screw.

Purplish color in pregnancy

See Table 11-3, Variations and Abnormalities of the Cervix (pp. 288–289).

Obtain Specimens for Cervical Cytology (Papanicolaou smears). Specimens from three sites are described here. Clinicians and pathologists vary in their preferences as to the numbers and sites of cytologic specimens. All agree on a cervical scrape, and most recommend one or both of the other two methods.

1. *The Endocervical Swab.* Insert the end of a cotton applicator stick into the cervical os. Roll it between your thumb and index finger, clockwise and counterclockwise. Remove it. Smear a glass slide with the cotton swab, gently, in a painting motion. (Rubbing hard on the slide will destroy the cells.) Either place the slide into an ether-alcohol fixative at once, or spray it promptly with a special fixative.

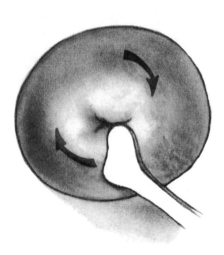

2. *Cervical Scrape.* Place the longer end of the scraper into the os of the cervix. Press, turn, and scrape. Smear on a second slide as before.

3. *Vaginal Pool.* Roll a cotton applicator stick on the floor of the vagina below the cervix. Prepare a third slide as before. If the vaginal mucosa is dry, as it may be in an elderly woman, for example, moisten the cotton tip with saline before gathering the specimen.

If the cervix has been removed, do a vaginal pool and a scrape from the cuff of the vagina.

Inspect the Vagina. Withdraw the speculum slowly while observing the vagina. As the speculum clears the cervix, release the thumb screw and maintain the speculum in its open position with your thumb. Close the blades as the speculum emerges from the introitus, avoiding both excessive stretching and pinching of the mucosa. During withdrawal inspect the vaginal mucosa, noting its color and any inflammation, discharge, ulcers, or masses.

See Table 11-4, Inflammations of and Around the Vagina (pp. 290–291).

Cancer of the vagina

Perform a Bimanual Examination. From a *standing position* introduce the index and middle finger of your gloved and lubricated hand into the vagina, again exerting pressure primarily posteriorly. Your thumb should be abducted, your ring and little fingers flexed into your palm. Note any nodularity or tenderness in the vaginal wall, including the region of the urethra and bladder anteriorly.

Identify the cervix, noting its position, shape, consistency, regularity, mobility, and tenderness. Normally the cervix can be moved somewhat without pain. Palpate the fornix around the cervix.

See Table 11-5, Changes in Pregnancy (p. 292).

Pain on movement of the cervix, together with adnexal tenderness, suggests pelvic inflammatory disease.

Place your abdominal hand about midway between the umbilicus and symphysis pubis and press downward toward the pelvic hand. Your pelvic hand should be kept in a straight line with your forearm, with inward pressure exerted on the perineum by your flexed fingers. Support and stabilize your arm by resting your elbow either on your hip or on your knee, which is elevated by placing your foot on a stool. Identify the uterus between your hands and note its size, shape, consistency, and mobility. Note any tenderness or masses.

See Table 11-6, Abnormalities and Displacements of the Uterus (pp. 293–294).

Uterine enlargement suggests pregnancy or benign or malignant tumors.

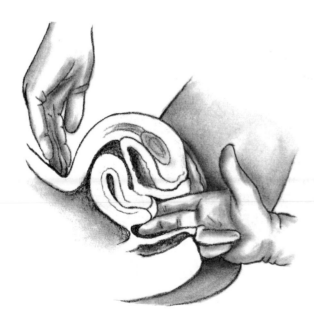

Place your abdominal hand on the right lower quadrant, your pelvic hand in the right lateral fornix. Maneuver your abdominal hand downward and, using your pelvic hand for palpation, identify the right ovary and any masses in the adnexa.

VIEW FROM THE RIGHT SIDE

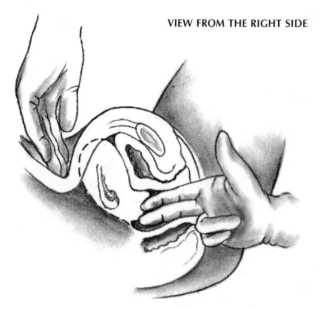

Three to five years after menopause the ovaries have usually atrophied and are no longer palpable. If you can feel an ovary in a postmenopausal woman, suspect an ovarian tumor.

Note the size, shape, consistency, mobility,and tenderness of any palpable organs or masses. (The normal ovary is somewhat tender.) Repeat the procedure on the left side.

See Table 11-7, Adnexal Masses (p. 295).

Withdraw your fingers. Lubricate your gloves again if necessary. (See note below on using lubricant.) Then slowly reintroduce your index finger into the vagina, your middle finger into the rectum. Ask the patient to strain down as you do this so that her anal sphincter will relax. Tell her

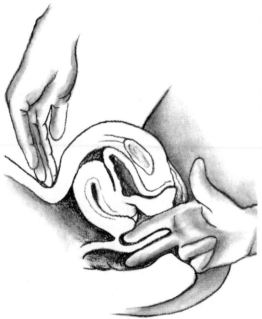

that this examination may make her feel as if she has to move her bowels—but she will not. Repeat the maneuvers of the bimanual examination, giving special attention to the region behind the cervix that may be accessible only to the rectal finger. In addition, try to push the uterus backward with your abdominal hand so that your rectal finger can explore as much of the posterior uterine surface as possible.

Proceed to the rectal examination (see Chap. 12). After your examination, wipe off the external genitalia and anus or offer the patient some tissue with which to do it herself.

A Note on the Small Introitus. Many virginal vaginal orifices will readily admit a single examining finger. Modify your technique so as to use your index finger only. A small Pedersen speculum or even a nasal speculum may make inspection possible. When the vaginal orifice is even smaller, a fairly good bimanual examination can be performed by placing one finger in the rectum rather than in the vagina.

An imperforate hymen occasionally delays menarche. Be sure to check for this possibility when menarche seems unduly late in relation to the development of a girl's breasts and pubic hair.

Similar techniques may be indicated in elderly women in whom the introitus has become tight.

A Note on Using Lubricant. When performing either a pelvic or rectal examination, you should never contaminate the tube of lubricant by touching it with your gloved hand after touching the patient. Develop the following habit: Always allow the lubricant to drop onto your gloved fingers without touching the tube with your fingers.

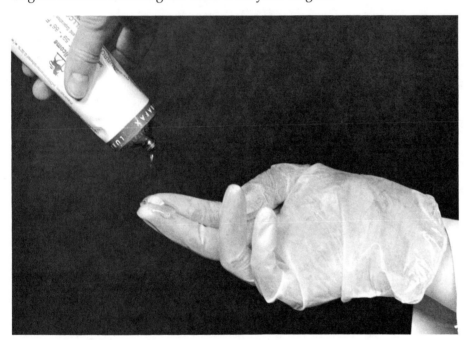

If you should accidentally contaminate the tube, discard it. Small disposable tubes for use with one patient circumvent this problem.

The Risk of Spreading Infection Between Vagina and Rectum. Gonorrhea may infect the rectum as well as the female genitalia. This fact, together with the rising prevalence of gonorrhea, has led to the recommendation that gloves be changed between vaginal and rectal examination in order to avoid spreading gonococcal infection. In order to avoid fecal soiling, gloves should always be changed if for some reason the practitioner examines the vagina after the rectum.

Table 11-1

Table 11-1 Lesions of the Vulva

SEBACEOUS CYST

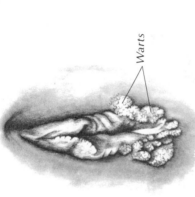

Cystic nodule in skin

Small, firm, round cystic nodules in the labia suggest sebaceous cysts. They are sometimes yellowish in color. Look for the dark punctum marking the blocked opening of the gland.

VENEREAL WART
(Condyloma Acuminatum)

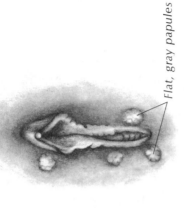

Warts

Warty lesions on the labia and within the vestibule suggest condylomata acuminata. Like warts elsewhere, they are reactions to a viral infection.

SECONDARY SYPHILIS
(Condyloma Latum)

Flat, gray papules

Slightly raised, flat, round or oval papules, covered by a gray exudate, suggest condylomata lata. These constitute one manifestation of secondary syphilis and are contagious.

SYPHILITIC CHANCRE

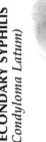

A firm, painless ulcer suggests the chancre of primary syphilis. Since most chancres in women develop internally, they often go undetected.

HERPES INFECTION

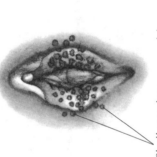

Shallow ulcers on red bases

Shallow, small, painful ulcers on red bases suggest a herpes infection. Initial infection may be extensive, as illustrated here. Recurrent infections are usually confined to a small local patch.

CARCINOMA OF THE VULVA

An ulcerated or raised red vulvar lesion in an elderly woman may indicate vulvar carcinoma.

Table 11-2

Table 11-2   Bulges and Swellings of Vulva and Vagina

CYSTOCELE

A cystocele is present when the anterior wall of the vagina, together with the bladder above it, bulges into the vagina and sometimes out the introitus. Look for the bulging vaginal wall as the patient strains down.

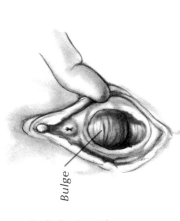

Bulge

RECTOCELE

Bulge

A rectocele is formed by the anterior and downward bulging of the posterior vaginal wall together with the rectum behind it. To identify it, spread the patient's labia and ask her to strain down.

INFLAMMATION OF BARTHOLIN'S GLAND

Inflammation of Bartholin's glands may be acute or chronic. It is commonly but not necessarily caused by gonococcal infection. Acutely, it presents as a tense, hot, very tender abscess. Look for pus coming out of the duct or erythema around the duct opening. Chronically, a nontender cyst occupies the posterior labium. It may be large or small.

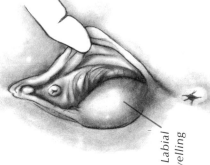

Labial swelling

URETHRAL CARUNCLE

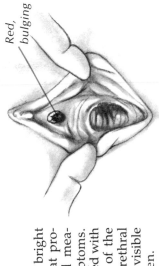

Red, bulging

A urethral caruncle is a bright red, polypoid growth that protrudes from the urethral meatus. Most cause no symptoms. A caruncle may be confused with simple outward pouting of the posterior aspect of the urethral mucosa, which is often visible in postmenopausal women.

Table 11-3 Variations and Abnormalities of the Cervix

NORMAL NULLIPAROUS CERVIX

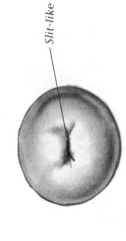

Round or oval

The nulliparous cervical os is small and either round or oval. The cervix is covered by smooth pink epithelium.

NORMAL PAROUS CERVIX

Slit-like

After childbirth, the cervical os presents a slitlike appearance.

LACERATIONS OF THE CERVIX

UNILATERAL TRANSVERSE

BILATERAL TRANSVERSE

STELLATE

The trauma of difficult deliveries may tear the cervix, producing permanent transverse or stellate lacerations.

Continued

Table 11-3

Table 11-3 (Cont'd)

ECTROPION (EROSION)

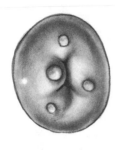

The mucosa around the central os is at times a plush red rather than the usual shiny pink. It may bleed easily when touched. This appearance is usually due to an ectropion (*i.e.,* the presence of columnar epithelium like that lining the cervical canal). An ectropion is not abnormal but may be difficult to distinguish from early carcinoma without further study (*e.g.,* by cytology, colposcopy, or biopsy). The term erosion is also used for this condition but is misleading because the mucosa has not actually been eroded away.

NABOTHIAN OR RETENTION CYSTS

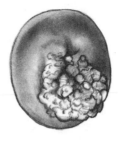

Retention or nabothian cysts may accompany or follow chronic cervicitis. Variable in size, single or multiple, they appear as translucent nodules on the cervical surface.

CERVICAL POLYP

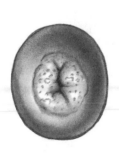

Cervical polyps usually arise from the endocervical canal, becoming visible when they protrude through the cervical os. They are bright red, soft, and rather fragile. When only the tips are seen they cannot be clinically differentiated from polyps originating in the endometrium.

CARCINOMA OF THE CERVIX

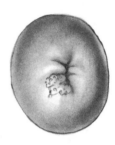
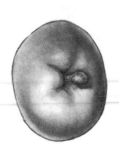

Carcinoma of the cervix usually begins at or near the cervical os. It presents a hard granular surface which bleeds easily, proceeding later to an extensive irregular cauliflower type of growth. Early carcinomas are clinically indistinguishable from ectropions and may even be present in a cervix that appears normal.

Table 11-4

Table 11-4 Inflammations of and Around the Vagina

	TRICHOMONAS VAGINITIS*	MONILIA (CANDIDA) VAGINITIS*
	Red spots / Inflamed mucosa	White patches / Inflamed mucosa
DISCHARGE	Thin or thick; white, yellowish, or green; often bubbly; often pooled in the vaginal fornix; profuse; malodorous	May be thin but is characteristically thick, white, and curdy; not so profuse as in Trichomonas vaginitis
VULVA	May be reddened, especially the vestibule and labia minora. Pruritus, though possibly present, is not usually so severe as in Monilia infection.	Often reddened, itchy, sometimes swollen, varying in extent from the vestibule alone to extension outward to involve the labia and the skin around them. Vulvar changes may occur without vaginal inflammation.
URETHRITIS	Usually absent, but a Trichomonas urethrocystitis occurs occasionally.	Absent
BARTHOLIN'S GLAND INFECTION	Absent	Absent
VAGINAL MUCOSA	In acute infection the mucosa is red, inflamed, with red granular or petechial spots in the fornix. In mild or chronic infections the mucosa may look normal.	In severe cases red, inflamed, with white or grayish, often tenacious patches of discharge. May bleed when plaques of discharge are scraped off. In mild cases the vaginal mucosa may look normal.
CERVIX	May show red spots ("strawberry" spots)	May show patches of discharge

*Many patients present less typical signs. Definitive diagnosis depends on identification of the causative organism.

Continued

Table 11-4

Table 11-4 (Cont'd)

	EARLY GONORRHEA*	NONSPECIFIC VAGINITIS (Associated with Gardnerella [Corynebacterium] Vaginalis)	ATROPHIC VAGINITIS (Associated with Aging)
	Purulent exudate from os; Urethritis and Skene's gland infection; Bartholin's gland infection		Small introitus; Small cervix; Atrophic mucosa
DISCHARGE	Greenish yellow	Gray, thin, homogeneous, malodorous, occasionally somewhat frothy; not so profuse as in Trichomonas or Monilia infections	Variable in color, consistency, and amount. May be whitish, gray, yellow, green, or blood-tinged; thick or watery; rarely profuse
VULVA	Often inflamed	Usually normal	Atrophic
URETHRITIS	Often present. The urethral orifice is red and swollen. Pus may be milked from the urethra and sometimes from Skene's glands.	Absent	Absent
BARTHOLIN'S GLAND INFECTION	May be present	Absent	Absent
VAGINAL MUCOSA	Usually normal in the adult	Usually normal; occasionally may be red or swollen	Atrophic, dry, pale, though may become reddened and develop petechiae, ecchymoses, and superficial erosions. May show filmy adhesions. Bleeds easily.
CERVIX	May be inflamed; pus exudes from os	Normal	Small

*Many patients present less typical signs. Definitive diagnosis depends on identification of the causative organism.

Table 11-5

Table 11-5   Changes in Pregnancy

6th WEEK FROM THE LAST MENSTRUAL PERIOD

3rd THROUGH 10th MONTHS

(Read from the bottom up.)

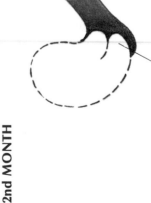

The height of the fundus drops slightly during the 10th month as the fetus settles deeper into the pelvis in preparation for labor and delivery.

Fetal movements become palpable after the 5th month and fetal parts may be discernible.

By the 5th month the fundus is at the level of the umbilicus. The fetal heart becomes audible, giving the first absolute proof of pregnancy obtainable by physical examination. Listen for it at this stage just above the symphysis pubis.

By the 3rd month, the uterus has become globular in shape and first rises above the symphysis pubis.

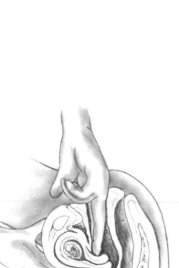

The isthmus of the uterus softens. Its soft consistency contrasts with the firm cervix below and the somewhat doughy or elastic uterus above. This phenomenon is called Hegar's sign. It is the first clinical manifestation of pregnancy but is not absolutely diagnostic. The uterine fundus tends to feel more globular and may become asymmetrical at the site of fetal implantation.

2nd MONTH

Soft and purplish

The cervix itself softens. In consistency it begins to resemble lips rather than a nose. Its color and that of the adjacent vaginal mucosa become purplish.

Table 11-6

Table 11-6   Abnormalities and Displacements of the Uterus

PROLAPSE OF THE UTERUS

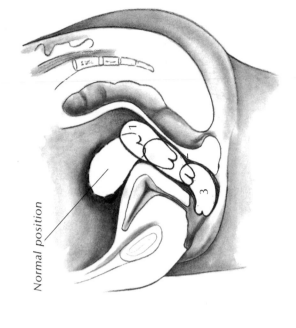

Normal position

Prolapse of the uterus results from weakness of the supporting structures of the pelvic floor and is often associated with a cystocele and rectocele. In progressive stages the uterus becomes retroverted and descends down the vaginal canal to the outside. In first degree prolapse the cervix is still well within the vagina. In second degree, it is at the introitus. In third degree prolapse, also called procidentia uteri, the cervix and vagina are outside the introitus.

MYOMAS OF THE UTERUS (FIBROIDS)

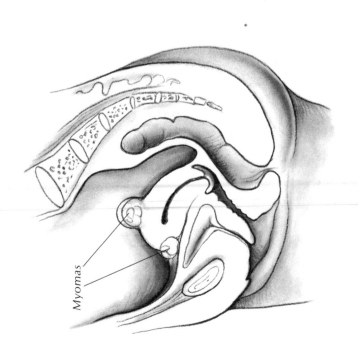

Myomas

Myomas are very common, benign, uterine tumors. They may be single or multiple and vary greatly in size, occasionally reaching massive proportions. They present as firm, irregular nodules in continuity with the uterine surface. Occasionally a myoma projecting laterally can be confused with an ovarian mass; a nodule projecting posteriorly can be mistaken for a retroflexed fundus. Submucous myomas project toward the endometrial cavity and are not themselves palpable, although they may be suspected because of an enlarged uterus.

Continued

Table 11-6

Table 11-6 (Cont'd)

RETROVERSION OF THE UTERUS

MODERATE

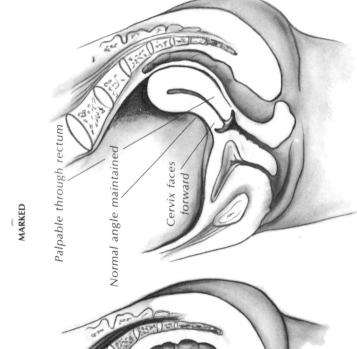

Fundus may not be palpable

Retroversion of the uterus refers to a tilting backward of the entire uterus, including both body and cervix. It is a common variant, occurring in about 1 out of 5 women. In moderate degrees of retroversion the fundus may not be accessible to either examining hand.

MARKED

Palpable through rectum

Normal angle maintained

Cervix faces forward

In marked retroversion, the fundus may often be felt through the rectum. The cervix faces forward rather than back.

RETROFLEXION OF THE UTERUS

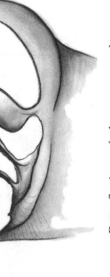

May be palpable through rectum

Angled back

Retroflexion of the uterus refers to a backward angulation of the body of the uterus in relationship to the cervix. The cervix maintains its usual position. The fundus may be palpable through the anterior rectal wall. This position is a variant of normal.

Table 11-7

Table 11-7   Adnexal Masses

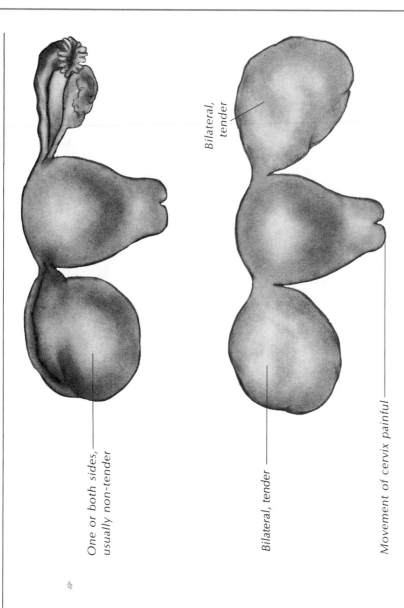

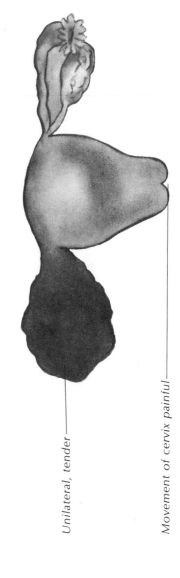

Bilateral, tender

One or both sides, usually non-tender

Bilateral, tender

Movement of cervix painful

Unilateral, tender

Movement of cervix painful

OVARIAN CYSTS AND TUMORS

Ovarian cysts and tumors may be detected as adnexal masses on one or both sides. Later they may grow up out of the pelvis. Cysts tend to be smooth and compressible, tumors more solid and often nodular. Uncomplicated cysts and tumors are not usually tender.

PELVIC INFLAMMATORY DISEASE

Acute pelvic inflammatory disease is associated with very tender, bilateral adnexal masses, although pain and muscle spasm usually make it impossible to delineate them. Movement of the cervix produces pain. *Chronic* pelvic inflammatory disease is manifested by bilateral, tender, usually irregular, and fairly fixed adnexal masses.

RUPTURED TUBAL PREGNANCY

Typically a ruptured tubal pregnancy presents with signs of hemorrhage into the peritoneal cavity: marked pelvic tenderness, and tenderness and rigidity of the lower abdomen. Motion of the cervix produces pain. A tender, unilateral adnexal mass may indicate the site of the pregnancy. Tachycardia and shock reflect the hemorrhage.

Chapter 12

THE ANUS AND RECTUM

Anatomy and Physiology

The gastrointestinal tract terminates in a short segment, the anal canal. Its external margin is poorly demarcated, but generally the skin of the anal canal can be distinguished from the surrounding perianal skin by its moist, hairless appearance. The anal canal is normally held in a closed position by action of the voluntary external muscular sphincter and the involuntary internal sphincter, the latter an extension of the muscular coat of the rectal wall.

The direction of the anal canal on a line roughly between anus and umbilicus should be carefully noted. Unlike the rectum above it the canal is liberally supplied by somatic sensory nerves, so that a poorly directed finger or instrument will produce pain.

The anal canal is demarcated from the rectum superiorly by a serrated line marking the change from skin to mucous membrane. This anorectal junction (often called the pectinate or dentate line) also denotes the boundary between somatic and visceral nerve supplies. It is readily visible on proctoscopic examination but is not palpable.

Above the anorectal junction, the rectum balloons out and turns posteriorly into the hollow of the coccyx and sacrum, forming almost a right angle with the anal canal. In the male, the prostate gland is palpable anteriorly as a rounded, heart-shaped structure about 2.5 cm in length. Its two lateral lobes are separated by a shallow median sulcus or groove. The seminal vesicles, shaped like rabbit ears above the prostate, are not normally palpable.

Through the anterior wall of the female rectum the uterine cervix can usually be felt.

The rectal wall contains three inward foldings, called *valves of Houston*. The lowest of these can sometimes be felt, usually on the patient's left.

Most of the rectum that is accessible to digital examination does not have a peritoneal surface. The anterior rectum usually does, however, and you may reach it with the tip of your examining finger. You may thus be able to identify the tenderness of peritoneal inflammation or the nodularity of peritoneal metastases.

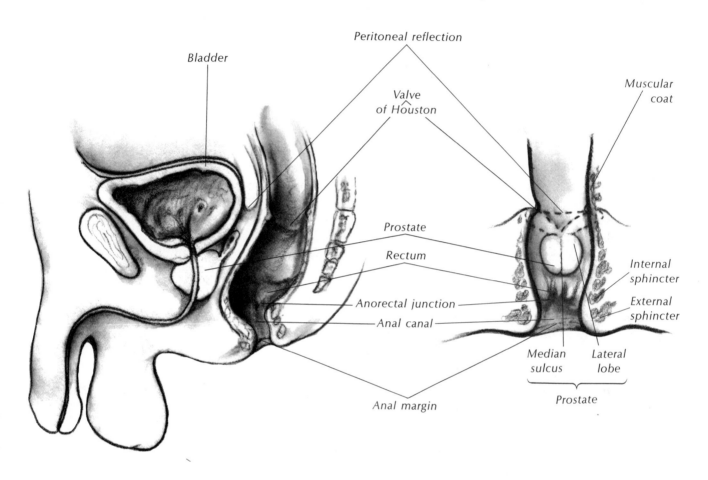

CROSS SECTION, SIDE VIEW

ANTERIOR WALL

ANUS AND RECTUM—MALE

Techniques of Examination

For most patients the rectal examination is probably the least popular segment of the entire physical examination. It may cause discomfort for the patient, perhaps embarrassment, but, if skillfully done, should not be truly painful in most circumstances. Although you may choose to omit a rectal examination in adolescents who have no relevant complaints, you should do one in adult patients. In middle-aged and older persons omission risks missing an asymptomatic carcinoma. A successful examination requires gentleness, slow movement of your finger, a calm demeanor, and an explanation to the patient of what he or she may feel.

MALE

The anus and rectum may be examined with the patient in one of several positions. For most purposes, the side-lying position is satisfactory and allows good visualization of the perianal and sacrococcygeal areas. This is the position described below. If you suspect a cancer high in the rectum, the lithotomy position may help to bring it into reach. By placing your opposite hand on the patient's abdomen you can also perform a bimanual examination in this position, thus delineating a pelvic mass. Some clinicians prefer to examine a patient while he stands with his hips flexed and his upper body resting across the examining table.

Ask the patient to lie on his left side with his buttocks close to the edge of the examining table near you. He should flex his legs at hips and knees. Drape the patient appropriately and adjust the lighting for good visualization of the anus and surrounding area. Put a glove on your right hand. With your left hand spread the buttocks apart.

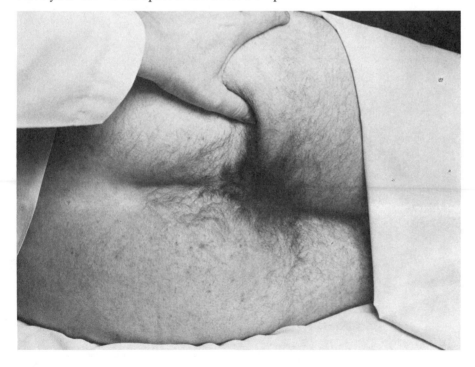

Inspect the sacrococcygeal and perianal areas for lumps, ulcers, inflammation, rashes, or excoriations. Adult perianal skin is normally more pigmented and somewhat coarser than the skin over the buttocks. Palpate any abnormal areas, noting lumps or tenderness.

Swollen, thickened, fissured skin with excoriations in pruritus ani

Tenderness of a perianal abscess

Lubricate your gloved index finger, explain to the patient what you are going to do, and tell him that the examination may make him feel as if he were moving his bowels but that he will not do so. Ask him to strain down. Inspect the anus, noting any lesions.

Venereal warts, syphilitic chancres, anal herpes, and, rarely, anal carcinoma

As the patient strains, place the pad of your lubricated and gloved index finger over the anus. As the sphincter relaxes, gently insert your fingertip into the anal canal, in a direction pointing toward the umbilicus.

See Table 12-1, Abnormalities of the Anus, Surrounding Skin, and Rectum (pp. 301–302).

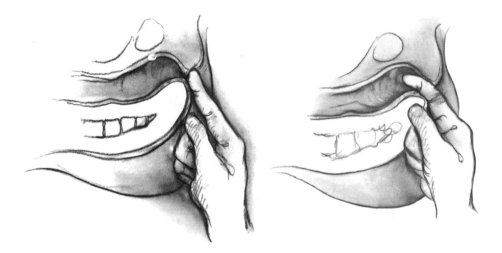

If you feel the sphincter tighten, pause, reassure the patient, and, when in a moment the sphincter relaxes, proceed. Occasionally an acutely tender lesion such as an anal fissure prevents you from completing your examination. Do not try to force it. Local anesthesia or consultation may be necessary.

Note:

The sphincter tone of the anus. Normally the muscles of the anal sphincter close snugly around your finger.
Tenderness
Irregularities or nodules

Sphincter tightness in anxiety, inflammation, or scarring; laxity in some neurological diseases

Insert your finger farther into the rectum so that you can examine as much of the rectal wall as possible. Palpate in sequence the right lateral, posterior, and left lateral surfaces, noting any nodules or irregularities.

Then turn your hand so that your finger can examine the anterior surface and the prostate gland. Tell the patient that you are going to feel his prostate gland and that it may make him want to urinate but he will not. Identify the lateral lobes of the prostate and the median sulcus between them. Note the size, shape, and consistency of the prostate, feel for any nodules, and note any tenderness.

See Table 12-2, Abnormalities of the Prostate (p. 303).

If possible, extend your finger above the prostate to the region of the seminal vesicles and peritoneal cavity. Note nodules or tenderness.

Rectal lesions just beyond your fingertip can sometimes be felt by asking the patient to strain down again. Use this maneuver if there is any suspicion of cancer.

Gently withdraw your finger, and wipe the patient's anus or give him tissues to do it himself. Note the color of any fecal matter on your glove, and test it for occult blood.

FEMALE

The rectum is usually examined after the female genitalia, while the patient is in the lithotomy position. This position is essential for bimanual palpation. If a rectal examination alone is indicated, the lateral position offers a satisfactory alternative and affords much better visualization of the perianal and sacrococcygeal areas.

The technique is basically similar to that described for males. The cervix is usually readily felt through the anterior rectal wall. Sometimes a retroverted uterus is also palpable. Neither of these, nor a tampon, should be mistaken for a tumor.

Table 12-1

Table 12-1 Abnormalities of the Anus, Surrounding Skin, and Rectum

PILONIDAL CYST AND SINUS

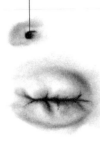

— Location

A pilonidal cyst is a fairly frequent, probably congenital abnormality located in the midline superficial to the coccyx or lower sacrum. It is clinically identified by the opening of a sinus tract. This opening may exhibit a small tuft of hair and be surrounded by a halo of erythema. Although pilonidal cysts are generally asymptomatic, except perhaps for slight drainage, abscess formation and secondary sinus tracts may complicate the picture.

Continued

ANORECTAL FISTULA

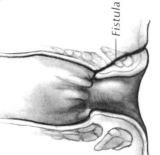

— Fistula

— Opening

An anorectal fistula is an inflammatory tract or tube that opens at one end into the anus or rectum and at the other end onto the skin surface (as shown here) or into another viscus. An abscess usually antedates such a fistula. Look for the fistulous opening or openings anywhere in the skin around the anus.

ANAL FISSURE

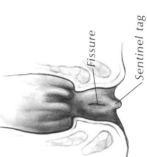

— Fissure

— Sentinel tag

An anal fissure is a very painful oval ulceration of the anal canal, most commonly found in the midline posteriorly, less commonly in the midline anteriorly. Its long axis lies longitudinally. Inspection may reveal a "sentinel" skin tag just below it, and gentle separation of the anal margins may reveal the lower edge of the fissure. The sphincter is spastic; the examination painful. Local anesthesia may be required.

Table 12-1

Table 12-1 (Cont'd)

EXTERNAL HEMORRHOID

Hemorrhoids are varicose veins. External hemorrhoids originate below the anorectal line and are covered by anal skin. When uncomplicated they may not be visible at rest, but a thrombosed hemorrhoid presents as a painful, bluish, shiny, ovoid mass at the anal margin. Flabby or fibrotic skin tags may mark the location of previously thrombosed or inflamed hemorrhoids.

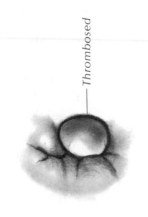

Thrombosed

INTERNAL HEMORRHOID

Internal hemorrhoids originate above the anorectal junction and are covered by mucous membrane, not skin. They are not visible unless they prolapse through the anus, nor are the soft swellings normally identifiable by palpation. Proctoscopic examination is usually required for diagnosis.

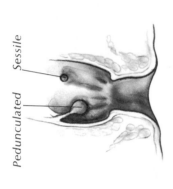

Soft

PROLAPSE OF THE RECTUM

On straining for a bowel movement the rectal mucosa, with or without its muscular wall, may prolapse through the anus, presenting as a doughnut or rosette of red mucosa. A prolapse involving only mucosa is shown here. When the entire bowel wall is involved the prolapse is larger, and circular rather than radiating folds are seen.

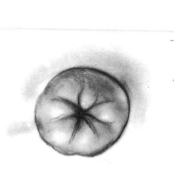

POLYPS OF THE RECTUM

Polyps of the rectum are fairly common. Varying considerably in size and number, they can develop on a stalk (pedunculated) or lie close to the mucosal surface (sessile). They are soft and may be difficult or impossible to feel even when in reach of the examining finger. Proctoscopy is usually required for diagnosis, as is biopsy for the differentiation of benign from malignant lesions.

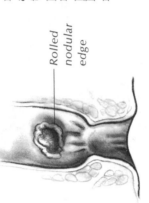

Sessile

Pedunculated

CARCINOMA OF THE RECTUM

Asymptomatic carcinoma of the rectum makes routine rectal examination mandatory for virtually all adults. As noted above, polypoid masses may be malignant. Another common form of presentation is the firm, nodular, rolled edge of an ulcerated malignancy.

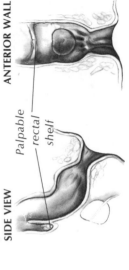

Rolled nodular edge

PERITONEAL METASTASES

SIDE VIEW   **ANTERIOR WALL**

Palpable rectal shelf

Widespread peritoneal metastases from any source may develop in the area of the peritoneal reflection anterior to the rectum. A firm to hard nodular rectal "shelf" may be just palpable with the tip of the examining finger.

Table 12-2

Table 12-2 Abnormalities of the Prostate

THE NORMAL PROSTATE GLAND

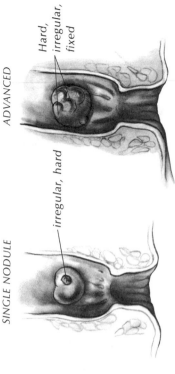

Smooth, elastic, symmetrical

As palpated through the anterior rectal wall, the normal prostate is a rounded, heart-shaped structure about 2.5 cm in length, projecting less than 1.0 cm into the rectal lumen. The median sulcus can be felt between the two lateral lobes. Only the posterior surface of the prostate is palpable. Anterior lesions, including those that may obstruct the urethra, may not be detectable by physical examination.

BENIGN PROSTATIC HYPERTROPHY

A very common condition in men over 50 years of age, benign prostatic hypertrophy presents as a firm, smooth, symmetrical, and slightly elastic enlargement of the gland. It may bulge more than a centimeter into the rectal lumen. The hypertrophied tissue tends to obliterate the median sulcus.

CARCINOMA OF THE PROSTATE

SINGLE NODULE

irregular, hard

ADVANCED

Hard, irregular, fixed

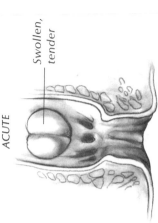

A hard, irregular nodule, producing asymmetry of the gland and a variation in its consistency, is especially suggestive of carcinoma. Prostatic stones and chronic inflammation can produce similar findings, and differential diagnosis often depends upon biopsy. Later in its course the carcinoma grows in size, obliterates the median sulcus, and may extend beyond the confines of the gland, producing a fixed, hard, irregular mass.

PROSTATITIS

ACUTE

Swollen, tender

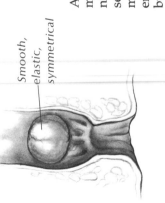

The acutely inflamed prostate gland is swollen, tender, and often somewhat asymmetrical.

The gland of chronic prostatitis is variable: it may (1) feel normal, (2) be somewhat enlarged, tender, and boggy, or (3) contain scattered firm areas of fibrosis.

Chapter 13
THE PERIPHERAL VASCULAR SYSTEM

Anatomy and Physiology

ARTERIES

The carotid arteries have been described in Chapters 5 and 7, the abdominal aorta in Chapter 9. This section will focus on the arteries supplying the arms and legs.

In the arms, arterial pulses are clinically accessible in two or perhaps three locations: (1) the *brachial artery* just medial to the biceps muscle above the elbow, (2) the *radial artery*, and (3) the less easily felt *ulnar artery* at the wrist.

The radial and ulnar arteries are interconnected by two vascular arches within the hand. Circulation to the hand and fingers is thereby doubly protected against possible arterial occlusion.

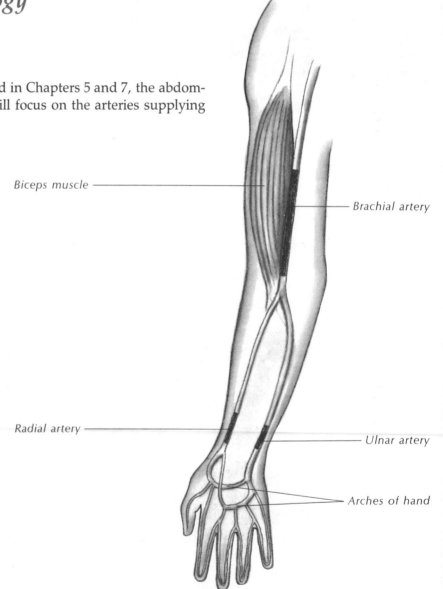

RIGHT ARM

Biceps muscle

Brachial artery

Radial artery

Ulnar artery

Arches of hand

Pulses in the legs can be identified in the following locations: the *femoral artery*, below the inguinal ligament midway between the anterior superior iliac spine and symphysis pubis; the *popliteal artery*, behind the knee; the *dorsalis pedis artery*, on the dorsum of the foot; and the *posterior tibial artery*, just behind the medial malleolus.

Like the hand, the foot is protected by an interconnecting arch between the two chief arterial branches supplying it.

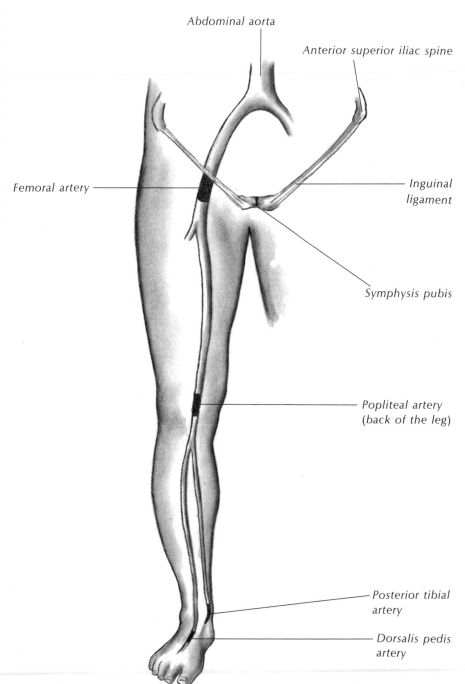

RIGHT LEG

Abdominal aorta

Anterior superior iliac spine

Femoral artery

Inguinal ligament

Symphysis pubis

Popliteal artery (back of the leg)

Posterior tibial artery

Dorsalis pedis artery

VEINS

The jugular veins have been discussed in Chapters 5 and 7. They are the principal veins from the head and, together with veins from the arms and upper trunk, drain into the superior vena cava. Veins from the legs and lower trunk drain into the inferior vena cava. Since venous disease most commonly affects the legs, special attention should be paid to the structure and function of the leg veins.

The *deep veins* of the legs carry about 90% of the venous return from the lower extremities. They are well supported by surrounding tissues.

In contrast, the *superficial veins* are located subcutaneously where they are supported relatively poorly. The superficial veins include 1) the *great saphenous vein*, which originates on the dorsum of the foot, passes just in front of the medial malleolus, and then continues up the medial aspect of the leg to join the deep venous system (the femoral vein) below the inguinal ligament; and 2) the *small saphenous vein*, which begins at the

FRONT

BACK

LEFT SIDE

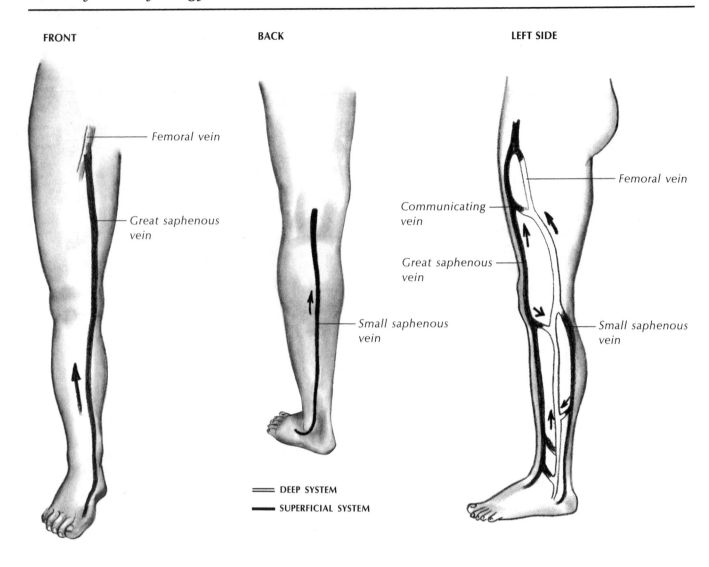

Femoral vein

Great saphenous vein

Communicating vein

Great saphenous vein

Femoral vein

Small saphenous vein

Small saphenous vein

═══ DEEP SYSTEM

▬▬▬ SUPERFICIAL SYSTEM

side of the foot and passes upward along the back of the leg to join the deep system in the popliteal space. Anastomotic channels join the two saphenous veins, and *communicating,* or *perforating,* veins connect the saphenous system with the veins of the deep system along its entire course.

Deep, superficial, and communicating veins all have thin valves along their courses, about 10 cm to 12 cm apart. These are so arranged that venous blood can flow from the superficial to the deep system and toward the heart but not in the opposite directions. Muscular activity provides the driving force behind venous blood flow. As muscles contract in walking, for example, blood is squeezed upward against gravity and kept from falling back by competent valves.

THE LYMPHATIC SYSTEM
AND LYMPH NODES

The lymphatic system consists of a series of channels that begin peripherally in blind lymphatic capillaries. These capillaries remove excess fluid from the tissues. The lymph so formed is carried centrally through lymphatic vessels and collecting ducts to empty into the venous system at the root of the neck. In its passage, lymph is filtered through lymph nodes that are interposed along the way.

The lymphatics draining the head and neck have been described in Chapter 5, the lymph nodes of the axilla in Chapter 8.

Recall that the axillary lymph nodes drain most of the arm. Lymphatics from the ulnar surface of the forearm, the little and ring fingers, and the adjacent surface of the middle finger drain first into the *epitrochlear node.* This node is located on the medial surface of the arm above the elbow. Most of the rest of the arm sends lymphatics directly to the axillary nodes. Some lymphatics may go directly to the infraclaviculars.

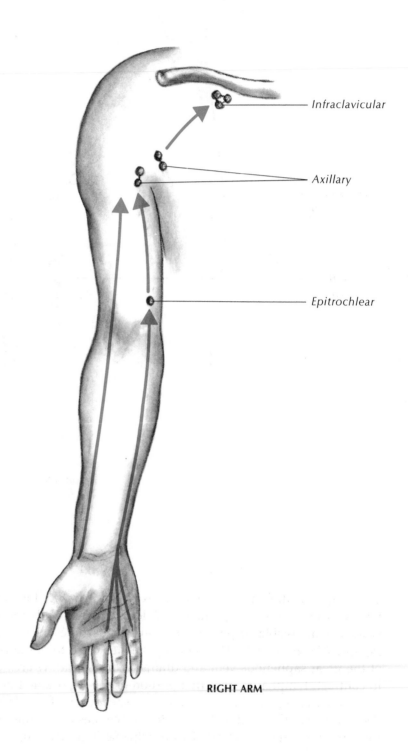

Infraclavicular

Axillary

Epitrochlear

RIGHT ARM

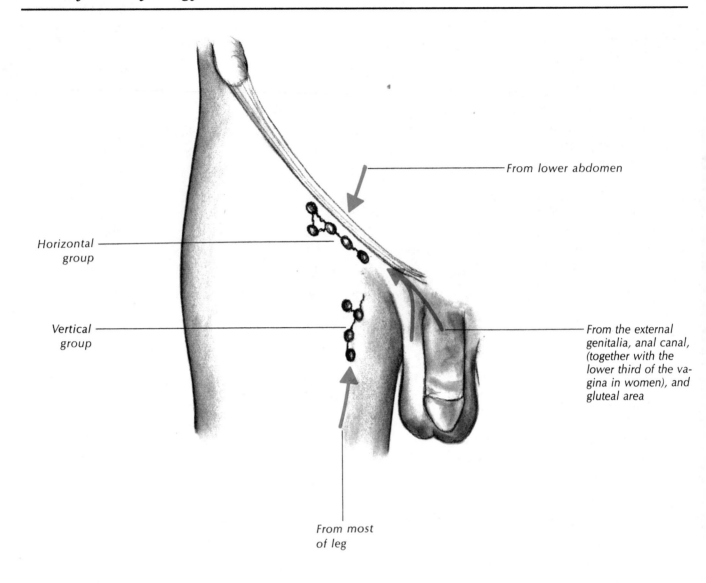

Horizontal group

Vertical group

From lower abdomen

From the external genitalia, anal canal, (together with the lower third of the vagina in women), and gluteal area

From most of leg

The lymphatic drainage of the lower extremity parallels the venous supply, consisting of both superficial and deep systems. Only the superficial system is accessible to physical examination. There are two groups of *superficial inguinal nodes.* The *vertical group* lies close to the upper portion of the great saphenous vein and drains a corresponding area of the leg. In contrast, lymphatics from that portion of the leg drained by the small saphenous vein (*i.e.,* the heel and outer aspect of the foot) drain into the deep system at the level of the popliteal space. Lesions in this area, therefore, are not usually associated with palpable inguinal lymph nodes.

A *horizontal group* of superficial nodes lies just below the inguinal ligament. This group drains the skin of the lower abdominal wall, the external genitalia (excluding the testes), the anal canal, the lower vagina, and the gluteal area.

FLUID EXCHANGE AND THE CAPILLARY BED

Blood circulates from arteries to veins through the capillary bed. Here fluids diffuse across the capillary membrane, maintaining a dynamic equilibrium between the vascular and interstitial spaces. Blood pressure (or hydrostatic pressure) within the capillary bed, especially near the arteriolar end, forces fluid out into the tissue spaces. In effecting this movement, it is aided by the relatively weak osmotic attraction of proteins within the tissues (interstitial colloid osmotic pressure) and is opposed by the hydrostatic pressure of the tissues.

As blood continues through the capillary bed toward the venous end its hydrostatic pressure falls, and another force gains dominance. This is the colloid osmotic pressure of plasma proteins, which pulls fluid back into the vascular tree. Net flow of fluid, which was directed outward on the arteriolar side of the capillary bed, reverses itself and turns inward on the venous side. Lymphatic capillaries, which also play an important role in this equilibrium, remove excessive fluid, including protein, from the interstitial space.

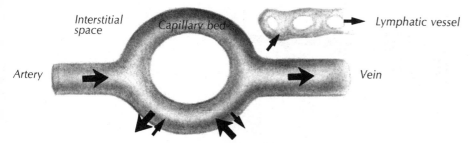

Lymphatic dysfunction or disturbances in hydrostatic or osmotic forces can all disrupt this equilibrium. The most common clinical result is the increased interstitial fluid known as edema. (See Table 13-3, Mechanisms and Patterns of Edema, pp. 320–321.) Secondary renal and hormonal forces that increase total body water and salt in most edematous states will not be discussed here.

CHANGES WITH AGE

Aging itself brings relatively few clinically important changes to the peripheral vascular sytem. Although arterial and venous disorders, especially atherosclerosis, do afflict older people more frequently, they probably cannot be considered part of the aging process. Age lengthens the arteries, makes them tortuous, and typically stiffens their walls, but these changes develop with or without atherosclerosis and therefore lack diagnostic specificity. Loss of arterial pulsations is not a part of normal aging, however, and demands careful evaluation. Skin may get thin and dry with age, nails may grow more slowly, and hair on the legs often becomes scant. Since these changes are common they are not specific for arterial insufficiency, although they are classically associated with it.

Techniques of Examination

Although this chapter focuses on the peripheral vascular system, you should integrate this examination with your assessment of the skin and of the musculoskeletal and neurological systems. See Chapter 2 for a method of doing this. Throughout your assessment compare one side with the other.

ARMS

Inspect both arms from the fingertips to the shoulders. *Note:*

Their size and symmetry
The color and texture of the skin and nail beds
The venous pattern
Edema

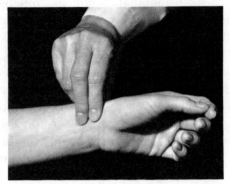

Radial pulse

With the pads of your index and middle fingers, *palpate the radial pulse* on the flexor surface of the wrist laterally. Compare the volume of the pulses on each side.

Pulses may be described as normal, diminished, or absent. A finer numerical classification is based on a 0 to 4 scale:

0—completely absent
1—markedly impaired
2—moderately impaired
3—slightly impaired
4—normal

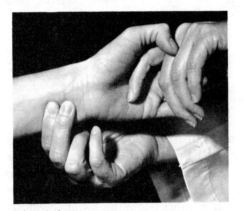

Ulnar pulse

If arterial insufficiency is suspected, palpate also (1) for the *ulnar pulse,* on the flexor surface of the wrist medially, and (2) for the *brachial pulse,* in the groove between the biceps and triceps muscle above the elbow.

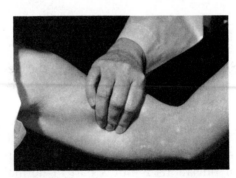

Brachial pulse

Pallor or cyanosis of the fingers in Raynaud's phenomenon

Edema and prominent veins in venous obstruction

Arterial occlusion in the arms is much less common than in the legs. If pulses are markedly diminished or absent, however, consider thromboangiitis obliterans (Buerger's disease), scleroderma, or, possibly, a cervical rib.

Since the normal ulnar artery is frequently not palpable, the *Allen test* may be useful. It tests the patency of the ulnar and radial arteries in turn. Ask the patient to rest his hands in his lap. Place your thumbs over his radial arteries and ask him to clench his fists tightly. Compress the radial arteries firmly, then ask the patient to open his hands into a relaxed position. Observe the color of the palms. Normally they should turn pink promptly. Repeat, occluding the ulnar arteries.

Persistence of pallor when one artery (*e.g.*, the radial) is manually compressed indicates occlusion of the other (*e.g.*, the ulnar).

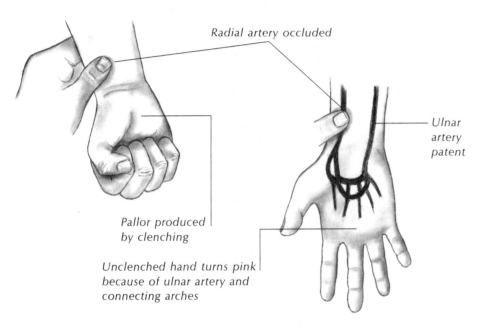

Radial artery occluded

Ulnar artery patent

Pallor produced by clenching

Unclenched hand turns pink because of ulnar artery and connecting arches

Medial aspect of left arm

Right hand of examiner

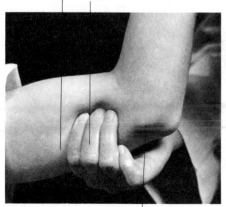

Medial epicondyle of humerus

Palpate for the *epitrochlear node*. With the patient's elbow flexed to about 90° and the forearm supported by your hand, reach around behind the arm and feel in the groove between the biceps and triceps muscles, about 3 cm above the medial epicondyle. If a node is present, note its size, consistency, and tenderness.

An enlarged epitrochlear node may be secondary to a lesion in its drainage area or may be associated with generalized lymphadenopathy.

LEGS

Drape the patient so that the external genitalia are covered and the legs fully exposed. A good examination is impossible through stockings or socks!

Inspect both legs from the groin and buttocks to the feet. *Note:*

Their size and symmetry
The color and texture of the skin and nail beds, and the hair distribution on the lower legs, feet, and toes
Pigmentation, rashes, scars, and ulcers
The venous pattern and evidence of venous enlargement
Edema

See Table 13-1, Chronic Insufficiency of Arteries and Veins (p. 318).

See Table 13-2, Common Ulcers of the Feet and Ankles (p. 319).

Palpate the superficial inguinal lymph nodes, both the horizontal and the vertical groups. Note their size, consistency, and tenderness. (Small, mobile, nontender inguinal nodes are frequently present.)

Tenderness suggests lymphadenitis.

Note any tenderness in the region of the femoral vein.

Venous tenderness together with other signs of venous obstruction suggests ileofemoral thrombophlebitis.

Palpate the pulses:

1. *The Femoral Pulse.* Press deeply, below the inguinal ligament and about midway between the anterior superior iliac spine and the symphysis pubis. As in deep abdominal palpation, the use of two hands, one on top of the other, may facilitate this examination, especially in obese patients.

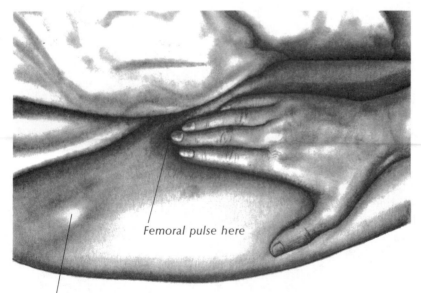

Femoral pulse here

Anterior superior iliac spine

2. *The Popliteal Pulse.* The patient's knee should be somewhat flexed, the leg relaxed. Press the fingertips of both hands deeply into the popliteal fossa, slightly lateral to the midline. The popliteal pulse is frequently more difficult to find than other pulses. It is deeper and feels more diffuse.

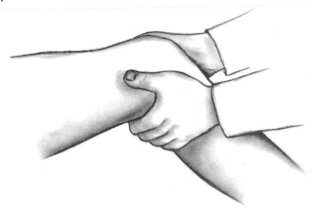

If you cannot feel the popliteal pulse with this approach, ask the patient to roll onto his abdomen. With the patient's leg flexed to 90° at the knee, palpate deeply for the popliteal pulse.

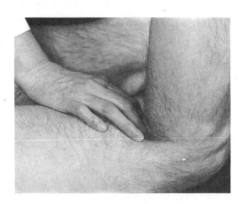

3. *The Dorsalis Pedis Pulse.* Feel the dorsum of the foot (not the ankle) just lateral to the extensor tendon of the great toe. If you cannot feel a pulse, explore the dorsum of the foot more laterally.

4. *The Posterior Tibial Pulse.* Curve your fingers behind and slightly below the medial malleolus of the ankle. (This pulse may be hard to feel in a fat or edematous ankle.)

Diminished or absent posterior tibial, popliteal, or femoral pulses suggest occlusive arterial disease. The dorsalis pedis pulse, however, may be congenitally absent. Its absence, therefore, is not diagnostic. Sometimes another artery in a more lateral position supplies the dorsum of the foot.

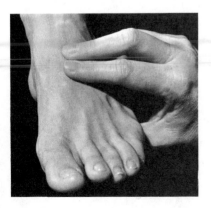

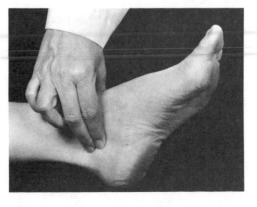

Note: Some pulses may be difficult to feel. Here are some aids: (1) Keep you own body and examining hand comfortable; awkward positions decrease your tactile sensitivity. (2) Place your hand properly and linger there, varying the pressure of your fingers to pick up a weak pulsation. If unsuccessful, then explore the area deliberately. Avoid flitting about. (3) Do not confuse the patient's pulse with your own pulsating fingertips. If you are unsure, count your own heart rate and compare it with the patient's. The rates are usually different. Your carotid pulse is convenient for this comparison.

Using the backs of your fingers, *note the temperature of the feet and legs,* comparing one side with the other.

Coldness may suggest arterial insufficiency, especially when it is unilateral. When bilateral, however, it is more frequently due to a cold environment or anxiety.

If all pulses below the femorals are diminished or absent, *listen* over the femoral arteries *for bruits.* If the femoral pulses are also absent, listen for bruits in the abdomen.

A localized systolic bruit may indicate the point of partial arterial occlusion.

Look for *edema* of the legs and check for *pitting edema.* Press firmly with your thumb for at least 5 seconds behind each medial malleolus, over the dorsum of each foot, and over the shins. Look for pitting, a depression in the skin caused by your pressure.

See Table 13-3, Mechanisms and Patterns of Edema (pp. 320–321).

See Table 13-4, Some Peripheral Causes of Edema (p. 322).

If you note edema involving much of one leg, look for an increase in the venous pattern of the leg or a diffuse reddish cyanosis of the leg.

A painful swollen leg with an increased venous pattern, increased warmth, and a normal or faintly reddish cyanotic hue suggests ileofemoral thrombophlebitis.

Palpate the calf for signs of deep phlebitis. Squeeze the calf muscles by compressing them against the tibia. Note any tenderness. Feel for any increased firmness or tension of the calf muscles.

Tenderness, increased firmness, and tension suggest thrombophlebitis in the calf. Unfortunately, however, phlebitis here usually has no signs.

Look for any signs of superficial phlebitis, such as redness or discoloration overlying the saphenous veins. If you see any or suspect phlebitis, palpate for tenderness or cords.

A tender, indurated, subcutaneous cord with warmth, redness, or discoloration indicates superficial thrombophlebitis.

Ask the patient to stand, and *inspect the saphenous system for varicosities.* The standing posture allows any varicosities to fill with blood and makes them visible. You can easily miss them when the patient is in a supine position. Feel for any varicosities, noting any signs of thrombophlebitis.

Varicose veins are dilated and tortuous. Their walls may feel somewhat thickened.

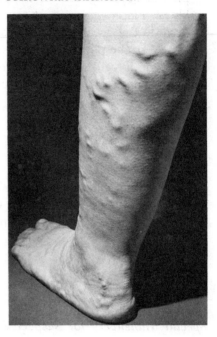

Special Maneuvers for Evaluating the Competency of Venous Valves in Varicose Veins. Assessing the competency of valves in varicose veins tests the functional sufficiency of the venous system. Two tests are useful:

Incompetent valves increase the hydrostatic pressure in the lower legs and lead to venous insufficiency.

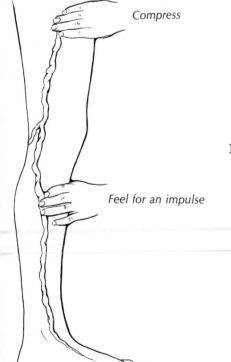

Compress

Feel for an impulse

1. *The manual compression test.* With the fingertips of one hand, feel the dilated vein. With your other hand compress the vein firmly at least 20 cm higher in the leg. Feel for an impulse transmitted to your lower hand. Competent saphenous valves should block the transmission of any impulse.

A palpable transmitted impulse indicates incompetency of the valve(s) in that portion of the vein between your two hands.

2. *The retrograde filling (Trendelenburg) test.* This test helps to assess valvular competency in the communicating veins as well as in the saphenous system. Elevate the patient's leg to 90° to empty it of venous blood. Place a tourniquet around the upper thigh, tightly enough to occlude the great saphenous vein without occluding the femoral artery. Ask the patient to stand. Watch for venous filling. Normally the saphenous vein fills slowly from below, taking about 35 seconds, as blood flows from arteries through the capillary bed into the venous system.

See Table 13-5, The Retrograde Filling Test for Incompetent Venous Valves (p. 323).

Rapid filling of superficial veins while the tourniquet is applied indicates incompetent valves in the communicating veins. Blood flows quickly in a retrograde direction from the deep to the superficial saphenous system.

After the patient has stood for 20 seconds, release the tourniquet and look for any sudden effect on venous filling. Normally there is none, since competent valves block retrograde flow.

Sudden additional filling of superficial veins after the release of the tourniquet indicates incompetent valves in the saphenous vein. Blood flows backward, unchecked by valves.

Special Maneuvers for Suspected Chronic Arterial Insufficiency. If you suspect chronic arterial insufficiency, elevate both of the patient's legs so that the feet are well above the level of venous pressure—at least 30 cm, or 12 inches, above the examining table. Ask the patient to move his feet up and down at the ankles for 30 to 60 seconds. These maneuvers drain the feet of venous blood, unmasking the color produced by the arterial supply. Inspect the feet for pallor. Mild pallor is normal.

Increased or deathly pallor in arterial insufficiency

Then have the patient sit up on the edge of the examining table with his legs dangling down. Note the time required for

1. Return of color to the skin, normally about 10 seconds or less
2. Filling of the veins of the feet and ankles, normally about 15 seconds

Delayed color return and venous filling in arterial insufficiency

Look for any unusual rubor (redness) or cyanosis of the dependent feet. Pinkness is normal, at least in the skin of white persons.

Dusky or cyanotic rubor in arterial insufficiency

When veins are incompetent, rubor, color return, and venous filling are unreliable in assessing arterial insufficiency.

SPECIAL EXAMINATION OF THE BED PATIENT

People who are confined to bed, especially when they are emaciated, elderly, or have neurologic impairment, are particularly susceptible to skin damage and ulceration. *Pressure sores* result when sustained compression obliterates arteriolar and capillary blood flow to the skin. Sores may also occur when, for example, a person slides down in bed from a partially sitting position, thus distorting the soft tissues of his buttocks and obstructing the small arteries or arterioles within.

The assessment of every susceptible patient should include careful inspection of the skin overlying the sacrum, buttocks, greater trochanters, knees, and heels. Roll the patient onto his side to get a good view of the sacrum and buttocks.

Local redness of the skin warns of impending necrosis, although some deep pressure sores develop without antecedent redness. Ulcers may be seen.

Use this position also to evaluate a patient for *sacral edema*. Press firmly for at least 5 seconds in the sacral area and look for any pitting. If you find it, check other areas higher on the back.

Dependent edema may accumulate in the back of a bed patient and not be apparent in the legs.

Table 13-1

Table 13-1 Chronic Insufficiency of Arteries and Veins

	CHRONIC ARTERIAL INSUFFICIENCY (Advanced)	CHRONIC VENOUS INSUFFICIENCY (Advanced)
PULSES	Decreased or absent	Normal, though may be difficult to feel through edema
COLOR	Pale, especially on elevation; dusky red on dependency	Normal, or cyanotic on dependency
TEMPERATURE	Cool	Normal
EDEMA	Absent or mild	Present, often marked
SKIN CHANGES	Thin, shiny, atrophic skin; loss of hair over foot and toes; nails thickened and ridged	May show brown pigmentation around ankles, stasis dermatitis
ULCERATION	If present, involves toes or points of trauma on feet	If present, develops at sides of ankle
GANGRENE	May develop	Does not develop

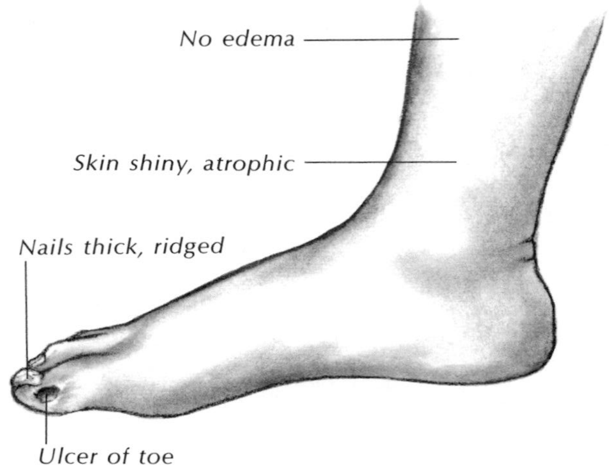

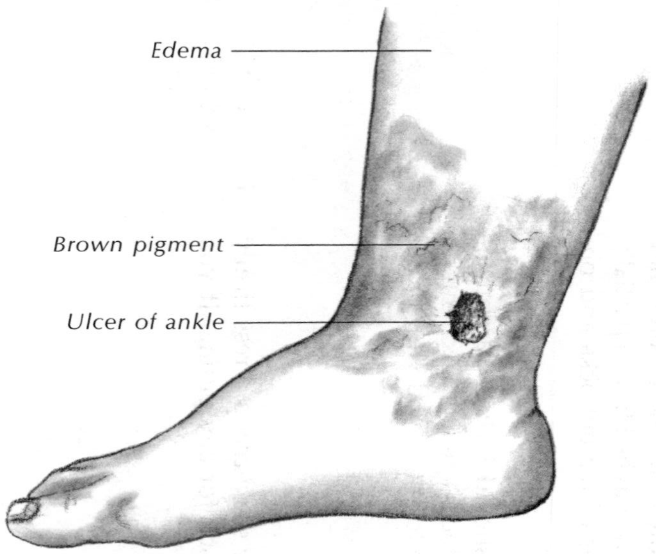

Table 13-2

Table 13-2 Common Ulcers of the Feet and Ankles

	CHRONIC VENOUS INSUFFICIENCY	ARTERIAL INSUFFICIENCY	TROPHIC ULCER
	Pitting · *Ulcer* · *Pigment*	*Ulcer* · *Shiny, atrophic skin* · *Gangrenous toe*	*Thickened skin* · *Ulcer*
LOCATION	Inner, sometimes outer ankle	Toes, feet, or possibly in areas of trauma (*e.g.*, the shin)	Pressure points in areas with diminished sensation, as in diabetic polyneuropathy
SKIN SURROUNDING THE ULCER	Pigmented, sometimes fibrotic	No callus or excess of pigment, may be atrophic	Calloused
PAIN	Not severe	Often severe, unless neuropathy masks it	Absent (and therefore the ulcer may go unnoticed)
ASSOCIATED GANGRENE	Absent	May be present	In uncomplicated trophic ulcer, absent
ASSOCIATED SIGNS	Stasis dermatitis, pigmentation, edema, and, possibly, cyanosis of the foot on dependency	Atrophic skin with decreased hair, pallor of foot on elevation, dusky or cyanotic rubor on dependency	Decreased sensation, ankle jerks absent

Table 13-3

Table 13-3 Mechanisms and Patterns of Edema

Causes of edema may be divided roughly into two groups: (1) *general or systemic causes,* including congestive heart failure, hypoalbuminemia, and excessive renal retention of salt and water; and (2) *local causes,* such as venous stasis, lymphatic stasis, and prolonged dependency. Increased capillary permeability may be either local or general in distribution.

	MECHANISM OF EDEMA	DISTRIBUTION OF EDEMA	OTHER SIGNS MAY INCLUDE—
RIGHT-SIDED CONGESTIVE HEART FAILURE	Decreased ability of the heart to accept venous blood increases the hydrostatic pressure in the veins and capillaries, producing congestion and loss of fluid into the tissues.	Edema first appears in the dependent areas of the body where hydrostatic pressure is highest (*i.e.,* the feet and the legs). When the patient is bedridden, the low back is dependent.	Increased jugular venous pressure, an enlarged and often tender liver, an enlarged heart, S_3
HYPOALBUMINEMIA	Decreased colloid osmotic pressure in the plasma allows excessive fluid to escape into the interstitial space. Causes include cirrhosis, the nephrotic syndrome, and severe malnutrition.	Edema may appear first in the loose subcutaneous tissues of the eyelids, especially after the patient lies down at night, but may also show first in the feet and legs. In cirrhosis, ascites often appears first. When cirrhosis is more advanced, edema may become generalized.	Signs of chronic liver disease such as ascites, spider angiomas, and jaundice. Signs of the nephrotic syndrome vary with its causes. Serum albumin is low, of course.
EXCESSIVE RENAL RETENTION OF SALT AND WATER	The kidneys may initiate edema by retaining excessive amounts of salt and water, some of which pass into the interstitial space. Drugs such as corticosteroids, estrogens, and some antihypertensives may be responsible.	Edema usually starts in the dependent areas and may become generalized.	Usually none

Continued

Table 13-3

Table 13-3 (Cont'd)

	MECHANISM OF EDEMA	DISTRIBUTION OF EDEMA	OTHER SIGNS MAY INCLUDE—
VENOUS STASIS SECONDARY TO OBSTRUCTION OR INSUFFICIENCY	Thrombophlebitis may block venous drainage. Venous valves may be damaged by thrombophlebitis or become incompetent because of varicose veins. Less commonly, veins may be compressed from the outside, as by a tumor or fibrosis. In any case hydrostatic pressure rises in the veins and capillaries, producing excessive loss of fluid into the tissues.	Edema is limited to the area of blockage, often one leg or, less commonly, both legs or an arm. A blocked superior vena cava may cause edema in the entire upper part of the body.	Local swelling and increased tissue turgor. When large veins such as the superior vena cava or the ileofemoral veins are involved, an increased venous pattern of dilated veins may be visible. Tenderness sometimes accompanies phlebitis. Signs of venous insufficiency
LYMPHATIC STASIS (LYMPHEDEMA)	Lymph channels may be congenitally abnormal or they may be obstructed by tumor, fibrosis, or inflammation.	Local, often involving one or both legs. Lymphedema of an arm may follow radical mastectomy.	Indurated skin in the involved area. Except in the early phases, lymphedema is characteristically nonpitting.
ORTHOSTATIC EDEMA	Prolonged sitting or standing, without sufficient muscular activity to promote venous flow, increases the pressure in the veins and capillaries and thus increases the flow of fluid into the interstitial spaces.	The dependent areas (*e.g.*, the legs)	None. Get a good history including long bus or train trips. People who get up after prolonged bedrest are at first especially susceptible to orthostatic edema.
INCREASED CAPILLARY PERMEABILITY	When capillary permeability increases, protein leaks into the interstitial spaces and, by increasing the interstitial colloid osmotic pressure, draws excessive fluid with it. Causes vary, including burns, snake bite, and allergy.	Usually local, depending on the cause; may be general	Variable

Table 13-4

Table 13-4   Some Peripheral Causes of Edema

	ORTHOSTATIC EDEMA	LYMPHEDEMA	LIPEDEMA	CHRONIC VENOUS INSUFFICIENCY
PROCESS	Edema from prolonged sitting or standing	Lymphatic obstruction	Fatty deposition in legs	Deep venous obstruction or valvular incompetence
NATURE OF EDEMA	Soft, pits on pressure	Soft early, becomes hard and nonpitting	Minimal if any	Soft, pits on pressure, later may become brawny
SKIN THICKENING	Absent	Marked	Absent	Occasional
ULCERATION	Absent	Rare	Absent	Common
PIGMENTATION	Absent	Absent	Absent	Common
FOOT INVOLVEMENT	Present	Present	Absent	Present
BILATERALITY	Always	Often	Always	Occasionally

Table 13-5

Table 13-5 The Retrograde Filling Test for Incompetent Venous Valves

	NORMAL	SAPHENOUS VEIN INCOMPETENT AND COMMUNICATING VEINS INCOMPETENT	SAPHENOUS VEIN INCOMPETENT BUT COMMUNICATING VEINS COMPETENT
ON STANDING WITH THE TOURNIQUET FASTENED	Slow venous filling from below *Saphenous* *Deep*	Rapid filling through communicating veins *Saphenous* *Deep*	Slow venous filling from below *Saphenous* *Deep*
ON RELEASE OF THE TOURNIQUET	No additional filling from above *Saphenous* *Deep*	Sudden additional filling from above *Saphenous* *Deep*	Sudden additional filling from above *Saphenous* *Deep*

323

Chapter 14
THE MUSCULOSKELETAL SYSTEM

Anatomy and Physiology

This section will review briefly the structure and function of joints and will describe the anatomical landmarks of several clinically important joints. Identify these landmarks first on yourself or on other normal people. Range of motion at each joint varies greatly with age and health. The figures given here are intended to be general guides, not absolute standards.

STRUCTURE AND FUNCTION OF JOINTS

A typical *freely movable joint* is diagrammed at the right.

Note that the bones themselves do not touch each other within a joint but are covered by articular cartilage that forms a cushion between the bony surfaces. At the margins of the articular cartilage is attached the synovial membrane. This membrane is pouched or folded to allow for joint movement. It encloses the synovial cavity and secretes into it a small amount of viscous lubricating fluid—the synovial fluid.

The synovial membrane is surrounded by a fibrous joint capsule, which in turn is strengthened by ligaments extending from bone to bone.

Some joints, such as those between the vertebral bodies illustrated here, are *slightly movable joints.* Here the bones are separated not by a synovial cavity but by a fibrocartilaginous disc. At the center of each disc is the nucleus pulposus, fibrogelatinous material that forms a cushion or shock absorber between the vertebral bodies.

Bursae develop at points of friction around joints, for example between tendons and cartilage or bone, or between the convex surface of a joint and the skin. A bursa is a disc-shaped, fluid-filled synovial sac that decreases friction and promotes ease of motion.

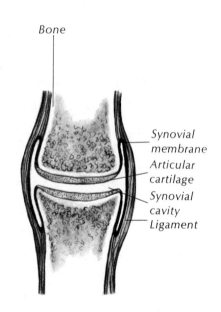

Bone

Synovial membrane
Articular cartilage
Synovial cavity
Ligament

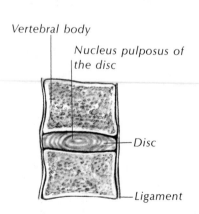

Vertebral body

Nucleus pulposus of the disc

Disc

Ligament

SPECIFIC JOINTS

Temporomandibular Joint. The temporomandibular joint forms the articulation between mandible and skull. Feel for it just in front of the tragus of each ear as the jaw is opened and closed.

Wrists and Hands. Identify the bony tips of the radius (on the lateral or thumb side) and the ulna (medially). On the dorsum of the wrist, palpate the groove of the radiocarpal or wrist joint.

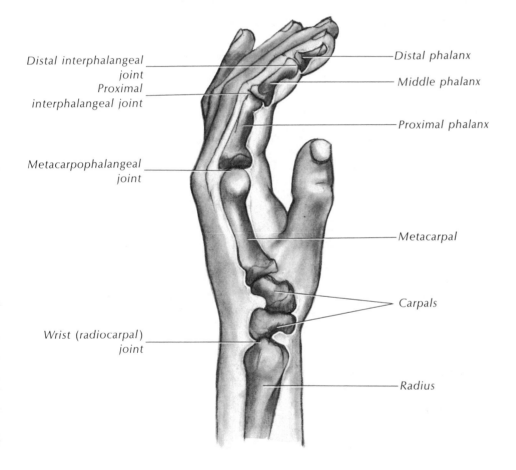

Distal interphalangeal joint — Distal phalanx
Proximal interphalangeal joint — Middle phalanx
— Proximal phalanx
Metacarpophalangeal joint
— Metacarpal
— Carpals
Wrist (radiocarpal) joint
— Radius

The carpal bones within the hand cannot be readily identified clinically. However, palpate each of the five metacarpals and the proximal, middle, and distal phalanges. (The thumb lacks a middle phalanx.) Flex the hand somewhat and find the groove marking the metacarpophalangeal joint of each finger. It is distal to the knuckle and can be felt best on either side of the extensor tendon.

Many tendons pass across the wrist and hand to insert on the fingers. Through much of their course these tendons travel in synovial sheaths or tunnels. Although not normally palpable, these sheaths may become swollen or inflamed.

Ilustrated below and at the right is the *range of motion at the wrists:*

And *at the joints of the fingers:*

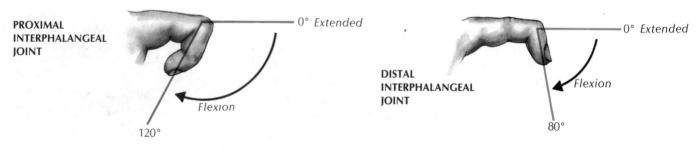

Elbows. Identify the medial and lateral epicondyles of the humerus and the olecranon process of the ulna. A bursa lies between the olecranon process and the skin. The synovial membrane is most accessible to examination between the olecranon and the epicondyles. Neither bursa nor synovium is normally palpable, however.

The sensitive ulnar nerve can be felt posteriorly between olecranon and medial epicondyle.

Movements at the elbow are illustrated here:

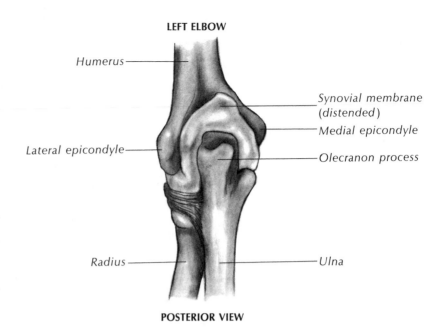

LEFT ELBOW

Humerus

Synovial membrane (distended)

Medial epicondyle

Lateral epicondyle

Olecranon process

Radius

Ulna

POSTERIOR VIEW

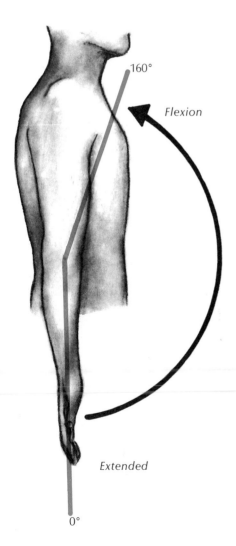

160°

Flexion

Extended

0°

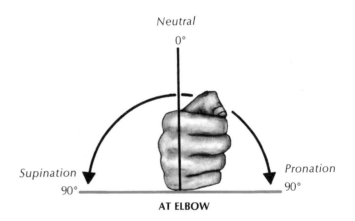

Neutral
0°

Supination
90°

Pronation
90°

AT ELBOW

Shoulders and Environs. Identify the following landmarks: (1) the manubrium of the sternum, (2) the sternoclavicular joint, and (3) the clavicle. With your finger trace the clavicle laterally to its distal end. Now, from behind, identify the triangular scapula and follow its bony spine laterally and upward to the acromion. Place a dot of ink on its anterior tip. With your finger firmly on top of the acromion feel medially for the slightly elevated clavicle. This junction marks the acromioclavicular joint. Below and medial to this joint lies the coracoid process, a part of the scapula. Mark it with ink. Below and lateral to the joint find the greater tubercle of the humerus. Mark this also. The triangle formed by these points—the tip of the acromion, the coracoid process, and the greater tubercle of the humerus—orients you to the anatomy of the shoulder.

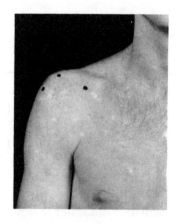

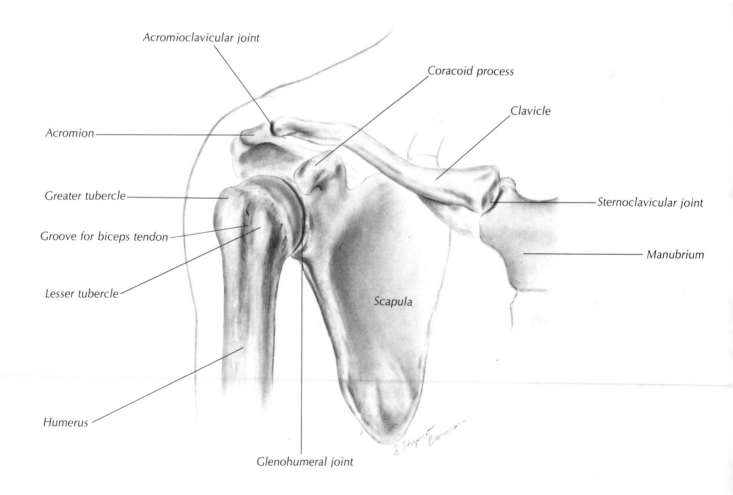

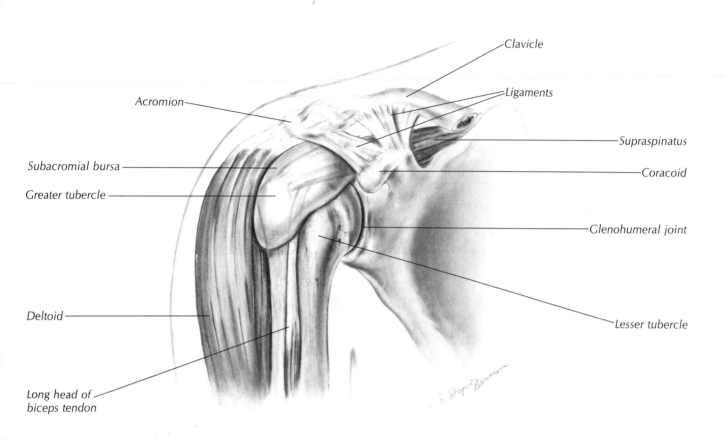

Clavicle

Ligaments

Acromion

Supraspinatus

Subacromial bursa

Coracoid

Greater tubercle

Glenohumeral joint

Deltoid

Lesser tubercle

Long head of
biceps tendon

While the arm is rotated externally, find the tendinous cord that runs just medial to the greater tubercle. Roll it under your fingers. This is the tendon of the long head of the biceps. It runs in a groove between greater and lesser tubercles.

The arch formed by the acromion, the coracoid, and the ligament between them protects the more deeply situated glenohumeral joint, between the scapula and humerus. Although not normally palpable, the clinically important subacromial bursa lies deep to the deltoid muscle between this arch above and the humeral head below. The supraspinatus muscle, important in abducting the arm at the shoulder, inserts on the greater tubercle just deep to this bursa.

The normal *range of motion at the shoulder joint* is illustrated below.

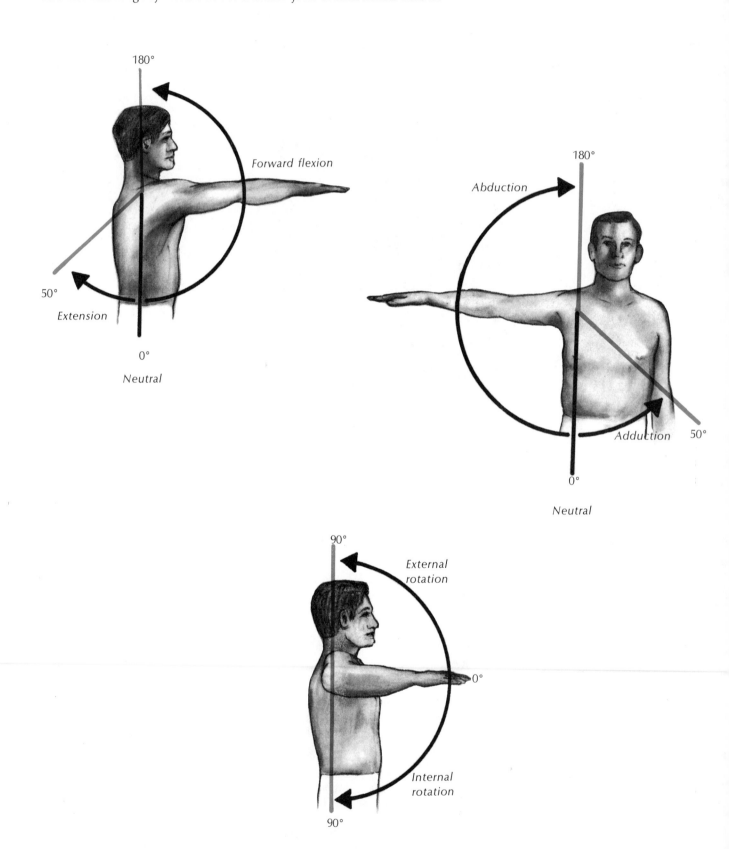

Ankles and Feet. The principal landmarks of the ankle are (1) the medial malleolus, the bony prominence at the distal end of the tibia, and (2) the lateral malleolus, the distal end of the fibula. Ligaments extend from each malleolus onto the foot. The strong Achilles tendon inserts on the heel posteriorly.

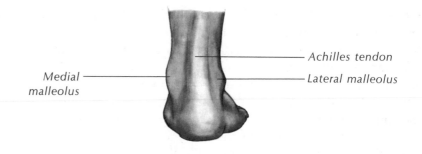

Medial malleolus

Achilles tendon

Lateral malleolus

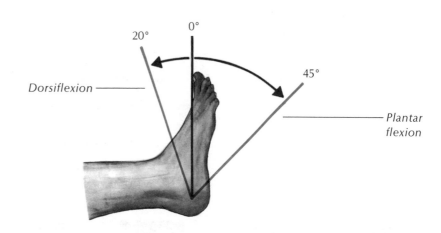

Motions at the ankle joint itself (the tibiotalar joint) consist of dorsiflexion and plantar flexion.

Dorsiflexion

Plantar flexion

20° 0° 45°

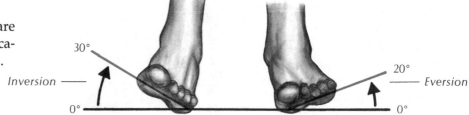

Inversion and eversion of the foot are functions of the subtalar (talocalcaneal) and transverse tarsal joints.

Inversion

Eversion

30° 0° 0° 20°

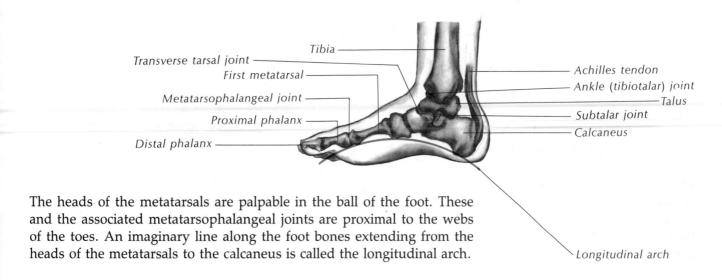

Transverse tarsal joint
First metatarsal
Metatarsophalangeal joint
Proximal phalanx
Distal phalanx

Tibia

Achilles tendon
Ankle (tibiotalar) joint
Talus
Subtalar joint
Calcaneus

Longitudinal arch

The heads of the metatarsals are palpable in the ball of the foot. These and the associated metatarsophalangeal joints are proximal to the webs of the toes. An imaginary line along the foot bones extending from the heads of the metatarsals to the calcaneus is called the longitudinal arch.

The Knee. Identify the flat medial surface of the tibia—the shin. Follow its anterior border upward to the tibial tuberosity. Mark this point with a dot of ink. Now follow the medial border of the tibia upward until it merges into a bony prominence—the medial condyle of the tibia. This is somewhat higher than the tibial tuberosity. In a comparable location on the other side of the knee, find a similar prominence—the lateral condyle. Mark both condyles with ink. These three points form an isosceles triangle. On the lateral surface of the knee, somewhat below the level of the lateral tibial condyle, find the head of the fibula.

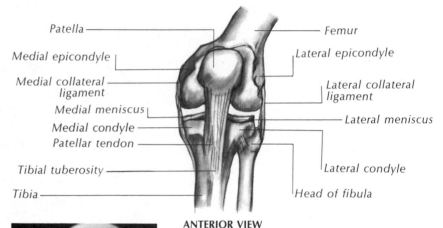

Patella — Femur

Medial epicondyle | Lateral epicondyle

Medial collateral ligament — Lateral collateral ligament

Medial meniscus | Lateral meniscus

Medial condyle — Patellar tendon —

Lateral condyle

Tibial tuberosity — Head of fibula

Tibia —

ANTERIOR VIEW

Now bring your fingertips firmly down the medial surface of the thigh along a line analogous to the inner seam of a pant leg. Your fingers will run up against an abrupt bony prominence that forms an important landmark of the knee. This is the adductor tubercle of the femur. Just below this is the medial epicondyle of the femur. The lateral epicondyle can be found comparably situated on the other side.

LEFT KNEE

With the knee moderately flexed, you can now place both thumbs—one on each side of the patellar tendon—in the groove of the knee joint itself, between femur and tibia. The patella, located within the tendon of the quadriceps, lies just above this joint line. It articulates with the femur behind it.

Quadriceps femoris

Femur — Adductor tubercle — Medial epicondyle — Synovial cavity (distended) — Medial collateral ligament — Fibula —

Suprapatellar pouch
Prepatellar bursa
Patella
Medial meniscus
Patellar ligament
Medial condyle
Tibial tuberosity

Tibia

MEDIAL ASPECT

Above the patella the quadriceps muscle, when contracted, can be easily identified. Observe the normal concavities on either side and above the patella. Occupying these areas is the synovial cavity of the knee joint, including an extension up behind the quadriceps called the suprapatellar pouch. Although the synovium is not normally visible or palpable, these areas may become swollen when the joint is inflamed. Below the patella the quadriceps inserts on the tibial tuberosity through its patellar tendon (technically termed the patellar ligament because it connects bone with bone).

Several other structures in the knee have clinical importance. The collateral ligaments give medial and lateral stability to the knee while the two cruciate ligaments (not illustrated), which cross obliquely within the knee, add anteroposterior stability. Two crescent-shaped fibrocartilaginous pads—the medial and lateral menisci—form cushions between the tibia and femur. Several bursae lie near the knee. The prepatellar bursa, for example, lies between the patella and the overlying skin, while the superficial infrapatellar bursa lies anterior to the patellar tendon. The soft tissue palpable in front of the joint space, on either side of the patellar tendon, is the infrapatellar fat pad.

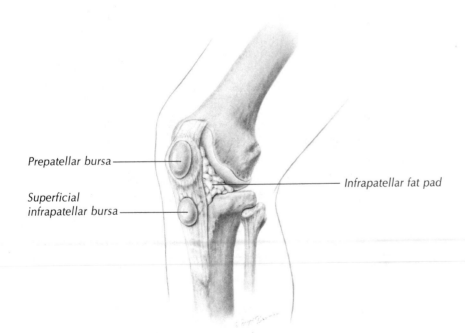

Prepatellar bursa

Superficial
infrapatellar bursa

Infrapatellar fat pad

The principal *movements of the knee* are extension, flexion, and sometimes hyperextension.

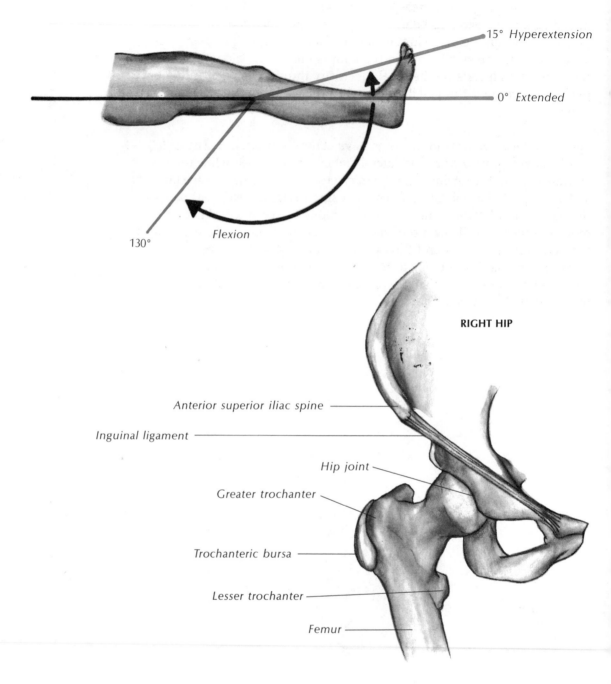

15° *Hyperextension*

0° *Extended*

130°

Flexion

RIGHT HIP

Anterior superior iliac spine

Inguinal ligament

Hip joint

Greater trochanter

Trochanteric bursa

Lesser trochanter

Femur

ANTERIOR VIEW

Pelvis and Hips. The hip joint lies deep and is not directly palpable. The greater trochanter of the femur can be felt about a palm's breadth below the iliac crest. The superficial trochanteric bursa lies on its posterolateral surface.

Movements of the hip are illustrated below.

WITH KNEE STRAIGHT

WITH KNEE FLEXED

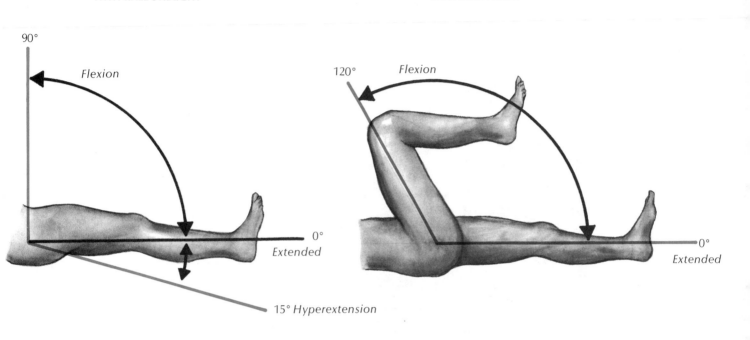

90°

Flexion

0°
Extended

15° *Hyperextension*

120°

Flexion

0°
Extended

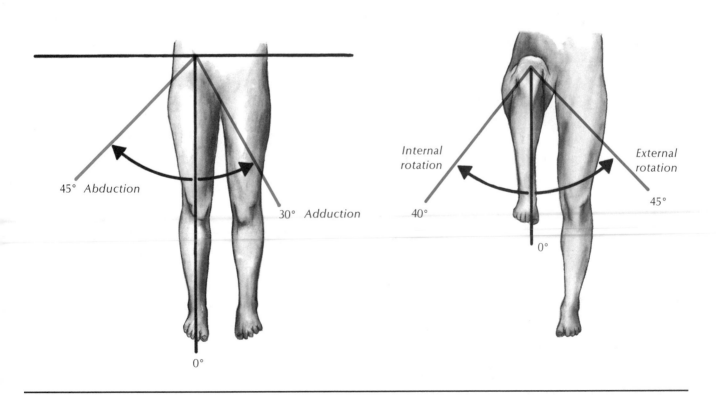

45° *Abduction*

30° *Adduction*

0°

Internal rotation

External rotation

40°

45°

0°

Spine. Viewing the patient from behind, identify the following landmarks: (1) the spinous processes, which become more evident on forward flexion, (2) the paravertebral muscles on either side of the midline, (3) the scapulae, (4) the iliac crests, and (5) the posterior superior iliac spines, usually marked by skin dimples. The spinous processes of C7 and often T1 are unusually prominent. A line between the iliac crests crosses the spinous process of L4.

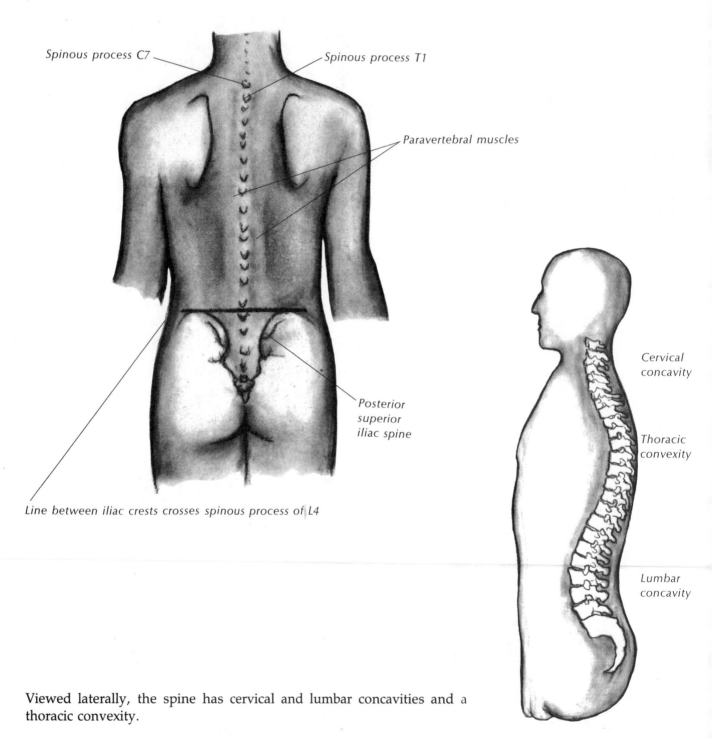

Spinous process C7

Spinous process T1

Paravertebral muscles

Posterior superior iliac spine

Line between iliac crests crosses spinous process of L4

Cervical concavity

Thoracic convexity

Lumbar concavity

Viewed laterally, the spine has cervical and lumbar concavities and a thoracic convexity.

The most mobile portion of the spine is the neck. Flexion and extension occur chiefly between the head and the 1st cervical vertebra, rotation occurs primarily between the 1st and 2nd vertebrae, and lateral bending involves the cervical spine from the 2nd to the 7th vertebrae.

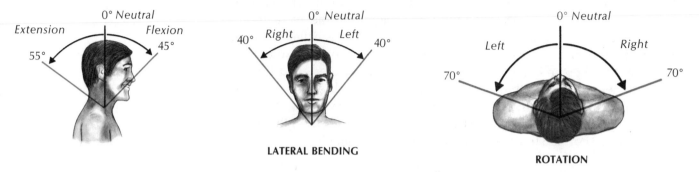

LATERAL BENDING

ROTATION

Movements of the rest of the spine (*i.e.*, from the sacrum to the base of the neck) are more difficult to measure than those in the neck and are subject to considerable individual variation. The ranges of motion illustrated here must be considered approximate. Some examiners prefer to measure forward flexion not by the angle but by the distance from fingertips to floor. Whichever method you use, watch the lumbar area as the patient flexes forward. The lumbar concavity should be replaced by a smooth convex curve.

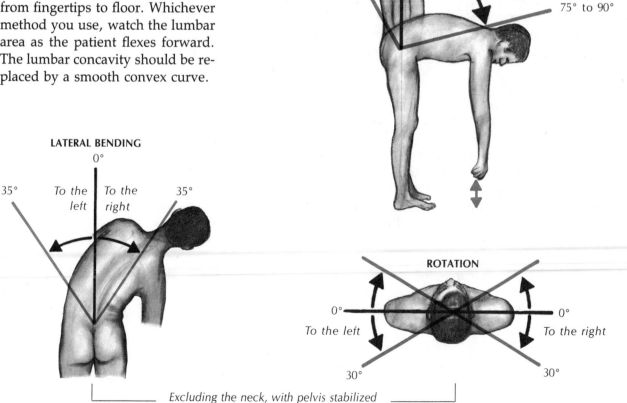

LATERAL BENDING

ROTATION

Excluding the neck, with pelvis stabilized

CHANGES WITH AGE

The musculoskeletal system changes importantly during adolescence—in size, proportion, and strength. Between the approximate ages of 12.5 and 15 years boys undergo an adolescent growth spurt, gaining an average of 8 inches in height and over 40 pounds in weight. On the average the growth spurt in girls occurs about 2 years earlier and is smaller in magnitude. Bodily proportions change in fairly regular sequence: the legs elongate, the hips and chest widen, the shoulders broaden, and finally the trunk lengthens and the chest deepens. Shoulders broaden more in boys, while in girls an increase in the bony pelvis produces relatively greater widening of the hips. Muscles increase in size and strength, especially in boys. For illustrations of these changes see page 36.

As in sexual maturation, adolescents vary widely in their musculoskeletal development. Those who mature relatively late in relation to their peers face competitive disadvantages even though they are entirely normal. Adolescent changes in height, musculoskeletal development, and sex maturity correlate well with each other and provide a better basis for counselling teenagers than does a normative concept based on chronologic age alone.

Musculoskeletal changes continue through the adult and aging years. Soon after maturity adults begin to lose height subtly, and significant shortening becomes obvious in old age. Most loss of height occurs in the trunk as intervertebral discs become thinner and the vertebral bodies shorten or even collapse because of osteoporosis. Flexion at the knees and hips may contribute to the shortened stature. The limbs of an elderly person thus tend to look long in proportion to the trunk.

The alterations in discs and vertebrae contribute too to the kyphosis of aging and increase the anteroposterior diameter of the chest, especially in women. For illustrations of these changes see page 37.

Skeletal muscles decrease in bulk and power. The hands of an aged person often look thin and bony because the small muscles of the hands have atrophied. Look for such muscular wasting in the backs of the hands where atrophy of the dorsal interosseous muscles leaves concavities or grooves. As illustrated on the facing page, this change is often most evident between thumb and hand (1st and 2nd metacarpal) but may also be seen between the other metacarpals. Atrophy of small muscles may also flatten the thenar and hypothenar eminences of the palms.

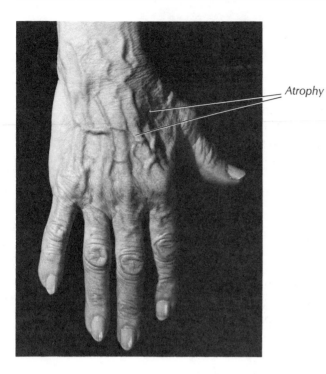 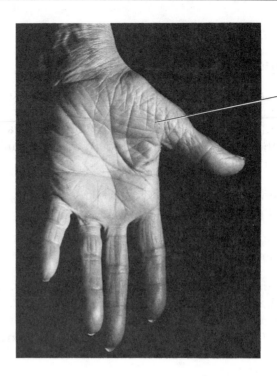

Atrophy

Flattening
of mild
atrophy

Although this kind of wasting would suggest neurologic disease in a younger person, it is normal in many elderly persons, and strength, although somewhat diminished, is relatively well maintained. Arm and leg muscles also show atrophy, sometimes exaggerating the apparent size of the joints.

Range of motion diminishes with age, partly because of degenerative joint disease, a condition that usually accompanies the repetitive and accumulated stresses of the passing years.

Techniques of Examination

GENERAL APPROACH

While examining the musculoskeletal system, direct your attention not only to structure but also to function. During the interview you should have evaluated the patient's ability to carry out normal activities of daily living. Keep these in mind too during your physical examination, including the patient's ability to:

1. Walk, stand, lean over, sit, sit up, rise from a sitting position, climb, pinch, and grasp

2. Comb his hair, brush his teeth, feed, wash, and dress himself, clean his perineum, and turn a page

During your initial survey of the patient you have assessed his general appearance, bodily proportions, and ease of movement. Now, using inspection and palpation, you will examine individual joints or groups of joints, their range of motion, and the tissues surrounding them.

Note particularly:

1. Any *limitation* in the normal *range of motion* or any unusual *increase* in the *mobility* of a joint (instability). Range of motion varies among individuals and decreases with aging.

   Decreased range of motion in arthritis, inflammation of tissues around the joint, fibrosis in or around a joint, or bony fixation (ankylosis)

2. Any *swelling* in or around the joint. Swelling may involve the synovial membrane, which then feels boggy, or doughy, to your fingers, or may be produced by excessive synovial fluid within the joint space. Swelling sometimes originates not in the joint itself but in tissues around it, such as bones, tendons, tendon sheaths, bursae, and fat.

   Palpable bogginess, or doughiness, of the synovial membrane indicates synovitis. Palpable joint fluid indicates an effusion in the joint. Synovitis and joint fluid often coexist.

3. *Tenderness* in or around the joint. Try to define the specific anatomic structure that is tender.

   Arthritis, tendonitis, bursitis, osteomyelitis

4. Increased *heat*. Use the backs of your fingers to compare the joint with the symmetrical joint on the opposite side or, if both joints are involved, with the tissues near them.

   Tenderness and warmth over a thickened synovium suggest rheumatoid arthritis.

5. *Redness* of the overlying skin

   Redness of the skin over a tender joint suggests septic or gouty arthritis, or possibly rheumatic fever.

6. *Crepitation*, a palpable or even audible crunching or grating sensation produced by motion of the joint

   Crepitation suggests roughening of articular cartilages, and is also felt in stenosing tenosynovitis.

7. *Deformities*, such as bony enlargement, subluxation (partial dislocation), or contracture

Bony enlargement suggests degenerative joint disease

8. *Condition of the surrounding tissues*, including muscle atrophy, subcutaneous nodules, and skin changes

Subcutaneous nodules in rheumatoid arthritis or rheumatic fever

9. Muscular *strength*. Testing of muscular strength is described in Chapter 15.

Muscular weakness and atrophy in rheumatoid arthritis

10. *Symmetry* of involvement. Note whether arthritic changes involve several joints symmetrically on both sides of the body or affect only one or perhaps two joints.

Involvement of only one joint increases the likelihood of bacterial arthritis. Rheumatoid arthritis typically involves several joints, symmetrically distributed.

When handling a person with painful joints, be gentle and move slowly. Often the patient can move more comfortably by himself. Let him show you how he manages.

The detail with which you examine the musculoskeletal system will vary widely from patient to patient. In an asymptomatic adolescent, for example, simple inspection of bodily proportions and major joints, together with careful assessment of the spine, may suffice. This chapter will describe a fairly detailed examination such as you might perform on a patient with joint complaints.

Scoliosis is an important problem in adolescents, especially girls, and is frequently asymptomatic in its early stages.

WITH THE PATIENT SITTING UP

HEAD AND NECK

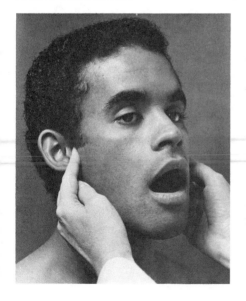

To palpate the temporomandibular joint, place the tip of your index finger just in front of the tragus of each ear and ask the patient to open his mouth. The tips of your fingers should drop into the joint spaces as the mouth opens. Observe the range of motion, feel for swelling, and note any tenderness. Snapping or clicking may be felt and heard in normal people.

Swelling, tenderness, and decreased range of motion suggest arthritis.

Inspect the neck for deformities and abnormal posture.

Palpate for tenderness of the cervical spine and the paravertebral and trapezius muscles.

See Table 14-1, Problems in the Neck (pp. 355–356).

Test the range of motion by asking the patient to:

Touch his chin to his chest (flexion)

Touch his chin to each shoulder (rotation)

Touch each ear to the corresponding shoulder (lateral bending)

Put his head back (extension)

HANDS AND WRISTS

Test the range of motion of the fingers and wrists by asking the patient to:

1. Extend and spread the fingers of both hands

2. Make a fist, with thumbs across the knuckles

Dupuytren's contracture may limit full extension of the fingers.

Arthritis may limit all movements of the fingers.

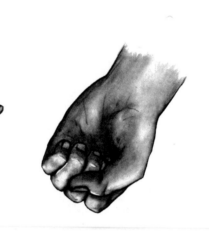

3. Flex and extend his wrists, abduct and adduct them

Inspect the hands and wrists, noting any swelling, redness, nodules, deformity, or muscular atrophy.

See Table 14-2, Swellings and Deformities of the Hands (pp. 357–359).

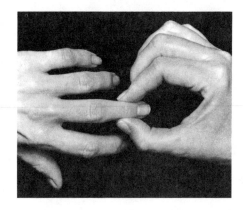

Palpate the medial and lateral aspects of each interphalangeal joint between your thumb and index finger, noting any swelling, bogginess, bony enlargement, or tenderness.

Bony enlargement of the interphalangeal joints suggests degenerative joint disease. It involves the distal joints more often than the proximals. Rheumatoid arthritis more commonly involves the proximal joints.

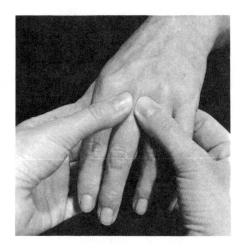

With your thumbs palpate the metacarpophalangeal joints, just distal to and on each side of the knuckle.

Note any swelling, bogginess, or tenderness.

Rheumatoid arthritis often involves the metacarpophalangeal joints; degenerative joint disease rarely does.

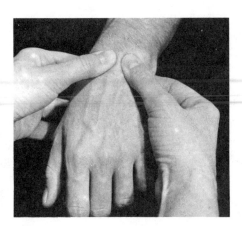

Palpate each wrist joint, with your thumbs on the dorsum of the wrist, your fingers beneath it. Note any swelling, bogginess, or tenderness.

Swelling suggests rheumatoid arthritis if it is bilateral and lasts for several weeks.

Gonococcal infection may involve the wrist joint (arthritis) or the tendon sheaths at the wrist (gonococcal tenosynovitis).

ELBOWS

Test the range of motion by asking the patient to bend and straighten his elbows. With his arms at his sides and elbows flexed, ask him to turn his palms up (supination) and down (pronation).

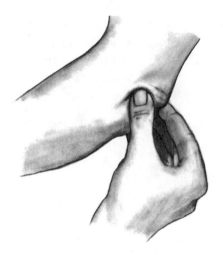

Support the patient's forearm with your opposite hand so that his elbow is flexed about 70°. Inspect and palpate the elbow, including the extensor surface of the ulna and the olecranon process, noting any nodules or swelling. Palpate the groove on either side of the olecranon as illustrated, noting any thickening, swelling, or tenderness.

Press on the lateral epicondyle, noting any tenderness.

Tender lateral epicondyle in tennis elbow

See Table 14-3, Swollen or Tender Elbows (p. 360).

SHOULDERS AND ENVIRONS

Test the range of motion by asking the patient to (1) raise both arms to a vertical position at the sides of his head, (2) place his hands behind his neck, with elbows out to the side (external rotation), and (3) place his hands behind the small of his back (internal rotation). By cupping your hand over the shoulder during these movements, note any crepitation.

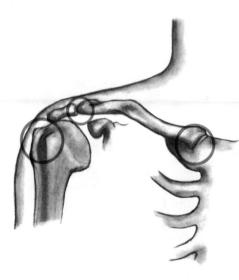

Inspect the shoulders and shoulder girdle anteriorly, noting any swelling, deformity, or muscular atrophy. Inspect the scapulae and related muscles posteriorly.

Palpate for tenderness in (1) the sternoclavicular joint, (2) the acromioclavicular joint, and (3) the shoulder itself, including the greater tubercle of the humerus and the biceps groove.

See Table 14-4, Painful Shoulders (pp. 361–362).

WITH THE PATIENT LYING DOWN

FEET AND ANKLES

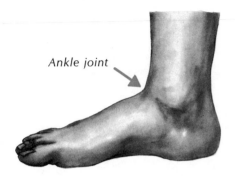

Ankle joint

Inspect the ankles and feet, noting any deformity, nodules, or swelling, any calluses or corns.

See Table 14-5, Abnormalities of the Feet and Toes (pp. 363–364).

Palpate the anterior surface of the ankle joint, noting any bogginess, swelling, or tenderness.

Arthritis of the ankle, but this may be difficult to differentiate from edema or cellulitis

Feel along the Achilles tendon for nodules.

Rheumatoid nodules

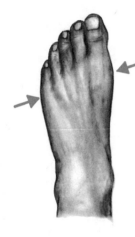

Test for tenderness of the metatarsophalangeal joints by compressing the fore part of the foot between your thumb and fingers.

Tenderness in the small metatarsophalangeal joints is an early sign of rheumatoid arthritis. Acute gout may produce severe pain, tenderness, swelling, and redness of the first metatarsophalangeal joint. A more common source of tenderness here is a bunion—an inflamed bursa overlying a hallux valgus deformity. (See p. 363.)

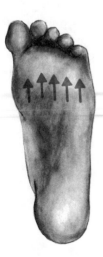

Each individual joint may be further evaluated by palpating the metatarsal heads in the sole of the foot and compressing each joint between thumb and finger.

Check the range of motion in ankles and feet:

1. Dorsiflex and plantar flex the foot at the ankle (the tibiotalar joint).

2. Stabilize the ankle with one hand, then grasp the heel with the other and invert and evert the foot at the subtalar joint.

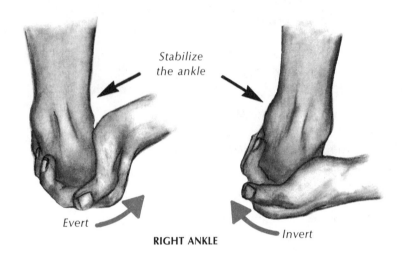

3. Stabilize the heel and invert and evert the forefoot, thereby testing the transverse tarsal joint.

These four maneuvers help to identify which joints of an arthritic foot are involved.

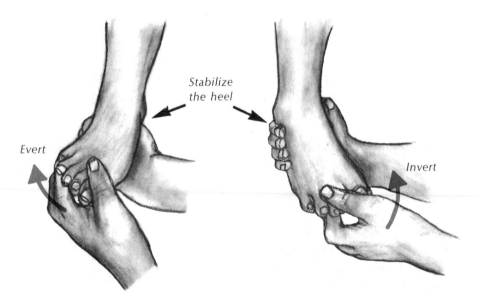

An arthritic joint is frequently painful when moved in any direction, while a ligamentous sprain produces maximal pain when the ligament is stretched. For example, in a common form of sprained ankle, inversion and plantar flexion of the foot cause pain while eversion and dorsiflexion are relatively pain-free.

4. Flex the toes on the metatarsophalangeal joints.

KNEES AND HIPS

Inspect the *knees,* noting their alignment and any deformity. Note any atrophy of the quadriceps muscles or loss of the normal hollows around the patella.

Bow legs (genu varum), knock knees (genu valgum), or flexion contracture (inability to extend fully)

Loss of normal hollows above and adjacent to the patella suggests synovial thickening or fluid in the knee joint.

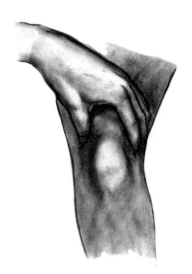

Palpate between your thumb and fingers the area of the suprapatellar pouch on each side of the quadriceps, noting any thickening, bogginess, or tenderness of the synovial membrane. Feel for any bony enlargement around the knee joint.

See Table 14-6, Swellings of the Knee (p. 365).

Thickening, bogginess, or tenderness suggests synovial inflammation of the knee joint.

Bony enlargement develops in advanced degenerative joint disease.

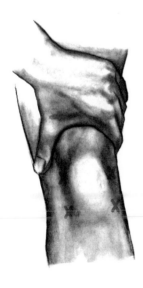

While compressing the suprapatellar pouch with one hand, palpate (1) on each side of the patella, and (2) over the tibiofemoral joint space itself. Identify any thickening, bogginess, or fluid. Note any tenderness of the joint space or of the areas near the femoral epicondyles. In an adolescent with knee pain, press on the tibial tuberosity and note any swelling or tenderness.

See Table 14-7, Local Tenderness in the Knee (pp. 366–367).

A tender, swollen tibial tuberosity in an adolescent suggests Osgood–Schlatter disease.

Palpate the popliteal space for swellings or cysts. (These are often found more easily when the patient stands with knees extended.)

If you suspect a small amount of fluid in the knee joint (because there is fullness, for example, in the usual hollows next to the patella),

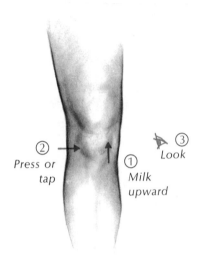

Look for a Bulge Sign

1. With the ball of your hand milk the medial aspect of the knee firmly upward two or three times to displace any fluid.

2. Then press or tap the knee just behind the lateral margin of the patella.

3. Watch for a bulge of returning fluid in the hollow medial to the patella. Normally none is seen.

A bulge indicates fluid within the knee joint. This sign can detect very small amounts of fluid but may be absent when a large amount of fluid is present under pressure.

Try to Ballotte a "Floating Patella." Firmly grasp the thigh just above the knee with one hand, thus forcing fluid out of the superior portion of the joint space into the space between the patella and femur. With the fingers of your other hand, push the patella sharply back against the femur. Feel for a palpable tap. In the absence of fluid none is felt.

A palpable tap indicates fluid within the knee joint. Ballottement is a less sensitive test than the procedure to detect a bulge sign, but it is useful when larger amounts of fluid are present.

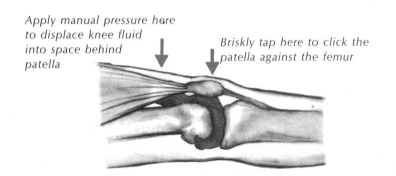

Apply manual pressure here to displace knee fluid into space behind patella

Briskly tap here to click the patella against the femur

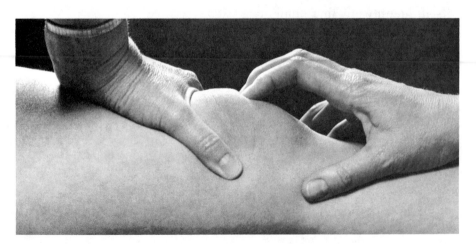

Range of Motion at Knees and Hips. Test rotation at the hip by rocking each of the patient's legs back and forth, in a rolling pin motion of the thigh.

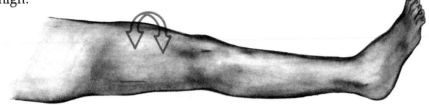

Estimate the range of motion by watching the patella and foot. Hip pain on this maneuver warrants great gentleness and caution with further tests.

Ask the patient to bend his knee up to his chest and pull it firmly against his abdomen.

Flexion of the opposite thigh indicates a flexion deformity of that hip.

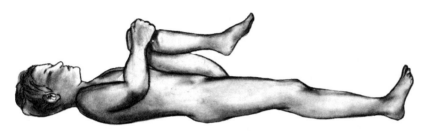

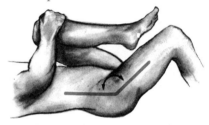

Observe the degree of flexion at the hip and knee. In addition, note whether the opposite thigh remains flat on the table.

Place the patient's foot on the opposite patella. Pull the knee laterally to rotate the leg externally at the hip. This maneuver combines flexion, abduction, and external rotation of the hip.

Pain in the hip or limitation of motion suggests an abnormality of the hip joint, such as arthritis.

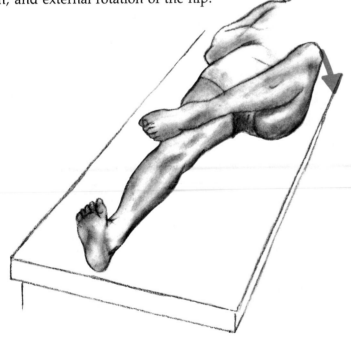

Then rotate the hip internally by pulling the knee medially, the foot laterally.

Pain in the hip or limitation of motion suggests an abnormality of the hip joint, such as arthritis.

As you return the patient's leg to its resting position, cup your hand over the knee to detect crepitation.

WITH THE PATIENT STANDING

THE SPINE

The gown should allow adequate visualization of the patient's spine.

Inspect the spinal profile, noting the normal cervical, thoracic, and lumbar curves.

See Table 14-8, Abnormal Spinal Curvatures (pp. 368–369).

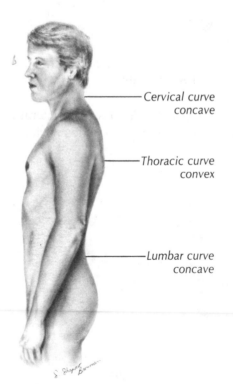

Cervical curve concave

Thoracic curve convex

Lumbar curve concave

Stand behind the patient and inspect the spine for lateral curvatures. Note any difference in height of the shoulders, the iliac crests, and the skin creases below the buttocks.

Unequal heights of the iliac crests (*i.e.*, a pelvic tilt) suggest that the legs may be unequal in length. Adduction or abduction deformities of the hip may also cause a tilt.

Note any knock-knee or bowleg deformity of the knees, swellings in the popliteal spaces, or flat feet.

Check the range of motion in the spine.

Ask the patient to bend forward to touch his toes (flexion). Note the symmetry of movement, the range of motion, the distance of his fingertips from the floor, and the curve in the lumbar area. As flexion proceeds, the lumbar concavity should become convex. A further way to test lumbar flexion is to place two or three fingers of the same hand on adjacent spinous processes and note their separation during flexion.

Persistence of the lumbar concavity and failure of the spinous processes to separate suggest spondylitis (arthritis of the spine).

Sit down, stabilize the patient's pelvis with your hands, and ask the patient to (1) bend sideways (lateral bending), (2) bend backwards toward you (extension), and (3) twist his shoulders one way and then the other (rotation).

Decreased spinal mobility in degenerative joint disease, ankylosing spondylitis

Now ask the patient to place his hands on the examining table, palms down and elbows straight, and rest his body weight there. Using your thumb, palpate the spinous processes for tenderness. You may also wish to percuss the spine for tenderness by thumping it (not too roughly) with the ulnar surface of your fist.

Percussion may produce pain when osteoporosis, malignancy, or infection involves the spine.

Inspect and palpate the paravertebral muscles for tenderness and spasm. Palpate for tenderness in any other areas that are suggested by the patient's symptoms. Try to identify the underlying structures involved. A skin dimple usually overlies the posterior iliac spine and guides you toward the sacroiliac area.

A paravertebral muscle in spasm looks prominent, feels tight, and is usually tender.

Remember that tenderness in the costovertebral angles may signify kidney infection rather than a musculoskeletal problem.

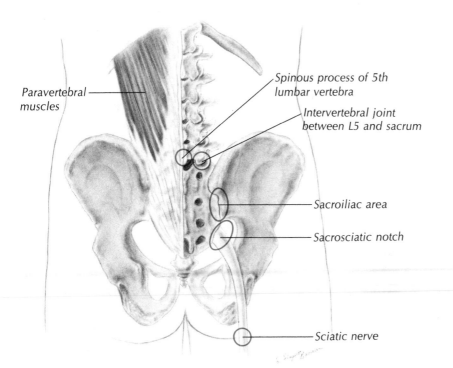

Paravertebral muscles

Spinous process of 5th lumbar vertebra

Intervertebral joint between L5 and sacrum

Sacroiliac area

Sacrosciatic notch

Sciatic nerve

Herniated intervertebral discs, most common between L5 and S1 or between L4 and L5, may produce tenderness of the spinous processes, the intervertebral joints, the paravertebral muscles, the sacrosciatic notch, and the sciatic nerve.

Rheumatoid arthritis may also cause tenderness of the intervertebral joints. Ankylosing spondylitis may produce sacroiliac tenderness.

See page 353 for further testing for a herniated lumbar disc.

If you suspect spondylitis, ask the patient to stand straight again, and measure his chest expansion in full inspiration and expiration. Use a nonelastic tape at the level of the nipple (or just above the nipples in women). Normal expansion in young adults is at least 5 cm or 6 cm.

Decreased chest expansion in spondylitis

SPECIAL MANEUVERS

For the Carpal Tunnel Syndrome. Pain and numbness in the hand, especially at night, suggest this syndrome. Hold the patient's wrists in acute flexion for 60 seconds.

If numbness and tingling develop over the distribution of the median nerve, (*e.g.,* the palmar surface of the thumb, index, middle, and part of the ring fingers) the sign is positive (a positive Phalen's sign). This indicates compression of the median nerve at the wrist.

For Stability of the Knee. When the patient reports that his knee buckles or gives way, test for stability. With the patient's knee extended, fix the femur in one hand, grasp the ankle with the other, and attempt to adduct and abduct the leg at the knee. Normally there is almost no motion.

Mobility on abduction indicates relaxation or tear of the medial collateral ligament; on adduction, of the lateral collateral ligament.

With the patient lying down, flex the knee to 90°. Stabilize the foot by gently sitting on it. Grasp the lower leg below the knee and try to push it forward and backward. Normally there is little or no movement.

Increased anterior mobility indicates anterior cruciate ligament instability; increased posterior mobility indicates posterior cruciate ligament instability.

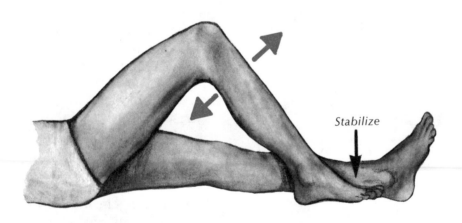

Stabilize

For a Torn Meniscus. A torn meniscus may be suspected because of local tenderness or because of pain on abduction or adduction of the leg at the knee. (See test for stability of the knee above.)

See Table 14-7, Local Tenderness in the Knee (pp. 366–367).

McMurray's test may also be helpful. Fully flex the knee of the supine patient so that the foot is close to the buttock. Place one hand on the knee so that your thumb and index finger lie on either side of the joint space. With your other hand grasp the heel and, using both hand and forearm, rotate the foot and lower leg laterally. Maintaining this rotation, extend the knee to a right angle. Feel and listen for a click.

A palpable or audible click that is recognized by the patient as one of his symptoms and is sometimes associated with transient pain suggests a torn medial meniscus.

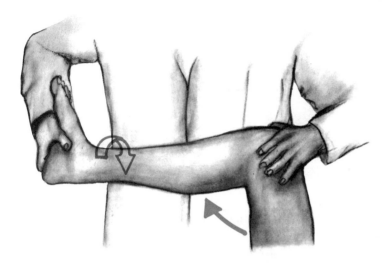

Repeat the maneuver, using medial rotation of the foot.

A click with similar characteristics suggests a torn lateral meniscus.

For a Herniated Lumbar Disc (Sciatica). If the patient has noted low back pain or sciatic pain, check straight leg raising. Raise the patient's relaxed leg until back pain occurs. Then dorsiflex his foot. Tight hamstrings may normally produce discomfort or pain behind the knees.

Back pain (not hamstring pain) is produced by straight leg raising and is increased by dorsiflexion of the foot when there is pressure on the lumbosacral nerve roots, as from a herniated disc. Be sure to check the legs for neurologic impairment such as sensory loss, weakness, or decrease in reflexes.

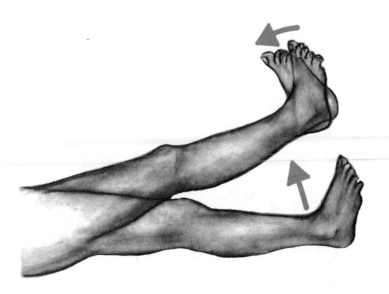

For Sacroiliac Pain. Move the patient to one side of the examining table. While he is clasping the opposite knee firmly flexed against his abdomen, carefully lower the patient's extended leg and thigh over the edge of the examining table, thus hyperextending the leg at the hip.

In sacroiliac disease, sacroiliac pain occurs on the hyperextended side.

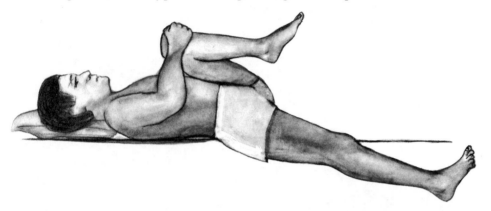

Move the patient to the other side of the table and repeat on the opposite side.

Measuring the Length of Legs. If you suspect that the patient's legs are unequal in length, measure them. Get the patient relaxed, flat on his back, and symmetrically aligned with legs extended. With a tape, measure the distance between anterior superior iliac spine and the medial malleolus. The tape should cross the knee on its medial side.

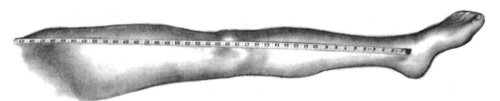

Describing Limited Motion of a Joint. The range of motion of a joint, when limited, should usually be described in degrees. Two examples follow. In the first the zero point of the joint cannot be reached and a flexion deformity results. The numbers in parentheses show abbreviated recordings.

A. The elbow flexes from 45° to 90° (45° → 90°),

-or-

The elbow has a flexion deformity of 45° and flexes further to 90° (45° → 90°).

B. Supination of elbow = 30° (0° → 30°)
Pronation of elbow = 45° (0° → 45°)

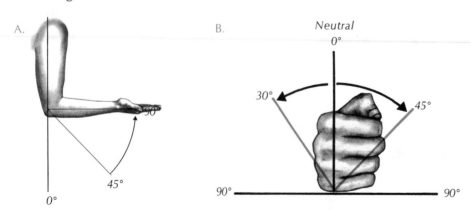

Table 14-1

Table 14-1 Problems in the Neck

MUSCLE SPASM

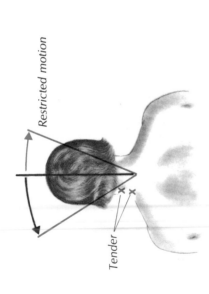

Restricted motion

Tender

Acute self-limited episodes of muscle spasm and pain in the neck produce the familiar "stiff neck." Its cause is unknown. The involved muscles, usually the trapezius, are tender and cordlike to the touch. Pain is often accentuated by lateral bending away from the painful side.

More chronic areas of aching pain and tightness of the neck muscles are also common. They may be associated with chronic postural strain, tension states, and depression. Look for tender muscular cords when the patient complains of chronic headache or neck pain.

HERNIATION OF A CERVICAL DISC

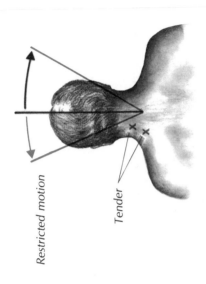

Restricted motion

Tender

Acute and recurrent neck pain may be caused by herniation of an intervertebral disc that presses on a nerve root in the neck. Muscles of the neck or near the scapula on the involved side are tender and spastic. Their location varies according to the disc involved. Movements of the neck, especially extension and lateral bending toward the involved side, are limited by pain. Examine the arms for evidence of nerve root involvement: areas of diminished or absent sensation and signs of lower motor neuron damage (*i.e.*, atrophy, fasciculations, and diminished reflexes).

Continued

Table 14-1

Table 14-1 (Cont'd)

CERVICAL SPONDYLOSIS

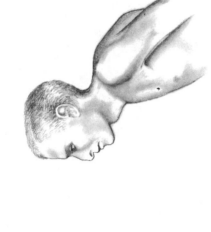

Restricted motion

Cervical spondylosis is a chronic problem, comprising degeneration of one or more intervertebral discs in the neck, narrowing of the joint spaces, and the bony spurring of degenerative arthritis. Some neck pain and limitation of neck movements are common. Two complications are important: (1) pressure on nerve roots with symptoms and signs like those of a herniated cervical disc, and (2) less commonly, pressure on the spinal cord itself. The latter may produce upper motor neuron signs (weakness, spasticity, and increased deep tendon reflexes) and sensory loss (especially vibration) in the legs.

ANKYLOSING SPONDYLITIS

Ankylosing spondylitis usually begins in the sacroiliac joints and low back, reaching the neck only relatively late in its course. Diagnosis of the neck problem, therefore, is not usually difficult. Limitation of motion and tender spastic muscles are common early signs. The late picture of extensive disease is shown here. The head and neck are thrust forward, contrasting with the kyphotic thoracic spine. Immobility of the neck may force the patient to turn his whole body in order to look sideways.

Table 14-2

Table 14-2 Swellings and Deformities of the Hands

DEGENERATIVE JOINT DISEASE (OSTEOARTHRITIS)

Nodules on the dorsolateral aspects of the distal interphalangeal joints are the hallmark of degenerative joint disease, or osteoarthritis, and are called Heberden's nodes. Usually hard and painless, they affect the middle-aged or elderly and often, although not always, are associated with arthritic changes in other joints. Flexion and deviation deformities may develop. Similar nodules on the proximal interphalangeal joints, called Bouchard's nodes, are less common. The metacarpophalangeal joints are spared.

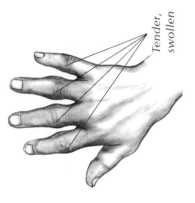

Radial deviation of distal phalanx

Heberden's node

Bouchard's node

Metacarpophalangeal joints uninvolved

ACUTE RHEUMATOID ARTHRITIS

Tender, painful, stiff joints characterize rheumatoid arthritis. Symmetrical involvement on both sides of the body is typical. The proximal interphalangeal, metacarpophalangeal, and wrist joints are frequently affected; the distal interphalangeal joints rarely so. Patients with acute disease often present with fusiform or spindle-shaped swelling of the proximal interphalangeal joints.

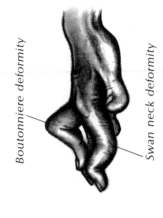

Tender, swollen

CHRONIC RHEUMATOID ARTHRITIS

As the arthritic process continues and worsens, chronic swelling and thickening of the metacarpophalangeal and proximal interphalangeal joints appear. Range of motion becomes limited and the fingers may deviate toward the ulnar side. The interosseous muscles atrophy. The fingers may show "swan neck" deformities (*i.e.*, hyperextension of the proximal interphalangeal joints with fixed flexion of the distal interphalangeal joints). Less common is a boutonniere deformity, (*i.e.*, persistent flexion of the proximal interphalangeal joint with hyperextension of the distal interphalangeal joint).

Rheumatoid nodules may accompany either the acute or chronic stage.

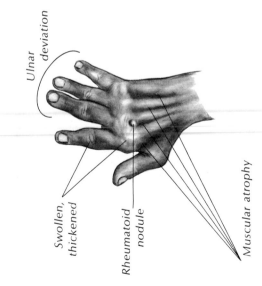

Ulnar deviation

Swollen, thickened

Rheumatoid nodule

Muscular atrophy

Boutonniere deformity

Swan neck deformity

Continued

Table 14-2

Table 14-2   (Cont'd)

GANGLION

Ganglia are cystic, round, usually nontender swellings located along tendon sheaths or joint capsules. The dorsum of the hand and wrist is a frequent site of involvement. Flexion of the wrist makes ganglia more prominent; extension tends to obscure them. Ganglia may also develop elsewhere on the hands, wrists, ankles, and feet.

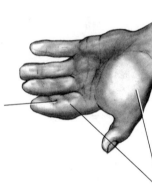

Cystic swelling

CHRONIC TOPHACEOUS GOUT

The deformities that develop in longstanding chronic tophaceous gout can sometimes mimic those of rheumatoid and osteoarthritis. Joint involvement is usually not so symmetrical as in rheumatoid arthritis. Acute inflammation may or may not be present. Knobby swellings around the joints sometimes ulcerate and discharge white chalklike urates.

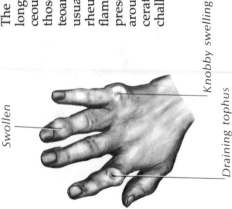

Swollen

Knobby swelling

Draining tophus

TENDON SHEATH AND PALMAR SPACE INFECTIONS

ACUTE TENOSYNOVITIS

Infection of the flexor tendon sheaths (acute tenosynovitis) may follow local injury, even of apparently trivial nature. Unlike arthritis, tenderness and swelling develop not in the joint but along the course of the tendon sheath, from the distal phalanx to the level of the metacarpophalangeal joint. The finger is held in slight flexion; attempts to extend it are very painful.

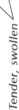

ACUTE TENOSYNOVITIS

Pain on extension

Swelling and tenderness along tendon sheath

Finger held in slight flexion

ACUTE TENOSYNOVITIS AND THENAR SPACE INVOLVEMENT

If the infection progresses, it may escape the bounds of the tendon sheath to involve one of the adjacent fascial spaces within the palm. Infections of the index finger and thenar space are illustrated.

Early diagnosis and treatment are important.

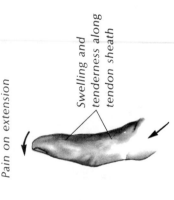

Puncture wound

Tender, swollen

Continued

Table 14-2

Table 14-2 (Cont'd)

DUPUYTREN'S CONTRACTURE

The first sign of a Dupuytren's contracture is a thickened plaque overlying the tendon of the ring finger and possibly the little finger at the level of the distal palmar crease. Subsequently the skin in this area puckers, and a thickened fibrotic cord develops between palm and finger. Flexion contracture of the fingers may gradually ensue.

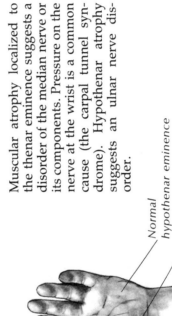

Flexion contraction

Cord

FELON

Injury to the fingertip may result in infection in the enclosed fascial spaces of the finger pad. Severe pain, localized tenderness, swelling, and dusky redness are characteristic. Early diagnosis and treatment are important.

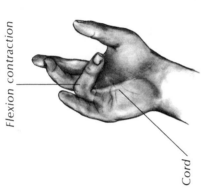

Puncture wound

Swollen, tender, dusky red

THENAR ATROPHY

Muscular atrophy localized to the thenar eminence suggests a disorder of the median nerve or its components. Pressure on the nerve at the wrist is a common cause (the carpal tunnel syndrome). Hypothenar atrophy suggests an ulnar nerve disorder.

Normal hypothenar eminence

Flattened thenar eminence

Table 14-3

Table 14-3 Swollen or Tender Elbows

OLECRANON BURSITIS

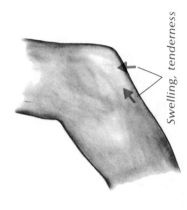

Swelling and inflammation of the olecranon bursa may result from trauma or may be associated with rheumatoid or gouty arthritis. The swelling is superficial to the olecranon process.

ARTHRITIS OF THE ELBOW

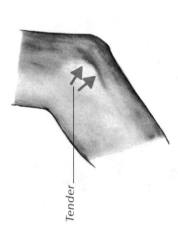

Swelling, tenderness

Synovial inflammation or fluid is best felt in the grooves between the olecranon process and the epicondyles on either side. Palpate for a boggy, soft, or fluctuant swelling and for tenderness.

RHEUMATOID NODULES

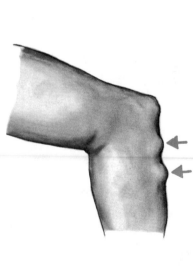

Subcutaneous nodules may develop at pressure points along the extensor surface of the ulna in patients with rheumatoid arthritis. They are firm and nontender, and are not attached to the overlying skin. They may or may not be attached to the underlying periosteum. Although they may develop in the area of the olecranon bursa, they often occur more distally.

TENNIS ELBOW

Tender

Tennis elbow is a painful musculoskeletal condition that may follow repetitive forceful pronation–supination of the forearm or extension of the wrist. Point tenderness is found at or just distal to the lateral epicondyle, where the extensor muscles of the forearm originate. The elbow joint itself and the olecranon process are not involved.

Table 14-4

Table 14-4 Painful Shoulders*

CALCIFIED DEPOSITS IN THE SUPRASPINATUS AND RELATED TENDONS (THE ROTATOR CUFF)

Calcified deposit in the supraspinatus tendon

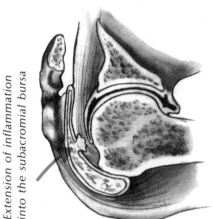

Extension of inflammation into the subacromial bursa

Compression with abduction

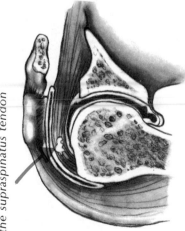

Acute inflammation associated with calcified deposits in the tendons around the shoulder (most often the supraspinatus) produces an acutely painful shoulder. The arm is held close to the side, and all motions, especially abduction and external rotation, are severely limited by pain. Tenderness is maximal below the acromion along the greater tubercle and lateral aspect of the humeral head.

Gradually the deposits work their way to the surface of the tendon, produce inflammation in the wall of the subacromial bursa, or rupture into the bursa itself. The term "bursitis," which is often loosely applied to all such painful shoulder syndromes, is then appropriate.

Less severe, chronic symptoms may also be seen with calcified deposits in the rotator cuff tendons. Protruding deposits may produce characteristic twinges of pain on abduction as they are compressed between the humerus and the ligamentous arch joining acromion and coracoid. Pain begins at about 60° or 70° of abduction and persists until the protrusion clears the arch at about 120°.

Continued

Table 14-4

Table 14-4   (Cont'd)

TENDONITIS OF THE BICEPS

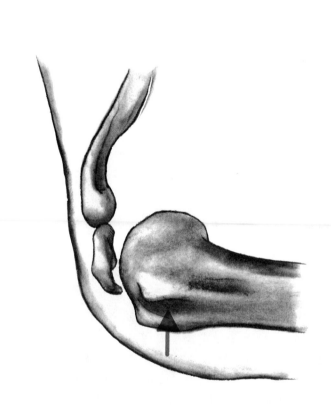

Pain and tenderness are maximal over the long head of the biceps tendon in the groove between the tubercles on the head of the humerus. Maneuvers which increase the tension in the biceps tendon produce localized pain in this area. To test for this, place the patient's arm at his side with elbow flexed to 90° and instruct him to supinate his forearm against your resisting hand.

RUPTURE OF THE SUPRASPINATUS TENDON

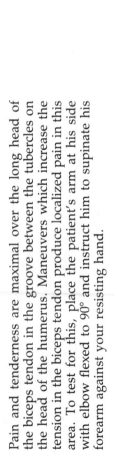

Shoulder shrugging effort

Tender

Normal abduction

Limited abduction

Because of injury, such as a fall, the supraspinatus tendon may rupture completely or partially. In addition to tenderness just below the acromion along the greater tubercle of the humerus, the patient is unable to abduct his arm. Efforts to do so produce a characteristic shoulder shrugging instead.

*For other causes of painful shoulders, refer to textbooks of arthritis or orthopedics.

Table 14-5

Table 14-5 Abnormalities of the Feet and Toes

ACUTE GOUTY ARTHRITIS

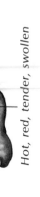

Hot, red, tender, swollen

The metatarsophalangeal joint of the great toe is often the first joint involved in acute gouty arthritis. It is characterized by a very painful and tender, hot, dusky red swelling which extends beyond the margin of the joint. It is easily mistaken for a cellulitis.

HALLUX VALGUS

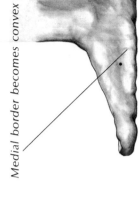

In hallux valgus the great toe is abnormally abducted in relationship to the first metatarsal, which itself is deviated medially. The head of the first metatarsal may enlarge on its medial side and a bursa may form at the pressure point. This bursa may become inflamed.

FLAT FEET

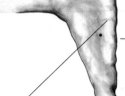

Medial border becomes convex

Sole touches floor

Signs of flat feet may be apparent only when the patient stands, or they may become permanent. The longitudinal arch flattens so that the sole approaches or touches the floor. The normal concavity on the medial side of the foot becomes convex. Tenderness may be present from the internal malleolus down along the medial-plantar surface of the foot. Swelling may develop anterior to the malleoli. Inspect the shoes for excess wear on the inner side of the soles and heels.

Continued

Table 14-5

Table 14-5   (Cont'd)

INGROWN TOENAIL

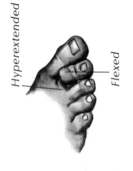

Red, tender

Granulation tissue

The sharp edge of the great toenail may dig into and injure the skin fold, resulting in inflammation and infection. A tender, reddened, overhanging nail fold, sometimes with granulation tissue and purulent discharge, results.

HAMMER TOE

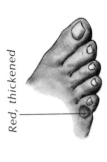

Hyperextended

Flexed

Most commonly involving the second toe, a hammer toe is characterized by hyperextension at the metatarsophalangeal joint with flexion at the proximal interphalangeal joint. A corn frequently develops at the pressure point over the proximal interphalangeal joint.

CORN

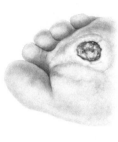

Red, thickened

A corn is a painful conical thickening of skin that results from recurrent pressure on normally thin skin. The apex of the cone points inward and causes pain. Corns characteristically occur over bony prominences (*e.g.,* the 5th toe). When located in moist areas (*e.g.,* at pressure points between the 4th and 5th toes), they are called soft corns.

CALLUS

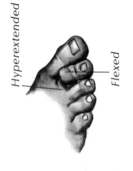

Like a corn, a callus is an area of greatly thickened skin that develops in a region of recurrent pressure. Unlike a corn, however, a callus involves skin that is normally thick, such as the sole, and is usually painless. If a callus is painful, suspect an underlying plantar wart.

PLANTAR WART

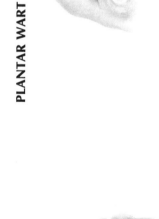

A plantar wart is a common wart (Verruca vulgaris) located in the thickened skin of the sole. It may look somewhat like a callus or even be covered by one. Look for the characteristic small dark spots that give a stippled appearance to a wart. Normal skin lines stop at the wart's edge.

NEUROTROPHIC ULCER

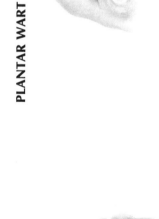

When pain sensation is diminished or absent (as in diabetic neuropathy, for example), neurotrophic ulcers may develop at pressure points on the feet. Although often deep, infected, and indolent, they are painless. Callus formation about the ulcer is diagnostically helpful. Like the ulcer itself, it results from chronic pressure.

Table 14-6

Table 14-6   Swellings of the Knee

SWELLING IN THE KNEE JOINT

SUPRAPATELLAR SWELLING

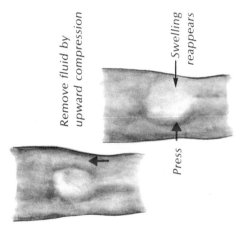

Mild to moderate

Marked

With synovial thickening or effusion the normal hollows above and on either side of the patella may be obliterated. Swelling of the suprapatellar pouch may produce fullness or even bogginess. Feel for bogginess above and beside the patella and in the tibiofemoral joint space. Look for associated atrophy of the quadriceps muscle.

BULGE SIGN

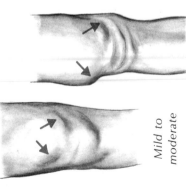

Remove fluid by upward compression

Press

Swelling reappears

Small amounts of fluid (4–8 ml) in the knee are demonstrable by the bulge sign. Stroke the medial aspect of the knee upward to displace the fluid, then press or tap the opposite side and watch for the fluid to return. This is a more sensitive sign of knee fluid than the patellar tap.

PREPATELLAR BURSITIS
(Housemaid's Knee)

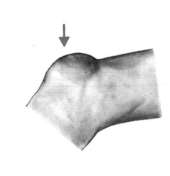

Superficial swelling sharply limited to the prepatellar area (including the upper part of the patellar tendon) indicates fluid in the prepatellar bursa.

Table 14-7

Table 14-7 Local Tenderness in the Knee

Tenderness in or near the knee may be caused by inflammation of the synovial membrane within the joint itself, but may also stem from other structures, such as the collateral ligaments, menisci, tibial tuberosity, bursae, and infrapatellar fat pad.

COLLATERAL LIGAMENTS AND MENISCI

POINTS OF MAXIMAL TENDERNESS

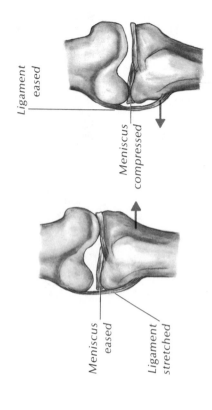

Medial collateral ligament

Lateral collateral ligament

Lateral meniscus

Medial meniscus

Tenderness maximal at the ligamentous attachment at one of the femoral epicondyles suggests a disorder of the collateral ligament. Tenderness localized below the epicondyle in the area of the joint space suggests a disorder of the meniscus.

DIFFERENTIATING MANEUVERS

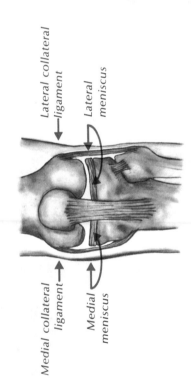

Ligament eased

Meniscus compressed

Meniscus eased

Ligament stretched

To help distinguish further between these two, stabilize the femur and try to abduct and adduct the lower leg, using the knee as a fulcrum. Movement that stretches a diseased collateral ligament produces pain. The opposite movement compresses the meniscus which, if torn, hurts.

Continued

Table 14-7

Table 14-7 (Cont'd)

OSGOOD–SCHLATTER DISEASE

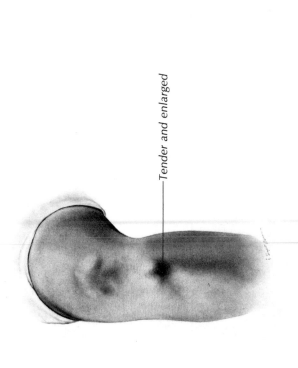

Tender and enlarged

A painful knee in an overweight adolescent boy, especially when he kneels or exercises, suggests Osgood–Schlatter disease. Examination of the knee joint is normal, but the tibial tuberosity is tender and enlarged.

BURSAE AND FAT PAD

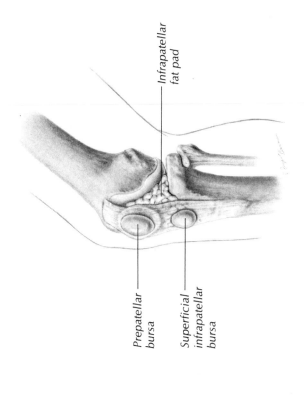

Infrapatellar fat pad

Prepatellar bursa

Superficial infrapatellar bursa

Other structures of the knee may become tender, especially when traumatized. They include the prepatellar bursa, the superficial infrapatellar bursa, and the infrapatellar fat pad.

Table 14-8

Table 14-8 Abnormal Spinal Curvatures

NORMAL SPINAL CURVA-TURES	FLATTENING OF THE LUMBAR CURVE	LUMBAR LORDOSIS	KYPHOSIS
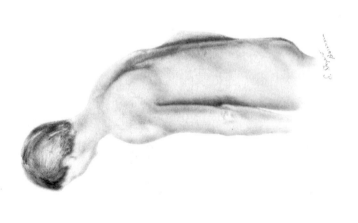	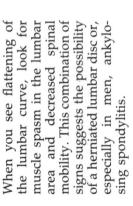	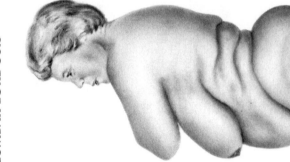	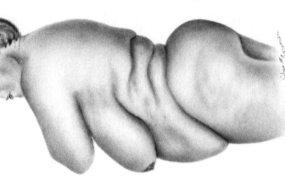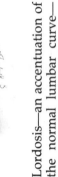
Note the gentle curves of the normal spine—concavities in the cervical and lumbar regions and a convexity in the thorax.	When you see flattening of the lumbar curve, look for muscle spasm in the lumbar area and decreased spinal mobility. This combination of signs suggests the possibility of a herniated lumbar disc or, especially in men, ankylosing spondylitis.	Lordosis—an accentuation of the normal lumbar curve—develops to compensate for the protuberant abdomen of pregnancy or marked obesity (as illustrated here). It may also compensate for kyphosis and flexion deformities of the hips. A deep midline furrow may be seen between the lumbar paravertebral muscles.	Kyphosis—a rounded thoracic convexity—is common in aging, especially in women. In adolescents consider Scheuermann's disease.

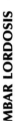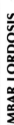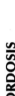

Continued

Table 14-8

Table 14-8 (Cont'd)

GIBBUS	LIST	SCOLIOSIS

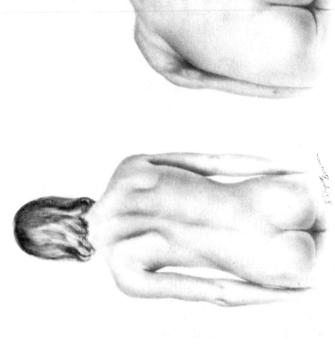

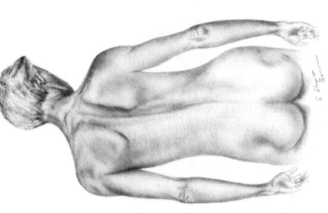

Gibbus is an angular deformity of a collapsed vertebra. Causes include metastatic cancer and tuberculosis of the spine.

List is a lateral tilt of the spine. When a plumb line dropped from the spinous process of T1 falls to one side of the gluteal cleft, a list is present. Causes include a herniated disc and painful spasms of the paravertebral muscles. Scoliosis (a lateral curve of the spine) is inherent in a list but has not been fully compensated for by a spinal deviation in the opposite direction.

Scoliosis—a lateral curvature of the spine—is shown here with a thoracic convexity to the right. Scoliosis may be structural, as illustrated, or functional, when it compensates for other abnormalities such as unequal leg lengths. Structural scoliosis is typically associated with rotation of the vertebrae upon each other, and the rib cage is accordingly deformed. When the patient bends forward, structural scoliosis is accentuated, the chest wall on the side of the thoracic convexity is prominent, and the scapula is elevated. Functional scoliosis does not involve vertebral rotation and disappears with forward flexion.

Chapter 15
THE NERVOUS SYSTEM

Anatomy and Physiology

It is impossible to review here all the anatomy and physiology relevant to the nervous system. This section deals briefly with the anatomy and physiology that relate directly to physical examination. First it outlines the simplest level of nervous response—the reflex arc. It then summarizes the motor pathways that initiate voluntary action, coordinate movements, and maintain posture and balance. Sensory pathways are considered next, then the cranial nerves, and the general structure of the brain itself. The section concludes with variations in neurologic findings that are associated with age.

THE REFLEX ARC

A reflex is an involuntary bodily response involving three basic components: a receiving apparatus, a nerve center, and a responding apparatus. Muscle stretch (or deep tendon) reflexes in the arms and legs illustrate this fundamental organization.

To elicit a muscle stretch reflex one briskly taps the tendon of a partially stretched muscle. By stretching the muscle further, such a tap stimulates special sensory endings in the muscle and generates an impulse that travels up each of many *sensory** nerve fibers* to the spinal cord. Each sensory fiber travels with other sensory and motor nerve fibers in a *peripheral nerve*.

---

*The word "sensory," as used here, does not necessarily imply conscious sensation, although many authors prefer to use the term in this restricted sense. It would be more precise to use the term "afferent," indicating the direction in which the nerve impulse travels (*i.e.*, toward the spinal cord or brain).

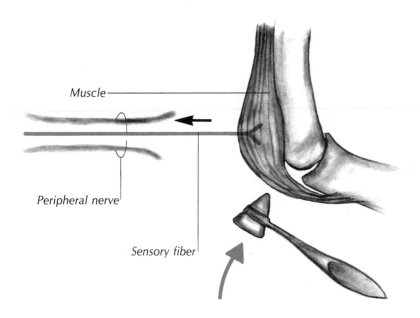

Muscle

Peripheral nerve

Sensory fiber

A peripheral nerve may carry nerve fibers supplying a fairly large area of the body. Centrally, peripheral nerves are reorganized on a segmental basis into 31 pairs of *spinal nerves* (8 cervical, 12 thoracic, 5 lumbar, 5 sacral, and 1 coccygeal). Within the vertebral canal, each spinal nerve separates into posterior (dorsal) and anterior (ventral) roots. The *posterior root* contains the sensory fibers. The sensory nerve impulse for the muscle stretch reflex is carried on through the sensory fiber into the spinal cord where it synapses with a *motor neuron,* or *anterior horn cell.*

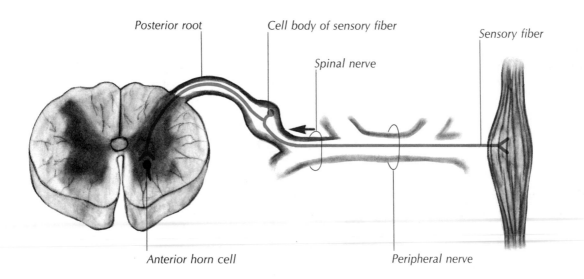

Posterior root

Cell body of sensory fiber

Sensory fiber

Spinal nerve

Anterior horn cell

Peripheral nerve

After stimulation across the synapse, an impulse is then transmitted down the motor neuron, traversing in turn the motor *anterior nerve root,* the spinal nerve, and the peripheral nerve. By transmitting an impulse across the neuromuscular junction, it then stimulates the muscle to a brisk contraction, completing the reflex arc.

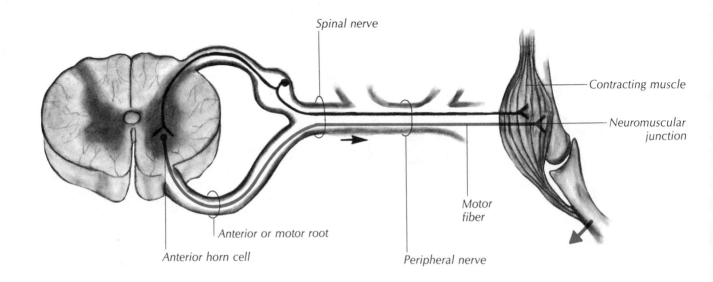

A muscle stretch reflex is thus dependent on (1) intact sensory nerve fibers, (2) functional synapses in the spinal cord, (3) intact motor nerve fibers, (4) functional neuromuscular junctions, and (5) competent muscle fibers.

Muscle stretch reflexes characteristically involve only a few spinal segments together with their sensory and motor fibers. An abnormality in such a reflex, therefore, helps to localize a pathologic lesion. You should know the segmental levels of the following muscle stretch reflexes:

Biceps reflex	Cervical 5,6
Supinator (brachioradialis) reflex	Cervical 5,6
Triceps reflex	Cervical 6,7,8
Knee reflex	Lumbar 2,3,4
Ankle reflex	Lumbar 5, Sacral 1,2

Reflexes may be initiated by stimulating skin as well as muscle. Such superficial, or cutaneous, reflexes depend not only on their spinal reflex arcs, however, but also on pathways to and from the cerebral cortex. Unlike muscle stretch reflexes they disappear when these higher pathways are destroyed. Learn the segmental levels of the following superficial reflexes:

Abdominal—Upper	Thoracic 8,9,10
—Lower	Thoracic 10,11,12
Plantar	Lumbar 4,5, Sacral 1,2

MOTOR PATHWAYS

Higher motor pathways of three kinds impinge on the anterior horn cells: (1) the corticospinal, or pyramidal, tract, (2) the extrapyramidal system, and (3) the cerebellar system.

1. *The Corticospinal or Pyramidal Tract.* Voluntary movements originate in the motor cortex of the brain. Fibers from nerve cells there travel down through the corticospinal tract to the brain stem. Here most of them cross over to the opposite side and then continue down the spinal cord where they synapse with anterior horn cells or with intermediate neurons. The corticospinal tracts not only mediate voluntary movement but also integrate skilled, complicated, or delicate movements by grading the motor responses and by stimulating selected muscular actions while inhibiting others. They also carry impulses that inhibit muscle tone, the slight tension maintained by a normal muscle even when it is relaxed. Fibers similar to corticospinal fibers connect with motor nerve cells in the cranial nerves and are then termed corticobulbar. Both corticospinal and corticobulbar neurons are often called "upper motor neurons."

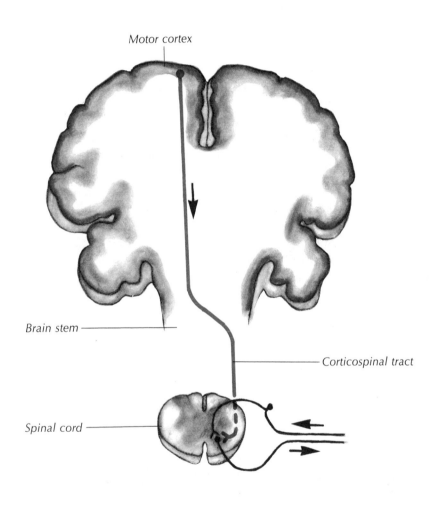

2. *The Extrapyramidal System.* This exceedingly complex system includes motor pathways between the cerebral cortex, basal ganglia, brain stem, and spinal cord but is outside the corticospinal or pyramidal tract system. It helps to maintain muscle tone and to control body movements, especially gross automatic movements such as walking.

3. *The Cerebellar System.* The cerebellum receives both sensory and motor input and coordinates muscular activity, maintains equilibrium, and helps control posture.

All three of these higher motor pathways affect motor activity only through the lower motor neuron—hence its name, "final common pathway." Any movement, whether initiated voluntarily in the cortex, "automatically" in the basal ganglia, or reflexly in the sensory receptor, must ultimately be translated into action via the anterior horn cell, the lower motor neuron. A lesion in any of these areas will produce effects on movement or reflex activity.

The type and distribution of motor deficit produced helps the examiner to determine where the causative lesion might be. A cerebellar lesion produces incoordination, for example, while disease of the basal ganglia increases muscle tone and diminishes the automatic movements associated with walking. Neither causes paralysis. In contrast, lesions of both upper and lower motor neurons cause weakness or paralysis. Interruption of lower motor neurons abolishes muscle stretch reflexes and decreases tone in the muscles that they innervate. These muscles, deprived of their motor nerve supply, lose bulk as well as tone, become wasted or atrophied, and may show spontaneous fine movements known as fasciculations (see p. 422). A lesion involving the corticospinal tracts, or upper motor neurons, in contrast, augments both muscle tone and muscle stretch reflexes because the normal inhibitory action is lost. There is relatively little associated atrophy in the muscles involved, and there are no fasciculations (see Table 15-7, pp. 423–424).

SENSORY PATHWAYS

Sensory impulses do not only participate in reflex activity, as previously described; they also give rise to conscious sensation.

Sensation is initiated by stimulation of sensory receptors located in skin, mucous membranes, muscles, tendons, and viscera. An impulse generated by one of these receptors travels along a sensory nerve fiber toward the spinal cord. In its course it usually travels with other sensory and motor nerve fibers in a peripheral nerve. The peripheral nerve is reorganized centrally on a segmental basis, divides into posterior and anterior roots, and enters the spinal cord. The sensory nerve fiber follows the posterior (or dorsal) root. After entry into the spinal cord, the sensory impulse proceeds along one of two courses: (1) the spinothalamic tracts, or (2) the posterior columns.

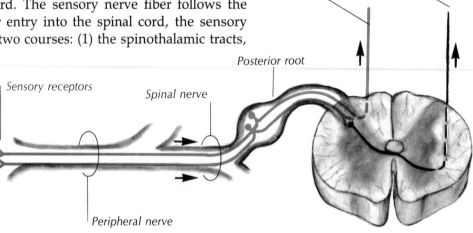

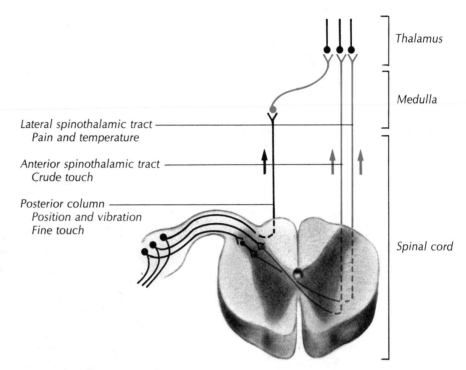

Within one or two spinal segments from their entry into the cord, fibers conducting the sensations of *pain* and *temperature* pass into the posterior horn of the spinal cord and synapse with secondary sensory neurons. These second neurons then cross to the opposite side just anterior to the central canal and pass upward in the lateral spinothalamic tract of the cord.

Fibers conducting the sensations of *position* and *vibration* pass directly into the *posterior columns* of the cord and travel upward to the medulla where they then synapse with secondary sensory neurons. These secondary neurons also cross over to the other side where they and the spinothalamic tracts continue on to the thalamus.

Lateral spinothalamic tract
Pain and temperature

Anterior spinothalamic tract
Crude touch

Posterior column
Position and vibration
Fine touch

Thalamus

Medulla

Spinal cord

Nerve fibers carrying the sensation of *light touch* take one of two pathways. Some fibers conduct *fine touch*—touch that is accurately localized and finely discriminating. These fibers travel in the posterior column together with fibers that carry position and vibration sense. A second group transmits *crude touch*—a sensation perceived as light touch but without accurate localization. These fibers synapse in the posterior horn with secondary neurons that cross to the opposite side and ascend in the anterior spinothalamic tract to the thalamus. Because touch impulses originating on one side of the body travel up both sides of the cord, touch sensation is often preserved despite partial damage to the cord.

At the thalamic level, the general quality of sensation is perceived (*e.g.*, pain, cold, pleasant and unpleasant), but fine distinctions are not made. For full perception, a third group of sensory neurons carries impulses from synapses in the thalamus to the sensory cortex of the brain. Here stimuli are localized and discriminations made between them.

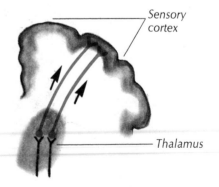

Sensory cortex

Thalamus

Lesions at different points in the sensory pathways produce different kinds of sensory loss. Patterns of sensory loss, together with their associated motor findings, are therefore helpful in figuring out where the causative lesions might be. Loss of position and vibration sense with preservation of other sensations points to disease of the posterior columns, for example, while the loss of all sensations from the waist down, together with paralysis and hyperactive reflexes in the legs, indicates transection of the spinal cord (see Table 15-8, pp. 425–426).

A knowledge of dermatomes also aids in localizing neurologic lesions. A dermatome is the band of skin innervated by the sensory nerve root of a single spinal segment. Dermatome patterns are mapped in the next two figures. Their levels are considerably more variable than the diagrams suggest, and dermatomes overlap each other. Do not try to memorize their details. It is useful, however, to remember the locations of the dermatomes outlined in red on the right side of the diagrams. The distribution of a few key peripheral nerves is shown in the inserts on the left.

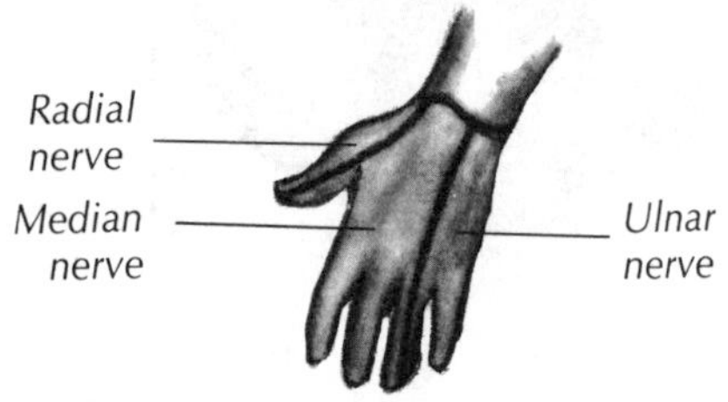

Radial nerve

Median nerve

Ulnar nerve

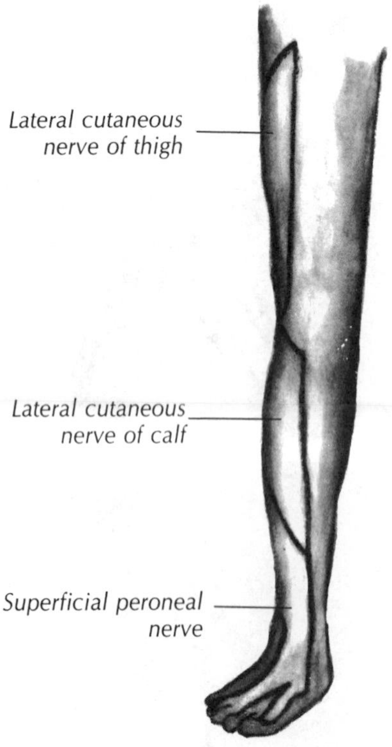

Lateral cutaneous nerve of thigh

Lateral cutaneous nerve of calf

Superficial peroneal nerve

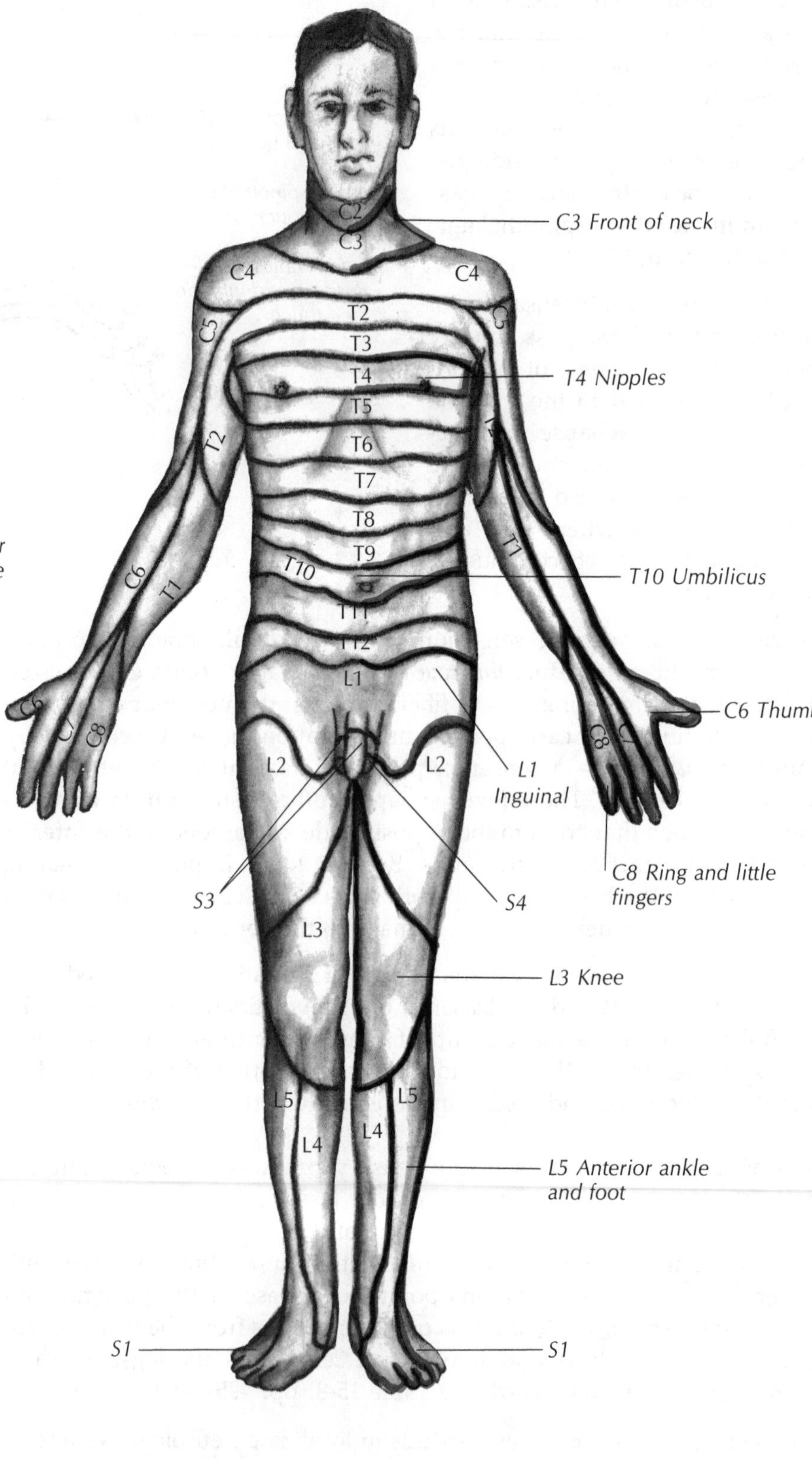

C2

C3

C4

C4

C5

C5

T2

T3

T4

T5

T6

T7

T8

T9

T10

T11

T12

L1

L2

L2

S3

S4

L3

L5

L5

L4

L4

S1

S1

C6

T1

T2

T1

C7

C8

C6

C8

C3 Front of neck

T4 Nipples

T10 Umbilicus

C6 Thumb

L1 Inguinal

C8 Ring and little fingers

L3 Knee

L5 Anterior ankle and foot

ANTERIOR

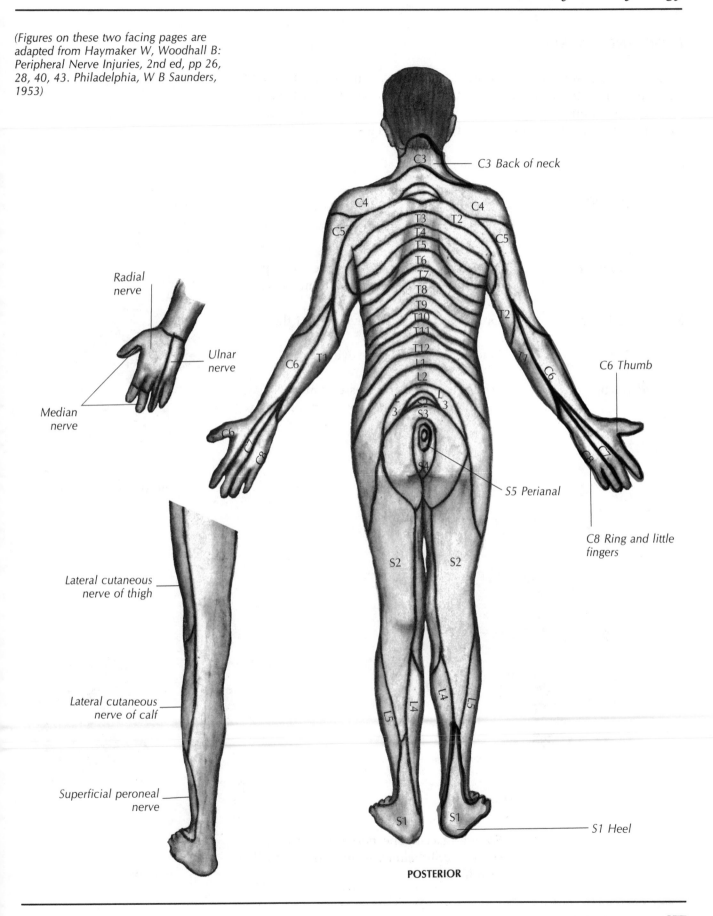

(Figures on these two facing pages are adapted from Haymaker W, Woodhall B: *Peripheral Nerve Injuries*, 2nd ed, pp 26, 28, 40, 43. Philadelphia, W B Saunders, 1953)

Radial nerve

Ulnar nerve

Median nerve

Lateral cutaneous nerve of thigh

Lateral cutaneous nerve of calf

Superficial peroneal nerve

C3 Back of neck

C6 Thumb

S5 Perianal

C8 Ring and little fingers

S1 Heel

POSTERIOR

THE CRANIAL NERVES

Nerves that emerge from the central nervous system within the head rather than from the vertebral column are called cranial nerves. There are 12 pairs. Functions of the cranial nerves most relevant to physical examination are summarized on these two facing pages.

No.	Nerve	Function
N_1	Olfactory	Sense of smell
N_2	Optic	Vision
N_3	Oculomotor	Pupillary constriction, elevation of upper eyelid, most of the extraocular movements
N_4	Trochlear	Downward, inward movement of the eye
N_6	Abducens	Lateral deviation of the eye
N_5	Trigeminal	*Motor*—temporal and masseter muscles (jaw clenching), also lateral movement of the jaw

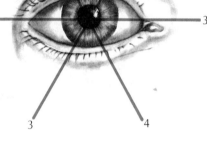

RIGHT EYE (N_3, N_4, N_6)

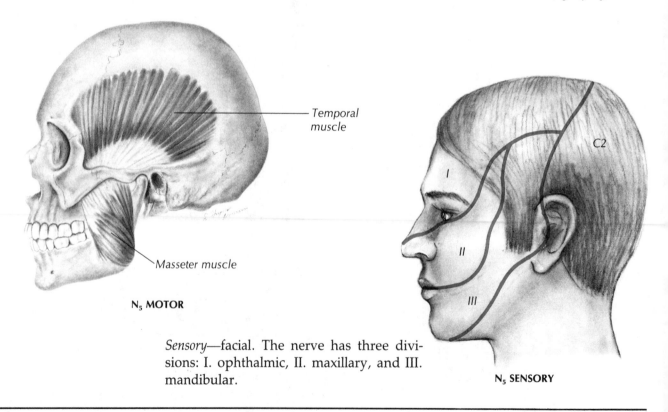

N_5 MOTOR

Sensory—facial. The nerve has three divisions: I. ophthalmic, II. maxillary, and III. mandibular.

N_5 SENSORY

N₇	Facial	*Motor*—muscles of the face, including those of the forehead and around the eyes and mouth
		Sensory—taste on anterior ⅔ of tongue
N₈	Acoustic	Hearing (cochlear division) and balance (vestibular division)
N₉	Glosso-pharyngeal	*Sensory*—posterior portion of eardrum and ear canal, pharynx, and posterior tongue, including taste
		Motor—pharynx
N₁₀	Vagus	*Sensory*—pharynx and larynx
		Motor—palate, pharynx, and larynx
N₁₁	Spinal accessory	*Motor*—the sternomastoid and upper portion of the trapezius

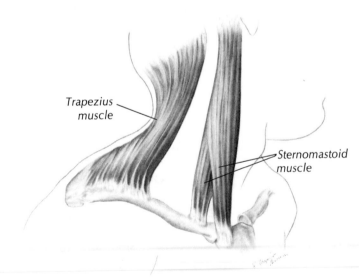

Trapezius muscle

Sternomastoid muscle

N₁₁ MOTOR

| N₁₂ | Hypo-glossal | *Motor*—tongue |

THE BRAIN

The brain has three regions: the brain stem, the cerebrum, and the cerebellum.

The brain stem is continuous with the spinal cord. It is traditionally divided into four sections: the diencephalon, the midbrain, the pons, and the medulla.

The paired cranial nerves 2 through 12 emerge from the brain stem. Their involvement by pathological processes sometimes helps to localize neurologic lesions. The relationships of the cranial nerves to the four parts of the brain stem are summarized in the diagram on the right.

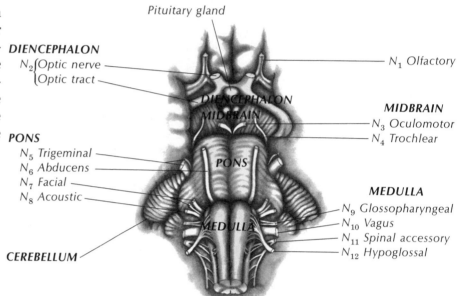

The cerebral hemispheres comprise the greatest mass of brain tissue. Their outer layers are formed by the cellular gray matter known as the cerebral cortex.

Consciousness depends upon interaction between intact cerebral hemispheres and the upper brain stem, where arousal or activating mechanisms reside. Either extensive disease of the cerebral cortex or lesions of the brain stem may impair consciousness to the point of coma.

The cerebellum is primarily concerned with coordination.

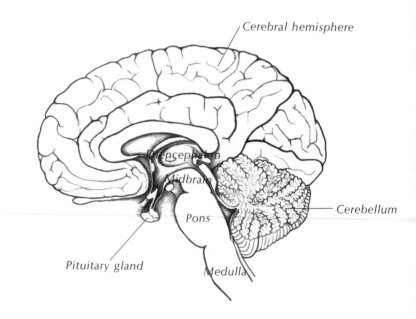

CHANGES WITH AGE

In assessing the nervous system of an elderly person it is sometimes difficult to distinguish the changes of normal aging from those of age-related disease. Some findings that you would consider abnormal in younger people, however, occur often enough in the elderly that you may attribute them to aging alone. Alterations in hearing, vision, extraocular movements, and pupillary size, shape, and reactivity have been described in Chapter 5 (see pp. 68–69). In addition, a person's ability to smell and taste may decline with age.

Muscular strength and agility begin to wane fairly early in adult life, as the relatively brief careers of professional athletes illustrate. Elderly persons move and react more slowly than younger ones. Muscle bulk decreases, and about half of elderly people will show some degree of muscular atrophy in their hands (see p. 389). Grip, though diminished, remains relatively strong. Ankle reflexes may be symmetrically decreased or absent, even when reinforced. Less commonly, knee reflexes are similarly affected. Abdominal reflexes may diminish or disappear, and partly because of musculoskeletal changes in the feet the plantar responses become less obvious and more difficult to interpret. Vibration sense is frequently decreased or lost in the feet and ankles. Less commonly, position sense may diminish or disappear and may contribute to unsteadiness in gait. Aged people occasionally become tremulous. Head, jaw, lips, or hands may tremble at a rate and amplitude suggesting Parkinson's disease, but without its muscular rigidity.

If changes such as those described are accompanied by other neurologic abnormalities, or if atrophy and reflex changes are asymmetrical, you should search for an explanation other than age alone.

Techniques of Examination

GENERAL APPROACH

Appropriate neurologic examination varies widely. In apparently healthy young adults simple screening is adequate. Screening procedures for the motor and sensory systems are included in this chapter and summarized in Chapter 2. If a person has symptoms such as headache, weakness, sensory changes, or loss of consciousness, however, you should evaluate his condition in greater depth. This chapter presents a practicable and reasonably inclusive neurologic examination. Be aware that many other techniques may be useful in specific situations. Consult textbooks of neurology as the need arises.

For efficiency you should integrate certain portions of your neurologic assessment with other parts of your examination. Make an initial survey of mental status and speech, for example, during the interview. Assess at least some of the cranial nerves as you examine the head and neck, and inspect the arms and legs for neurologic abnormalities while you also evaluate the peripheral vascular and musculoskeletal systems. Chapter 2 provides an outline for this kind of integrated approach. Think about and describe your findings, however, in terms of the nervous system as a unit.

Organize your thinking into five categories: (1) mental status and speech, (2) cranial nerves, (3) the motor system, (4) the sensory system, and (5) reflexes.

SURVEY OF MENTAL STATUS AND SPEECH

Note the patient's dress, grooming, and personal hygiene; his facial expression, manner, and affect; his manner of speech and his state of awareness or consciousness.

See Table 15-1, Abnormalities of Speech (p. 413).

See Table 15-2, Abnormalities of Consciousness (p. 413).

Make inquiries within the framework of interviewing that will give you information about the patient's orientation, memory, intellectual performance, and judgment.

If this survey suggests an abnormality, plan a more complete mental status examination as described in Chapter 16.

THE CRANIAL NERVES

First Cranial Nerve (Olfactory). Test the sense of smell by presenting the patient with one or more familiar odors. First be sure that each nasal passage is open by compressing one side of the nose and asking him to sniff through the other. Then ask him to close his eyes. Occlude one nostril and hold under his nose one of several nonirritating substances such as tobacco, coffee, soap, or vanilla. Ask him if he smells anything, and if so, what. Test the other side. A person should normally perceive odor on each side and can often identify it. The sense of smell may decrease with age.

Bilateral decrease or loss of smell has many causes, including nasal disease, excessive smoking, and the use of cocaine. It may be congenital. Unilateral loss of smell without nasal disease suggests a lesion in the frontal lobe of the brain.

Second Cranial Nerve (Optic). (See Chap. 5.)
Test visual acuity.

Inspect the optic fundi ophthalmoscopically, with special attention to the optic discs.

Optic atrophy, papilledema

Determine the visual fields by confrontation.

Now test for extinction of vision on one side. With both the patient's eyes open, wiggle your fingers simultaneously in both of the patient's upper temporal quadrants. Ask him to point to your movements. He should see both stimuli. Repeat in the lower temporal quadrants.

See Table 5-2, Visual Field Defects (p. 96). Perception of movement on only one side suggests a subtle visual loss, or extinction, on the other side. Like a hemianopsia or a quadrantic defect, extinction signifies a lesion of the parietal or occipital cortex.

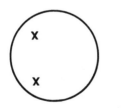 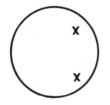   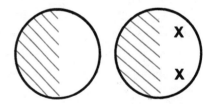

Third, Fourth, and Sixth Cranial Nerves (Oculomotor, Trochlear, and Abducens). (See Chap. 5.) Inspect the size and shape of the pupils, and compare one side with the other. Test the pupillary reactions to light and accommodation.

See Table 5-7, Pupillary Abnormalities (pp. 101–102).

Test the extraocular movements in the six cardinal fields of gaze, and look for loss of conjugate movements in any of the six directions. Check convergence of the eyes during accommodation. Identify any nystagmus, noting the field of gaze in which it appears, the plane in which movements occur (*e.g.,* horizontal, vertical), and the direction of the quick and slow components.

See Table 5-8, Deviations of the Eyes (p. 103).

See Table 15-3. Nystagmus (pp. 414–415).

Look for ptosis of the upper eyelids. A slight difference in the width of the palpebral fissures may be noted in about one third of all normal people.

Fifth Cranial Nerve (Trigeminal)

Motor. While palpating the temporal and masseter muscles in turn, ask the patient to clench his teeth. Note the strength of muscle contraction.

Weak or absent contraction of the temporal and masseter muscles on one side suggests a lesion of the 5th cranial nerve. Bilateral weakness may result from upper or lower motor neuron involvement. When the patient has no teeth, this test may be difficult to interpret.

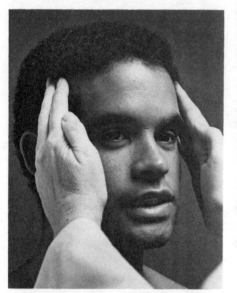

PALPATING TEMPORAL MUSCLES

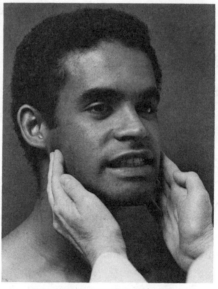

PALPATING MASSETER MUSCLES

Unilateral decrease or loss of facial sensation suggests a lesion of the 5th cranial nerve or of interconnecting higher sensory pathways. Such a sensory loss may also be associated with a conversion reaction.

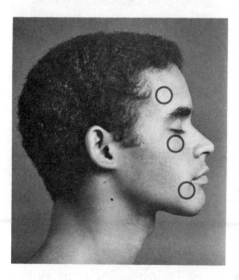

Sensory. With the patient's eyes closed, test the forehead, cheeks, and jaw on each side for pain sensation. Suggested areas are indicated by the circles. Use a safety pin, occasionally substituting the blunt end for the point as a stimulus. Ask the patient to report whether it is "sharp" or "dull" and to compare sides. (*Note:* You have tested for pain only in areas touched with the point of the pin. The dull end is a check on the patient's reliability.)

If you find an abnormality, confirm it by testing *temperature* sensation. Use two test tubes filled with hot and cold water. Touch the skin and ask the patient to identify "hot" or "cold."

Then test for *light touch*, using a fine wisp of cotton. Ask the patient to respond whenever you touch his skin.

Test the corneal reflex. Ask the patient to look up and away from you. Approaching from the other side, out of his line of vision, and avoiding his eyelashes, touch the cornea (not the conjunctiva) lightly with a fine wisp of cotton.

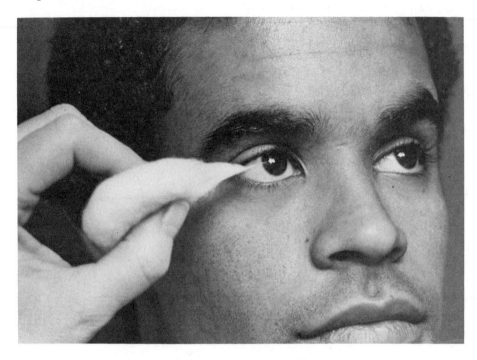

Look for blinking of the eyes, the normal reaction to this stimulus. (The sensory limb of this reflex is carried in the 5th cranial nerve, the motor response in the 7th).

Absence of blinking suggests a lesion of the 5th cranial nerve (as long as the 7th nerve is intact). Use of contact lenses may also diminish or abolish this reflex.

Seventh Cranial Nerve (Facial). Inspect the face, both at rest and during conversation with the patient. Note any asymmetry (*e.g.*, of the nasolabial folds), and observe any tics or other abnormal movements. Ask the patient to:

Flattening of the nasolabial fold and drooping of the lower eyelid suggest facial weakness.

1. Raise his eyebrows
2. Frown
3. Close his eyes tightly so that you cannot open them. Test his muscle strength by trying to open them.

4. Show his teeth
5. Smile
6. Puff out his cheeks

Note any weakness or asymmetry.

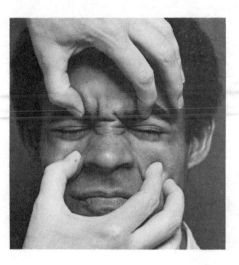

See Table 15-4, Types of Facial Paralysis (pp. 416–417).

In unilateral facial paralysis, the mouth is pulled away from the paralyzed side when the patient smiles or shows his teeth.

Eighth Cranial Nerve (Acoustic). *Assess hearing.* If hearing loss is present, (1) test for lateralization, and (2) compare air and bone conduction. (See Chap. 5.)

See Table 5-17, Patterns of Hearing Loss (p. 115).

Specific tests of *vestibular function* are seldom included in the usual neurologic examination, although nystagmus may indicate vestibular dysfunction. Consult textbooks of neurology or otolaryngology as the need arises.

Ninth and Tenth Cranial Nerves (Glossopharyngeal and Vagus). Listen for any hoarseness of the voice or a nasal quality to the patient's speech.

Hoarseness in vocal cord paralysis; a nasal voice in paralysis of the palate

Ask him to say "ah" or to yawn. Observe the upward motion of the soft palate and uvula and the inward "curtain" movement of the posterior pharynx. Identify any asymmetry. Except for the occasional slight curve in the uvula, the structures should be symmetrical.

The palate fails to rise with a bilateral lesion of the vagus nerve. In unilateral paralysis, one side of the palate fails to rise and, together with the uvula, is pulled toward the normal side. (See p. 123.)

Warn the patient that you are going to test his gag reflex. Stimulate the back of his throat lightly on each side in turn and note the gag reflex. It may be symmetrically diminished or absent in some normal people.

Unilateral absence of this reflex suggests a lesion of the 9th or perhaps the 10th cranial nerve.

Eleventh Cranial Nerve (Spinal Accessory). Look for atrophy or fasciculations in the trapezius muscles, and compare one side with the other. Ask the patient to shrug his shoulders upward against your hands. Note the strength and contraction of the trapezii.

Atrophy and fasciculations suggest lower motor neuron disease.

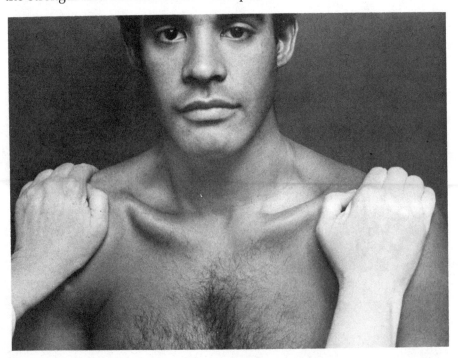

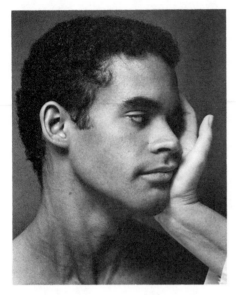

Ask the patient to turn his head to each side against your hand. Observe the contraction of the opposite sternomastoid and note the force of the movement against your hand.

Twelfth Cranial Nerve (Hypoglossal). Inspect the patient's tongue as it lies on the floor of the mouth. Look for any fasciculations. Some coarser restless movements are often seen in a normal tongue.

Atrophy and fasciculations suggest lower motor neuron disease.

Ask the patient to stick out his tongue. Look for asymmetry, atrophy, or deviation from the midline. Ask the patient to move his tongue from side to side, and note the symmetry of the movement.

The tongue deviates toward the paralyzed side. (See p. 122.)

THE MOTOR SYSTEM

SCREENING PROCEDURES, INCLUDING GAIT

Ask the patient to *walk* across the room or, preferably, down the hall, then turn, and come back. Observe his posture, balance, the swinging of his arms, and the movements of his legs. Normally balance is easy, the arms swing at the sides, and turns are smoothly accomplished.

See Table 15-5, Abnormalities of Gait and Posture (pp. 418–419).

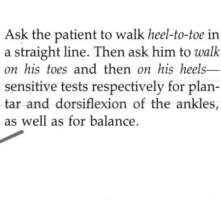

Ask the patient to walk *heel-to-toe* in a straight line. Then ask him to *walk on his toes* and then *on his heels*—sensitive tests respectively for plantar and dorsiflexion of the ankles, as well as for balance.

Done clumsily and uncertainly in cerebellar disease and during intoxicated states

Perform a Romberg test. Ask the patient to stand with his feet together and without support from his arms. Note his ability to maintain an upright posture first with his eyes open, then with his eyes closed. (Stand close enough to protect him should he lose his balance.) Normally only minimal swaying occurs.

When a patient has ataxia, or incoordination, from cerebellar disease, he may have difficulty standing with his feet together whether his eyes are open or closed. When a patient is ataxic because of decreased position sense, his vision can compensate for the sensory loss and he can stand fairly well with eyes open. With eyes closed, however, he loses his balance. This phenomenon constitutes a *positive Romberg's sign.*

When examining a reasonably healthy ambulatory patient, it is convenient to survey the patient further at this point by asking him to *hop in place* on each foot in turn. The ability to do this indicates an intact motor system in the legs, normal cerebellar function, and good position sense.

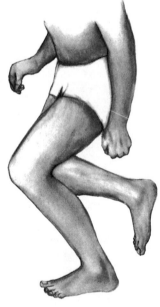

Ask him to do a shallow *knee bend*, first on one leg, then on the other.

Quadriceps weakness makes a knee bend difficult or impossible.

Screen the motor function of the arms by testing the patient's grip and asking him to *hold his arms forward, palms up.* (See pp. 391–392.)

FURTHER ASSESSMENT

If you detect abnormalities in screening or suspect them because of symptoms, proceed to a more detailed examination of the motor system. You may wish to alter the exact sequence of your examination to improve your efficiency or avoid tiring the patient. Keep in mind, however, the underlying organization of the assessment: inspection, assessment of muscle tone, testing of muscle strength, and assessment of coordination.

Inspection. Inspect the muscles of limbs and trunk, noting any *atrophy, fasciculations, involuntary movements,* or *abnormalities of position.* When looking for atrophy, pay particular attention to the shoulder and pelvic girdles and the hands. The thenar and hypothenar eminences should be full and convex, and the spaces between the metacarpals, where the dorsal interosseous muscles lie, should be full or only slightly depressed. Atrophy of hand muscles, however, may occur with normal aging, as shown below.

Atrophy and fasciculations suggest a lower motor neuron problem. Flattening of the thenar and hypothenar eminences and concavities or furrowing between the metacarpals suggest atrophy. Localized atrophy of the thenar and hypothenar eminences suggests damage to the median and ulnar nerves respectively.

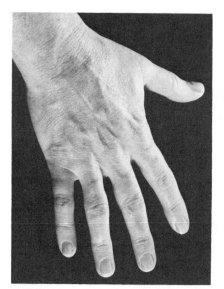

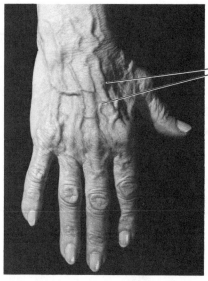

Atrophy

Hand of a 44-year-old woman

Hand of an 84-year-old woman

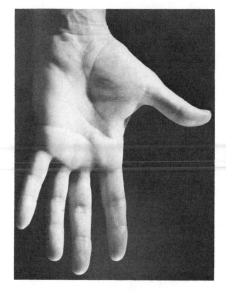

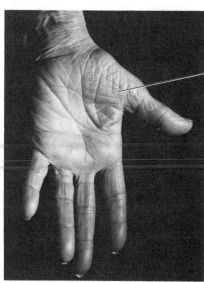

Flattening of mild atrophy

Hand of a 44-year-old woman

Hand of an 84-year-old woman

If you see any involuntary movements, note their location, quality, rate, rhythm, amplitude, and relation to posture, activity, fatigue, emotion, or other factors.

See Table 15-6. Involuntary Movements (pp. 420–422).

Assessment of Muscle Tone. When a normal muscle with an intact nerve supply is voluntarily relaxed, it maintains a slight residual tension known as muscle tone. This can be best assessed by feeling the muscle's resistance to passive stretch. Persuade the patient to relax. Take his hand with yours and, while supporting his elbow, flex and extend the patient's fingers, wrist, and elbow, and put his shoulder through a moderate range of motion. With practice, these actions can be combined into a single smooth movement. On each side note his muscle tone—the resistance offered to your movements. Tense patients may show increased resistance. You will learn the feel of normal resistance only with repeated practice.

Resistance to passive stretch is increased in upper motor neuron lesions and in parkinsonism. It is decreased when there is a lower motor lesion, when sensory neurons are destroyed, or when a cerebellar lesion is present. Hypotonic muscles are also called flaccid muscles.

If you suspect decreased resistance, hold the forearm and shake the hand loosely back and forth. Normally the hand moves back and forth freely but is not completely floppy.

Unusual floppiness suggests hypotonic, or flaccid, muscles.

While supporting the patient's thigh with one hand, flex and extend the patient's knee and ankle on each side. Note the resistance to your movements.

Testing Muscle Strength. Normal individuals vary widely in their strength, and your standard of normal, while admittedly rough, should allow for such variables as age, sex, and muscular training. A person's dominant side is usually stronger than the other side. Keep this difference in mind when you compare sides.

You usually test muscle strength by asking the patient to move actively against your resistance or to resist your movement. Watch for muscular contraction and feel for the strength exerted. Some muscles may be too weak to overcome resistance. You can then test them against gravity alone or with gravity eliminated. Finally, you may be able to see or feel a weak muscular contraction even if it fails to move the body part.

Impaired strength is called weakness or paresis. Absence of strength is called paralysis. *Hemiparesis* refers to weakness of one half of the body; *hemiplegia* refers to paralysis of one half of the body. *Paraplegia* means paralysis of the legs; *quadriplegia* means paralysis of all four limbs.

Muscle strength may be graded on a 0 to 5 scale:

0 No muscular contraction detected
1 A barely detectable flicker or trace of contraction
2 Active movement of the body part with gravity eliminated
3 Active movement against gravity
4 Active movement against gravity and some resistance
5 Active movement against full resistance without evident fatigue. This is normal muscle strength.

See Table 15-7, Differentiation of Motor Dysfunctions (pp. 423–424).

Ask the patient to close his eyes and, for 20 to 30 seconds, to hold his arms straight in front of him, with palms up. Watch how well he maintains this position. Normally a person maintains his arms in this position.

Tendency of one forearm to pronate suggests mild hemiparesis; downward drift of the arm with flexion of fingers and elbow may also occur. Such movements are called a pronator drift.

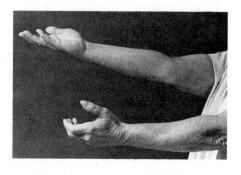

As you gain experience you may combine this maneuver with the Romberg test (p. 368).

On each side try to depress the patient's outstretched arms against his resistance. Note his strength. Then ask him to lower his arms slowly to his sides, and watch for "winging" of the scapula.

When a patient has a weak serratus anterior muscle, winging of the scapula appears as he lowers his arm or pushes against a wall. The inferior tip of the scapula juts backward and medially, simulating a wing.

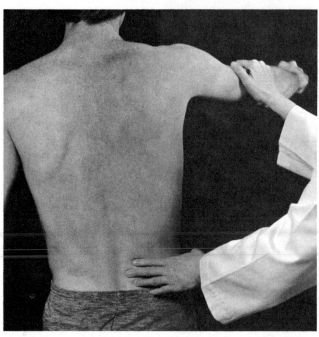

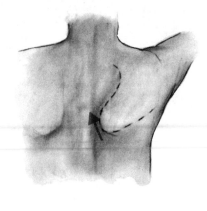

Alternatively, watch for winging as the patient pushes with his extended arms against a wall in front of him.

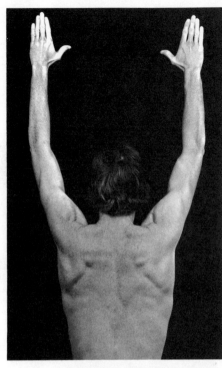

Then ask the patient to raise his arms over his head with palms forward for 20 to 30 seconds. Again, observe the maintenance of this position. Try to force his arms down to his sides against his resistance. Note any weakness.

Drifting or weakness on one side suggests hemiparesis or shoulder girdle disease.

Test flexion and extension at the elbow by having the patient pull and push against your hand.

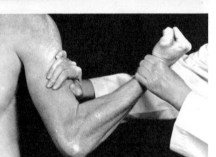

FLEXION

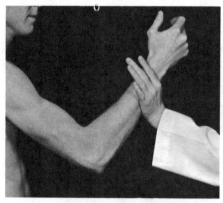

EXTENSION

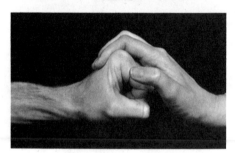

Test extension at the wrist by asking the patient to make a fist and resist your pulling it down.

Wrist drop (severe weakness of extensors) is associated with radial nerve disorders.

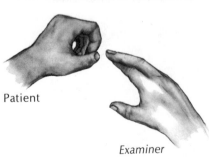

Patient

Examiner

Test the grip by asking him to squeeze your fingers as hard as he can. You can avoid painfully hard gripping by offering the patient only your index and middle fingers, with the middle finger on top of the index. You should normally have difficulty removing your fingers from the patient's grip.

A weak grip may come from weak forearm muscles or from painful disorders of the hands.

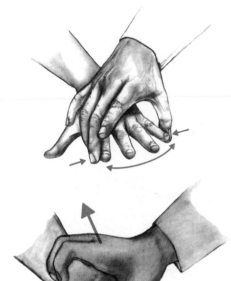

Ask the patient to spread his fingers. Check abduction by trying to force them together.

Weak abduction in ulnar nerve disorders

To test flexion of the fingers together with adduction and opposition of the thumb, instruct the patient to hold his thumb tightly against his fingertips. Pull your thumb between his thumb and fingers and note his strength.

Assessment of muscle strength of the trunk may already have been made in other segments of the examination. It includes:

1. Flexion, extension, and lateral bending of the trunk
2. Excursion of the rib cage and diaphragm during respiration

Test flexion at the hip by placing your hands on the patient's thigh and asking him to raise his leg against it.

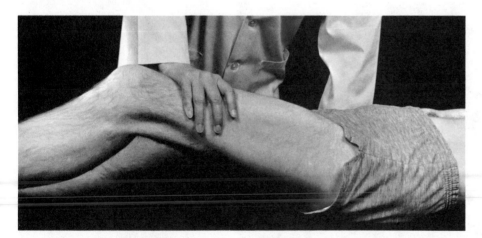

Test abduction at the hips. Place your hands firmly on the bed outside the patient's knees. Ask him to spread his legs against your hands.

Test adduction at the hips. Place your hands firmly on the bed between the patient's knees. Ask him to bring his legs together.

Symmetrical weakness of the proximal muscles suggests a myopathy; symmetrical weakness of distal muscles suggests a polyneuropathy.

Test flexion at the knee. Place the patient's leg so that the knee is flexed with his foot resting on the bed. Tell him to keep his foot down as you try to straighten his leg.

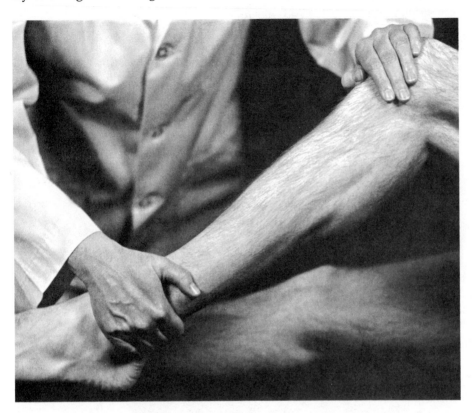

Test extension at the knee by supporting his knee and asking him to straighten his leg against your hand.

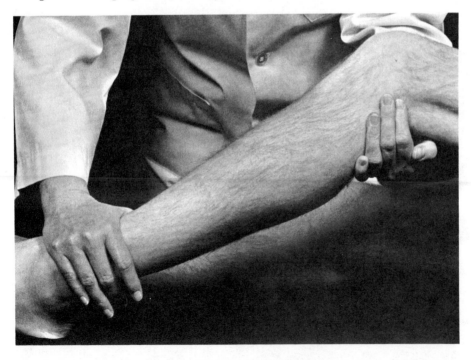

Test plantar flexion and dorsiflexion at the ankle by asking the patient to push down and pull up against your hand.

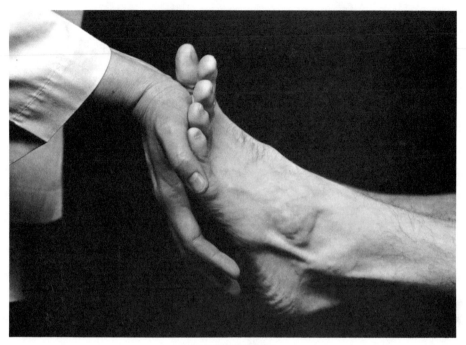

PLANTAR FLEXION

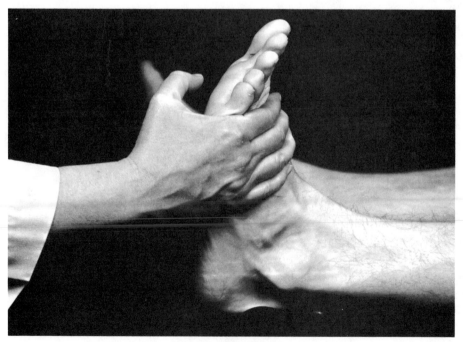

DORSIFLEXION

Assessing Coordination. You have already examined the coordination relevant to walking. Now test coordination in the arms and hands by two methods.

1. *Rapid Rhythmic Alternating Movements.* Testing each hand separately, ask the patient to (1) pat his leg as fast as he can with his hand, (2) turn his hand over and back as rapidly as he can, and (3) touch each of his fingers with his thumb in rapid sequence.

In cerebellar disease, movements tend to be slow, jerky, and awkward, with breaks in rhythm especially when the direction of movement changes.

Motor weakness, extrapyramidal disease, and gross sensory loss may also impair rapid rhythmic alternating movements.

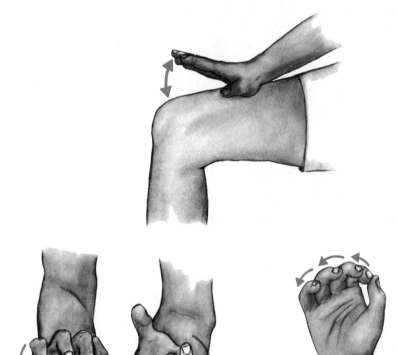

Note the speed, rhythm, smoothness, and accuracy of the movements. The nondominant hand often performs slightly less well.

2. *Point-to-Point Testing.* Ask the patient to touch your index finger and then his nose alternately several times. Move your finger about so that the patient has to alter directions and extend his arm fully to reach it. Observe the accuracy and smoothness of his movements and watch for any tremor.

In cerebellar disease movements tend to be clumsy and inaccurate. An intention tremor may appear, especially on reaching.

Now hold your finger in one place. After the patient has touched it and then touched his nose several times, ask him to close his eyes and continue his movements. Normally a person can find both your finger and his nose with eyes closed.

Assess coordination in the legs with

1. *Rapid Rhythmic Alternating Movements.* Ask the patient to tap your hand as quickly as possible with the ball of each foot in turn. Note any slowness or awkwardness. The feet normally perform less well than the hands.
2. *Point-to-Point Testing.* Ask the patient to place his heel on the opposite knee, then run it down his shin to his big toe. Note any tremor or awkwardness.

THE SENSORY SYSTEM

Sensory testing readily fatigues the patient and then produces unreliable and inconsistent results. To avoid this problem conduct an efficient and relatively rapid survey. In a patient with no neurologic symptoms or signs, a few *screening procedures* suffice. These include (1) assessment of pain and vibration sense in the hands and feet, (2) brief comparison of light touch over the arms and legs, and (3) assessment of stereognosis. Other patients need *more complete evaluation.* Examine in special detail those areas (1) where there are symptoms such as numbness or pain, (2) where there are motor or reflex abnormalities, and (3) where there are trophic changes (e.g., absent or excessive sweating, atrophic skin, or cutaneous ulceration). Repeated testing at another time is often required to confirm abnormalities.

In *testing a sensation:*

1. Note the patient's ability to perceive the stimulus.
2. Compare sensation in symmetrical areas on the two sides of the body.
3. When testing pain, temperature, and touch, compare distal and proximal areas of the extremities. When testing vibration and position, however, first test the fingers and toes. If these are normal, you may safely assume that more proximal areas will also be normal.
4. Scatter the stimuli so that you cover most of the dermatomes and major peripheral nerves.
5. Vary the pace of your testing so that the patient does not merely respond to your repetitive rhythm.

Inaccuracy that appears with eyes closed suggests loss of position sense. Repetitive and consistent deviation to one side, worse with the eyes closed, suggests cerebellar or vestibular disease.

Awkwardness in cerebellar disease or loss of position sense

Symmetrical distal sensory loss suggests a polyneuropathy or possibly a conversion reaction.

6. When you detect an area of sensory loss or hypersensitivity, map out its boundaries in detail. Stimulate first at a point of reduced sensation and move outward by progressive steps until the patient detects the change. For example:

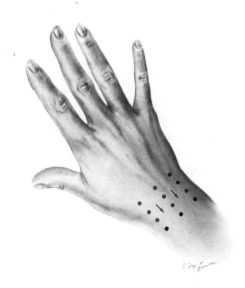

By identifying the distribution of sensory abnormalities and the kinds of sensations affected, you can infer where the causative lesion might be. Any motor deficit or reflex abnormality, of course, also helps in this localizing process.

Ask the patient to close his eyes. Test sensation on the arms, trunk, and legs, using the following stimuli:

1. *Pain.* Use a sharp safety pin, occasionally substituting the blunt end for the point as a stimulus. Stimulating in patterns suggested above, ask the patient, "Is this sharp or dull?" or, when you are making comparisons with a sharp stimulus, "Does this feel the same as this?" Use as light a stimulus as the patient can perceive, and try not to draw blood.

   There is some concern that pin pricks may transmit hepatitis and other diseases from one patient to another. Until the extent of this risk is clarified, it is prudent at least to discard all pins that have drawn blood accidentally and all pins used in testing patients with known past or present hepatitis.

2. *Temperature.* (This may be omitted if pain sensation is normal.) Use two test tubes, filled with hot and cold water. Touch the skin and ask the patient to identify "hot" or "cold."

Here pain, together with all other sensation, is lost at a sharp line around the wrist. This distribution of sensory loss does not fit any organic pattern such as peripheral nerve or dermatome. It is characteristic of the "glove and stocking" sensory loss associated with a conversion reaction. In polyneuropathy, the demarcation of sensory loss is less distinct.

See Table 15-8, Patterns of Sensory Loss (pp. 425–426).

Analgesia refers to absence of pain sensation, *hypalgesia* to decreased sensitivity to pain, and *hyperalgesia* to increased sensitivity.

3. *Light touch.* With a fine wisp of cotton touch the skin lightly, avoiding pressure, and ask the patient to respond whenever you touch his skin and to compare one side with another.

Anesthesia is absence of touch sensation, *hypesthesia* is decreased sensitivity, and *hyperesthesia* is increased sensitivity.

4. *Vibration.* Use a relatively low-pitched tuning fork, preferably of 128 Hz. Tap it on the heel of your hand and place it firmly over a distal interphalangeal joint of a finger and over the interphalangeal joint of the big toe. Ask the patient what he feels. If you are uncertain whether he feels pressure or vibration, ask him to tell you when the vibration stops, then touch the fork to stop it. If vibration sense is impaired, proceed to more proximal bony prominences (*e.g.*, wrist and elbow or medial malleolus, patella, anterior superior iliac spine, and spinous processes).

Vibration sense is often the first sensation to be lost in a peripheral neuropathy. Common causes include diabetes and alcoholism. Remember that aging may also be associated with decreased vibration sense.

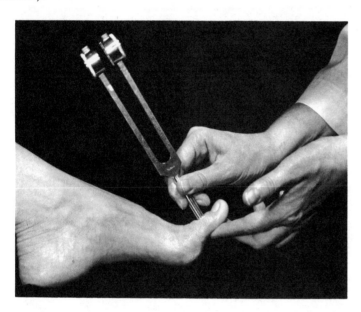

5. *Position.* Grasp the patient's big toe, holding it by its sides between your thumb and index finger and avoiding friction against the other

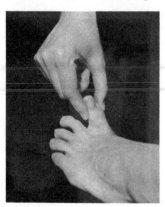

toes. Then move it and ask the patient to identify whether you are moving it up or down. If position sense is impaired, move proximally to test it at the ankle joint. In a similar fashion test position in the fingers, moving proximally if indicated to the metacarpophalangeal joints, wrist, and elbow.

Loss of position and vibration senses suggest posterior column disease.

6. *Discriminative Sensations.* Several additional maneuvers test the ability of the sensory cortex to correlate, analyze, and interpret sensations. Testing these discriminative functions is useful chiefly when other types of sensation are preserved or only mildly impaired, because a cortex receiving no stimuli would have nothing to interpret. Intact posterior columns with their fine touch and position sense are particularly important here.

Screen a patient with stereognosis, and proceed on to the other methods if indicated. The patient's eyes should be closed during all these maneuvers.

Stereognosis. Place a familiar small object in the patient's hand (e.g., a coin, paper clip, key, pencil, cotton ball). Ask him to identify it. Normally a patient will manipulate it skillfully and identify it correctly. Asking the patient to distinguish "heads" from "tails" on a coin is a sensitive test of stereognosis.

Damage to the sensory cortex may impair but does not abolish pain, temperature, and touch senses. It frequently impairs position sense but rarely affects vibration sense. Two-point discrimination and the ability to identify objects in the hand (stereognosis) are impaired in posterior column lesions as well as in cortical lesions.

Astereognosis refers to the inability to recognize objects placed in the hand.

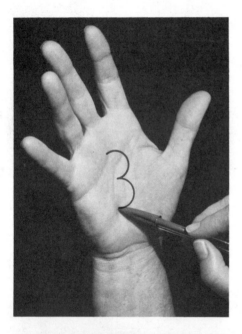

Number Identification. When motor impairment of the hand makes testing for stereognosis impractical, test the patient's ability to identify numbers. With the blunt end of a pen or pencil, draw a large number in his palm. A normal person can identify most such numbers.

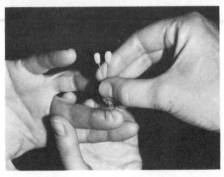

Two-point Discrimination. Using the sides of two pins or the two ends of an opened paper clip, touch a finger pad in two places simultaneously. Alternate the double stimulus irregularly with a one-point touch.

Find the minimal distance at which the patient can discriminate one from two points (normally about 2 mm or 3 mm on the finger pads). This test may be used on other parts of the body but normal distances vary widely from one region to another.

Lesions of the sensory cortex increase the distance between two recognizable points.

Point Localization. Briefly touch a point on the patient's skin. Then ask him to open his eyes and point to the place touched. Normally a person can do so accurately. This method, together with that for extinction, is especially useful on the trunk and legs.

Lesions of the sensory cortex impair the ability to localize points accurately.

Extinction. Simultaneously stimulate corresponding areas on both sides of the body. Ask the patient where he feels your touch. Normally he should feel both stimuli.

With lesions of the sensory cortex, only one stimulus may be recognized. The stimulus on the side opposite the damaged cortex is extinguished.

REFLEXES

To *elicit a muscle stretch reflex*, persuade the patient to relax, position the limbs properly and symmetrically, and strike the tendon briskly. Your strike should be quick and direct, not glancing. You may use either the pointed or the flat end of the hammer. The pointed end is useful in

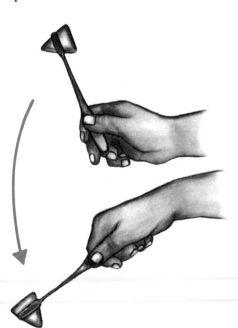

striking small areas, such as your finger as it overlies the biceps tendon, while the flat end gives the patient less discomfort over the brachioradialis. Hold the reflex hammer loosely between thumb and fingers, so that it swings freely in an arc yet is controlled in its direction. Note the speed, force, and amplitude of the reflex response. Always compare one side with the other.

If the patient's reflexes are symmetrically diminished or absent, use reinforcement, a technique involving isometric contraction of other muscles that may increase reflex activity. In testing arm reflexes, for example, ask the patient to clench his teeth or to squeeze his thigh with the opposite hand. If leg reflexes are diminished or absent, reinforce them by asking the patient to lock his fingers and pull one hand against the other. Tell the patient to pull just before you strike the tendon.

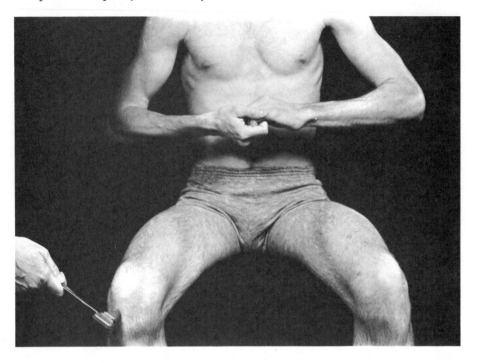

Reflexes are usually graded on a 0 to 4+ scale:

4+ Very brisk, hyperactive; often indicative of disease; often associated with clonus (rhythmic oscillations between flexion and extension)

Hyperactive reflexes suggest upper motor neuron disease. Sustained clonus confirms it.

3+ Brisker than average; possibly but not necessarily indicative of disease

2+ Average; normal

1+ Somewhat diminished; low normal ⎱ If you use reinforcement,
0   No response   ⎰ indicate it in the record.

Reflex response depends partly on the force of your stimulus. Use no more force than you need to provoke a definite response. Differences between sides are usually easier to assess than symmetrical changes.

Reflexes may be diminished or absent when sensation is lost, when the relevant spinal segments are damaged, or when the lower motor neurons are damaged. Diseases of muscles and neuromuscular junctions may also decrease reflexes.

The Biceps Reflex (C_5, C_6). The patient's arms should be partially flexed at the elbows with palms down. Place your thumb or finger firmly on the biceps tendon. Strike with the reflex hammer so that the blow is aimed directly through your digit toward the biceps tendon.

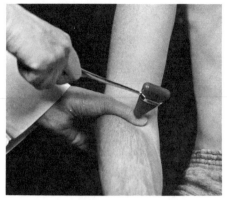
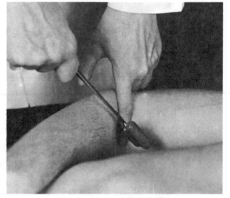

PATIENT SITTING　　　　　　　**PATIENT LYING DOWN**

Observe flexion at the elbow, and watch for and feel the contraction of the biceps muscle.

The Triceps Reflex (C₆, C₇, C₈). Flex the patient's arm at the elbow, with palm toward the body, and pull it slightly across the chest. Strike the triceps tendon above the elbow. Use a direct, not a glancing, blow. Watch for contraction of the triceps muscle and extension at the elbow.

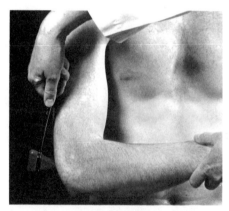
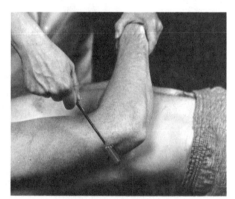

PATIENT SITTING　　　　　　　**PATIENT LYING DOWN**

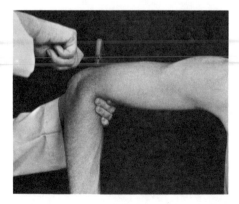

When it is difficult to get a sitting patient relaxed for a triceps reflex, an alternate method may help. Support the patient's upper arm as illustrated, and ask him to let it go limp as if it were "hung up to dry." Then strike the triceps tendon.

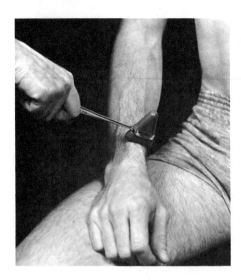

The Supinator or Brachioradialis Reflex (C₅, C₆). The patient's forearm should rest on the abdomen or in the lap, palm down. Strike the radius about 1 to 2 inches above the wrist. Observe flexion and supination of the forearm.

The Abdominal Reflexes. Test the abdominal reflexes by lightly but briskly stroking each side of the abdomen, above (T_8, T_9, T_{10}) and below (T_{10}, T_{11}, T_{12}) the umbilicus, in the directions illustrated. Use a key or a tongue blade, twisted so that it is split longitudinally. Note the contraction of the abdominal muscles and deviation of the umbilicus toward the stimulus. Obesity may mask an abdominal reflex. In this situation, use your finger to retract the patient's umbilicus away from the side to be stimulated. Feel with your retracting finger for the muscular contraction.

Abdominal reflexes may be absent in both upper and lower motor neuron disorders.

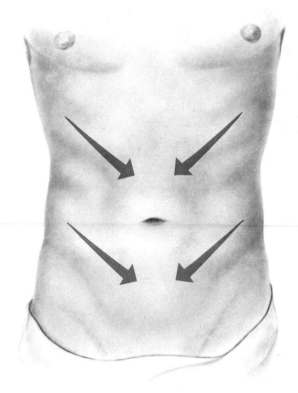

The Knee Reflex (L₂, L₃, L₄). The patient may be either (1) sitting or (2) lying down while you support his knees in a somewhat flexed position. Briskly tap the patellar tendon just below the patella. Note contraction of the quadriceps with extension at the knee.

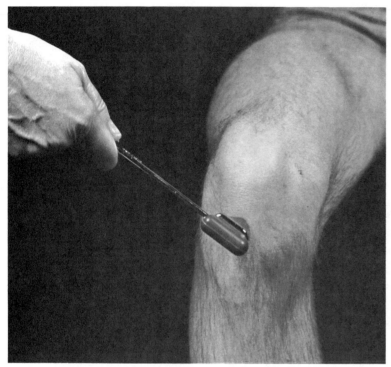

PATIENT SITTING

Two methods are useful in examining the supine patient. Supporting both knees at once, as shown below on the left, allows you to assess small differences between knee reflexes by repeated testing of one and then the other. Sometimes, however, supporting both legs is uncomfortable for both the examiner and the patient. A comfortable alternative method by which your supporting arm is in turn supported by the patient's opposite leg is shown below on the right. Some patients are better able to relax with this method.

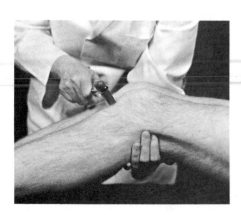 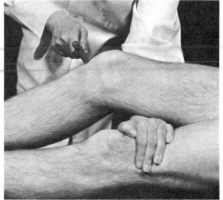

The Ankle Reflex (S₁, S₂). With the leg somewhat flexed at the knee, dorsiflex the foot at the ankle. Persuade the patient to relax. Strike the Achilles tendon. Watch for plantar flexion at the ankle. Note also the speed of relaxation after muscular contraction.

The slowed relaxation phase of reflexes in hypothyroidism is often easily seen and felt in the ankle reflex.

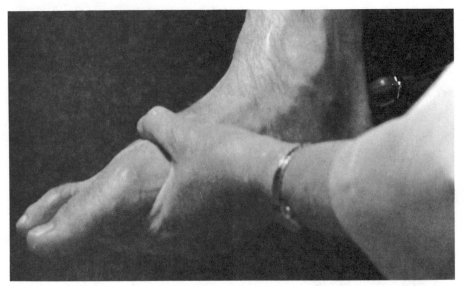

PATIENT SITTING

When the patient is lying down, flex one leg at both hip and knee and rotate it externally so that it rests across the opposite shin. Then dorsiflex the foot at the ankle and strike the Achilles tendon.

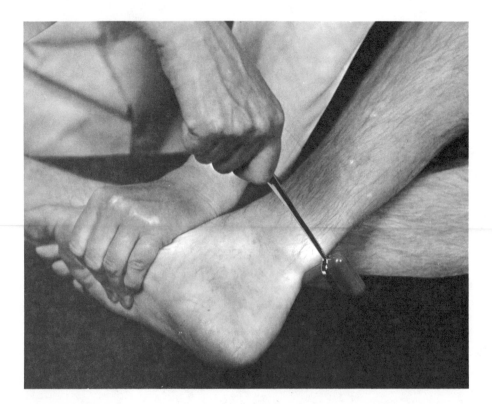

The Plantar Response (L₄, L₅, S₁, S₂). With a moderately sharp object such as a key, stroke the lateral aspect of the sole from the heel to the ball of the foot, curving medially across the ball. Use the lightest stimulus that will provoke a response. Note movement of the toes, normally flexion.

Dorsiflexion of the great toe with fanning of the other toes indicates upper motor neuron disease (Babinski response). It

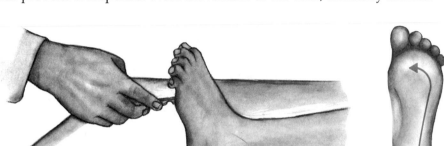

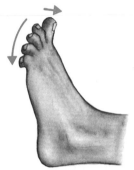

may also occur in unconscious states associated with drug and alcohol intoxication or following an epileptic seizure. A pronounced Babinski response is occasionally accompanied by reflex flexion at the hip and knee.

Some patients withdraw from this stimulus by flexing the hip and knee. Hold the ankle, if necessary, to complete your observation. It is sometimes difficult to distinguish withdrawal from a Babinski response.

If the reflexes are hyperreactive, *test for ankle clonus*. Support the knee in a partly flexed position. With your other hand, sharply dorsiflex the foot and maintain it in dorsiflexion. Look and feel for rhythmic oscillations between dorsiflexion and plantar flexion.

Sustained clonus indicates upper motor neuron disease.

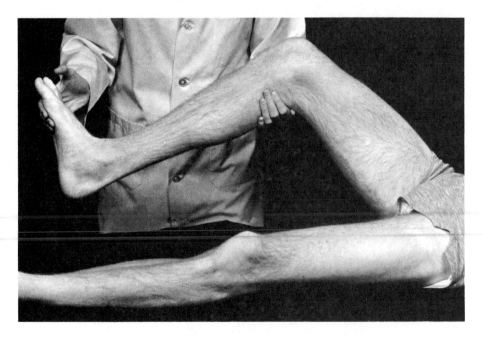

Clonus may also be elicited at other joints (*e.g.,* patellar clonus at the knee).

SPECIAL MANEUVERS

Meningeal Signs. Testing for meningeal signs is not part of a routine examination but should be done when you suspect inflammation of the meninges, by infection (meningitis), for example, or by blood (as in subarachnoid hemorrhage). (See also pp. 470–471 and 503.)

With the patient recumbent, place your hands behind his head and flex his neck forward. Note resistance or pain. Watch also for flexion of the patient's hips and knees in reaction to your maneuver *(Brudzinski's sign).*

Pain and resistance to flexion suggest meningeal inflammation but may be due to arthritis or neck injury. Flexion of hips and knees suggests meningeal inflammation.

Flex one of the patient's legs at hip and knee, then straighten the knee. Note resistance or pain *(Kernig's sign).*

Pain or resistance suggests meningeal inflammation or disc disease.

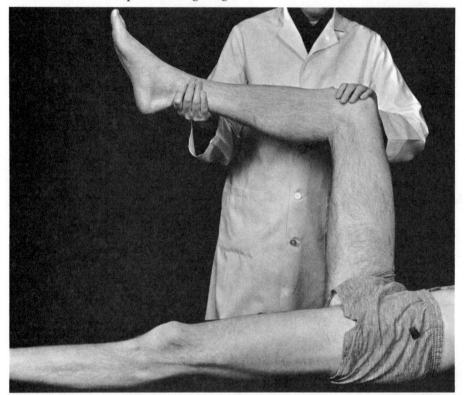

Frontal Release Signs. When you suspect widespread disease of the brain, because of bilateral hyperactive reflexes and Babinski responses, for example, or because of signs of dementia (see p. 444), look for frontal release signs. These include:

1. *The grasp reflex.* While you are talking with the patient, insert your fingers between the patient's thumb and fingers and gently touch or stroke his palm.

Slow flexion of the patient's fingers, often with closure around your fingers, constitutes a positive grasp reflex. Family members may mistake this reflex for a conscious response.

2. *The snout reflex.* Sweep a tongue depressor briskly and lightly across the lips from side to center. Alternatively, tap the lips lightly with a reflex hammer.

Puckering and protrusion of the lips constitute a positive snout reflex.

3. *The sucking reflex.* Use the same stimulus as in the snout reflex.

Sucking movements of the lips, tongue, and jaw constitute a positive sucking reflex.

All three of these reflexes are normal in early infancy but not in later life.

These three reflexes indicate diffuse brain disease, often involving the frontal lobes.

The Stuporous or Comatose Patient. Survey the patient quickly. Make sure that his airway is clear, and check for evidence of bleeding and shock. (Laboratory studies and emergency management are beyond the scope of this text.)

Check his vital signs, including pulse, blood pressure, and rectal temperature.

Despite the atmosphere of emergency, take several minutes and carefully observe:

His respirations

See Table 6-1, Abnormalities in Rate and Rhythm of Breathing (p. 149).

His posture and motor activity, noting especially his position in bed

See Table 15-9, Abnormal Postures in the Comatose Patient (p. 427).

The position of his head and eyes, and any spontaneous movements

Any odors

Any abnormalities of skin, including color, moisture, evidence of bleeding disorders, needlemarks or other lesions

Jaundice, cyanosis, cherry red color of carbon monoxide poisoning

As you go on with your examination, take two *important precautions:*

1. If there is any question of trauma to head or neck, do not bend the neck until x-ray examination has ruled out a fracture of the cervical spine.
2. In examining the ocular fundi do not use a mydriatic solution. It could mask important eye signs.

Proceed to a *general and neurologic examination,* with special attention to the following:

Examine the head carefully for signs of trauma.

Bruises, lacerations, local swelling

Techniques of Examination	Examples of Abnormalities
Test for meningeal signs.	Meningitis, subarachnoid hemorrhage
Examine the eyes, especially:	
The fundi	Papilledema, hypertensive retinopathy
The pupils and their reaction to light	See Table 5-7, Pupillary Abnormalities (pp. 101–102). In deep coma, the presence of pupillary reflexes favors a metabolic cause; their absence favors a structural cause.
The extraocular movements, if possible	
The corneal reflexes	
Inspect the ears and nose.	Bleeding or cerebral spinal fluid suggests a skull fracture; otitis media
Watch for facial asymmetry.	
Inspect the mouth and throat.	Tongue injury suggests a seizure.
Examine the heart, lungs, and abdomen.	
Complete a neurologic examination, insofar as you are able.	
Four additional maneuvers are especially helpful:	

1. *Assess response to stimuli,* increasing the strength of the stimulus as follows:

   a. Give a simple command.
   b. Call the patient's name.
   c. Produce pain—for example, by pressing the bony ridges above the eyes, or by pinching the sides of the neck or the inner portions of upper arms and thighs.

   (Examples of Abnormalities:) Avoidance movements persist in stupor and light coma but are lost in deeper coma.

   Observe how strong a stimulus is required to produce a response. Note whether:

   a. Motor responses are confined to one side of the body

   (Examples of Abnormalities:) Motor responses confined to one side suggest paralysis of the other side.

   b. Stimuli from both or only one side of the body produce a response

   (Examples of Abnormalities:) When a stimulus on one side of the body produces a response but a similar stimulus on the opposite side does not, suspect a sensory deficit on the latter side.

2. *Look for flaccid paralysis*, as in acute hemiplegia, by grasping each arm below the wrist and raising it to a vertical position. Note the position of the hand, usually only slightly flexed at the wrist.

The hemiplegia of sudden cerebral accidents is usually flaccid at first. A flaccid hand droops limply to form a right angle with the wrist.

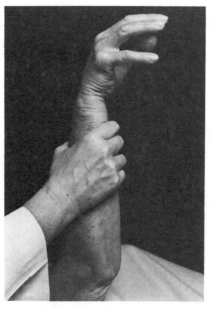

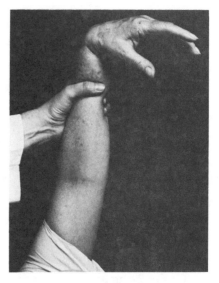

Then lower the arms to about 12 or 18 inches off the bed and drop them. Watch the way they fall. A normal arm drops, but somewhat slowly.

A flaccid arm drops rapidly in a flail-like manner.

Flex the patient's knees and support them on your arm. Then extend one leg at a time at the knee and drop it to the bed. Compare the speed with which each leg in turn falls.

In hemiplegia the flaccid leg falls more rapidly.

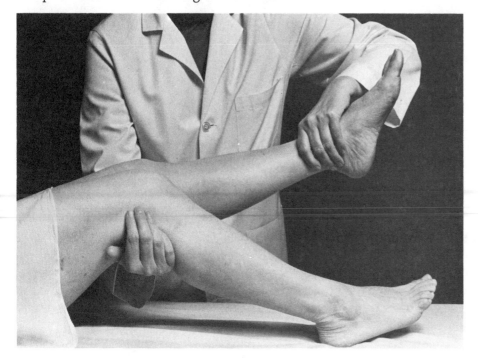

Flex the legs so that the heels rest on the bed and release them. The normal leg returns slowly to its original position.

In hemiplegia the flaccid leg falls rapidly into extension with external rotation at the hip.

3. *Test the oculocephalic reflex (doll's eye movements).* Holding open the upper eyelids so that you can see the eyes, turn the head quickly first to one side, then to the other. Flex the neck forward, then extend it.

In a comatose patient with an intact brain stem, the patient's eyes move in the opposite direction as if still gazing ahead in their initial position (doll's eye movements).

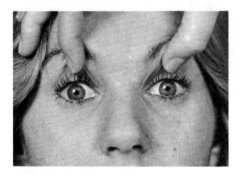 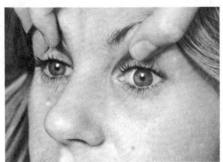

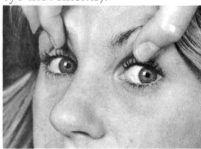

Observe the eye movements.

Unless consciously fixing their gaze, fully conscious patients move their eyes unpredictably or only slightly in a direction opposite to your movement. As illustrated above, for example, you have turned the patient's head to her right, and her eyes have moved slightly to her left.

Loss of doll's eye movements in a comatose patient suggests a lesion of midbrain or pons, or very deep coma.

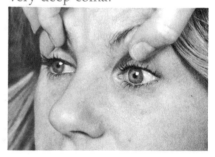

4. *Test the oculovestibular reflex with caloric stimulation.* Make sure that the eardrums are intact and the canals clear. Elevate the head to 30°. With a large syringe, inject icewater through a small catheter that is lying in (but not plugging) the ear canal. Use up to 200 ml of water in order to obtain a response. Repeat on the opposite side, waiting 3 to 5 minutes if necessary for the first response to disappear.

A comatose patient with an intact brain stem responds by conjugate deviation of the eyes toward the irrigated ear.

The normal awake patient (in whom a few milliliters of icewater is often an adequate stimulus) responds with nystagmus, with the quick component away from the irrigated ear.

Loss of this reflex (no response to stimulation) suggests a brain stem lesion.

Table 15-1 and Table 15-2

Table 15-1 Abnormalities of Speech

APHASIA OR DYSPHASIA

Defects in word formulation or power of expression secondary to damage of the cortical speech centers

Ranges from uncertainty or error in choice of words and syllables (dysphasia) to complete inability to speak (aphasia) despite adequate motor function of mouth and larynx

APHONIA OR DYSPHONIA

A disorder of the volume, quality, or pitch of the voice secondary to disease of the larynx or its innervation

Ranges from a rasping, hoarse voice (dysphonia) to a whisper (aphonia)

DYSARTHRIA

Defective articulation secondary to a motor deficit involving the lips, tongue, palate, or pharynx

Slurred speech, with difficulty especially in pronouncing the labial (m, b, p) and the lingual (t, d, l) consonants

PALATAL PARALYSIS

Nasal speech

CEREBELLAR DYSARTHRIA

Poorly coordinated, irregular speech with unnatural separation of syllables (scanning)

PARKINSONISM

A monotonous, slow, weak voice with slurring of words

Table 15-2 Abnormalities of Consciousness*

CONFUSION

A mild diminution of consciousness with mental slowness, inattentiveness, dulled perception of the environment, and incoherent thought patterns. The person may be disoriented.

STUPOR

Marked reduction in mental and physical activity; marked slowness and reduction in response to commands or stimuli; usually with preservation of reflexes

COMA

A complete loss of consciousness with unresponsiveness to stimuli and no voluntary movements. Muscle stretch reflexes may be hyperactive, and Babinski responses may appear. In deep coma, all reflexes are lost.

DELIRIUM

A state of confusion with agitation and hallucinations. This state is generally considered separate from the continuum of confusion–stupor–coma.

*Because these terms are not always used with sufficient precision to ascertain changes in a patient's state of consciousness, always describe your findings in some detail. Do not simply affix the appropriate label.

Table 15-3

Table 15-3   Nystagmus

Nystagmus is a rhythmic oscillation of the eyes. Analogous to a tremor in other parts of the body, it is essentially a disorder of ocular posture. Its causes are multiple, including impairment of vision in early life, disorders of the labyrinth and the cerebellar system, and drug toxicity. Nystagmus occurs normally when a person watches a rapidly moving object (*e.g.*, a passing train). Observe the three characteristics of nystagmus listed below and on the following page. Then refer to textbooks of neurology for differential diagnosis.

DIRECTION OF THE QUICK AND SLOW COMPONENTS
EXAMPLE: NYSTAGMUS TO THE LEFT

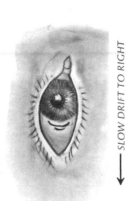

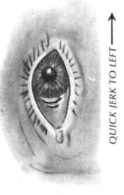

⟵ *SLOW DRIFT TO RIGHT*

QUICK JERK TO LEFT ⟶

Nystagmus is usually quicker in one direction than in the other, and is then defined by its quicker phase. For example, if the eyes jerk quickly to the left and drift back slowly to the right, the patient is said to have nystagmus to the left.

Occasionally nystagmus consists only of coarse oscillations without quick and slow components. It is then said to be *pendular*.

PLANE OF THE MOVEMENTS
HORIZONTAL NYSTAGMUS

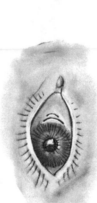

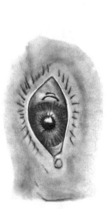

The movements of nystagmus may occur in one or more planes (*i.e.*, horizontal, vertical, or rotary).

VERTICAL NYSTAGMUS

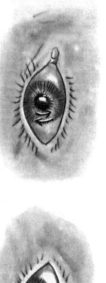

ROTARY NYSTAGMUS

Continued

Table 15-3

Table 15-3 (Cont'd)

FIELD OF GAZE IN WHICH NYSTAGMUS APPEARS
EXAMPLE: NYSTAGMUS ON RIGHT LATERAL GAZE

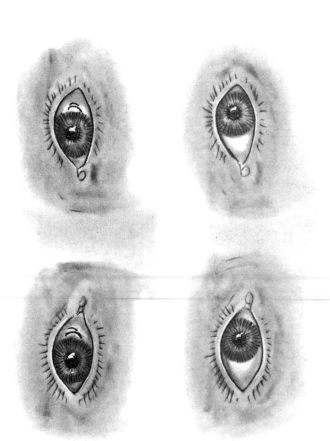

Although nystagmus may be present in all fields of gaze, it may instead appear or become accentuated only on deviation of the eyes (*e.g.*, to the side or upward). On extreme lateral gaze the normal person may show a few beats resembling nystagmus. Avoid such extreme movements and observe for nystagmus only within the field of full binocular vision.

Table 15-4

Table 15-4 Types of Facial Paralysis

LOWER MOTOR NEURON PARALYSIS
EXAMPLE: **BELL'S PALSY**

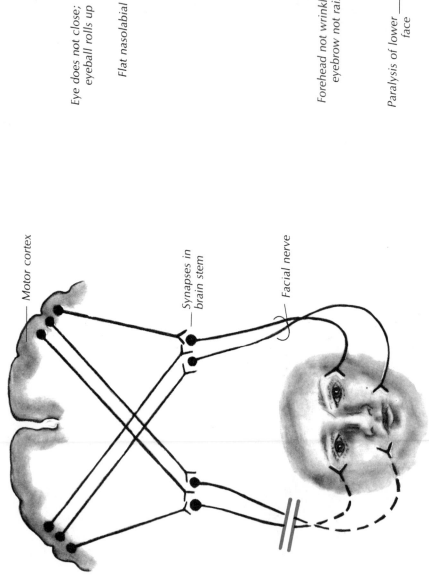

Motor cortex

Synapses in brain stem

Facial nerve

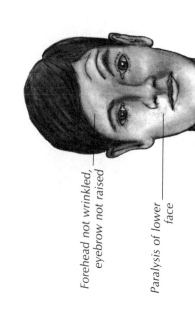

Eye does not close; eyeball rolls up

Flat nasolabial fold

CLOSING EYES

Forehead not wrinkled, eyebrow not raised

Paralysis of lower face

RAISING EYEBROWS

The nerve supply to the entire side of the face is affected.

Continued

Table 15-4

Table 15-4 (Cont'd)

UPPER MOTOR NEURON PARALYSIS

EXAMPLE: **HEMIPARESIS**

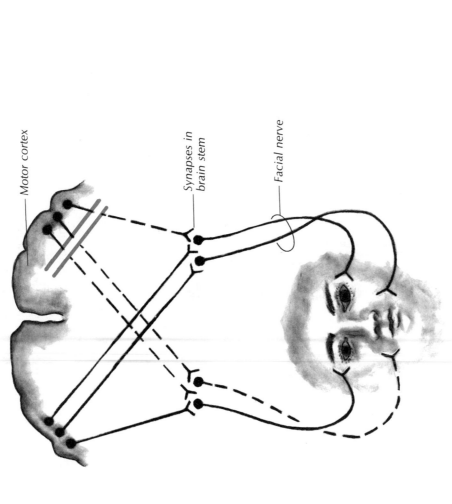

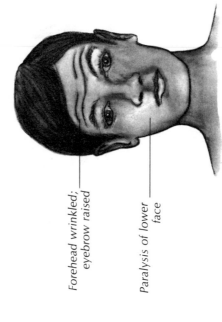

Eye closes perhaps
with slight weakness

Flat nasolabial fold

CLOSING EYES

Forehead wrinkled;
eyebrow raised

Paralysis of lower
face

RAISING EYEBROWS

Motor cortex

Synapses in
brain stem

Facial nerve

The muscles of the forehead and around the eye have an upper
motor neuron supply from both sides of the brain. A unilateral
cortical lesion therefore has relatively little effect on the upper
part of the face.

Table 15-5

Table 15-5   Abnormalities of Gait and Posture

	SPASTIC HEMIPARESIS	SCISSORS GAIT	STEPPAGE GAIT
	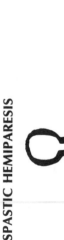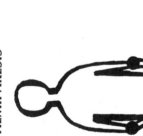	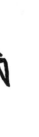	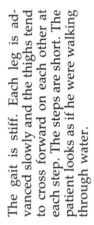
UNDERLYING DEFECT	Associated with unilateral upper motor neuron disease, as with a stroke	Associated with bilateral spastic paresis of the legs	Associated with foot drop, usually secondary to lower motor neuron disease
DESCRIPTION	One arm is held immobile and close to the side, with elbow, wrist, and interphalangeal joints flexed. The leg is extended with plantar flexion of the foot. On walking, the patient either drags his foot, often scraping his toe, or circles it stiffly outward and forward (circumduction).	The gait is stiff. Each leg is advanced slowly and the thighs tend to cross forward on each other at each step. The steps are short. The patient looks as if he were walking through water.	The patient either drags his feet or lifts them high, with knees flexed, and brings them down with a slap onto the floor. The patient then looks as if he were walking up stairs. He is unable to walk on his heels. The steppage gait may involve one or both sides.

Continued

Table 15-5

Table 15-5 (Cont'd)

	SENSORY ATAXIA	CEREBELLAR ATAXIA	PARKINSONIAN GAIT	GAIT OF OLD AGE
UNDERLYING DEFECT	Associated with loss of position sense in the legs, as from polyneuropathy or posterior column damage	Associated with disease of the cerebellum or associated tracts	Associated with the basal ganglia defects of Parkinson's disease	
DESCRIPTION	The gait is unsteady and wide-based (with feet wide apart). The patient throws his feet forward and outward and brings them down, first on the heel and then on the toes, with a double tapping sound. He watches the ground to guide his steps. When his eyes are closed, he cannot stand steadily with feet together (positive Romberg sign) and his staggering gait worsens.	The gait is staggering, unsteady, and wide-based, with exaggerated difficulty on the turns. The patient cannot stand steadily with feet together, whether eyes open or closed.	The posture is stooped with head and neck forward, hips and knees slightly flexed. Arms are flexed at elbows and wrists. The patient is slow in getting started. Steps are short and often shuffling. Arm swings are decreased and the patient turns around stiffly—"all in one piece."	Speed, balance, and grace decrease with aging. Steps become short, uncertain, and even shuffling. The legs may be flexed at hips and knees. A cane may bolster lost confidence.

Table 15-6

Table 15-6 Involuntary Movements

TREMORS

Tremors are relatively rhythmic oscillatory movements which may be roughly subdivided into three groups: resting (or static) tremors, intention tremors, and postural tremors.

RESTING (OR STATIC) TREMORS

These tremors are most prominent at rest, and may decrease or disappear with voluntary movement. Illustrated is the common, relatively slow, fine, pill-rolling tremor of parkinsonism, about 5 per second.

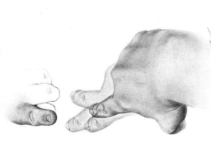

INTENTION TREMORS

Intention tremors, absent at rest, appear with activity and often get worse as the target is neared. Causes include disorders of cerebellar pathways, as in multiple sclerosis.

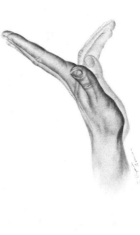

POSTURAL TREMORS

These tremors appear when the affected part is actively maintaining a posture. Examples include the fine, rapid tremor of hyperthyroidism and the tremors of anxiety and fatigue. Some postural tremors are familial.

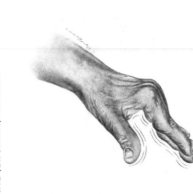

ASTERIXIS

Asterixis is a postural tremor characterized by nonrhythmic, flapping movements of wide amplitude. The extended wrist or fingers flex suddenly and briefly, then return to their original position. Watch 1 or 2 minutes for this sign while the patient holds his arms forward, with hands cocked up and fingers spread. Causes include liver failure, renal failure, and pulmonary insufficiency.

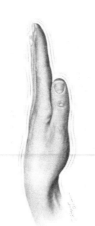

Continued

Table 15-6

Table 15-6 (Cont'd)

TICS

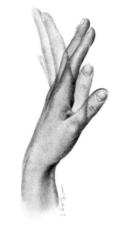

Tics are brief, repetitive, stereotyped, coordinated movements occurring at irregular intervals. Examples include repetitive winking, grimacing, and shoulder shrugging.

CHOREA

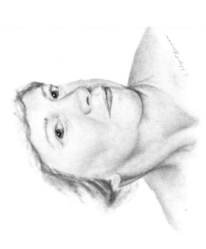

Choreiform movements are brief, rapid, jerky, irregular, and unpredictable movements which occur at rest or interrupt normal coordinated movements. Unlike tics, they seldom repeat themselves. The face, head, lower arms, and hands are often involved. Causes include Sydenham's chorea (with rheumatic fever) and Huntington's chorea.

ATHETOSIS

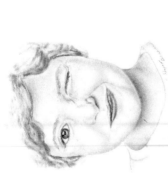
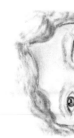

Athetoid movements are slower and more twisting and writhing than chorea, and have a larger amplitude. They most commonly involve the face and distal extremities. Athetosis is often associated with spasticity. Causes include cerebral palsy.

DYSTONIA

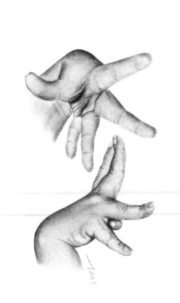

Dystonic movements are somewhat similar to athetosis, but often involve larger portions of the body, including the trunk. Grotesque, twisted postures may result. Causes include drugs such as phenothiazines, dystonia musculorum deformans, and, as illustrated, spasmodic torticollis.

Continued

Table 15-6

Table 15-6 (Cont'd)

FASCICULATIONS

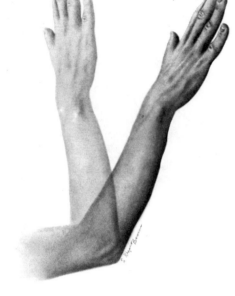

Fasciculations are fine, rapid, flickering or twitching movements originating in relatively small groups of muscle fibers (fascicles, or muscle bundles). They vary irregularly in frequency and extent, but rarely move a joint. When seen in muscles that are undergoing atrophy, they indicate lower motor neuron disease.

MYOCLONUS

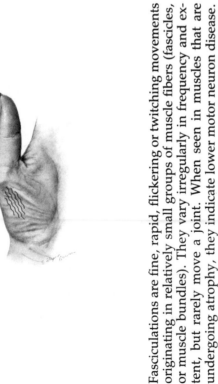

Myoclonic movements are sudden, brief, rapid, unpredictable jerks, usually involving the limbs or trunk. They may be single or repetitive. Myoclonus may occur in a normal person who is falling asleep, but is also associated with a variety of neurologic disorders.

ORAL–FACIAL DYSKINESIAS

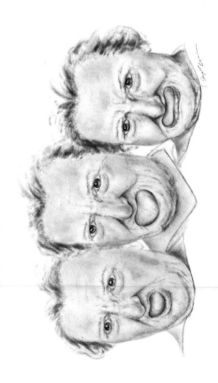

Oral–facial dyskinesias are repetitive, bizarre movements that chiefly involve the face, mouth, jaw, and tongue: grimacing, pursing of the lips, protrusions of the tongue, opening and closing of the mouth, and deviations of the jaw. The hands may show lesser involvement. These movements may be a late complication of psychotropic drugs such as phenothiazines, and have then been termed tardive (late) dyskinesias. They also occur in longstanding psychoses, in some elderly individuals, and in some edentulous persons.

Table 15-7

Table 15-7 Differentiation of Motor Dysfunctions

(4) extrapyramidal

(5) cerebellar

(3) corticospinal

(1) sensory

(2) lower motor neuron

	(1) SENSORY NEURON	(2) LOWER MOTOR NEURON	(3) CORTICOSPINAL TRACT
PROCESS	Loss of reflex activity and tone because of interruption of the sensory limb of the reflex arc; preservation of voluntary motion	All motor functions lost when the "final common pathway" is destroyed	Paralysis and spasticity are produced with hyperactive reflexes.
APPEARANCE	Normal	Atrophy, fasciculations	Relatively mild atrophy secondary to disuse; no fasciculations
MUSCLE TONE	Decreased	Decreased	Increased (spastic)*
VOLUNTARY MOVEMENT (STRENGTH)	Normal	Decreased or 0	Decreased or 0
COORDINATION	Normal with eyes open; poor with eyes closed	(Paralyzed or weak)	(Paralyzed or weak)
REFLEXES WHEN IN AFFECTED LOCATION—			
MUSCLE STRETCH	Absent	(Paralyzed or weak)	Increased
PLANTAR	Absent	Absent	Extensor (Babinski response)
ABDOMINALS	Absent	Absent	Absent

*Spasticity of upper motor neuron lesions is sometimes "clasp-knife" in character, with a gradual increase in tone followed by a sudden decrease in tone as a limb goes through its range of motion.

Continued

Table 15-7

Table 15-7 (Cont'd)

(4) extrapyramidal

(3) corticospinal

(1) sensory

(2) lower motor neuron

(5) cerebellar

	(4) EXTRAPYRAMIDAL SYSTEM	(5) CEREBELLAR SYSTEM
PROCESS	No paralysis; chief effects are on muscle tone and associated movement	No paralysis; chief effects are on coordination and balance
APPEARANCE	Tremor at rest, poverty of motion (*e.g.*, mask face)	Intention tremor
MUSCLE TONE	Increased (rigid)*	Decreased
VOLUNTARY MOVEMENT (STRENGTH)	Normal or decreased, slow	Normal or decreased, mainly uncoordinated
COORDINATION	Slowed	Poor; intention tremor
REFLEXES WHEN IN AFFECTED LOCATION—		
MUSCLE STRETCH	Normal	Swinging
PLANTAR	Flexor	Flexor
ABDOMINALS	Normal	Normal

*The *rigidity* of extrapyramidal disease is constant through the range of motion. It may be (1) steady or "lead-pipe," or (2) "cogwheel" when superimposed on a tremor.

Table 15-8

Table 15-8   Patterns of Sensory Loss

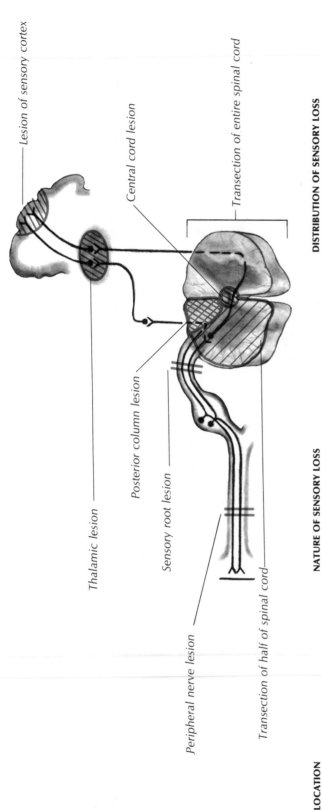

Lesion of sensory cortex

Central cord lesion

Transection of entire spinal cord

Thalamic lesion

Posterior column lesion

Sensory root lesion

Peripheral nerve lesion

Transection of half of spinal cord

LOCATION	NATURE OF SENSORY LOSS	DISTRIBUTION OF SENSORY LOSS
PERIPHERAL NERVE LESION	Usually all sensations	Distribution of a peripheral nerve
MULTIPLE PERIPHERAL NERVES (*Peripheral Polyneuropathy*)	Usually all sensations	Distal "glove-and-stocking" loss, with gradual shading from normal to diminished sensation
SENSORY ROOT LESION	Usually all sensations, but several roots must be affected to produce loss	One or more dermatomes
CENTRAL CORD LESION, AS IN SYRINGOMYELIA	Loss of pain and temperature	One or more dermatomes
POSTERIOR COLUMN LESION	Loss of position, vibration sense, also stereognosis and two-point discrimination	Below level of lesion and on same side

Continued

Table 15-8

Table 15-8   (Cont'd)

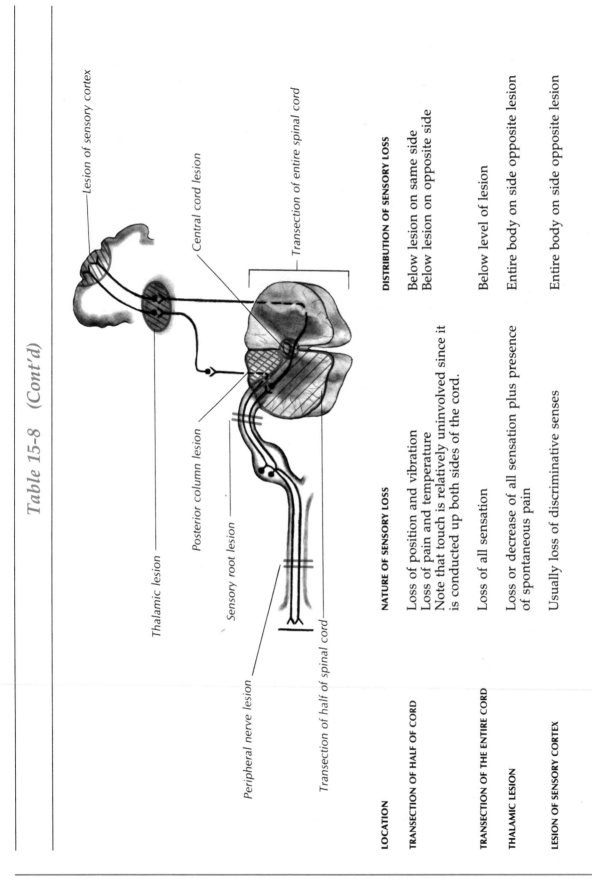

Lesion of sensory cortex

Central cord lesion

Transection of entire spinal cord

Thalamic lesion

Posterior column lesion

Sensory root lesion

Peripheral nerve lesion

Transection of half of spinal cord

LOCATION	NATURE OF SENSORY LOSS	DISTRIBUTION OF SENSORY LOSS
TRANSECTION OF HALF OF CORD	Loss of position and vibration	Below lesion on same side
	Loss of pain and temperature	Below lesion on opposite side
	Note that touch is relatively uninvolved since it is conducted up both sides of the cord.	
TRANSECTION OF THE ENTIRE CORD	Loss of all sensation	Below level of lesion
THALAMIC LESION	Loss or decrease of all sensation plus presence of spontaneous pain	Entire body on side opposite lesion
LESION OF SENSORY CORTEX	Usually loss of discriminative senses	Entire body on side opposite lesion

Table 15-9

Table 15-9 Abnormal Postures in the Comatose Patient

HEMIPLEGIA (EARLY)

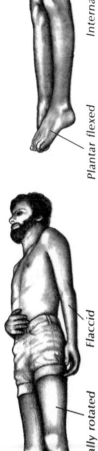

Externally rotated

Flaccid

Sudden unilateral brain damage involving the corticospinal tract may produce a hemiplegia or one-sided paralysis, which early in its course is flaccid. Spasticity will develop later. The paralyzed arm and leg are slack. They fall loosely and without tone when raised and dropped to the bed. Spontaneous movements or responses to noxious stimuli are limited to the opposite side. The leg may lie externally rotated. One side of the lower face may be paralyzed, and that cheek puffs out on expiration. Both eyes may be turned away from the paralyzed side.

DECORTICATE RIGIDITY

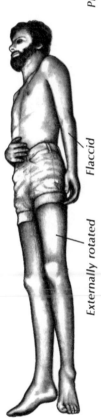

Flexed

Adducted

Flexed

Internally rotated

Plantar flexed

In decorticate rigidity the upper arms are held tight to the sides with elbows, wrists, and fingers flexed. The legs are extended and internally rotated. The feet are plantar flexed. This posture implies a destructive lesion of the corticospinal tracts within or very near the cerebral hemispheres. When unilateral, this is the posture of chronic spastic hemiplegia.

DECEREBRATE RIGIDITY

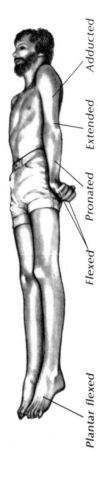

Adducted

Extended

Pronated

Flexed

Plantar flexed

In decerebrate rigidity the jaws are clenched and the neck extended. The arms are adducted and stiffly extended at the elbows, with forearms pronated, wrists and fingers flexed. The legs are stiffly extended at the knees with the feet plantar flexed. This posture may occur spontaneously or only in response to external stimuli such as light, noise, or pain. It is caused by a lesion in the diencephalon, midbrain, or pons, although severe metabolic disorders such as hypoxia or hypoglycemia may also produce it.

Chapter 16
MENTAL STATUS

Components of Mental Function

In every body system clinicians have selected certain readily observable characteristics with which to assess the structure and function of that system, to distinguish a healthy from a pathologic state, and to diagnose disease. While heart sounds, pressures, and pulse waves serve these purposes in the cardiovascular system, for example, various components of mental function do so for the mind. Although these components in no way encompass all the aspects of human thought and feeling, they serve as useful clinical tools.

Level of consciousness refers to a person's alertness and state of awareness of his or her environment. *Attention* refers to the ability to focus or concentrate over time on one task or activity. An inattentive or distractible person whose consciousness is clouded will be grossly impaired in giving a history or responding to questions. *Memory*, too, contributes importantly to such responses. A person first must *register* or record material in his mind—a function usually tested by asking for immediate repetition of material. Information must then be stored or retained in memory. *Recent memory*—a rather loosely defined term—refers to memory over an interval of minutes, hours, or days, while *remote memory* refers to intervals of years. *Orientation* depends on both memory and attention. It refers to a person's awareness of who or what he is in relation to time, place, and other people.

An individual becomes aware of objects in the environment and their qualities and interrelationships through sensory *perceptions*. While most perceptions are initiated by external stimuli, others, like dreams and hallucinations, arise in the mind itself.

Thought processes refer to the sequence, logic, coherence, and relevance of a person's thought as it leads to selected goals. While thought processes describe how a person thinks, *thought content* refers to what he or she thinks about. In contrast, affect and mood describe how an individual feels. *Affect* is an immediately observable, usually episodic feeling tone expressed through voice, facial expression, or demeanor, while *mood* is a more sustained emotion that may color a person's view of the world. As weather is to climate, so affect is to mood.

People communicate with each other through *language,* a complex symbolic system of expressing, receiving, and comprehending words. Like consciousness, attention, and memory, language is essential to other mental functions; significant impairment here makes assessment of certain other functions difficult or even impossible.

Higher intellectual functions include a person's *vocabulary,* fund of *information,* and capacity to reason abstractly and to make judgments. *Abstract reasoning* refers to the ability to think beyond concrete terms—to grasp, for example, the similarities or differences between them, or to understand the general meaning of literally worded proverbs. In making *judgments* a person compares and evaluates alternatives for purposes of deciding on a course of action. Inherent in judgment is a set of values that may or may not be based on reality and may or may not conform to societal norms.

None of the functions described in this chapter deals directly with an individual's personality, psychodynamics, or personal experiences. These other, very important aspects are explored during the interview. By integrating and correlating all the relevant data the clinician tries to understand the person as a whole.

CHANGES WITH AGE

Although psychologic research has demonstrated many alterations in mental function over the normal lifespan, clinical assessment identifies relatively few of these changes.

Adolescence marks a time of continuing intellectual maturation during which an individual's fund of information and vocabulary continue to grow—a process that began in childhood. At approximately 12 years of age adolescents begin to think abstractly—to use generalizations, make hypotheses, develop theories, reason logically, and consider future plans, risks, and possibilities. Given intelligence, education, and experience, among other requisites, judgment develops along with an underlying set of values. This maturational process, however, like height, weight, and puberty, varies in its time of onset, pace, and duration and cannot be predicted by chronologic age alone. Some individuals never achieve the levels customarily defined as normal adult function.

Most intellectual functions that are tested clinically hold up quite well in the later decades of life. Vocabulary and information, for example, decline relatively little, although they do diminish somewhat. Immediate memory persists well too, although in tests that require reorganization of data, such as repeating numbers backward, older people do less well than younger ones. Memory declines to some extent with age, and elderly people take longer to retrieve information from their minds.

Techniques of Examination

Most of the mental status examination should be done in the context of the interview. As you talk to the patient and listen to his story, you should assess his level of consciousness, his general appearance and affect, and his ability to pay attention, remember, understand, and speak. By noting the patient's vocabulary and general fund of information in the context of his cultural and educational background, you can often make a rough estimate of intelligence, while the patient's responses to his illness give you insight into his judgment. If the patient has unusual thoughts, preoccupations, beliefs, or perceptions, you should explore them as the subject arises. Moreover, if you suspect a problem in orientation or memory, you can check these too as part of the interview. "Let's see, your last clinic appointment was when? . . . and the date today is . . . ?"

For many patients such an evaluation is sufficient. For others, however, you need to go further. All patients with documented or suspected brain lesions, patients with psychiatric symptoms, and those in whom family members or friends have reported vague behavioral symptoms need further careful, specific assessment. So do many of those who cannot seem to take medications properly and those who act a little strangely after surgery or during an acute illness. Mental function, moreover, importantly influences a person's ability to find and hold a job and thus may constitute the critical component in evaluating disability.

For these kinds of patients, and others as well, you will need to supplement your interview with questions in specific areas. In doing so, give simple introductory explanations, be tactful, and show the same acceptance and respect for the patient as in other portions of the examination.

Many students feel insecure in performing mental status examinations and are reluctant to do them. They may worry about upsetting patients, invading their privacy, and labeling their thoughts or behavior as pathologic. It may be helpful to discuss these concerns or some of the issues they raise with your instructor or other experienced clinicians. As in other parts of the assessment process your skills and confidence will improve with practice, and rewards will follow. Many patients will appreciate an understanding listener, and some will owe their health, their safety, or even their lives to your attention.

The format that follows should help to organize your observations. Although it includes suggestions concerning technique, it is not intended as a step-by-step guide. When a full examination is indicated, you should be flexible in your approach while thorough in your coverage. In some situations such as organic brain disorders, however, sequence is important. Evaluate level of consciousness and attention first, since memory depends on them and defects here will influence much of the subsequent assessment. Similarly, a language problem such as dysphasia should be detected early because much of the remaining evaluation depends on comprehending and expressing words.

APPEARANCE AND BEHAVIOR

Use here all the relevant observations made throughout the course of your history and examination. Include:

Level of Consciousness. Is the patient awake and alert? Does he seem to understand your questions and respond appropriately and reasonably quickly, or does he lose track of the topic and fall silent or even asleep?

See Table 15-2, Abnormalities of Consciousness (p. 413).

Posture and Motor Behavior. Does the patient lie in bed, or prefer to walk about? Note his ability to relax and the way in which he holds his body. Observe the pace, range, and character of movements. Do they seem to be made under voluntary control? Are certain parts immobile? Do posture and motor activity change with topics under discussion or with activities or people around the patient?

Tense posture, restlessness, and fidgetiness of anxiety; crying, pacing, and handwringing of agitated depression; hopeless, slumped posture and slowed movements of depression; bizarre or sustained posture in schizophrenia; singing, dancing and expansive movements of the manic syndrome; oral–facial dyskinesias

Dress, Grooming, and Personal Hygiene. How is the patient dressed? Is clothing clean, pressed, and properly fastened? How does it compare with clothing worn by people of comparable age and social group? Note the patient's hair, nails, teeth, skin, and, if present, beard. How are they groomed? How do the person's grooming and hygiene compare with other people of comparable age, lifestyle, and socioeconomic group? Compare one side of the body with the other.

Deterioration in grooming and personal hygiene may occur in depression, schizophrenia, and organic brain syndromes, but always consider the norms of a person's group. Excessive fastidiousness may be seen in an obsessive–compulsive disorder. One-sided neglect may result from a lesion in the opposite parietal cortex, usually the nondominant side.

Facial Expression —both at rest and in interaction with others. Watch for variations in expression with topics under discussion. Are they appropriate? Or is the face relatively immobile throughout?

Expressions of anxiety, depression, apathy, anger, elation. Facial immobility of parkinsonism

Manner, Affect, and Relationship to Persons and Things. Using your observations of facial expression, voice, and bodily movements, assess the patient's affect. Does it vary appropriately with topics under discussion; does one consistent affect prevail; or is the affect labile, blunted, or flat? Does it seem inappropriate or extreme at certain points? If so, how? Note the patient's openness and approachability, his reactions to others and to the surroundings. Does he seem to hear or see things that you do not, or is he conversing with someone who is not there?

Anger, hostility, suspiciousness, or evasiveness of paranoid patients. Elation and euphoria of the manic syndrome. Flat affect and remoteness of schizophrenia. Apathy (dulled affect with detachment and indifference) in organic brain syndromes. Anxiety, depression

Speech. As the patient talks with you through the interview, note the characteristics of his speech:

Quantity. Is the patient talkative or relatively silent? Does he offer comments spontaneously or does he respond only to direct questions?

Rate and *rhythm* (*e.g.*, rapid, slow, or hesitant)

Volume or *loudness*

Slow speech of depression. Loud, rapid speech in manic syndrome

Quality, including fluency, inflection, and clarity of words. Does the patient search for the right word in a halting manner, use the wrong words, substitute letters, or use circumlocutions such as "what you drink out of" for "glass"?

Monotonous voice of parkinsonism. Halting speech with errors and circumlocutions in dysphasia

MOOD

You should assess mood during the interview by exploring the patient's own perceptions of it. Find out about his usual mood level and how it has varied with life events. "How did you feel about that?" for example, or, more generally, "How are your spirits?"

If you suspect depression, you must assess its depth and any associated risk of suicide. A series of questions such as the following is useful, proceeding as far as the patient's positive answers warrant.

See Table 16-1, Distinguishing Features of Depressive Disorders (p. 438).

> Do you get pretty discouraged (or depressed or blue)?
> How low do you feel?
> What do you see for yourself in the future?
> Do you ever feel that life isn't worth living? Or that you had just as soon be dead?
> Have you ever thought of doing away with yourself?
> How did (do) you think you would do it?
> What would happen after you were dead?

Although many student clinicians feel uneasy about exploring thoughts of suicide, most patients can discuss their thoughts and feelings about it freely with you, sometimes with considerable relief. By such discussion you demonstrate your interest and concern for what may well be the patient's most serious and threatening problem. By avoiding the issue, you may miss the most important feature of the patient's illness.

THOUGHT PROCESSES, THOUGHT CONTENT, AND PERCEPTIONS

Thought Processes. Assess the logic, relevance, organization, and coherence of the patient's thought processes as he reveals them in words and speech throughout the interview. Does speech progress in a logical man-

See Table 16-2, Variations and Abnormalities in Thought Processes (p. 439).

ner toward a goal? Here you are using the patient's speech as a window into the patient's mind.

Thought Content. You should ascertain most of the information relevant to thought content during the interview. Follow appropriate leads as they occur rather than using stereotyped lists of specific questions. For example, "You mentioned a few minutes ago that a neighbor was responsible for your entire illness. Can you tell me more about that?" Or, in another situation, "What do you think about at times like these?"

You may need to make more specific inquiries. If so, couch them in tactful and accepting terms. "When people are upset like this, they sometimes can't keep certain thoughts out of their minds," or ". . . things seem unreal," and so on. "Have you experienced anything like this?"

In these ways find out about any of the following:

Compulsions—repetitive acts that a person feels driven to perform in order to produce or prevent some future state of affairs, although expectation of such an effect is unrealistic

Obsessions—recurrent, uncontrollable thoughts, images, or impulses that a person considers unacceptable and alien

Phobias—persistent, irrational fears with a compelling desire to avoid the stimulus

Anxieties—apprehensions, fears, tensions, or uneasiness that may be focused (phobia) or free-floating (a general sense of ill-defined dread or pending doom)

Compulsions, obsessions, phobias, and anxieties are often associated with neurotic disorders. See Table 16-3, Irrational Anxiety and Avoidance Behaviors (pp. 440–441).

Feelings of unreality—a sense that things in the environment are strange, unreal, or remote

Feelings of depersonalization—a sense that one's self is different, changed, unreal, or has lost identity

Delusions—false, fixed, personal beliefs that are not shared by other members of the person's culture or subculture. Examples include:
    Delusions of persecution
    Grandiose delusions
    Delusional jealousy
    Delusions of reference in which a person believes that external events, objects, or people have a particular and unusual personal significance (for example, that the radio or television might be commenting on or giving instructions to the person)
    Delusions of being controlled by an outside force
    Somatic delusions
    Systematized delusions, a single delusion with many elaborations or a cluster of related delusions around a single theme, all systematized into a complex network

Delusions and feelings of unreality or depersonalization are more often associated with psychotic disorders. See Table 16-4, Distinguishing Features of Psychotic Disorders (pp. 442–443).

Perceptions. In a similar manner inquire about:

Illusions—misinterpretations of real external stimuli
Hallucinations—subjective sensory perceptions in the absence of relevant external stimuli. The person may or may not recognize the experiences as false. Hallucinations may be auditory, visual, olfactory, gustatory, tactile, or somatic. (False perceptions associated with dreaming, falling asleep, and awakening are not classified as hallucinations.)

Illusions and hallucinations are usually associated with psychotic disorders such as schizophrenia and delirium. See Table 16-4, Distinguishing Features of Psychotic Disorders (pp. 442–443).

COGNITIVE FUNCTIONS

Orientation. By skillful questioning you can often determine the patient's orientation in the context of the interview. For example, you can ask quite naturally for specific dates and times, for the patient's address, telephone number, the names of family members, or the route he took to the hospital. At times—when rechecking the status of a delirious patient, for example—simple direct questions may be indicated: "Can you tell me what time it is now?" In either of these ways, determine the patient's orientation for:

Disorientation occurs especially when memory and attention are impaired, as in organic brain syndromes. See Table 16-5, Distinguishing Features of Organic Brain Syndromes (pp. 444–445).

1. *Time* (*e.g.*, the time of day, day of the week, month, season, date and year, duration of hospitalization)
2. *Place* (*e.g.*, his residence, the name of the hospital, city, and state)
3. *Person* (*e.g.*, his own name, the names of relatives and professional personnel)

Attention. Tests of attention include:

Digit Span. Tell the patient that you would like to test his ability to concentrate, perhaps adding that people tend to have trouble with that when they are in pain, or ill, or feverish, or whatever. Read a series of digits, starting with the shortest set and enunciating each number clearly at a rate of about 1 per second. Ask the patient to repeat them back to you. If the patient makes a mistake, give him a second try with a series of the same length. Stop after a second failure in a series of any given length. In choosing digits avoid consecutive numbers and numbers that form easily recognized dates.

Poor performance of digit span is characteristic of organic brain syndromes such as delirium and dementia. Performance is also limited by mental retardation and by performance anxiety.

5,2	5,3,8,7	3,6,7,9,5,2	9,4,7,2,5,6,1,8
9,3	2,1,7,9	4,1,5,3,7,9	3,5,8,1,4,9,7,6
6,1,7	4,7,2,9,3	7,2,4,8,3,5,9	6,1,9,8,2,5,4,3,7
8,4,1	5,3,8,7,1	3,6,1,5,8,4,2	3,8,7,2,4,9,1,6,5

Now, (starting again with the shortest series) ask the patient to repeat the numbers to you backwards.

Normally a person should be able to repeat correctly at least five to eight digits forward and four to six backwards.

Serial 7s or Serial 3s. Instruct the patient, "Starting from a hundred, subtract 7, and keep subtracting 7. . . ." Note the effort required and the speed and accuracy of the responses. (Writing down the answers helps you keep up with the arithmetic.) Normally, a person can complete serial 7s in 1½ minutes, with fewer than four errors. If the patient cannot do serial 7s, try serial 3s, or ask him to count backward. Still easier tests are counting forward or reciting the alphabet.

Memory. Most questions relevant to remote and recent memory can be asked in the context of the interview. Evaluate:

Remote memory (*e.g.*, birthdays, anniversaries, names of schools attended, jobs held, past historical events such as presidents or wars relevant to the patient's past)

Recent memory (*e.g.*, the events of the day). Ask questions with answers that you can check against other sources so that you will know whether or not the patient is confabulating (making up facts to compensate for a defective memory). These might include the day's weather, today's appointment time in the clinic, and medications or laboratory tests taken during the day.

In addition, test *new learning ability*. Give the patient three or four words such as "83 Water Street and blue," or "table, flower, green, and hamburger." Ask him to repeat them so that you know that he has heard and registered the information. (This step, like digit span, tests registration and immediate recall.) Then proceed to other parts of the examination. After about 3 to 5 minutes ask him to repeat the words. Note the accuracy of his response, his awareness of whether he is correct, and any tendency to confabulate. Normally a person should be able to remember the words.

Language and Copying

Word Comprehension. Ask the patient to point to objects in the room or to specific body parts. For example, "Will you please point to your nose . . . the telephone . . . the bedspread. . . ."

Naming. Ask the patient to name a series of objects or colors as you point them out. Gradually increase the difficulty of the questions—from "hat" and "red," for example, to "belt buckle" and "purple." Note the patient's fluency and accuracy, and listen for evidence of dysphasia such as halting, searching language or substitutions of words and letters. For example, when shown a pen, a dysphasic person might reply, "It's . . . it's . . . you write . . . it's a den."

Reading. Write a simple command on a paper in large clear print—for example, "CLOSE YOUR EYES" or "RAISE YOUR HAND."

Poor performance may be secondary to organic brain syndromes such as delirium and dementia, but also occurs with mental retardation, anxiety, and depression.

Remote memory may be impaired in the late stages of dementia.

Recent memory, including new learning ability, is impaired in organic brain syndromes such as dementia, delirium, and the amnestic syndrome. Impairments in attention produced by anxiety, depression, and mental retardation also impair recent memory. See Table 16-5, Distinguishing Features of Organic Brain Syndromes (pp. 444–445).

Dysphasias and aphasias refer to specific disturbances in understanding or expressing language, whether written or spoken. They result from cortical disease, not from disorders of vision, hearing, or the organs of articulation, nor from general intellectual deficiency.

Impairment in these tests also may occur in mental retardation and organic brain syndromes such as dementia, but these impairments lack the qualitative attributes of dysphasia.

Writing. Ask the patient to write a sentence—one that he makes up on his own. Note whether the sentence makes sense, has a subject and verb, or contains misspelled words.

Copying Figures. Show him some figures of increasing complexity, one at a time, and ask him to copy each as well as he can on a piece of blank unlined paper.

If vision and motor ability are intact, poor performance in copying suggests organic brain disease such as dementia or parietal lobe damage. Mental retardation may also impair performance.

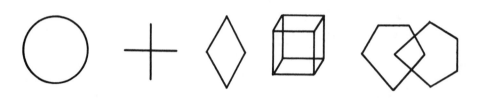

Higher Intellectual Functions

Information. You can explore a person's fund of information in the context of the interview. Ask a student, for example, about his favorite courses, or inquire about a person's work or hobbies, or about current events. More directly, you can ask the patient to name the last five presidents or five big cities in the country. Alternatively, ask a series of specific questions such as the following:

1. How many days are there in a week?
2. What must you do to water to make it boil?
3. How many things are there in a dozen?
4. Name the four seasons of the year?
5. What do we celebrate on the 4th of July?
6. How many pounds are there in a ton?
7. What does the stomach do?
8. What is the capital of Greece?
9. Where does the sun set?
10. Who invented the airplane?
11. Why does oil float on water?
12. What do we get turpentine from?
13. When is Labor Day?
14. How far is it from New York to Chicago?
15. What is a hieroglyphic?
16. What is a barometer?
17. Who wrote "Paradise Lost?"
18. What is a prime number?
19. What is *habeas corpus*?
20. Who discovered the South Pole?

If considered against the patient's cultural and educational background, information is a good indicator of underlying intelligence. It is relatively unaffected by any but the most severe psychiatric disorders and may be helpful in distinguishing mentally retarded adults (whose information is poor) from those with mild or moderate dementia (whose information is relatively good).

Persons of average ability should be able to answer correctly from 8 to 13 of these questions. Take into consideration, however, the patient's cultural and educational background.

Vocabulary. Ask the patient to give you the meaning of the following words or to use each word in a sentence.

1. Apple	9. Tint	17. Seclude
2. Donkey	10. Armory	18. Spangle
3. Diamond	11. Fable	19. Recede
4. Nuisance	12. Nitroglycerine	20. Affliction
5. Join	13. Microscope	21. Chattel
6. Fur	14. Stanza	22. Dilatory
7. Shilling	15. Guillotine	23. Flout
8. Bacon	16. Plural	24. Amanuensis

Persons of average intellectual ability should be able to define or use from 8 to 16 of these words. Again, keep in mind the patient's cultural and educational background.

If considered against the patient's cultural and educational background, vocabulary is probably the best indicator of underlying intelligence. It is relatively unaffected by any but the most severe psychiatric disorders. It may be helpful in distinguishing mentally retarded adults (whose vocabulary is limited) from those with mild or moderate dementia (whose vocabulary is fairly well preserved).

Abstract Reasoning. The capacity to reason abstractly is tested in two ways:

Proverbs. Ask the patient what people mean when they use some of the following proverbs:

1. A stitch in time saves nine.
2. Don't count your chickens before they're hatched.
3. The proof of the pudding is in the eating.
4. A rolling stone gathers no moss.
5. The squeaking wheel gets the grease.

Note the relevance of the answers and their degree of concreteness or abstractness. For example, "You should sew a rip before it gets bigger" is concrete, while "Prompt attention to a problem prevents trouble" is abstract. Average patients should give abstract or semi-abstract responses.

Concrete responses are often given by persons with mental retardation, delirium, or dementia, but may also, however, be simply a function of little education. Schizophrenics may respond concretely or with personal, bizarre interpretations.

Similarities. Ask the patient to tell you how the following are alike:

1. An orange and an apple	4. A church and a theater
2. A cat and a mouse	5. A piano and a violin
3. A child and a dwarf	6. Paper and coal

Note the accuracy and relevance of the answers and their degree of concreteness or abstractness. For example, "A cat and a mouse are both animals" is abstract, while "A cat chases a mouse" is neither abstract nor relevant to the question.

Judgment. You can usually assess the patient's judgment during the interview by noting, for example, his or her responses to family situations, jobs, use of money, and interpersonal conflicts. Note whether decisions and actions are based on reality or, for example, on impulse, wish ful-

Judgment may be poor in organic brain disease, mental retardation, and psychotic states.

(Text continues on p. 446.)

Table 16-1

Table 16-1 Distinguishing Features of Depressive Disorders

SYMPTOMS	HISTORY	POSSIBLE DIAGNOSIS
Clinical depression is manifested by several of the following:	*What preceded the present depressive state?*	*Then consider:*
	A psychiatric diagnosis	Primary degenerative dementia with depressive features
		Organic affective syndrome
		Psychotic disorder with depression (*e.g.,* schizophrenia)
1. Poor appetite or significant weight loss, or increased appetite or significant weight gain	A serious medical diagnosis	Depression associated with cancer, heart disease, or other life-threatening or life-changing illness
2. Sleep disturbance (*e.g.,* insomnia, hypersomnia)		
3. Fatigue, loss of energy	Previous episode(s) of depression lasting at least 2 weeks	Major affective disorder—depressive
4. Psychomotor agitation or retardation		
5. Loss of interest in stimulating activities	Previous episode(s) of manic syndrome with or without depressive episodes	Major affective disorder—bipolar (manic–depressive)
6. Decreased ability to think and concentrate		
7. Feelings of worthlessness, self-reproach, or guilt		
8. Recurrent thoughts of death or suicide	Over the past 2 years numerous episodes of manic and depressive symptoms that were shorter and less severe than in a major depression. No psychotic features	Cyclothymic disorder
Four, or preferably, five of the above, occurring nearly every day for at least 2 weeks, constitute a major depression.		
	Over the past 2 years (1 year for adolescents), recurrent or persistent depressive symptoms that were shorter or less severe than in a major depression. No psychotic features	Dysthymic disorder

Table 16-2

Table 16-2   Variations and Abnormalities in Thought Processes

CIRCUMSTANTIALITY	Speech characterized by indirection and delay in reaching the point because of unnecessary detail, although the components of the description have a meaningful connection. Circumstantiality is observed in many people without mental disorders and in persons with compulsive personality disorders.
LOOSENING OF ASSOCIATIONS	Speech in which a person shifts from one subject to others that are unrelated or only obliquely related without realizing that the subjects are not meaningfully connected. Loosening of associations is observed in schizophrenia, manic episodes, and other psychotic disorders.
FLIGHT OF IDEAS	An almost continuous flow of accelerated speech in which a person changes abruptly from topic to topic. Changes are usually based on understandable associations, plays on words, or distracting stimuli, but the ideas do not progress to sensible conversation. Flight of ideas is most frequently noted in manic episodes, but may also be present in organic mental disorders and schizophrenia.
NEOLOGISMS	Invented or distorted words, or words with new and highly idiosyncratic meanings. Neologisms are used by schizophrenics and by persons who have other psychotic disorders.
INCOHERENCE	Speech that is mostly incomprehensible because of illogic, lack of meaningful connections, abrupt changes in topic, disordered grammar or use of words. When severe, both loosening of associations and flight of ideas may produce incoherence. Incoherence is observed in severely disturbed psychotic patients who are usually schizophrenic.
BLOCKING	Sudden interruption of speech in mid-sentence or before completion of an idea. The person attributes this to losing his thought. Blocking occurs in normal people and is striking in schizophrenia.
CONFABULATION	Fabrication of facts or events in response to questions, to fill in the gaps in an impaired memory. Patients with the organic amnestic syndrome characteristically confabulate.
PERSEVERATION	Persistent repetition of words or ideas. Perseveration occurs in organic mental disorders, schizophrenia, and other psychotic disorders.
ECHOLALIA	The repetition of the words or phrases of others. Echolalia is observed in organic mental disorders and schizophrenia.
CLANGING	Speech in which a person chooses a word on the basis of sound rather than meaning, as in rhyming and punning speech. Clanging is found characteristically in schizophrenia and manic episodes.

Table 16-3

Table 16-3 Irrational Anxiety and Avoidance Behaviors

	ORGANIC MENTAL DISORDER	PSY-CHOTIC DISORDER	SEPARA-TION ANXIETY DISORDER*	AVOIDANT DISORDER OF CHILD-HOOD AND ADOLES-CENCE*	OVER-ANXIOUS DISORDER*	AGORAPHOBIA WITH PANIC ATTACKS	WITHOUT PANIC ATTACKS
Known organic cause	Yes, see Table 16-5	No	No	No	No	No	No
Psychotic features		Yes, see Table 16-4	No	No	No	No	No
Excessive anxiety about separation from those to whom person is attached			Yes, for at least 2 weeks	No	No		
Persistent shrinking from contact or familiarity with strangers				Yes, for at least 6 weeks	No		
Generalized, persistent anxiety or worry					Yes, for at least 6 months		
Irrational avoidance— of objects or situations						Yes, fear of being alone or in a public place where escape seems impossible	
of leaving home						Yes. Fears and avoidance increase to constrict normal life.	
of special social situations, with overconcern about humiliation or embarrassment							
Recurrent panic attacks						Yes	No
Obsessions or compulsions							
Relation of stress to anxiety							
Repeated reexperiencing of traumatic events							

*Pay special attention to these three possibilities when the patient is a child or adolescent.

Table 16-3

Table 16-3   (Cont'd)

SOCIAL PHOBIA	PANIC DISORDER	SIMPLE PHOBIA	OBSESSIVE COMPULSIVE DISORDER	GENERALIZED ANXIETY DISORDER	POST-TRAUMATIC STRESS DISORDER	ADJUSTMENT DISORDER WITH ANXIOUS MOOD
No	No	No	No	No	No	No
No	No	No	No	No	No	No
				Yes, with tension, autonomic symptoms, apprehensive expectations, dysfunctional vigilance		
No	Not specifically	Yes, specific (*e.g.,* dogs, heights)	No	No	No	No
No	Not specifically	No	No	No	No	No
Yes	Not specifically	No	No	No	No	No
	Yes, without consistent stimulus					
		Yes	No	No	No	No
				Generalized anxiety for at least a month without specific stressor	Unusually severe stress (*e.g.,* rape, combat) preceded symptoms	Stressor present within 3 months but less severe
					Yes	No

441

Table 16-4

Table 16-4 Distinguishing Features of Psychotic Disorders*

Psychotic manifestations include delusions, hallucinations, incoherence, a marked loosening of associations, markedly illogical thinking, and bizarre, grossly disorganized, or catatonic behavior.

	ORGANIC BRAIN SYNDROME (e.g., *DELUSIONAL HALLUCINOSIS*)	MALINGERING OR FACTITIOUS DISORDERS	BRIEF REACTIVE PSYCHOSIS
PSYCHOTIC MANIFESTATIONS	Present	Present	Present
KNOWN ORGANIC FACTOR CAUSALLY RELATED	*Present,* See Table 16-5	Absent	Absent
SYMPTOMS DELIBERATE, PURPOSEFUL, VOLUNTARY	No	*Yes*	No
DURATION			From a few hours to *less than 2 weeks*
PROFOUNDLY UPSETTING ENVIRONMENTAL EVENT JUST BEFORE ILLNESS			*Yes*
MOOD AND AFFECT			
DELUSIONS			
HALLUCINATIONS, INCOHERENCE, OR MARKED LOOSENING OF ASSOCIATIONS	Hallucinations, if present, are often visual.		

*Abnormalities are printed in red, key features in italics.

Table 16-4

Table 16-4 (Cont'd)

MAJOR AFFECTIVE DISORDERS	SCHIZO– AFFECTIVE DISORDER	SCHIZO– PHRENIA	PARANOID DISORDERS
Present	Present	Present	Present
Absent	Absent	Absent	Absent
No	No	No	No
		At least 6 months	
Full depressive or manic syndrome		Blunt, flat, or inappropriate affect; but depressive or manic syndrome is absent, relatively brief, or follows psychotic syndrome.	Depression or manic syndrome is absent, relatively brief, or follows psychotic symptoms.
May be present	Differentiation between major affective disorders and schizophrenia cannot be made in these individuals.	*Often present*	*Present, predominantly delusions of persecution or jealousy*
May be present		*Often present*; hallucinations are usually auditory	Not present

Table 16-5

Table 16-5 Distinguishing Features of Organic Brain Syndromes*

	DELIRIUM	DEMENTIA	AMNESTIC SYNDROME
LEVEL OF CONSCIOUSNESS	*Clouded; reduced awareness of environment*	*Not clouded (unless delirium coexists)*	*Not clouded*
MAJOR INTELLECTUAL ABILITIES	General loss	*Significant general loss*	*No significant general loss*
MEMORY	Impaired	Impaired	*Impaired (recent and remote)*
ORIENTATION	Disorientation	May become impaired	Often impaired
THOUGHT PROCESSES AND PERCEPTIONS	Often shows illusions, misinterpretations, hallucinations		May confabulate
MOOD			
PERSONALITY CHANGE		Alteration or accentuation of pre-morbid traits	
TIME COURSE	Develops over short period, fluctuates; duration usually brief	Varies with cause but often slow and progressive	Varies with cause but often has rapid onset, chronic course
ORGANIC FACTOR JUDGED CAUSAL	Present	Present or presumed	Present
EXAMPLES OF CAUSE	Many, such as drug intoxications, hypoglycemia, post-operative states, systemic infections; chronic renal, liver, and pulmonary disease; heart failure	Many, often involving diffuse brain disease, such as Alzheimer's disease, cerebrovascular disorders, brain trauma	Head trauma, thiamine deficiency associated with alcohol abuse

*Abnormalities are printed in red, key features in italics.

Table 16-5

Table 16-5 (Cont'd)

ORGANIC DELUSIONAL SYNDROME	ORGANIC HALLUCINOSIS	ORGANIC AFFECTIVE SYNDROME	ORGANIC PERSONALITY SYNDROME
Not clouded	*Not clouded*	*Not clouded*	*Not clouded*
Intact	*Intact*	*Intact*	*Intact*
Delusions, often persecutory. Hallucinations, if present, not prominent.	*Hallucinations.* Delusions, if present, relate to hallucinations.	Delusions and hallucinations, if present, relate to mood and are not predominant.	
		Depressive or *manic*	
			A marked change of behavior such as lability, impaired impulse control, marked apathy, or suspiciousness
Varies with cause	Varies		
Present	Present	Present	Present
Amphetamines, cannabis, hallucinogens; brain damage	Chronic alcohol abuse, sensory deprivation, epilepsy	Depressive—reserpine, methyldopa, other drugs, viral illnesses. Manic—adrenocortical steroids, stimulants	Most often brain damage of frontal or temporal lobes; toxic and metabolic factors

(Text continued from p. 437)

fillment, or disordered thought content. What values seem to underlie the patient's decisions and behavior? Allowing for cultural variations, how do these compare with mature adult standards? Some additional hypothetical questions may help you evaluate the patient's judgment and comprehension of other circumstances. For example:

1. What should you do if you are stopped for speeding?
2. What should you do if you lose a library book?
3. What should you do if you see a train approaching a broken track?
4. What would you do if you found a stamped, addressed, and sealed letter lying in the street?
5. Why are criminals put in prison?

Since judgment is part of the maturational response, it may be variable and unpredictable during adolescence.

A NOTE ON MENTAL ASSESSMENT

As in other portions of the interview and examination, you should vary your focus according to the nature of the patient's problems. The tables on pages 438–445 may help to guide your approach.*

While all human observations are inherently subject to error, assessments of mental status are especially susceptible to bias based on such factors as age, race, sex, class, cultural background, personal appearance, and even body weight. For example, most adults of any age have at some time lost track of the date, forgotten the name of an acquaintance, or allowed a pot to boil dry on the stove. Just because a person is elderly such lapses do not by themselves justify the label of "senility" or organic brain disease. Neither teenage pregnancy nor rejection of medical treatment necessarily means poor judgment; each may well be quite appropriate to the patient's cultural milieu or personal situation. A person who displays anger, suspiciousness, or depression may be responding fittingly to an oppressive, restrictive, or discriminatory environment; it may be society, not the man or woman, that is "abnormal" or inappropriate. A patient, moreover, may remind you of someone such as your parents or grandparents, and your reactions and perceptions may be colored accordingly. As you develop your skills in evaluating mental status, try to be sensitive to sources of bias such as these, monitor your judgments, and modify them as necessary.

---

*The terminology and differential points used in these tables are based primarily on the third edition of *Diagnostic and Statistical Manual of Mental Disorders,* published by the American Psychiatric Association in 1980.

Chapter 17

THE PHYSICAL EXAMINATION OF INFANTS AND CHILDREN

Robert A. Hoekelman

The anatomy and physiology, the techniques of examination, and the normal and abnormal findings presented in the foregoing sections of this book are focused primarily on the adult patient. Most of what is presented is also applicable to infants and children. In the process of development, however, children are anatomically and physiologically unique. Consequently, many of the techniques of examination, the physical findings, and their significance are altered in younger patients.

The purpose of this section is to describe how to conduct those parts of the physical examination of infants and children that require different approaches and techniques than those used for the physical examination of adults. No attempt will be made to discuss or describe findings other than the normal, variations of normal, and those accompanying common pathologic conditions of infancy and childhood. Uncommon pathologic conditions will not be presented except for those few that require specific examination techniques for detection. The texts listed in the bibliography should be consulted for complete differential diagnoses of abnormal physical findings.

When assessing an infant or a child, always consider where the patient is on the continuum of growth and development, as well as the age range in which that point is normally reached. You must also reflect upon the different rates of growth of the various systems of the body. For example, growth and development of the central nervous system, the lymphatic system, and the reproductive system parallel neither general somatic growth nor each other. The figure at the right illustrates these differences.

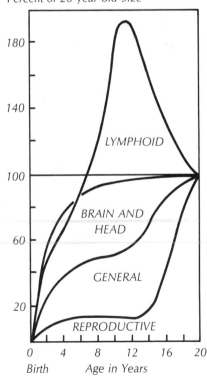

GROWTH PATTERNS OF VARIOUS SYSTEMS

Percent of 20-year-old Size

LYMPHOID

BRAIN AND HEAD

GENERAL

REPRODUCTIVE

Birth   *Age in Years*

It is essential, therefore, that, in examining infants and children, you are well acquainted with the normal and abnormal patterns of growth and development. You should be aware, for example, that a physical finding such as a Babinski response is abnormal beyond the age of 2 years, but may be found in normal subjects prior to that age. The scope of this text does not allow for inclusion of this kind of information in any sequential form, nor for description of the systematic methods of testing developmental levels. Texts dealing with this information are also listed in the bibliography.

In this discussion of each part of the pediatric physical examination, beginning with the approach to the patient, it will be useful to consider *three developmental levels:* **infancy (the first year), early childhood (1 year through 5 years), and late childhood (6 years and over). Because treatment of individual systems here is brief, sections on** *techniques of examination* **are set off in boldface rather than presented separately as in the earlier chapters.**

APPROACH TO THE PATIENT

INFANCY

The newborn should be examined briefly, immediately after birth, to determine the general condition of his cardiorespiratory, neurologic, and gastrointestinal systems and to detect any gross congenital abnormalities.

Newborn infants may be classified according to their birth weight, their gestational age (maturity), or a combination of these two dimensions.

Classification by Birth Weight
   Premature = Birth weight < 2500 grams
   Full-term = Birth weight ≥ 2500 grams

Classification by Gestational Age
   Pre-term = Gestation ≤ 37 weeks
   Term = Gestation 38 to 42 weeks
   Post-term = Gestation ≥ 42 weeks

Classification by Birth Weight and Gestational Age
   Weight Small for Gestational Age (SGA) = Birth weight < 10th percentile on the intrauterine growth curve

   Weight Appropriate for Gestational Age (AGA) = Birth weight within the 10th and 90th percentile on the intrauterine growth curve

   Weight Large for Gestational Age (LGA) = Birth weight > 90th percentile on the intrauterine growth curve

The figure below, devised by Battaglia and Lubchenco of the University of Colorado, depicts nine possible categories of maturity for newborn infants based upon birth weight and gestational age: pre-term SGA, AGA, and LGA; term SGA, AGA, and LGA; and post-term SGA, AGA, and LGA.

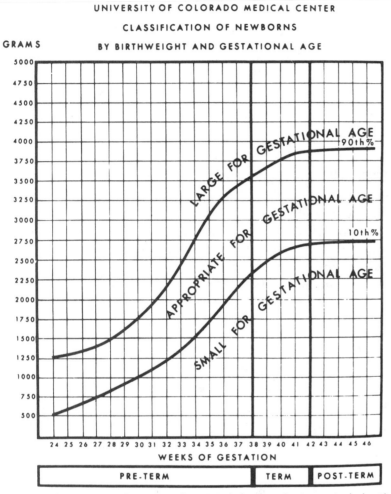

UNIVERSITY OF COLORADO MEDICAL CENTER

CLASSIFICATION OF NEWBORNS

BY BIRTHWEIGHT AND GESTATIONAL AGE

(Reproduced with permission from Battaglia FC, Lubchenko LO: A practical classification of newborn infants by weight and gestational age. J Pediatr 71:161, 1967)

Several physical and neurological characteristics of newborns, defined by Dubowitz, Dubowitz, and Goldberger, can also be used to estimate an infant's gestational age fairly accurately. (See the bibliography.)

The infant's immediate adaptation to extrauterine life can be assessed with a set of five clinical signs developed by Dr. Virginia Apgar, each scored on a 3-point scale (0, 1, or 2). The Apgar scores may range from 0 to 10, using the method of scoring shown in Table 17-1. Each infant should be scored at 1 minute and 5 minutes following birth. If at 5 minutes the Apgar score is 8 or more, a more complete examination can then be conducted.

Each of these categories has a different mortality rate, highest for pre-term SGA and AGA infants and lowest for term AGA infants. Furthermore, pre-term AGA infants are more prone to hyaline membrane disease, apnea, patent ductus arteriosus with left-to-right shunt, and infection, while pre-term SGA infants are more likely to experience asphyxia, hypoglycemia, and hypocalcemia.

One-minute Apgar scores of 7 or less usually indicate nervous system depression. Scores of 4 or less indicate severe depression requiring immediate resuscitation.

Table 17-1   The Apgar Scoring System

CLINICAL SIGN	ASSIGNED SCORE		
	0	1	2
HEART RATE	Absent	<100	>100
RESPIRATORY EFFORT	Absent	Slow and irregular	Good and crying
MUSCLE TONE	Flaccid	Some flexion of the arms and legs	Active movement
REFLEX IRRITABILITY*	No responses	Crying	Crying vigorously
COLOR	Blue, pale	Pink body, blue extremities	Pink all over

*Reaction to insertion of a soft rubber catheter into the external nares.

Listen to the anterior thorax with your stethoscope, palpate the abdomen, and inspect the head, face, oral cavity, extremities, and perineum. Pass a small tube through the nose, nasopharynx, and esophagus into the stomach to establish their patency. To be sure that the tube is in the stomach, palpate the epigastrium for the tip itself; alternatively, feel or listen there for the emergence of a bubble of air blown through the tube into the stomach. Aspirate the gastric contents in premature babies and babies born by cesarean section in order to prevent regurgitation and aspiration.

Failure to pass the tube through the nasopharynx suggests posterior nasal (choanal) atresia. Failure to pass the tube into the stomach suggests esophageal atresia, usually with an associated tracheoesophageal fistula.

A more extensive examination of the newborn should be conducted within 12 hours of birth, and again at approximately 72 hours of age when the effects of anesthesia and shock of birth have subsided.

Observe the baby, at first lying undisturbed in his bassinet and then completely undressed on an examining table.

Best results, in terms of responsiveness, are obtained 2 or 3 hours after a feeding when the baby is neither too satiated (and therefore less responsive) nor too hungry (and therefore more agitated).

Observe the baby's color, size, body proportions, nutritional status, and posture as well as respirations and movements of the head and extremities.

Normal newborns lie in a symmetrical position with the limbs semiflexed and the legs partially abducted at the hip. The head is slightly flexed and positioned in the midline or turned to one side. In normal newborns there is spontaneous motor activity of flexion and extension alternating between the arms and legs. The forearms supinate with flexion at the elbow and pronate with extension. The fingers are usually flexed in a tight fist, but may be seen to extend in slow athetoid posturing movements. Low amplitude and high frequency tremors of the arms, legs, and body are

In breech babies, the legs and head are extended, and the legs of a frank breech baby are abducted and externally rotated.

seen with vigorous crying and even at rest during the first 48 hours of life.

Most newborn infants are cooperative during the examination unless it is close to a feeding time.

Make sure that the baby is quiet when you auscultate the heart and lungs and palpate the abdomen, since these maneuvers are more difficult to perform if the baby is crying. Place a sugar nipple, a bottle of formula, or the tip of one of your fingers in a crying baby's mouth to silence him long enough to complete these portions of the examination.

Beyond this, the order of examination is of little importance except that hip abduction should be performed at the end because it usually causes the baby to cry.

After the newborn period and throughout the rest of infancy, little difficulty should be encountered in the performance of the complete physical examination. The key to success is distraction, since infants seem to be able to attend to only one thing at a time. It is relatively easy to bring the baby's attention to something other than the examination being performed.

Use a moving object, a flashing light, a game of peek-a-boo, tickling, or any sort of noise to distract the baby.

Infants usually do not object to removal of their clothing. Indeed, most seem to prefer the nude state, perhaps because it allows for greater tactile stimulation. It is wise, however, to leave the diaper in place throughout the examination, removing it only to examine the genitalia, rectum, lower spine, and hips.

You can perform much of the examination with the infant lying or sitting in the parent's lap or held in an upright position against the parent's chest, although this is usually not necessary except with tired, hungry, or acutely ill babies. Occasionally almost the entire physical examination can be completed without waking a sleeping infant.

Observation of the parent–infant interaction is important. The mother's (or father's) affect in talking about her infant, the manner in which she holds, moves, and dresses the baby, and her response to situations that may produce discomfort for her child should be noted. A breast or a bottle feeding should be observed.

With older infants, before performing the general physical examination you should test for attainment of developmental milestones, such as the ability to reach for a toy, transfer a cube from one hand to the other, and use the thumb and forefinger pincer grasp in picking up a small object.

By 4 days after birth, however, tremors occurring at rest signal central nervous system disease. Asymmetrical movements of the arms or legs at any time should alert the clinician to the possibility of central or peripheral neurologic deficits, birth injuries, or congenital anomalies.

This may give some indication of maladaptive nurturing patterns on the parent's part. These observations are important in assessing malnutrition, colic, chronic regurgitation, and suspected maternal deprivation.

EARLY CHILDHOOD

One of the most difficult challenges facing the professional who cares for children in this age group is completing the examination without producing a physical struggle, a crying child, or a distraught parent. When this is accomplished successfully it provides a great measure of satisfaction to all involved, and comes as close to "art" in practice as any other pursuit.

Gaining the child's confidence and dispersing his or her fears begins at the moment of encounter and continues throughout the entire visit. The approach may vary with the place and circumstances of the visit; however, a health supervision visit for a well child will allow greater development of rapport than will a visit at home or in the hospital emergency room when the child is acutely ill.

During the interview, the child should usually remain dressed. This may prolong the visit time, but avoids apprehension on the child's part and affords the opportunity later to observe his response to being undressed or his ability to undress himself. Children are also more apt to play quietly and interact with the parent and examiner more appropriately if fully clothed.

Engage the child in conversation appropriate to his age and ask simple questions concerning his health or illness. Make complimentary remarks about the child's appearance, dress, or performance, tell a story, or play a simple trick to help "break the ice."

This dialogue will indicate the child's level of receptive and expressive function and will give direction for approach by the examiner.

If the child responds to conversation and questions directed to him with silence, shielding of the eyes, or apprehension, it is wise to ignore him temporarily.

Include in your observations during the interview a general assessment of the degree of sickness or wellness, mood, state of nutrition, speech, cry, respiratory pattern, facial expression, apparent chronological and emotional age, posture (particularly as it may reflect discomfort), and developmental skills. In addition, closely observe the parent–child interaction, including the amount of separation tolerated, displays of affection, and response to discipline.

Abusing parents pay little or no attention to their abused child, treating him or her more like a piece of property than a person. By the same token, an abused child usually demonstrates no separation anxiety when physically and environmentally removed from the parents.

Specific developmental testing (such as building towers with blocks, playing ball with the examiner, and performing hop, skip, and jump maneuvers) is best accomplished at the end of the interview, just prior to the formal physical examination. This "fun and games" interlude is likely to improve the child's view of the examiner and his behavior at the time of the examination.

The actual performance of the physical examination, with certain exceptions, need not take place on the examining table. In fact, some parts of the examination can best be accomplished with the child standing, sitting on the parent's lap, or even sitting on the examiner's lap. Also, it is not essential that the child be completely undressed throughout the course of the examination; often, exposing only the part of the body being examined will suffice and most likely avert objection by the child. Occasionally a child's reluctance to undress stems from the coolness of the examining room and the coldness of the examining table and instruments (including the examiner's hands), rather than from apprehension or modesty. When there are two or more siblings to be examined, it is wise to begin with the oldest, who is most likely to be cooperative and set a good example for the younger children.

Actually, only a few children resist undressing. Most will allow themselves to be stripped to their underpants and placed upon the examining table in a sitting position without objection.

During the examination, ask the parent to stand at the head of the examining table, to the right of the child and to your left as you face the examining table. As with infants, distraction is the key to gaining the patient's cooperation. The child in this age group, however, is not as easily distracted as the infant; therefore, approach the patient pleasantly and, whenever possible, explain each step of the examination prior to performing it. Demonstrate the procedure on yourself or on a doll or toy animal. This is also very helpful to the child in gaining understanding of what is to be done. For example, you can place the otoscope in your ear, flash the light into your open mouth, or place the stethoscope on your chest. Allow the child to play with the examining instruments prior to their use to create an atmosphere of trust. Play at blowing out the examining light or use the stethoscope bell as a telephone to create attractive diversions.

The initial "laying on of the hands" is the most crucial point of the examination; if resistance is to be encountered, it will most likely be at this point. Therefore the first contact should be in nonvulnerable areas.

Hold the patient's hand, count his fingers, and palpate his wrist and elbow while talking to him gently in order to place him at ease.

Having both of the examiner's hands in contact with the patient's body whenever possible has a comforting effect on the patient and is less apt to produce involuntary withdrawal than is the use of one hand or a few probing fingers.

For example, when examining the heart, place your left hand on the patient's right shoulder while your right hand, holding the stethoscope, makes contact with the chest wall.

In a sense, the left hand acts as both a distracting and comforting force. The examiner who moves in an unhesitating, firm, and graceful manner and who talks with a friendly, pleasant, reassuring voice throughout the examination is not apt to provoke apprehension.

Use a firm tone of voice and unequivocal instructions when asking a child to perform an act pertaining to the examination. Tell him what to do rather than asking him to do it. For example, say "Roll over on your belly" rather than "Will you roll over on your belly for me?"

Some children will cease to resist when spoken to sharply, but usually this will produce increased resistance. Often the child will sit or lie passively on the examining table, covering both eyes with his hands, because (to his way of thinking), if he cannot see the examiner, the examiner cannot see him. This posture can certainly be tolerated, since it does not interfere with the examination. The eyes in this instance are easily examined after the child has dressed.

Base the order of your examination on performing the least distressing procedures first and the most distressing last. Thus, perform those parts of the examination that can be accomplished in the sitting position—for example, palpation, percussion, and auscultation of the heart and lungs—before the child lies down. Since lying down may make the child feel more vulnerable and provoke resistance to further examination, accomplish this with great care. Often you can avert apprehension by supporting the head and back with your arm while the child lies down. Once the child is in the supine position, examine the abdomen first, the throat and ears next to last, and the genitalia and rectum last. Examination of the genitalia and perineum, when a rectal examination is not performed, is usually less disturbing to the child than is the examination of the throat. However, in light of the fastidious and perhaps modest nature of some parents, leave these portions of the examination to last.

The child's comfort should be paramount in conducting the examination. Immediately before an examination maneuver he should be told kindly, but matter-of-factly, of the likelihood of pain or other unpleasant sensations that might result from the maneuver. In instances where the child is extremely apprehensive about one portion of the examination (*e.g.*, the examination of the throat) it is helpful to do this first. Indeed, it may be necessary to complete the entire physical examination before obtaining the history to ensure a reasonable interview. Distasteful portions of the examination should be accomplished quickly so as to minimize the child's discomfort. The examiner should remember, however, that the physical examination is designed to gather essential information, and that the child's comfort may need to be sacrificed to some extent to achieve this end. A completed examination is a comfort and reassurance to the parent and examiner, while an incomplete examination is a frustration and a source of dissatisfaction to both.

Obviously, there will be instances where resistance to the examination will be encountered. Some children will scream and yell throughout the examination but offer no physical resistance. Most, however, will fight the examination and strive to gain an upright position and the comfort and security of a parent's arms. The parent can be helpful here in orally reassuring the child and in actually restraining his movements for certain portions of the examination. It is sometimes necessary to ask a parent who is overly sympathetic and ineffective in calming the child to leave the room. Surprisingly, the parent may be happy to leave, but if the request to leave is refused the examiner should obtain the assistance of another neutral person to aid in restraining the child, and make the best of it.

The use of another person, in addition to the parent, to restrain the child is often helpful under ordinary circumstances; however, using other kinds of restraints or mummying methods has no place in the physical examination procedure.

The examiner should not convey feelings of frustration or anger, but should reassure the parent that the child's resistance is not unexpected. Embarrassment may cause the parent to compound the problem by scolding the child. Some parents feel that the examiner is at fault when their child is uncooperative while being examined. Others feel that such resistance is a reflection of the child's level of development of independence.

The neophyte examiner is apt to be less successful in examining very young children than in examining older ones. However, with practice, perseverance, and patience, he should succeed. It is difficult to teach "how to approach a reluctant child." Each examiner must learn which techniques work best for him and which approach he finds most comfortable.

LATE CHILDHOOD

There is usually little difficulty in examining most children after they reach school age. Some, however, may have unpleasant memories of previous encounters with examiners and offer resistance.

Question the child to determine his orientation to time and place, his factual knowledge, and his language and number skills. Use intelligence screening tests, such as the Goodenough draw-a-man, the Durrell, and the Bender, when there is some element of doubt concerning the child's intellectual capacity. Keep these tests to a minimum, however, to avoid familiarity-of-content errors should formal psychological testing be necessary. Observe motor skills involved in writing, tying shoelaces, buttoning shirt fronts, and using scissors, and determine right–left discrimination for self (attained at age 6 or 7 years) and for the examiner (attained at age 8 or 9 years).

Modesty on the child's part may be the greatest deterrent to a successful examination. Therefore, girls, as early as age 6 or 7, should be gowned.

Rarely, for the child's sake or the parent's, it is necessary to discontinue the examination before it is completed and return to it another time.

If this resistance is inappropriate for the child's age, then the examiner should consider the possibility of underlying developmental or emotional difficulties.

For both boys and girls, leave underpants on until their removal is required, even if the lower half of the body is draped. It is usually wise for examiners who are of the opposite sex from their preadolescent and adolescent patients to leave the room while the patient disrobes. Younger children often request that siblings of the opposite sex depart, and older boys frequently prefer that their mothers leave during the examination.

The order of examination in late childhood can follow that used with adults. At any age it is important to withhold examination of painful areas until last.

THE GENERAL SURVEY

The rewards of careful and continuous observation have already been discussed, as has the importance of noting general physical and behavioral signs. This section will cover the measurement of vital signs and body size, which is of particular importance in infants and children because deviations from the normal in this regard are apt to be the first and often the only indicators of the presence of disease.

For example, *maternal deprivation, chronic renal disease,* and *hyperthyroidism*

TEMPERATURE

For infants and children younger than 7 years, rectal temperatures should be used almost exclusively, because accurate oral temperature readings are difficult to obtain. For premature infants, axillary temperatures are satisfactory for close monitoring of temperature regulation, although electronic thermometers for continuous temperature recordings are used in neonatal intensive care units. Otherwise, electronic thermometers are rarely used with infants and children because of their expense and fragility.

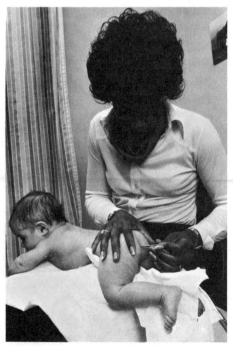

The technique of obtaining the rectal temperature is relatively simple. Place the infant or child in a prone position on the examining table, on his parent's lap, or on your own lap. While you separate the buttocks with the thumb and forefinger of one hand, with the other hand gently insert a well-lubricated rectal thermometer (inclined approximately 20° from the table or lap) through the anal sphincter approximately one inch into the rectum. One method for holding a child while obtaining the rectal temperature is demonstrated in the illustration on the right.

Body temperature in infants and children is less regular than in adults. The average rectal temperature is higher in infancy and early childhood, usually not falling below 99.0°F (37.2°C) until after the third year. At 18 months, 50% of children will have mean rectal temperatures of 100°F (37.8°C) or higher. Ranges in body temperature in individual children may be as much as three or more degrees Fahrenheit during the course of a single day. Rectal temperature recordings may approach 101°F (38.3°C) in normal children, particularly in late afternoon after a full day of activity.

Anxiety may elevate the body temperature, as witnessed by the frequency with which elevated temperatures are found on elective hospital admissions in children.

In the face of overwhelming infection, the temperature in infants may be normal or subnormal. On the other hand, during early childhood, extremely high temperature recordings (103° to 105°F, 39.5° to 40.5°C) are not uncommon, even with minor infections.

PULSE

The heart rate in infants and children is quite labile and more sensitive to the effects of illness, exercise, and emotion than that in adults. The average heart rates for pediatric patients, according to age, are shown in Table 17-2.

Obtain the heart rate in infants by observing the pulsations of the anterior fontanelle, by palpating the carotid or the femoral arteries, or by directly auscultating the heart if the rate is very rapid. Palpate the radial artery at the wrist in older children and in young children who are cooperative.

Beyond the neonatal period, a pulse greater than 180 usually indicates *paroxysmal auricular tachycardia*.

Table 17-2   Average Heart Rate of Infants and Children at Rest

AGE	AVERAGE RATE	TWO-STANDARD DEVIATIONS
Birth	140	50
1st 6 months	130	50
6–12 months	115	40
1–2 years	110	40
2–6 years	103	35
6–10 years	95	30
10–14 years	85	30

RESPIRATORY RATE

As with the heart rate, the respiratory rate in infants and children has a greater range and is more responsive to illness, exercise, and emotion than that in adults. The rate of respirations per minute ranges between 30 and 80 in the newborn, 20 and 40 during early childhood, and 15 and 25 during late childhood, reaching adult levels at age 15 years.

The respiratory rate may vary appreciably from moment to moment in premature and full-term newborn infants, with periods of rapid breathing alternating with spells of apnea. Therefore the respiratory pattern in these circumstances should be observed for more than the usual 30 to 60 seconds to determine the true rate.

In infancy and early childhood, diaphragmatic breathing is predominant and thoracic excursion is minimal; therefore, you can more easily ascertain the respiratory rate by observing abdominal rather than chest excursions. Auscultation of the chest and placement of the stethoscope in front of the mouth and external nares are also useful for counting respirations in this age group. In older children, observe the thoracic movement directly or palpate the thorax to determine the respiratory rate.

BLOOD PRESSURE

The level of systolic blood pressure increases gradually throughout infancy and childhood. Measured in mm Hg, normal systolic pressures are in the vicinity of 50 (mm Hg) at birth, 60 at 1 month, 70 at 6 months, 95 at 1 year, 100 at 6 years, 110 at 10 years, and 120 at 16 years. The values for infants represent pressures obtained by using the flush method (see description following). The diastolic pressure reaches about 60 mm Hg at 1 year of age and gradually increases throughout childhood to approximately 75 mm Hg.

Measurement of the blood pressure in infants and children is omitted more often than not from the physical examination because it has been erroneously judged to be too difficult to obtain from an active child. However, when the procedure is explained and demonstrated beforehand, most children beyond the age of 3 years are fascinated by the sphygmomanometer and are very cooperative.

Variations of blood pressure levels in normal individuals are brought on by exercise, crying, and emotional upset. Because children may be anxious about the entire physical examination procedures as well as the blood pressure procedure *per se*, some clinicians prefer to obtain the blood pres-

Respiratory rates that exceed 100 per minute are seen in diseases associated with lower respiratory tract obstruction (for example, *bronchiolitis* and *bronchial asthma*).

Apnea of greater than 20 seconds duration can occur in both premature infants and seemingly healthy newborns. These infants may be at risk for *Sudden Infant Death Syndrome (SIDS)*.

Anxiety may produce elevated systolic blood pressure readings.

sure near the end of the examination. Others will repeat the determination at the end of the formal examination if the initial pressure was high. For anxious children with elevated blood pressures in examinations repeated over time, a sedative can be prescribed to allay apprehension, since most sedatives have no primary effect on the blood pressure.

Use the sphygmomanometer in determining blood pressures of children as you would in an adult. The width of the cuff should be one half to two thirds the length of the upper arm or leg. The width of the inflatable rubber bag should be approximately 40% of the circumference of the arm, while the bag's length should be approximately twice its width. A narrower cuff will elevate the pressure reading, while a wider cuff will lower it and will interfere with the technique of the procedure by partially covering the brachial artery as it traverses the antecubital space.

With children, unlike adults, the point at which the sounds first become muffled (Phase IV) is recorded as the diastolic pressure. At times, especially in early childhood, the heart sounds are not audible due to a narrow or deeply placed brachial artery; in such instances, palpate the radial artery at the wrist to determine the blood pressure. The point at which the pulse is first felt is recorded as the systolic pressure. This is approximately 10 mm Hg lower than the systolic pressure determined by auscultatory means. The diastolic pressure cannot be determined by using the radial pulse method.

In infants and very young children, smallness of the extremity and lack of cooperation preclude the use of auscultatory and palpation techniques to determine the blood pressure. However, a value lying somewhere between the systolic and diastolic pressures can be obtained by using the *flush technique.*

With the cuff in place, wrap an elastic bandage snugly around the elevated arm, proceeding from the fingers to the antecubital space. This essentially empties the capillary and venous network. Inflate the cuff to a pressure above the expected systolic reading, remove the bandage, and place the pallid arm at the patient's side. Allow the pressure to fall slowly until the sudden flush of normal color returns to the forearm, hand, and fingers. The endpoint is strikingly clear. This method may be used in the leg with equally good results.

For infants and young children, a specific cause of hypertension can usually be determined. In older children and adolescents, however, the etiology may be obscure, and in many instances observed elevated blood pressure may be a developmental phenomenon that disappears over time.

Renal disease (78%), renal arterial disease (12%), *coarctation of the aorta* (2%), and *pheochromocytoma* (0.5%) are the most common causes of hypertension in children.

Children who demonstrate hypertension without apparent cause should be monitored on a long-term basis using percentile charts, as shown below. Patients with blood pressure levels sustained above the 95th percentile should have extensive evaluations performed.

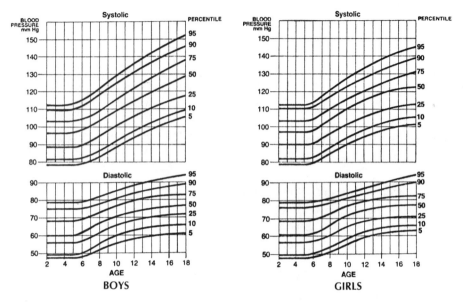

Percentiles of blood pressure measurement in boys and girls (right arm, seated). (Reproduced with permission from the Report of the Task Force on Blood Pressure Control in Children of the National Heart, Lung and Blood Institute. Pediatrics (Suppl) 59:797-820, 1977)

SOMATIC GROWTH

Growth, as reflected in increases in body weight, length, and girth along expected pathways and within certain limits, is probably the best indicator of health. The significance of any measure is determined by relating it to prior measurements of the same dimension, to mean values and standard deviations for that dimension as they occur in other individuals, and to measures of other dimensions in the same patient. Measures of somatic growth in infants and children, therefore, should be plotted on standard growth charts so they can be seen in these relationships.

Height. **Measure the body length of infants by placing them in the supine position on a measuring board or in a measuring tray, as illustrated. If these are not available, determine the length by measuring the distance between marks made on the examining table paper that indicate the crown and the heel of the infant. Direct measurement of the infant with a tape is inaccurate, unless accomplished with an assistant holding the baby still with the legs extended. Measure the height in older children by standing the child with his heels, back, and head against a wall marked with a centimeter or inch rule. Hold a small board flat against the top of the child's head and at right angles to the rule to complete the measure.**

Measurements of height and weight above the 97th percentile or below the 3rd percentile on standard growth charts may indicate a growth disturbance and require investigation.

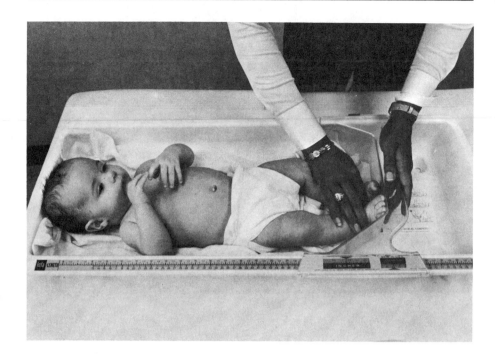

Weighing scales equipped with a height measure are not as satisfactory, since children are not as likely to stand erect when not against a wall; many younger children are also fearful of standing on the scale's slightly raised, unsteady base.

Weight. **Weigh infants directly with an infant scale, rather than indirectly by holding them and subtracting your weight from the total weight registered. Remove all clothing, except for underpants in children beyond infancy and dressing gowns provided for girls in late childhood. Use balance rather than spring scales, and whenever possible weigh the child on the same scale at each visit.**

Head Circumference. The head circumference should be determined at every physical examination during the first 2 years of life, at least biennially thereafter, and at any initial examination at whatever age, to determine the rate of growth and absolute growth of the head.

A cloth or soft plastic centimeter tape is preferred for this procedure, but disposable paper tapes are satisfactory.

Place the tape over the occipital, parietal, and frontal prominences to obtain the greatest circumference. During infancy and early childhood, this is best done with the patient supine.

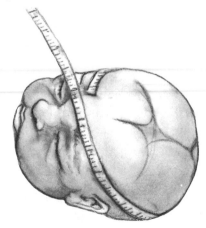

The measurement of the head circumference reflects the rate of growth of the cranium and its contents.

If growth is delayed, *premature closure of the sutures* or *microcephaly* should be considered. When growth is too rapid, *hydrocephalus, subdural hematoma,* or *brain tumor* should be suspected.

Chest Circumference. This measure is obtained with the patient supine.

Pass the tape around the thorax at the level of the nipples and take the measurement midway between inspiration and expiration.

The chest circumference and the abdominal circumference (obtained similarly with the tape at the level of the umbilicus) are often referred to in pediatric circles, but in fact are of little value. The chest circumference, however, is sometimes used as a comparative measure for head size, in that the circumference of the head is supposed to exceed that of the chest until age 2 years and be smaller than the circumference of the chest thereafter.

THE SKIN

INFANCY

The skin of the newborn infant has many unique characteristics. The texture is soft and smooth. An erythematous flush, giving the entire surface of the skin the appearance of a "boiled lobster," is present during the first 8 to 24 hours, after which the normal pale pink coloring predominates. Vasomotor changes in the subcutaneous tissue—a response to cooling or chronic exposure to radiant heat—produce a mottled appearance *(cutis marmorata),* particularly on the trunk, arms, and legs. In normal newborns, a striking color change is often seen: one side of the body is red, the other pale, and an abrupt border separates the two sides at the midline. This phenomenon *(harlequin dyschronica)* is transient and of unknown etiology. Blueness of the hands and feet *(acrocyanosis)* is present at birth and may remain for several days. It may recur throughout early infancy under chilling conditions. After 4 or 5 hours the cyanosis in the hands becomes less marked than in the feet.

Generalized pallor indicates either anoxia, in which case the pulse will be slowed, or severe anemia, in which case the pulse will be very rapid.

This marbled, or dappled, reticular pattern is especially prominent in premature infants and *cretins* and in infants with *Down's syndrome.*

If acrocyanosis does not disappear within 8 hours, cyanotic congenital heart disease should be considered.

Melanotic pigmentation of the skin is not intense in most black newborns, with the exception of the nailbeds and the skin of the scrotum. Ill-defined blackish blue areas located over the buttocks and lower lumbar regions are often seen, especially in black, Native American, and oriental babies. These areas, called *Mongolian spots,* are due to the presence of pigmented cells in the deeper layers of the skin. The spots become less noticeable as the pigment in the overlying cells becomes more prominent, and they eventually disappear in early childhood.

There is a fine, downy growth of hair called *lanugo* over the entire body, but mostly on the shoulders and back. The amount and length vary from baby to baby, being unusually prominent in prematures. Most of this hair is shed within 2 weeks. The amount of hair on the head of a newborn varies considerably, being absent entirely in some and abundant in others. All of the original hair is shed within a few months and replaced with a new crop, sometimes of a different color.

Desquamation of the skin may be present normally at birth, varying in degree from a scattered flakiness to complete shedding of entire areas in large sheets of cornified epidermis. Also, a cheesy white material, composed of sebum and desquamated epithelial cells and called *vernix caseosa*, covers the body in varying degrees at birth. It is always present in the vaginal labial folds and under the fingernails. A certain amount of puffiness and edema, even to the point of pitting over the hands, feet, lower legs, pubis, and sacrum, may be present normally, but usually disappears by the second or third day.

Normal "physiologic" jaundice, which occurs in approximately 50% of all babies, appears on the second or third day and usually disappears within a week, but may persist for as long as a month.

In general, jaundice which appears within 24 hours of birth should alert one to the possible presence of hemolytic disease, and jaundice which appears or persists beyond 2 weeks of age should raise suspicions of biliary obstruction. Jaundice may indicate severe infection at any time in infancy, particularly in the newborn period.

Use natural daylight rather than artificial light when evaluating for the presence of jaundice at any age. In borderline cases, press a glass slide against the infant's cheek. This will help you detect the presence of jaundice by producing a blanched background for contrast.

Older infants who are fed yellow vegetables (carrots, sweet potatoes, and squash) may develop a pale, yellow orange color to the skin, which is sometimes mistaken for jaundice. However, the pigmentation in this condition, called *carotenemia*, is limited to the palms, soles, nose, and nasolabial folds.

Three dermatologic conditions are seen in newborns with enough frequency to deserve description. None is of clinical significance. *Milia*, pinhead-sized, smooth, white, raised areas without surrounding erythema, on the nose, chin and forehead, are caused by retention of sebum in the openings of the sebaceous glands. These areas may be present at birth, but more often appear within the first few weeks of life and disappear spontaneously over the course of several weeks. *Miliaria rubra* consists of scattered vesicles on an erythematous base, usually on the face and trunk, caused by obstruction of the ducts of the sweat glands. *Erythema toxicum*, which usually appears on the second or third day of life, consists of erythematous macules with central urticarial wheals or vesicles scattered diffusely over the entire body, appearing much like flea bites. Eosinophiles may be seen on smear of the vesicular fluid. The cause is unknown and the lesions disappear spontaneously within a week.

Irregular, reddened areas are frequently found over the nape of the neck ("stork's beak" mark) and on the upper eyelids, the forehead, and the upper lip ("angel kisses"). The redness is due to proliferation of the capillary bed of the skin. These lesions are variously called *capillary hemangioma*, *nevus flammeus*, *nevus vasculosus*, and *telangiectatic nevus*. They invariably disappear at about a year of age, although they may occasionally reappear, even in adulthood, when the skin flushes in anger or embarrassment. When these lesions appear on other areas of the skin, they are larger, darker (purplish), more sharply demarcated, and may involve the mucosa of the mouth or vagina. These "port-wine stains" are not likely to fade.

When a port-wine stain affects the skin innervated by the ophthalmic portion of the trigeminal nerve, the vascular network of the meninges and ocular orbit may also be affected, this can result in epicortical or meningeal calcifications, seizures, hemiparesis, mental retardation, and glaucoma—the *Sturge–Weber syndrome.*

The ridges on the palms of the hands formed by the raised apertures of the sweat glands create patterns called *dermatoglyphics*. These are often helpful in diagnosing certain chromosomal defects. Finger and hand prints are usually used to study dermatoglyphic patterns.

Characteristic patterns may be found in patients with *leukemia* and *schizophrenia.*

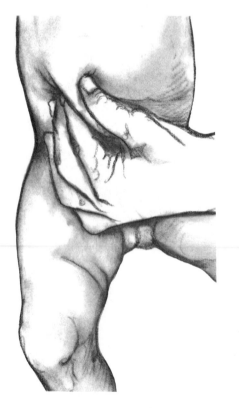

The examination of the skin should go beyond observation and include palpation.

Roll a fold of loosely adherent skin on the abdominal wall between your thumb and forefinger to determine its consistency, the amount of subcutaneous tissue present, and the degree of hydration.

The skin in well-hydrated infants and children will return to its normal position immediately upon release.

Delay in return, a phenomenon called tenting, usually occurs in dehydrated patients.

EARLY AND LATE CHILDHOOD

The skin in the normal child beyond the first year does not present any variations worthy of note. The techniques of examination and the general classification of pathologic lesions for this age are as with the adult.

THE HEAD AND NECK

INFANCY

The *head* accounts for one fourth of body length and one third of body weight at birth, whereas at full maturity it only accounts for one eighth of body length and, for most, one tenth of body weight. The bones of the skull are separated from one another by membranous tissue spaces called *sutures*. The areas where the major sutures intersect in the anterior and posterior portions of the skull are known as *fontanelles*. The sutures and fontanelles, shown in this figure, form the basis for much of the physical assessment of the head in infancy.

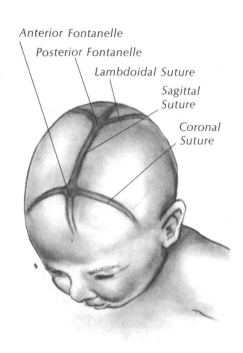

Anterior Fontanelle
Posterior Fontanelle
Lambdoidal Suture
Sagittal Suture
Coronal Suture

The sutures can be felt as slightly depressed ridges, and the fontanelles as soft concavities. The anterior fontanelle measures 4 cm to 6 cm in its largest diameter at birth, and normally closes between 4 and 26 months; 90% close between 7 and 19 months of age. The posterior fontanelle measures 1 cm to 2 cm at birth, and usually closes by 2 months of age. The intracranial pressure is reflected in the amount of tenseness and fullness seen and felt in the anterior fontanelle. Increased intracranial pressure produces a bulging, full anterior fontanelle. This is normally seen when a baby cries, coughs, or vomits. Pulsations of the fontanelle reflect the peripheral pulse.

For best results, examine the anterior fontanelle for tenseness and fullness while the baby is quietly sitting or being held in an upright position.

The degree to which the anterior fontanelle is held to be an indicator of intracranial pressure and a barometer of serious central nervous system illness can be appreciated by noting that seasoned clinicians palpate the anterior fontanelle before proceeding with any other part of the physical examination on an acutely ill baby.

Increased intracranial pressure is found in infectious and neoplastic diseases of the central nervous system, and with obstruction to the ventricular circulation. Decreased intracranial pressure, reflected in a depressed fontanelle, is a sign of dehydration in infants.

Dilated scalp veins are indicative of long-standing increased intracranial pressure.

The cranial bones of the newly born infant may overlap at the sutures to a certain degree. This phenomenon, called *molding*, results from passage of the head through the birth canal, and disappears within 2 days. It is not seen in babies born by cesarian section.

Newborn babies often have a soft swelling with edema and bruising of the scalp over a portion of the occipitoparietal region. This is the *caput succedaneum*, which is caused by that presenting portion of the scalp being drawn into the cervical os at the time the amniotic sac ruptures. The negative pressure or vacuum effect caused by the loss of amniotic fluid produces distention of capillaries with extravasation of blood and fluid locally. These findings subside within the first 24 hours of life.

A second type of localized swelling involving the scalp, the *cephalohematoma*, is seen with reasonable frequency in the newborn infant (see Table 17-3, p. 468).

In examining the infant's head, ascertain the shape and symmetry of the skull and face.

Asymmetry of the cranial vault *(plagiocephaly)* will occur when an infant sleeps constantly on one side when in the supine position. Such positioning results in a flattening of the occiput on the dependent side and a prominence of the frontal region on the opposite side. It disappears as the baby becomes more active and spends less time in one position. In almost all instances, symmetry is restored when the position of the head becomes less constant. *In utero* positioning may result in transient facial asymmetries. If the head is flexed on the sternum, this may produce a shortened chin *(micrognathia)*; pressure of the shoulder on the jaw may create a temporary lateral displacement of the mandible.

Plagiocephaly is apt to be more prominent in infants with *torticollis* secondary to injury to the sternomastoid muscle at birth, in the mentally and physically handicapped, and in understimulated infants secondary to maternal neglect.

The head of the premature infant at birth is relatively long in the occipitofrontal diameter and narrow in the bitemporal diameter. This relationship continues for most of the first year of life. An abnormally large head *(hydrocephaly* or *megacephaly)* and an abnormally small head *(microcephaly)* should be recognized easily in classical presentation, but either condition will initially require frequent observation, including measurements, for early diagnosis and treatment (see Table 17-3, p. 468).

The shape of the head may be altered by premature closure of one or more of the cranial sutures *(craniosynostosis)*. The nature of the resultant deformity of the skull depends on the sutures involved. Although palpation of affected sutures may reveal a raised bony ridge in the final stages, early diagnosis is made by roentgenographic means.

If, in palpating the skull of the newborn, you press your thumb or forefinger firmly over the temporo parietal or parieto–occipital areas, you may feel the underlying bone give momentarily, much as a ping-pong ball would respond to similar pressure.

This condition, known as *craniotabes,* is due to osteoporosis of the outer table of the involved membranous bone. It may be found in some normal infants.

Craniotabes may result from increased intracranial pressure, as in *hydrocephaly,* from metabolic disturbances such as *rickets,* and from infection such as *congenital syphilis.*

Percuss the head by tapping your index or middle finger directly against its surface. Percussion over the parietal bone in this manner will produce a cracked-pot sound prior to closure of the sutures. In the normal newborn, similar direct percussion at the top of the cheek just below the zygomatic bone will produce contraction of the facial muscle in the immediate area *(Chvostek's sign).*

This sign may persist through infancy and early childhood in some.

Chvostek's sign is often present in hypocalcemic and hyperventilation *tetany* and in *tetanus.* It is obviously of no use in the diagnosis of neonatal tetany.

Transillumination of the skull is a useful procedure and should be part of every initial examination of an infant.

In a completely darkened room, place a standard, 3-battery flashlight, with a soft rubber collar attached to the lighted end, flush against the skull at various points (see Table 17-3, p. 468). In normal infants, a 2 cm halo of light is present around the circumference of the flashlight when it is placed over the frontoparietal area, and a 1 cm halo is present when the flashlight is placed over the occipital area.

Uniform transillumination of the entire head occurs when the cerebral cortex is partially absent or thinned. Localized bright spots may be seen with *subdural effusion* and *porencephalic cysts.*

Routine auscultation of the skull to detect the presence of a *bruit* is of little use until a child reaches late childhood, since a systolic or continuous bruit may be heard over the temporal areas in normal children until the age of 5. Similar findings may be found in older children who have a significant anemia.

Bruits heard in nonanemic older children suggest increased intracranial pressure or an intracranial arteriovenous shunt or aneurysm.

The *neck* of the newborn is relatively short.

While the infant is in the supine position, palpate the neck with your thumb and forefinger, feeling for masses, lymph nodes, cysts, and the position of the thyroid cartilage and the trachea. Move the head through its full range of motion at the neck (extension, forward and lateral flexion, and rotation 90° to the left and right).

A *thyroglossal duct fistula* or *cyst* may be seen or felt in the midline immediately superior to the thyroid cartilage. Thyroglossal duct cysts are rarely found at birth, but may appear in early infancy. They are usually small, rounded, and firm, and can be differentiated from midline subcutaneous lesions in that they move with swallowing.

Table 17-3

Table 17-3   Abnormal Enlargement of the Head in Infancy

CEPHALOHEMATOMA

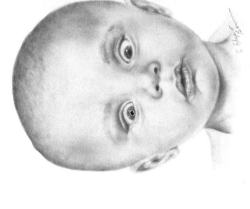

HYDROCEPHALY

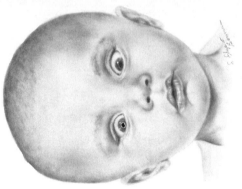

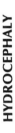

Although not present at birth, cephalohematomas appear within the first 24 hours and are due to subperiosteal hemorrhage involving the outer table of one of the cranial bones. The swelling (see illustration above, which shows a cephalohematoma overlying the left parietal bone), unlike the *caput succedaneum* and hematomas associated with skull fractures, does not extend across a suture. It may be small and well localized or may involve the entire bone. Occasionally bilateral, symmetrical swellings occur after difficult deliveries. Although initially soft, the swellings develop a raised bony margin within 2 to 3 days, due to the rapid deposition of calcium at the edges of the elevated periosteum. The entire process usually disappears within a few weeks, but may remain as a residual osteoma which is not resorbed for a year or two.

In hydrocephaly the eyes are deviated downward, revealing the upper sclerae and creating the *"setting sun" sign* as shown in the figure above. The setting sun sign is also seen briefly in some normal newborns. (Redrawn from Paine RS: Neurological examination of infants and children. Pediatr Clin North Am 7:476, 1960)

Transillumination of the skull in advanced cases of hydrocephaly produces a glow of light over the entire cranium, as illustrated above.

Table 17-4

Table 17-4 Diagnostic Facies in Childhood

DOWN'S SYNDROME	CRETINISM	BATTERED-CHILD SYNDROME	PERENNIAL ALLERGIC RHINITIS
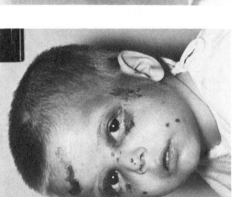 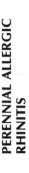	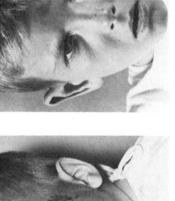	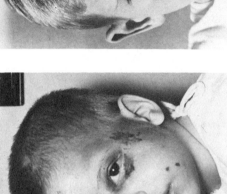	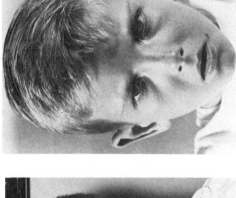

The child with Down's syndrome (Trisomy 21) usually has a small, rounded head, a flattened nasal bridge, oblique palpebral fissures, prominent epicanthal folds, small, low-set, shell-like ears, and a relatively large tongue. (A black and white print of a color photograph, reproduced with permission from Dynski–Klein M: Color Atlas of Pediatrics, p 309. London, Year Book Medical Publishers/Wolfe Medical Publications, 1975)

The child with cretinism (congenital hyperthyroidism) has coarse facial features, a low-set hair line, sparse eyebrows, and an enlarged tongue. (A black-and-white print of a color photograph, reproduced with permission from Gellis S, Feingold M: Syndromes in Pediatrics, Part I. In Famous Teachings in Modern Medicine. Medcom, Inc, 1969)

The child who has been physically abused (battered) usually has old and fresh bruises about the head and face as well as a sad, forlorn facial expression.

The child suffering from perennial allergic rhinitis has an open mouth (cannot breath through his nose), and edema and discoloration of the lower orbitopalpebral grooves ("allergic shiners"). Such a child is often seen to push his nose upward and backward with his hand ("allergic salute") and to use facial grimaces (wrinkling of the nose and mouth) to relieve nasal itching and obstruction. (Illustration reproduced with permission from Marks MB: Allergic shiners: Dark circles under the eyes in children. Clin Pediatr 5:656, 1966)

The neck is supple and easily mobile in all directions throughout infancy. Its musculature is not sufficiently developed to enable the infant to turn his head from side to side until 2 weeks of age, to lift his head 90° when lying in a prone position until 2 months of age, or to hold his head upright when placed in a sitting position until 3 months of age.

Remnants of the three lower branchial clefts may be seen as skin tags, cysts, or fistulae along the anterior border of the sternomastoid muscle.

The neck may retain its mobility in infants, even at times when meningeal irritation, as with meningitis, is present.

Injury to the sternomastoid muscle with bleeding into the muscle belly as it is stretched during the birth process results in wry neck (*torticollis*). The head is tilted and twisted toward the injured side, and in 2 or 3 weeks a firm fibrous mass may be felt within the muscle.

EARLY AND LATE CHILDHOOD

Beyond infancy the examination of the head and neck, except as previously mentioned, should follow the procedures used in examining the adult. There are diagnostic facies in childhood that reflect chromosomal abnormalities, endocrine defects, social disease, chronic illness, and other categories of disease (see Table 17-4, p. 469, for examples).

Swelling of the parotid gland may be difficult to detect during the early stages of *mumps*. Mumps should be strongly suspected if tenderness over the parotid gland is detected.

With your index finger, palpate along a line extending from the outer canthus of the eye to the lower tip of the pinna. Tenderness will be elicited when mumps is present.

Inspect the orifice of the parotid (Stenson's) duct, which emerges from the midportion of the buccal mucosa, for redness and swelling, which are usually present with mumps.

Parotid gland swelling, from any cause, extends above and below the mandible at the angle of the jaw, while the swelling due to *cervical adenitis* occurs only below these landmarks.

Neck mobility is an important determinant in considering central nervous system diseases, especially meningitis, because they may cause the neck to be less supple than normal.

With the child in the supine position, cradle his head in your hands so that you provide its complete support. Move the head gently in all directions to determine the presence of any resistance to motion, especially to flexion.

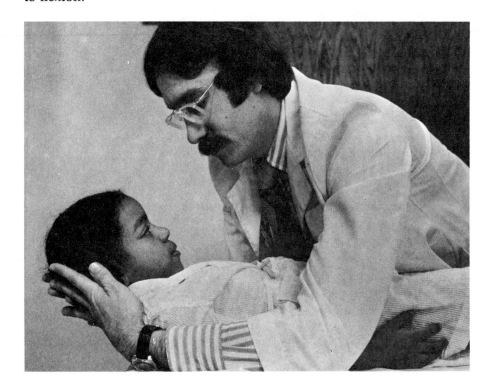

In infancy and early childhood, this is a more reliable test for nuchal rigidity and meningeal irritation than *Brudzinski's sign* or *Kernig's sign* (see p. 408).

To detect nuchal rigidity in early and late childhood, ask the child to sit with his legs extended on the examining table. Normally he should be able to sit upright and voluntarily touch his chin to his chest. Younger children may be persuaded to flex their necks forward by getting them to look at a small toy or a light beam placed on their upper sternum.

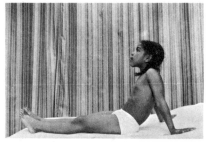

When meningeal irritation is present, the child assumes the *tripod position* and is unable to assume a full upright position to perform the chin-to-chest maneuver.

THE EYE

INFANCY

It is somewhat difficult to examine the eyes of the newborn because the lids are ordinarily held tightly closed. Attempts at separating the lids usually increase the contraction of the orbicularis oculi muscles. Since bright light causes the infant to blink his eyes, the newborn's eyes should be examined in subdued lighting.

Hold the baby upright in your extended arms, fixing the head in the midline with your thumbs as illustrated below. Rotate slowly in one direction. This usually causes the eyes to open, providing a clear view of the sclerae, pupils, irides, and extraocular movements. The eyes will look in the direction you are turning. When the rotation stops, the eyes look in the opposite direction, following a few unsustained nystagmoid movements.

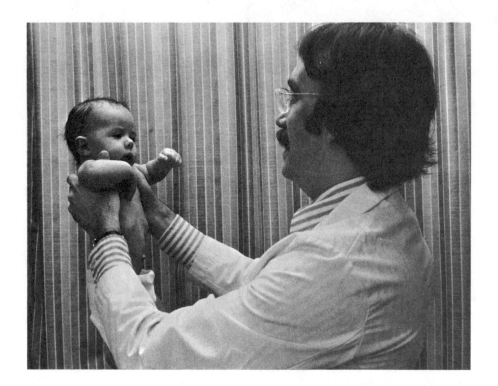

Conjugate eye movements develop rapidly after birth, but definitive following movements are not seen for a few weeks. Searching nystagmus is common immediately after birth. During the first 10 days of life, the eyes do not move but remain fixed, staring in one direction, as the head is slowly moved through the full range of motion (*doll's eye test*). Intermittent alternating convergent strabismus is frequently seen or reported by parents during the first 6 months of life. Should it persist beyond that time or become unilateral sooner, of if divergent strabismus is observed at any time, the baby should be referred to an ophthalmologist.

Nystagmus present after a few days may be indicative of blindness.

Small subconjunctival, scleral, and retinal hemorrhages are common in newborns. Because the pupillary reactivity to light is poor during the first 4 to 5 months, reactions are best observed by first shading one eye and then uncovering it. The *optical blink reflex*, wherein the infant blinks his eyes and dorsiflexes his head in response to a bright light, is normally

If retinal hemorrhages are extensive, severe anoxia or *subdural hematoma* should be suspected.

present in all newborns and may be used to test light perception. In-equality of the size of the pupils in both bright and subdued light is not uncommon, but should be considered significant if it is constant over time and associated with other ocular or central nervous system findings. In all babies the corneal reflex is present at birth.

The irides should be inspected for the presence of a cleft (*coloboma*) and for *Brushfield's spots*. The latter appear as white specks scattered in a linear fashion, usually around the entire circumference of the iris; although present in some normal infants, they strongly suggest *Down's syndrome*. The presence of prominent inner epicanthal folds along with an upward outer slant to the eyelids is also suggestive of this malady. Chemical conjunctivitis, due to instillation of silver nitrate into the eyes at birth as a prophylaxis against gonorrheal conjunctivitis (*ophthalmia neonatorum*), occurs frequently in normal infants and is characterized by edema of the lids and inflammation of the conjunctivae with a purulent discharge.

Dacryocystitis and *nasolacrimal duct obstruction* with ocular discharge and tearing may follow chemical conjunctivitis due to silver nitrate instillation.

Demonstrate the red retinal (or fundus) reflex by setting the ophthalmoscope at "0" diopters and viewing the pupil at a distance of approximately 10 inches. Normally a red or orange color is reflected from the fundus through the pupil.

A *funduscopic examination* should be performed on all infants. Normally the examination can be postponed until between 2 and 6 months of age, when the infant is most cooperative, unless the ocular or neurologic examination indicates that it be done immediately.

Instill a mydriatic (10% phenylephrine with 1% mydriacyl—2 drops in each eye every 15 minutes over a 45-min period) for proper visualization. Place the baby in a supine position on the examining table or on the parent's lap, or have the parent hold him upright over the shoulder. If the baby needs calming, use a sugar nipple. Lid retraction can be accomplished, if necessary, with your thumb and first finger. The method of funduscopic examination is otherwise the same as with adults. The cornea can ordinarily be seen at +20 diopters, the lens at +15 diopters, and the fundus at "0" diopters.

Both retinal anomalies and opacities of the cornea, anterior chamber, or lens will interrupt the light pathway and give a partial red reflex or a completely dark reflex. In infants, *cataracts*, a *persistent posterior lenticular fibrovascular sheath*, and *retrolental fibroplasia* may cause a dark light reflex. Beyond infancy, *retinal detachment*, *chorioretinitis*, and *retinoblastoma* should be suspected when an abnormal retinal reflex is encountered.

The optic disc is paler in infants, the peripheral vessels are not well developed, and the foveal light reflection is absent. *Papilledema* is rarely seen, even with markedly increased intracranial pressure, because the fontanelles and open sutures absorb the increased pressure. Until age 3 years the sutures will separate sufficiently to prevent papilledema. If vascular or optic disc anomalies are found, the parents' fundi should be examined to determine a possible genetic origin and prognosis for the findings.

Retinal hemorrhages associated with intracranial bleeding are accompanied by dilated, congested, tortuous retinal veins.

The development of central vision progresses from birth, when only light perception is thought to be present, to adult visual levels attained at approximately 6 years of age.

The assessment of vision in the newborn is based on the presence of visual reflexes—direct and consensual pupillary constriction in response to light, and blinking in response to bright light and to an object moved quickly toward the eyes.

Those visual reflexes imply that both light perception and some degree of visual acuity are present shortly after birth. Opticokinetic nystagmus (produced by the rapid movement of vertical black lines across the visual fields), used as a test of vision on one group of newborns $1\frac{1}{2}$ to 5 days after birth, demonstrated a visual acuity of at least 20/670 in 93% of the group. That this acuity improves is evident even without refractive measurement references. At 2 to 4 weeks of age, fixation on objects occurs; at 5 to 6 weeks, coordinated eye movements in following an object are seen; at 3 months the eyes converge and the baby begins to reach for various sized objects at various distances as eye–hand coordination and the ability to focus are accomplished. At the age of 1 year, normal visual acuity is in the range of 20/200.

Failure to progress along these lines may indicate mental deficiency as well as diminished or absent vision.

EARLY CHILDHOOD

When examining a child in this age group, the most important condition the examiner must detect is *amblyopia exanopsia*. This is not the most serious ophthalmologic disease, but in comparison with others of significance it is the most prevalent and offers, with early intervention, the best prognosis. Improvement in this condition is unlikely if treatment is instituted after the sixth year of life. Amblyopia means reduced vision in an otherwise normal eye, and the reduced vision in this situation is caused by disuse. In essence, because of disconjugate fixation, one of the two images received by the optic cortex is suppressed to avoid diplopia or images of unequal clarity. One eye then becomes "lazy" and stops functioning to its full capacity; visual acuity in that eye is reduced markedly by suppression of central (foveal) vision. Since the two most common causes of amblyopia exanopsia are *strabismus* and *anisometropia* (an eye with a refractive error 1.5 diopters or more greater than its pair), it is important to be able to test for muscle weakness and visual acuity accurately.

Obstructive amblyopia is secondary to a *cataract, corneal opacity*, or severe *ptosis*.

Muscle weakness causing deviation of one eye inwardly (*esotropia*) or outwardly (*exotropia*) may be detected by the *Hirschberg test*, the *prism test*, or the *cover test*.

The *Hirschberg test* requires the reflection of a light on the cornea of each eye. Attract the patient's attention to a light held at your midforehead. While the patient's eyes are fixed upon the light, note the light's reflection on each cornea. First, hold the patient's head fixed in the midline and then turn it to the left and right while fixation is maintained.

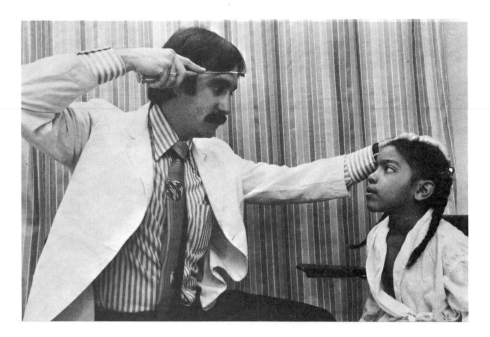

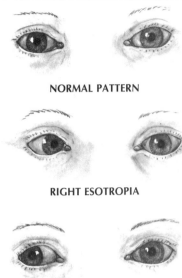

NORMAL PATTERN

RIGHT ESOTROPIA

RIGHT EXOTROPIA

Look for a change in the corneal reflection pattern of lateral gaze. The reflections on each cornea should be symmetrically placed; thus, the type and degree of tropia can be determined by noting the pattern of asymmetrical placement of the reflections. The normal pattern and those with esotropia and exotropia are shown to the right.

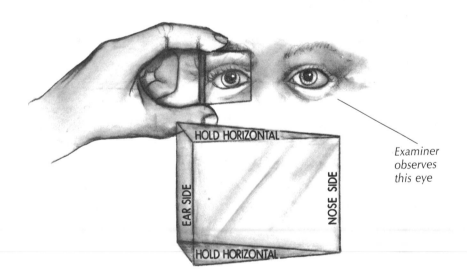

HOLD HORIZONTAL

EAR SIDE

NOSE SIDE

HOLD HORIZONTAL

Examiner observes this eye

The *prism test* is conducted in much the same way as the Hirschberg test.

Again, attract the patient's attention to a light held at your midforehead. While the patient's eyes are fixed upon the light, hold a 4-diopter prism,

base out, in front of one eye while observing the other eye. If the observed eye moves inward or outward and remains in whichever position it has moved, strabismus is present. The opposite eye is tested in the same way. An amblyopic (lazy) eye will not move when the prism is placed in front of it.

The *cover test* is the most sophisticated of the three tests for strabismus because it detects frank strabismus, differentiates the type of deviation, and determines the characteristics of any latent deviation.

Attract the patient's attention once more to the midforehead light. Place your hand on the top of the child's head and your thumb in front of one eye while observing the other for movement. Then remove your thumb and observe both eyes for movement. If either or both eyes move, a strabismus is present. Repeat the test, covering and uncovering the other eye with your thumb.

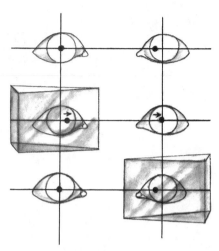

PRISM TEST IN LEFT ESOTROPIA

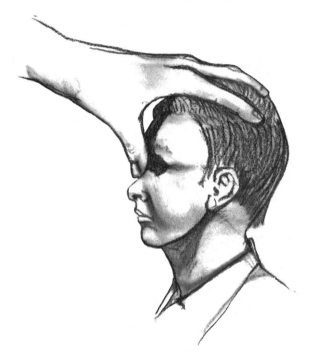

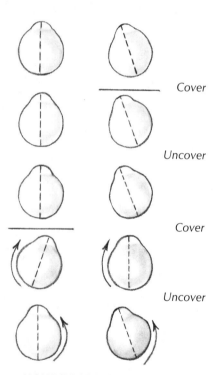

Cover

Uncover

Cover

Uncover

MONOCULAR RIGHT ESOTROPIA

The combination of movements observed allows for differential diagnosis of the strabismus in question. The results of using the cover test, or what is more properly called the cover–uncover test, in monocular right esotropia are shown at the right.

Testing visual acuity in early childhood is not a simple matter. The variables of the child, the examiner, the testing environment, and the test itself all contribute significantly to the outcome and should be given careful attention if valid results are to be obtained. Unfortunately, there is no testing method that accurately measures visual acuity in children under the age of 3 years. Since each eye must be tested separately to detect amblyopia, one eye must be covered by an elastoplast bandage to ensure complete occlusion. Resistance to placement of the patch may be overcome by calling it a "pirate's patch." A child with amblyopia might accept the patch on the amblyopic eye, but not on the good eye.

Opticokinetic testing is the most accurate method for testing visual acuity in this age group; however, this method requires too much technical equipment to use in most settings. Two other simpler *tests of visual acuity* are, however, of some worth.

The *miniature toy test* uses identical sets of small toys representing familiar objects. Give the child one set and keep the other. Ask the child to match each toy as it is shown to him at a distance of 10 feet. *Worth's test* uses five balls ranging from $\frac{1}{2}$ to $1\frac{1}{2}$ inches in diameter. Beginning with the largest, throw each on the floor and ask the child to retrieve it. These tests, at best, detect only grossly impaired vision rather than the degree of such impairment.

In children over the age of 3 years, the *Snellen E chart* (a form of direct visual testing) is very adequate. Most youngsters will cooperate in indicating, either orally or by positioning of the fingers, in which direction the E is pointing. For those who initially have difficulty with this test, a single E card can be sent home with the child for practice purposes. Charts with pictures instead of Es are often used but have no special advantage, nor do any other testing methods generally available. The normal visual acuity at age 3 years is ±20/40, at age 4 to 5 years, ±20/30, and at 6 to 7 years, 20/20.

Visual field examination in infants and young children can be done with the child sitting on the parent's lap.

Hold the head in the midline while bringing a dangling object, such as a measuring tape case or a small toy, into the child's field of vision from several points behind, above, and below him. Deviation of the eyes in its direction indicates that the child has seen the object.

LATE CHILDHOOD

The eye problems and methods of examining the eye for this age group have been covered in the adult section. In general, vision testing machines used for mass screening in schools tend to underrate visual acuity and produce over-referrals.

You can distinguish a simple refractive error from organic causes of diminished vision by asking the child to take his vision test looking through a pinhole punched in a card. Visual acuity improves using the pinhole card when refractive errors are present, but not when organic ocular disease exists.

THE EAR

INFANCY

Note the position of the ears in relation to the eyes. Normally the ear joins the scalp on or above the extension of a line drawn across the inner and outer canthus of the eye.

Small, deformed, or low-set auricles may indicate associated congenital defects, especially renal agenesis or anomalies.

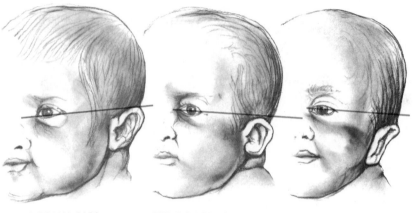

NORMAL EARS   PSEUDO LOW-SET EARS   TRUE LOW-SET EARS

Examination of the ear in the immediate neonatal period establishes the patency of the external auditory canal only, because the tympanic membranes are obscured by accumulated vernix caseosa for the first 2 or 3 days of life. In infancy the external auditory canal is directed downward from the outside; therefore, the pinna should be pulled gently downward for the best visualization of the ear drum. The light reflex on the tympanic membrane is diffuse and does not assume the cone shape for several months.

Inspect the ear and surrounding skin. Test the hearing in infants by observing a blinking of the eyes in response to a sudden sharp sound, which should be produced at a distance of 12 inches from the ear by snapping the fingers, clapping the hands, or using a bell or other kinds of mechanical noise-making devices. Be sure that in generating the sound you do not produce an airstream that could evoke the blink reflex.

A small skin tab, cleft, or pit is frequently found just forward of the tragus and represents a remnant of the first branchial cleft.

The *acoustic blink reflex* is difficult to elicit during the first 2 or 3 days of life, and may disappear temporarily after it is elicited a few times. This is a crude test at best, and the absence of blinking in response to sound is not diagnostic of deafness nor does its presence assure normal hearing. At 2 weeks of age, the infant may jump in response to a sudden noise; at 10 weeks he may respond by momentary cessation of body movements. Between 3 and 4 months of age, the eyes and head will turn toward the source of sound. Even before this, an increase in respiratory rate may occur when familiar sounds are heard.

Because the parents' impression of the baby's auditory acuity is usually correct, when parents believe that their baby cannot hear it should be assumed that he cannot hear until proven otherwise.

EARLY CHILDHOOD

The examination of the ear becomes more difficult as the child grows older. Greater resistance is encountered because the ear canals are sensitive and the child cannot observe the procedure.

Often it is helpful if you initially place the otoscopic speculum gently into the external auditory canal of one ear, removing it instantly and repeating the procedure on the other. Then you can begin again, taking the necessary time in the actual examination with a child whose apprehensions have been allayed.

The ears can be successfully examined even in a struggling child if care is taken in restraining him and in manipulating both ear and otoscope gently.

Place the patient in the supine position. Ask the parent or an assistant to hold his arms extended, close to the sides of his head, thus limiting movement from side to side. Approach the child from the right side and lean across his lower chest and upper abdomen to restrict movements of the trunk. A third person may be required to hold the feet and legs if the child struggles unduly; however, this is rarely necessary.

This same restraining procedure may be used in examining the eyes, nose, and throat, as illustrated below.

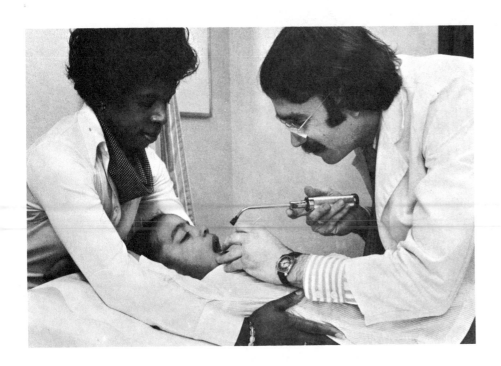

When examining the right ear, turn the child's head to the left and hold it firmly in this position by the lateral aspect of your right hand. Hold the otoscope in your right hand in an inverted position and manipulate the auricle with your left hand. In this age group, the external auditory canal is directed upward and backward from the outside, and the pinna must be pulled upward and backward to afford the best visualization. The thumb and forefinger of your right hand, which holds the otoscope, should be buffered from sudden movements of the child's head by your restraining right hand and your forearm, which rests firmly on the examining table. See the illustration below.

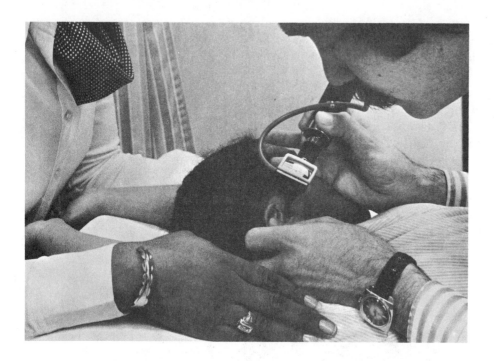

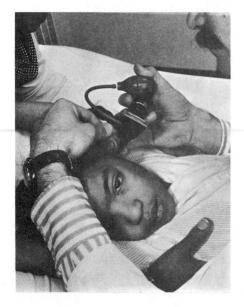

When examining the left ear, turn the patient's head to the right and hold it firmly in this position by the lateral aspect of your left hand and wrist. The thumb and forefinger of your left hand should manipulate the auricle, and your right hand should hold the otoscope in an inverted position. The lateral aspect of the fifth finger of your right hand is held against the patient's head to provide a buffer against sudden movement by the patient. This procedure is demonstrated in this figure.

The speculum of the otoscope should be as large in diameter as will allow for comfortable $\frac{1}{4}$ to $\frac{1}{2}$ inch penetration into the external auditory canal. This provides maximum visualization of the canal and drum and a reasonable seal to observe the effects of pneumatic otoscopy. Some examiners attach a rubber tip to the end of the speculum to gain a tighter, more comfortable seal.

Pneumatic otoscopy is accomplished by observing the tympanic membrane as the pressure in the external auditory canal is increased or decreased. You can do this by introducing and removing air from the canal—by applying positive and negative pressures with a rubber squeeze bulb (as shown in the figure here and the second figure on p. 480), or by blowing and sucking on a rubber tube attached to the otoscope (shown in the first figure on p. 480).

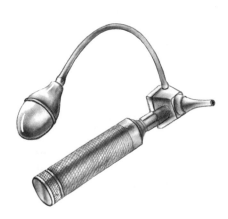

When air is introduced into the normal ear canal, the tympanic membrane and its light reflex are seen to move inward. When air is removed, the tympanic membrane moves outward, toward the examiner. This to and fro movement of the tympanic membrane has been likened to the luffing of a sail.

This movement is absent in chronic middle ear infection (*serous otitis media*), and diminished in some cases of *acute otitis media.*

Cerumen accumulation within the ear canal commonly obscures the view of the tympanic membrane in children. Very often this is unilateral. There are several instruments and ear washing techniques that may be used to remove ear wax comfortably, but they will not be described here.

Accumulation of purulent material and debris in the ear canal is found both in *otitis externa* and in *otitis media* with a ruptured tympanic membrane. Washing out the ear canal is contraindicated, in the first instance because of the pain incurred by the procedure, and in the second instance because the cleansing fluid and canal debris will be forced into the middle ear through the perforated tympanic membrane.

Otitis media and *otitis externa* may be differentiated clinically by gentle movement of the pinna, which will cause exquisite pain in otitis externa but no discomfort in purulent otitis media.

Simple auditory screening in this age group can be accomplished by whispering at a distance of 8 feet.

Ask the child questions or give commands, taking care that lip reading is not allowable. In addition you can use a tuning fork to screen for hearing, using your own auditory acuity as the control.

Acute *mastoiditis* in children is accompanied by a forward protrusion of the pinna of the ear on the affected side, in addition to the redness, swelling, and tenderness overlying the mastoid bone.

If these screening methods reveal any diminution of hearing, a full audiometric testing should be performed. Furthermore, all children should be given a full-scale acoustic screening test with an audiometer prior to beginning school, as should any child, at whatever age, with delayed speech development. Because of their complexity, audiometric screening devices used for older children are often unsatisfactory for use in early childhood; when delayed or defective speech is present, direct referral to a hearing and speech center may be more appropriate.

Significant, temporary hearing loss for as long as 4 months may follow an episode of otitis media.

LATE CHILDHOOD

As the child grows older, the ease and techniques of examining the ears and testing the hearing approach the levels and methods for adults. There are no unique abnormalities, or variations from the normal, concerning the ear and its function in this age group, as compared with older age groups, including the "selective deafness" some children and adolescents demonstrate in hearing only what they choose when spoken to in either soft or loud voices by their parents and teachers.

THE NOSE AND THROAT

INFANCY

Obstruction to the *nasal passages* in newborn infants occurs with *choanal atresia* and with displacement of the nasal cartilage during delivery.

Pass a number 14 French catheter through each nostril into the posterior nasopharynx to detect these anomalies. You may also test the patency of the nasal passages by holding the infant's mouth closed and occluding each nostril alternately.

This will not cause stress in a normal baby, since most newborns are nasal breathers. On the other hand, occluding both nares simultaneously and allowing the mouth to open will cause considerable distress. Indeed, some infants are unable to breathe through their mouths at all (*obligate nasal breathers*).

The *mouth* of the newborn is edentulous. The gums are smooth with a raised, 1-mm, serrated fringe of tissue on the buccal margins. Occasionally, pearl-like retention cysts are seen along the ridges and are often mistaken for teeth—they disappear spontaneously within a month or two.

Rarely, *supernumerary teeth* are found. These are soft, without enamel, and shed within a few days. However, they should be removed to prevent their aspiration into the lower respiratory tract.

Petechiae are commonly found on the soft palate after birth.

The frenulum of the upper lip may be quite thick and extend from the superior aspect of the inner lip to the posterior portion of the upper gum, creating a deep notch in the midline of the gum. The frenulum of the tongue varies in consistency from a thin, filamentous membrane to a thick, fibrous cord. Its length varies, so that it may attach midway on the undersurface of the tongue or at its very tip. A heavy fibrous frenulum that extends to the tip of the tongue may interfere with its protrusion (*tongue tie*). However, there will be no difficulties encountered with nursing or speech if the tongue can be extended as far as the alveolar ridge, which is so in almost all instances.

Epstein's pearls, pinhead-sized, white or yellow, rounded elevations which are located along the midline of the hard palate near its posterior border, are caused by retained secretions and disappear within a few weeks or months.

Visualization of the *pharynx* is best accomplished while a baby is crying. This is true throughout infancy and early childhood. A tongue blade produces strong reflex elevation of the base of the tongue and obstructs the view of the infant's pharynx. Tonsillar tissue is not seen in the newborn.

Oral moniliasis (*thrush*) is a common malady in infants, usually contracted from mothers with vaginal moniliasis. In thrush, a lacy white material with an erythematous base is seen on the surface of the oral mucous membranes. It is difficult to remove, distinguishing it from milk curds, which wipe away.

There is little saliva produced during the first 3 months of life. As the infant begins to produce saliva, drooling occurs, because there are no lower teeth to provide a dam for retention.

The presence of large amounts of saliva in the newborn suggests a *tracheoesophageal fistula.*

Listen to the infant's *breathing* and the *quality of his cry*.

A shrill or high-pitched cry in infancy may indicate increased intracranial pressure. A hoarse cry should make one suspect hypocalcemic *tetany* or *cretinism*, while absence of any cry suggests severe illness or profound mental retardation. A continuous inspiratory and expiratory stridor may be caused by a relatively small larynx (*infantile laryngeal stridor*), or by delay in the development of the cartilage in the tracheal rings (*tracheomalacia*).

EARLY AND LATE CHILDHOOD

Visualize the anterior portion of the *nose* by pushing up its tip. Use a large-bored speculum attached to the otoscope to look deeper into the nostrils.

Examination of the *mouth* may present difficulties in early childhood, and restraints are usually needed (see figure on p. 479). The young child may be more comfortable sitting in the parent's lap, as shown here.

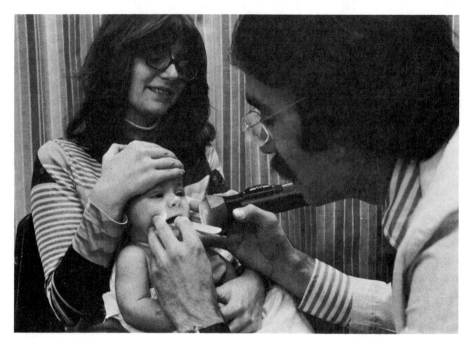

If the child clamps his teeth and purses his lips, gently push the tongue blade through the lips along the buccal mucosa and between the alveolar ridges behind the molars. This produces a gag reflex and, with it, complete visualization of the *pharynx*.

A direct assault on the front teeth will only meet with failure and a splintered tongue blade. Most children, however, are not that resistant and can be easily enticed to open their mouths, especially if they do not see a throat stick in the examiner's hand. A child who can stick out his tongue and say "ahhh!" does not require further manipulation for complete visualization of the pharynx. A good examiner can determine all that needs to be known with one quick look. Older children will permit placement of the tongue blade on one side of the base of the tongue and then the other. A transilluminator attachment to the oto–ophthalmoscopic handle is more useful than the standard penlight or flashlight in that its giraffe-like configuration allows for delivery of concentrated light in the recesses of the oral cavity and the pharynx.

The transilluminator may also be used, of course, to transilluminate the sinuses when sinusitis is suspected. This requires a completely dark room and a cooperative child.

The presence of *Koplik's spots*, although a diagnostic sign now rarely seen, deserves description. Their appearance on the buccal mucosa opposite the first and second molars in a child with fever, coryza, and cough is proof positive of prodromal measles (*rubeola*), and the appearance of a generalized maculopapular rash within 24 hours can be predicted with certainty. Koplik's spots appear as grains of salt on individual erythematous bases. Their number varies according to when in the course of the illness they are observed. When three or more appear in a particular spot, they should be easily recognized.

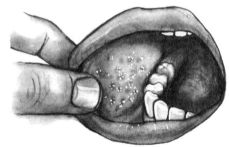

Transilluminate the frontal sinuses by firmly placing the tip of the light above each eye against the inner aspect of the supraorbital ridge of the frontal bone.

Normally one sees a faint glow of light transmitted through the bone outlining the frontal sinus on the same side.

Transillumination is absent or diminished when *sinusitis* is present.

Transilluminate the maxillary sinuses by placing the neck and head of the light in the patient's mouth, and pressing the tip against first one side and then the other of the hard palate. Instruct the patient to seal his lips around the shaft of the transilluminator attachment while you look for the maxillary sinus glow on the corresponding side of the face.

The appearance of the *tongue* may indicate disease. The *coated* tongue is nonspecific, the *smooth* tongue is found in avitaminosis, the *geographic* tongue in many allergic conditions, and the *strawberry* and *raspberry* tongues at specific stages of scarlet fever. The *scrotal* and *fissured* tongues have no significance (see Table 5–22, p. 122).

The *teeth* should be examined for timing and sequence of eruption, number, character, condition, and position. Abnormalities of the enamel may reflect past or present, general or localized disease. Malocclusion should be looked for in late childhood. Most malocclusion and misalignment of teeth due to thumb sucking in early childhood are reversible if the habit is substantially arrested by age 6 or 7 years. When examining for maxillary protrusion (*overbite*) or mandibular protrusion (*underbite*), one should be careful not to fall into the trap of asking the child to "show his teeth," because the upper and lower teeth are aligned reflexly when they are presented for inspection.

Green coloration of the teeth is seen following severe *erythroblastosis fetalis*; grayish mottling of the enamel may result from administration of tetracycline in infancy and early childhood; caries reflect poor nutrition and oral hygiene; and black lines along the gingival margins signal the ingestion of heavy metals.

Rather, ask the child to bite down as hard as possible. Upon parting the lips you will observe the true bite. In normal children the upper teeth slightly override the lower teeth.

Malocclusion is most often due to hereditary predisposition, but may be due to chronic mouth breathing secondary to obstruction of the nasal airway. Maxillary overgrowth is associated with *chronic hemolytic anemia*. Mandibular overgrowth occurs rarely in the initial stages of *juvenile rheumatoid arthritis* affecting the temporomandibular joint; micrognathia eventually ensues, however, in chronic cases.

The *primary teeth* erupt in a more predictable fashion in contrast to when they are shed or when the secondary teeth arrive. At age 7 months, most infants have two upper and two lower central incisors. From that point on, four teeth are added every 4 months, so there are eight at 11 months, 12 at 15 months, 16 at 19 months, and a full complement of 20 at 23 months. Normally, the shedding of primary teeth begins at about age 5 years; it precedes the eruption of corresponding *secondary teeth*, which begins at the end of early childhood between 6 and 7 years of age and ends in early adulthood at age 17 to 22 years.

When the *throat* is examined, the size and appearance of the *tonsils* should be noted. In both early and late childhood the tonsils are relatively larger than in infancy and adolescence, as demonstrated by the abundance of lymphoid tissue at this time of life (see figure on p. 447). They appear even larger as they move out of their fossae toward the midline and forward when the gag reflex is elicited or when the tongue is voluntarily protruded and the traditional "ahhh!" is sounded. The tonsils usually have deep crypts on their surface, which often have white concretions or food particles protruding from their depths. This is no indication of disease current or past.

The *adenoids* are not ordinarily visible unless extremely enlarged or unless the soft palate is elevated with the tongue blade to expose them in the nasopharynx. Adenoidal size can be determined indirectly by noting the degree of posterior nasal obstruction present when the patient sniffs through each nostril, and by the nasal quality they produce in the voice. Their size may also be determined directly by palpation. Adenoidal palpation should be carried out when there is a history of recurrent fever, headaches, and cough, and thus the diagnosis of *chronic adenoiditis* and *adenoidal abscess* are entertained.

During this examination, position the child and restrain as for examination of the throat (see p. 479). Tape three tongue blades together, place them, with your left hand, between the molars, and turn them on edge to ensure wide exposure. Place your plastic-gloved right index finger through the mouth into the nasopharynx behind the soft palate, and very rapidly palpate and thoroughly massage the adenoidal and surrounding lymphoid tissue. The procedure is accomplished with three or four quick strokes of the finger.

The child and parents should be warned that this procedure is uncomfortable and is likely to be followed by vomiting.

The same method may be used to palpate a peritonsillar abscess to determine the presence or absence of fluctuation and the posterior pharyngeal wall to determine the presence and state of a retropharyngeal abscess.

A white exudate over the surface of the tonsils suggests *streptococcal tonsillitis;* a thick, gray, adherent exudate suggests *diphtheritic tonsillitis;* and necrosis of the tonsillar tissue without exudate suggests *infectious mononucleosis.* All three conditions produce a fetid odor, but no one odor is distinguishable from the others. When one tonsil appears inflamed and unilaterally protrudes toward the midline and forward, *peritonsillar abscess* is an almost certain diagnosis.

In cases of chronic adenoiditis and adenoidal abscess, palpation will reveal enlarged and boggy adenoidal tissue, and massage will produce copious amounts of bloody mucus and purulent material.

Absence or asymmetry of movement of the soft palate in response to gagging and phonation, which is indicative of paralysis or weakness, should be noted. Asymmetry and corresponding voice change are often observed for varying periods following tonsillectomy.

Often overlooked in the examination of the throat is the presence of a submucosal cleft palate in which the muscles of the medial portion of the soft palate are missing. The mucosa is intact, however, and the underlying defect is easily missed. This condition is usually associated with notching of the posterior margin of the hard palate and a bifid uvula. Children with this anatomic variation may have hypernasal speech, but many have no voice changes. Adenoidectomy should be avoided, since difficulties with regurgitation of liquids and food into the nasal passages and nasality of speech will surely occur.

The child who has a croupy cough, hoarseness, difficulty swallowing, and signs of upper respiratory tract obstruction may have acute *epiglottitis*. In such a case, the epiglottis is markedly swollen and cherry red. Invoking the gag reflex in this instance could produce complete laryngeal obstruction and a fatal outcome. Therefore, great care must be taken in examining the throat. It should be done only once, if at all, and then deftly and gently with the child in the upright position, with a tracheostomy set at hand for use in the event that complete upper airway obstruction results from the examination procedure. The danger of such obstruction is sufficiently great that many clinicians prefer to omit direct examination of the throat in suspected cases of acute epiglottitis, and to rely upon lateral x-rays of the neck to establish the diagnosis.

THE THORAX AND LUNGS

INFANCY

The configuration of the infant's *thorax* is rounded, with the anteroposterior diameter being equal to the transverse diameter. The *thoracic index,* which is the ratio of the transverse diameter to the anteroposterior diameter, is 1 at birth. At 1 year of age it is 1.25, and it reaches 1.35 at 6 years without much change thereafter.

The chest wall in infancy is thin with little musculature, and the bony and cartilaginous rib cage is very soft and pliant. The tip of the xiphoid process is often seen protruding anteriorly immediately beneath the skin at the apex of the costal angle.

The *breasts* of the newborn in both male and female are often enlarged and engorged with secretion of a white liquid called "witch's milk." This is due to maternal estrogen effect and usually lasts only a week or two.

Pectus excavatum may be manifested in early infancy by marked midline substernal retractions with normal respirations, but it and other asymmetric thoracic deformities such as *pectus carinatum* ("chicken breast" deformity) do not ordinarily become evident until early childhood (see p. 150).

The respiratory rate and patterns in infancy and early childhood are discussed on page 458. The predominantly diaphragmatic breathing produces a simultaneous drawing in of the lower thorax and protrusion of the abdomen on inspiration and the reverse on expiration—termed *paradoxical breathing*.

Feel for tactile fremitus in infants by placing your hand on the baby's chest when he cries. Place your whole hand, palm and fingertips, over the anterior, lateral, or posterior thorax to detect gross changes in transmission of sound through the parenchyma of the lung, pleura, and chest wall of the infant. Percuss the infant's chest directly by tapping the thoracic wall with one finger, or indirectly by using the finger-on-finger method.

The percussion note is normally hyperresonant throughout. Any decrease in hyperresonance detected over the lung fields has the same significance as dullness or flatness in the adult.

Use the bell or small diaphragm stethoscope when auscultating the infant's chest, to allow for maximum localization of findings.

The breath sounds are louder and harsher than in adults because the stethoscope is closer to the origin of the sounds. Breathing in newborns is usually intermittently slow and shallow, then rapid and deep, so the examiner must be both patient and opportunistic. Breath sounds will often be diminished on the side of the chest opposite the direction in which the head is turned. There may be fine crackles at the end of deep inspiration in normal newborns and older infants. Crying, fortunately, will produce all of the deep breaths one could want and actually enhances auscultation, except in the unusual baby who cries on inspiration as well as expiration. Because of the smallness of the thoracic cage and the ease of sound transmission within, breath sounds are rarely entirely absent. Even with atelectasis, effusion, empyema, and pneumothorax, breath sounds are diminished rather than absent. In infants, pure bronchial breathing is rarely heard, even when consolidation is present. Wheezes, which are palpable and audible vibrations caused by air rushing through a narrowed segment of the lumen, occur more frequently in infancy and early childhood than in older children and adults because the small lumen of the tracheobronchial tree is easily narrowed by slight swelling of the mucous membrane or by small amounts of mucus.

EARLY AND LATE CHILDHOOD

Breast development for girls may begin normally as early as 8 years of age. Asymmetrical growth with resulting differences in size of the breasts during preadolescence is the rule; symmetrical breast growth is the exception. Completion of growth through adolescence corrects these inequalities in most instances. It is often helpful to explain this both to parents and to the young person herself, even if no mention of the subject is made by them.

When paradoxical breathing changes to predominantly thoracic breathing, intra-abdominal or intrathoracic pathology, which restricts the use of the diaphragm, should be suspected. On the other hand, an *increase* in abdominal breathing suggests pulmonary disease.

Extension or other movement of the head with inspiration indicates use of accessory muscles of respiration, and usually accompanies severe respiratory disease.

Both dullness and flatness may be elicited in infants when consolidation of the lung, an intrathoracic mass, or pleural fluid is present.

An inspiratory wheeze is indicative of narrowing high in the tracheobronchial tree, while an expiratory wheeze indicates narrowing lower down.

The breath sounds on auscultation of the lungs in early and late childhood, as in infancy, are louder and harsher than in adults because of the continued relative lack of musculature and subcutaneous tissue overlying the thorax. Respiratory patterns are more regular than in infancy, and increasing cooperation in taking deep breaths and conducting other breathing maneuvers during auscultation of the lungs is obtained with increasing age.

The stethoscope may be a threatening instrument to the very young child; therefore, your success in placing it upon the chest will be enhanced if you tell the child what it is and if you allow him to manipulate it or even listen through it.

You can usually generate tactile and vocal fremitus easily by feeling the chest wall while carrying on a conversation with the child. A surprising number will go the spoken "99" and "1, 2, 3" routes. You can usually gain the child's cooperation in deep breathing and breath holding by demonstrating each maneuver to him. If this is not successful, ask the child to blow out a match held too far away for immediate success. This seldom fails to produce full inspiration.

THE HEART

The examination of the heart in infants and children is, with few exceptions, conducted in the same manner as with the adult. The femoral pulses assume greater importance, since their diminution (as compared to the radial pulse) or their absence may be the only findings to raise suspicion of *coarctation of the aorta* in infancy and early childhood.

Feel along the inguinal ligament midway between the iliac crest and the symphysis pubis for the femoral pulse.

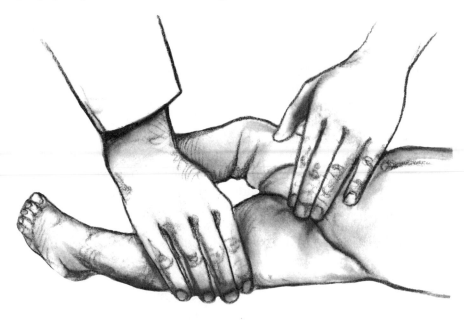

Because the respiratory rate may approximate the heart rate in infancy, breath sounds may be thought to be murmurs.

Occlude the nares momentarily to interrupt the respirations long enough to clarify this issue.

There are some distinct characteristics of the cardiac findings in normal infants and children that are not found in adults. The apical impulse (PMI), which is often visible, is at the level of the 4th interspace until age 7 years, when it drops to the 5th interspace. It is to the left of the midclavicular line until age 4 years, is at the midclavicular line between ages 4 and 6, and moves to the right of it at age 7. On percussion the heart appears larger than it actually is because of its more horizontal position and the overlying thymus gland at its base. *Sinus arrhythmia* is almost always present, and *premature ventricular contractions* are quite common. The heart sounds are louder because the chest wall is thinner, and they are of higher pitch and shorter duration. S_1 is louder than S_2 at the apex. Splitting of S_2 at the apex is found in 25% to 33% of children. S_2 is louder than S_1 in the pulmonic area.

In the pediatric cardiac examination, the *murmur* assumes great significance in differential diagnosis, because more than 50% of all children (indeed, some say all) develop an innocent murmur at some time during childhood, and because significant heart disease in the pediatric age group is infrequent in the absence of a murmur. The examiner must therefore distinguish between the innocent and the organic murmur. The intensity of murmurs is graded on a scale of 1 to 6, as shown on page 179.

The *innocent murmur* has received over 120 labels indicative of its benign or functional nature, its origin, or its auscultatory characteristics. It is systolic in timing, is usually of short duration and of grade 3 or less in intensity, and has an empty, low-pitched, vibratory, musical groaning quality to its sound. It is usually loudest along the left sternal border, either in the 2nd or 3rd intercostal spaces or in the 4th or 5th intercostal spaces medial to the apex. It is poorly transmitted and is heard best in the supine position. Its intensity may vary with change in position, with the phase of respiration, with exercise, and from day to day. The most important characteristic of the innocent murmur is that it is heard in the absence of any other demonstrable evidence of cardiovascular disease.

The physical indications of severe heart disease include those not found with the stethoscope. Poor weight gain, delayed development, tachypnea, tachycardia, a prominent, active, heaving or thrusting precordium, cyanosis, and clubbing of the fingers and toes all signal cardiac disease. Heart failure is marked by venous engorgement, pulsus alternans, gallop rhythm, and hepatic enlargement. Pulmonary and peripheral edema appear late in the course of heart failure. (Peripheral edema, when it occurs in children, is more likely to be caused by renal failure.)

When S_2 is equal to or greater than S_1 at the apex, prolongation of the P–R interval on the electrocardiogram should be suspected. Splitting of S_2 in the pulmonic area may be found normally, but is frequently present in *mitral stenosis* and *right bundle branch block.*

Murmurs of grade 3 or higher usually indicate the presence of heart disease.

In *atrial septal defect,* a grade 1 to 3 coarse systolic murmur is heard at the 2nd and 3rd left interspaces. It is less coarse than the murmur of a ventricular septal defect, is rarely accompanied by a thrill, and is not widely distributed. The murmur of *coarctation of the aorta* (adult type) is heard in the same area, is louder, is transmitted to the back medial to the scapula, and may be accompanied by a visible

The noninnocent or *organic murmurs* are caused by congenital or acquired heart disease. Almost all acquired heart disease productive of murmurs in childhood is caused by acute rheumatic fever. An organic murmur first appearing before 3 years of age is almost always caused by a congenital cardiac defect, and one first appearing after that age is usually caused by rheumatic valvulitis.

The murmurs of congenital cardiac defects are caused either by abnormal communications between the arterial and venous circuits of the heart and great vessels or by valvular deformities. For the most part, they are coarse in character, systolic in timing, and usually heard best at the base of the heart. The murmurs of *ventricular septal defect* and of *patent ductus arteriosus* have been described on pages 204 and 207. Those of *aortic stenosis* and *pulmonic stenosis* are described on page 202.

The presence or absence of cyanosis may be helpful to the examiner in differentiating the various types of congenital heart disease that present with similar murmurs (see Table 17-5).

More often than not, the final diagnostic impression must await the results of electrocardiograms, chest x-rays, fluoroscopic examinations, cardiac catheterization, echocardiograms, and more sophisticated studies.

The murmurs associated with acquired rheumatic heart disease include those of mitral stenosis (see p. 206), mitral regurgitation (see p. 204), aortic stenosis (see p. 202), and aortic regurgitation (see p. 206). Stenosis and regurgitation of the same valve usually occur concomitantly. Mitral valvular disease occurs in 90% of children who develop heart disease following acute rheumatic carditis, either alone or in combination with aortic valvular disease. Aortic valve involvement occurs in approximately 25% of cases. The tricuspid and pulmonic valves are rarely involved in the rheumatic process.

The examiner of a child's heart should be able to differentiate normal from abnormal findings. Final decisions regarding specific abnormalities must often be left to the pediatric cardiologist, whose experience and access to special diagnostic tools will be more likely to bring accurate diagnoses and appropriate management. Therefore, early referral of the infant or child found to have evidence of congenital or acquired heart disease should be made to a pediatric cardiologist.

pulsation and palpable thrill at the suprasternal notch. It is also associated with decreased to absent femoral pulses and elevated blood pressure in the upper extremities. The murmurs associated with *tetralogy of Fallot*, *pure pulmonic stenosis, tricuspid atresia, transposition of the great vessels*, and *Eisenmenger's syndrome* are grades 3 to 5 in intensity, are systolic in timing, may be heard best at the left 2nd and 3rd interspaces, are not well transmitted, may or may not be accompanied by a thrill, and have no individual distinguishing characteristics. These murmurs may be absent in infancy. In addition, palpable liver pulsations may be present with tricuspid atresia and pure pulmonic stenosis.

Table 17-5 Cyanosis and Congenital Heart Disease

NO CYANOSIS	Septal defects—small
	Patent ductus arteriosus
	Pure pulmonic stenosis—mild
	Coarctation of the aorta
	*Right coronary artery
	*Subendocardial fibroelastosis
	*Glycogen storage disease
EARLY CYANOSIS	Tetralogy of Fallot—severe
	Tricuspid atresia
	Transposition of the great vessels
	Two- and three-chambered hearts
	Severe pulmonic stenosis with intact ventricular septum
LATE CYANOSIS	Eisenmenger complex
	Pure pulmonic stenosis—mild
	Tetralogy of Fallot
	Septal defects—large

*Present with cardiac enlargement, tachycardia, and tachypnea, but without a heart murmur

THE ABDOMEN

INFANCY

The abdomen in infants is protuberant, due to poorly developed abdominal musculature.

A newborn with a concave abdomen should be immediately investigated for *diaphragmatic hernia* with displacement of some of the abdominal organs into the thoracic cavity.

The *umbilical cord* should be checked routinely at birth for the number of vessels present. Normally, two umbilical arteries and one umbilical vein are present.

A high correlation exists between a *single umbilical artery* and a variety of congenital anomalies.

The umbilicus in the newborn may have a relatively long cutaneous portion (*umbilicus cutis*) or a relatively long amniotic portion (*umbilicus amnioticus*). In either event, the amniotic portion dries up within a week and falls off within two. The cutaneous portion retracts to become flush with the abdominal wall during the same period.

Failure of the *navel* to heal, with granulomatous tissue formation at its base, occurs frequently.

Infants are prone to *umbilical hernias, ventral hernias,* and *diastasis recti.* However, these are not usually discernible until 2 or 3 weeks of age. All are easily detected with crying.

The defect in the abdominal wall at the umbilicus may be as large as 1½ inches in diameter, and the hernia itself may protrude 3 to 4 inches from the abdominal wall when intra-abdominal pressure is increased. Most umbilical hernias disappear by 1 year of age.

The presence of diastasis recti may reflect a congenital weakness of the abdominal musculature (rare), or result from a chronically distended abdomen. Most, however, are normal variants and disappear in early childhood.

A superficial abdominal venous pattern is observable until puberty. Abdominal reflexes are usually absent until after the first year of life.

Dilated veins may indicate portal vein obstruction. In veins below the umbilicus the direction of venous flow in *portal hypertension* is downward.

Palpation of the infant's abdomen is relatively easy.

Obtain relaxation by holding the infant's legs flexed at the knees and hips with one hand, and palpate with the other.

The *liver edge* and *spleen tip* are more often palpable than not, and frequently both *kidneys* can be felt by using the technique described for adults. The *bladder* is often felt and normally percussed to the level of the umbilicus. The *descending colon* is easily felt and may present as a sausagelike mass in the left lower quadrant. Any abdominal masses of other origin are easily outlined.

Differentiate *cysts*, which occur rarely, from solid *tumors* by transillumination.

Avoid the spasm and rigidity encountered in palpating the abdomen of a crying infant with the administration of a bottle feeding or a sugar nipple.

Percussion of the infant's abdomen is accomplished as in the adult, but the examiner must allow for a greater amount of air within the stomach and the intestinal lumen because infants frequently swallow air when feeding and crying.

Auscultation of the abdomen should be accomplished before palpation. During auscultation, metallic tinkling every 10 to 30 seconds is heard normally.

The abdominal examination technique is altered when *pyloric stenosis* is suspected.

Place the infant, unclothed, in the supine position and stand at the foot of the table. Direct a bright light at table height across the abdomen from the patient's right side. Feed the infant a bottle of sugar water or milk and observe the abdomen closely. When pyloric stenosis is present, peristaltic waves are seen to go across the upper abdomen from left to right. These become increasingly large and frequent as the feeding progresses, as shown in the figure at the right.

Inevitably, the baby will vomit with projectile force. At this point, palpate deeply in the right upper quadrant. This will most likely reveal the presence of an olive-sized pyloric mass. Similar palpation with the baby in the prone position may prove more successful.

In *Hirschsprung's disease* (congenital megacolon), a midline suprapubic mass representing a feces-filled rectosigmoid is often found.

An increase in pitch or frequency of bowel sounds, or marked diminution, is indicative of *intestinal obstruction* and *ileus*, respectively. A venous hum is a sign of *portal hypertension.*

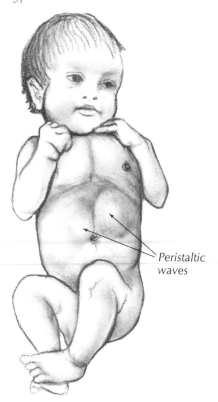

Peristaltic waves

EARLY AND LATE CHILDHOOD

Protuberance of the abdomen, apparent when the child is in upright position and disappearing when the child lies down, is noted in most children until adolescence.

Children are almost universally ticklish when you first place your hand on the abdominal wall. This disappears in most cases, particularly if you distract the child by conversation and by placing your whole hand flush on the surface for a few moments without making initial probing movements with your fingers. With those children who persist in their sensitivity, placement of the child's hand under yours, as shown in the illustration below, will reduce apprehension and increase relaxation of the abdominal musculature. Precede deep palpation with light superficial palpation of all quadrants. The last area you should examine is that which the history suggests as the site of pathology.

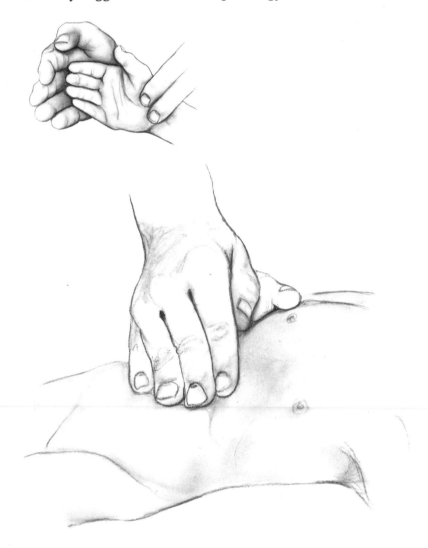

Tenderness may be determined by direct response of the child or may be detected by a change in the facial expression or a change in the pitch of the child's cry.

The *liver* and *spleen* are easily palpated in most children. The edge of the liver is normally felt 1 cm to 2 cm below the right costal margin. It is sharp and soft and moves easily when pushed from below upward during deep inspiration. The size of the liver is better determined by percussion than palpation. Table 17-6 shows the expected liver span by percussion for male and female patients by age.

A pathologically enlarged liver is usually palpable at more than 2 cm below the costal margin and has a rounded, firm edge.

Table 17-6   Expected Liver Span of Infants, Children, and Adolescents by Percussion

| AGE, YR | MEAN ESTIMATED LIVER SPAN (CM) | |
	MALES	FEMALES
6 mo	2.4	2.8
1	2.8	3.1
2	3.5	3.6
3	4.0	4.0
4	4.4	4.3
5	4.8	4.5
6	5.1	4.8
8	5.6	5.1
10	6.1	5.4
12	6.5	5.6
14	6.8	5.8
16	7.1	6.0
18	7.4	6.1
20	7.7	6.3

As a rule the spleen, like the liver, is felt easily in most children. It too is soft with a sharp edge, and presents as a downward, tonguelike projection along the lateral aspect of the left upper quadrant.

You can often palpate the spleen between the thumb and forefinger of your right hand, and will find it to be freely moveable.

Epigastric pulsations are seen normally, but also may be caused by enlargement of the right ventricle with its pulsations transmitted through the diaphragm.

Deeply palpate the abdomen to the left of the midline to feel the *aorta* and its pulsations.

Because the omentum is poorly developed in early childhood, localization of intra-abdominal infection or other inflammatory reaction is less apt to occur than in late childhood and adolescence. Whenever serious pathology occurs within the abdomen, tenderness and spasm are usually diffuse, indicating *generalized peritonitis.*

The examination for *inguinal hernia* in this age group is similar to that performed on the adult and should be done with the patient standing.

Because the child's cough may be of insufficient strength to demonstrate a reduced hernia, the hernia can sometimes be demonstrated if the child attempts to lift a heavy object, such as the end of the examining table or the chair in which you are sitting.

In *acute appendicitis* in this age group, localization of the inflammation may be demonstrated by eliciting pain in the right lower quadrant. This is accomplished in the case of an appendix lying anteriorly by having the patient attempt to raise his head while the examiner's hand pushes down on the forehead. When the appendix lies retrocecally over the psoas and obturator muscles, positive *psoas* and *obturator signs* are present (see pp. 248–249).

THE GENITALIA AND RECTUM

INFANCY

Examining the genitalia in the male infant presents no difficulties. The *foreskin* adheres to the *glans penis,* covers it completely, and has a tiny orifice at its distal end. It does not retract over the glans until the infant is several months old, and then only if it has been stretched on a regular basis.

Most male infants in our society are circumcised in the immediate neonatal period, so that the glans is exposed to its base.

The *testes* are normally found in the scrotum, or in the inguinal canal, from which they can easily be milked down into the scrotum.

In the newborn female the *labia minora* are prominent. They quickly atrophy and become almost nonexistent until puberty. More often than not there is a bloody, mucoid vaginal discharge during the first week of life, due to the maternal estrogen influence on the vaginal mucosa. A serosanguinous vaginal discharge may supplant this for a week or two more.

Visualize the perineal structures, the urethral orifice, the hymen, and the vaginal mucosa by separating the labia with the thumb and forefinger of one hand while you press forward and downward from within the rectum with the index finger of your other hand.

The genitalia of both male and female breech babies may be markedly edematous and bruised for several days following delivery.

The *rectal examination* of infants (and of patients in early and late childhood) should be accomplished with the patient in the supine position.

Hypospadias is present when the urethral orifice presents at some point along the ventral surface of the glans or the shaft of the penis. The foreskin in these instances is incompletely formed ventrally.

Hydroceles of the testes and the spermatic cord are common in infancy and often associated with actual or potential *inguinal hernias.* Hydroceles may be differentiated easily from hernias in that the former transilluminate and are not reducible.

Hold the feet together and flex the knees and hips upon the abdomen with one of your hands while the index finger of your other hand is introduced into the rectum. Once this is done, place your first hand upon the abdomen to conduct a bimanual examination. The index finger is preferred for the rectal examination, even in infancy, because of its greater tactile sensitivity. Regardless of the size of your examining finger, slight bleeding and protrusion of the rectal mucosa will occur upon its removal.

EARLY AND LATE CHILDHOOD

The size of *the penis* in early childhood and prepubescence is of little significance unless it is very large. In obese boys the fatpad over the symphysis pubis may envelop the penis, obscuring it completely. The testes in young boys are quite retractile and are often found in the inguinal canal rather than in the scrotum.

Enlargement of the penis to adolescent or adult size occurs in *precocious puberty,* due to an excess in circulating androgens of adrenal or testicular origin. This occurs with tumors of these organs or of the pituitary gland. Other signs of virilization—pubic and axillary hair, increased testicular size, increased somatic growth and muscle mass, hirsutism, and deepening of the voice—usually accompany the penile enlargement.

Cryptorchidism, or undescended testicle, may occur unilaterally or bilaterally, with the testicle remaining in the abdomen or within the inguinal canal.

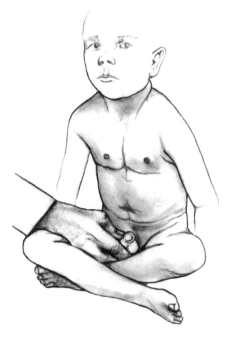

You can overcome testicular retractibility by having the child sit in a crosslegged squatting position on the examining table, as illustrated here. A diagnosis of undescended testicle should not be made until you have palpated the inguinal canal and scrotum with the patient in this position.

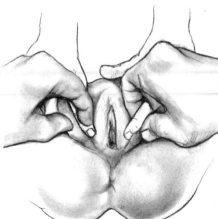

You can enhance the examination of the female genitalia in this age group by using the child's own hands to distract and reassure her, as shown here.

You can obtain greater relaxation and cooperation during the rectal examination if you first demonstrate and then ask the child to try breathing in and out rapidly "like a puppy dog."

Perianal skin tabs are common and have no significance. Bimanual rectoabdominal palpation in females will reveal a small midline mass, which is *the cervix*. Any other mass that is palpable on this examination should be considered abnormal, since none of the other anatomical structures are normally palpable until adolescence. Vaginoabdominal palpation as a method of examining the pelvic structures, and direct visualization of the vagina and cervix, are not considered as part of the ordinary physical examination in childhood. When these procedures are indicated on the basis of the history or abdominal or perineal findings, they are best accomplished with an otoscope equipped with a vaginal speculum.

Fusion of the labia minora is commonly seen. It may be partial, with only the posterior portion of the labia fused, or it may be complete. A thin membrane that joins the labial edges is easily lysed with a cotton swab or a probe. The labia will also separate if an estrogen-containing cream is applied to the labia once or twice daily for several days.

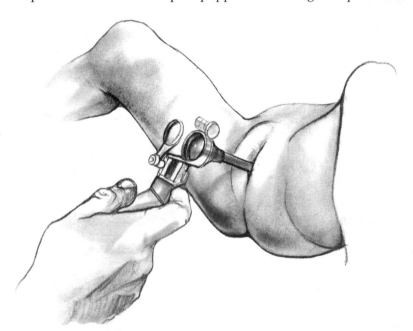

Secondary sexual *hair growth* parallels the development of other secondary sexual characteristics. Pubic hair may appear sparsely as early as the eighth year. Axillary, facial, body, arm, and leg hair proliferate in sequence before and during puberty.

THE MUSCULOSKELETAL SYSTEM

INFANCY

The *range of motion* at all joints is greatest in infancy and gradually lessens throughout childhood to adult levels.

At birth, *the feet* may appear deformed if they retain their intrauterine positioning. Such positional deformities can be distinguished by the ease with which the affected foot can be manipulated to neutral and over-

True deformities do not return to even the neutral position through manipulation.

corrected positions. Scratching or stroking along the outer edge of the positionally deformed foot will cause it to assume a normal position. Adduction of the forefoot distal to the metatarsal–tarsal line (*metatarsus adductus deformity*) is commonly found. Correction occurs spontaneously within the first 2 years of life.

During infancy there is a distinct *bowlegged growth pattern.* This begins to disappear at 18 months of age, when a transition from bowlegs to knock-knees occurs. The *knock-knee pattern* usually persists from 2 until 6 to 10 years of age, when a balancing takes place and, for most, the legs straighten. Some babies exhibit a twisting or torsion of the tibia inwardly or outwardly on its longitudinal axis. This invariably corrects itself during the second year of life.

When the forefoot is twisted inward on its longitudinal axis (inverted) in addition to being adducted, *metatarsus varus* exists, as shown in the figure below.

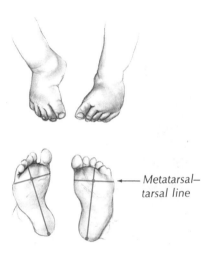

Metatarsal–tarsal line

When the infant stands, his legs are set wide apart and the weight is borne on the inside of the feet. When walking is accomplished, a wide-based gait is used for the first year or two. This causes a certain degree of *pronation of the feet* and incurving of the Achilles tendons when they are viewed from behind.

The longitudinal arch in infancy is obscured by adipose tissue, giving the foot the appearance of being flat. This is accentuated by pronation of the foot so that the infant is often misdiagnosed as being flatfooted.

Normally, a straight line drawn forward from a point at the center of the back of the heel through a point at the center of the metatarsal–tarsal line will bisect the second toe or the space between the second and third toes. With *metatarsus varus,* the point of bisection is placed more laterally, as shown above (lower pair of feet). *Talipes varus* is present when the forefoot is adducted and the entire foot is inverted. Both of these foot deformities require orthopedic correction.

The hips of all infants should be examined for signs of dislocation.

Place the baby in the supine position with the legs pointing toward you. Flex the legs to right angles at the hips and knees, and abduct them until the lateral aspect of each knee touches the examining table. When a congenitally dislocated hip is present, you will see, feel and sometimes hear a "click" as the femoral head, which in this condition lies posterior

to the acetabulum, enters the acetabulum at some point in the 90° abduction arc. This maneuver and finding are known as *Ortolani's test* and *sign*. The test is more sensitive if your middle fingers are placed over the greater trochanters of the femur and your thumbs over the lesser trochanters as shown in the accompanying figures.

Beyond the newborn period, as the muscles surrounding the hip increase in strength, the "click" of the Ortolani sign is less obtainable; then decreased abduction of the legs (at the hip, on one or both sides) becomes the significant finding in detecting unilateral or bilateral *congenital dislocation of the hip*.

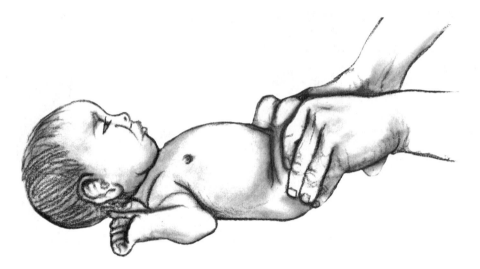

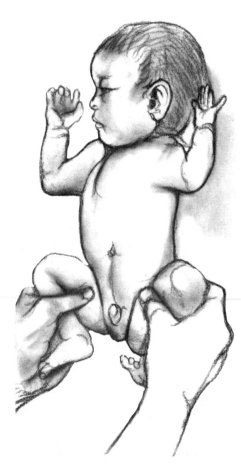

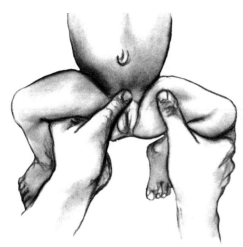

Lifting of your middle finger with the thigh held at mid-abduction will cause reduction of the dislocated hip. The test is more sensitive if the pelvis is steadied with one hand, applying pressure from above downward, while the other hand performs the maneuver shown.

You can detect unstable (nondislocated but potentially dislocatable) hips by exerting backward and outward pressure with your thumb placed medially over the lesser trochanter. You can then feel the femoral head slipping onto the posterior lip of the acetabulum and, when the pressure is placed over the greater trochanter with your middle finger, back into the hip socket (*Barlow's sign*), as shown in the figures below.

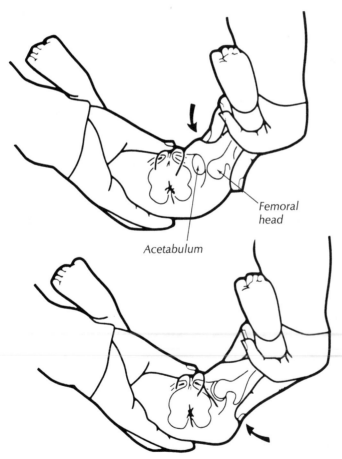

Femoral head

Acetabulum

(Reproduced with permission from Burnside JW: Physical Diagnosis: An Introduction to Clinical Medicine, 16th ed, p 246. Baltimore, Williams & Wilkins, 1981)

EARLY AND LATE CHILDHOOD

From both in front of and behind, watch the child as he stands upright. You can often detect the presence of musculoskeletal difficulties in this age group by closely observing the child in various postures (*e.g.,* from the front and rear standing upright with the feet together, walking, stooping to obtain an object from the floor, rising from the supine position, and touching the toes or shins while standing).

In childhood, the thoracic convexity is decreased and the lumbar concavity is increased.

You can detect severe hip disease with its associated weakness of the gluteus medius muscle by observing the child from behind as he shifts his weight from one leg to the other. The pelvis is seen to tilt toward the unaffected hip when weight is borne on the affected side, and to remain level when the weight is borne on the unaffected side (*Trendelenburg's sign*).

Normal hip abductors   Weak hip abductors

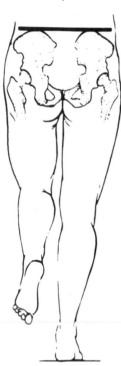 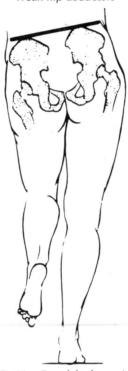

Negative Trendelenburg sign   Positive Trendelenburg sign
(Reproduced with permission from Chung SMR: Hip Disorders in Infants and Children, p 65. Philadelphia, Lea & Febiger, 1981)

You can determine *shortening of the leg* in hip disease by comparing the distance from the anterior superior spine of the ilium to the medial malleolus on each side.

When you suspect *scoliosis,* ask the child to bend forward. Mark the spinous processes with a felt tip pin. After he stands again, look for a curve in the line of ink dots.

THE NERVOUS SYSTEM

INFANCY

The findings during the neurologic examination in infancy, especially in the newborn period, differ markedly from those present in children and adults.

The central nervous system at birth is underdeveloped and functions at subcortical levels. Cortical function develops slowly after birth and cannot be tested in its entirety until early childhood. Thus, in the newborn period and early infancy, findings of normal brainstem and spinal functioning do not ensure an intact cortical system, and abnormalities of the brainstem and spinal cord may exist without concomitant cortical difficulties. There are a number of specific reflex activities (*infantile automatisms*) found in the normal newborn that disappear in early infancy.

The absence of infantile automatisms in the neonate or the persistence of some beyond their expected time of disappearance may indicate severe central nervous system dysfunction.

The neurologic examination in infancy, for the most part, will enable the clinician to detect extensive disease of the central nervous system, but will be of little use in pinpointing minute lesions and specific functional deficits.

The general appearance, positioning, activity, cry, and alertness of the newborn baby should be noted, as these observations are an important part of the neurologic assessment of this age group.

Test for *motor function* by putting each major joint through its range of motion to determine whether normal muscle tone, spasticity, or flaccidity are present.

Beyond the newborn period, throughout infancy, specific *gross and fine motor coordination testing* can be accomplished by using an age-appropriate protocol, such as the *Denver Developmental Screening Test.* This test also assesses social and language development. Discrepancies in achievement in the motor and communication areas may suggest whether the deficit is in the motor, sensory, or intellectual spheres. Knowledge of when developmental landmarks are normally achieved is essential in assessing the function of the infant's nervous system.

Postural indications of severe intracranial disease include persistent asymmetries, predominant extension of the extremities, and constant turning of the head to one side. Marked retroflexion of the head, stiffness of the neck, and extension of the arms and legs (*opisthotonus*) indicate severe meningeal irritation, seen in intracranial infection or hemorrhage and in brainstem irritation (see figure below).

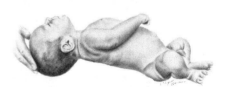

(Redrawn from Paine RS: Neurological examination of infants and children. Pediatr Clin North Am 7:477, 1960)

The *sensory examination* in infants is rather limited in terms of defining neurologic disease. Thresholds of touch, pain, and temperature are higher than in older children, and reactions to these stimuli are relatively slow.

Gently touch the baby's arms and legs with a pin, and observe movement of the stimulated extremity or change in the facial expression. If the pin is used vigorously enough, crying will result.

The *cranial nerves* are tested in infancy as in the adult. The difficulties encountered in assessing the function of the 2nd and 8th nerves have already been mentioned.

Absence of withdrawal when a painful stimulus is applied to an extremity indicates anesthesia or paralysis. If a change in facial expression or a cry is elicited in the absence of withdrawal, paralysis is indicated rather than anesthesia. With spinal cord lesions, the extremity will withdraw reflexly in response to pain, but there will be no concomitant change in the baby's facial expression or cry.

The 12th nerve is easily tested. Pinch the nostrils of the infant. This produces a reflex opening of the mouth and raising of the tip of the tongue.

If *12th nerve paresis* is present, the tongue tip will deviate toward the affected side.

Because the corticospinal pathways are not fully developed in infants, the *spinal reflex mechanisms* (deep tendon reflexes and plantar response) are variable in infancy. Their presence in exaggerated form, or their absence, has very little diagnostic significance unless there is asymmetry of response or change in response from a previous testing.

The technique for eliciting these reflexes is similar to that used with adults, except that your semiflexed index or middle finger can substitute for the neurologic hammer, its tip acting as the striking point. Your thumbnail may be used to elicit the plantar response.

The *Babinski response* to plantar stimulation can be elicited in most normal infants, and until 2 years of age in many children. The *triceps reflex* is usually not present until after 6 months of age. Rapid, rhythmic plantar flexion of the foot in response to eliciting the ankle reflex (*ankle clonus*) is a common finding in newborns; as many as eight to ten such contractions in response to one stimulus may occur normally (*unsustained ankle clonus*).

When the contractions are continuous (*sustained ankle clonus*), severe central nervous system disease should be suspected.

You can also elicit ankle clonus by pressing the thumb over the ball of the infant's foot and abruptly dorsiflexing the foot.

The *abdominal reflexes* are absent in the newborn but appear within the first 6 months of life. The *anal reflex*, however, is normally present in newborns.

The anal reflex is elicited by straightening and raising the lower legs with the baby in a supine position, scratching the perianal region with a pin, and observing contracture of the external anal sphincter.

Infantile Automatisms

The infantile automatisms are reflex phenomena that are present at birth or appear shortly thereafter. Some remain only a few weeks while others persist well into the second year of life. Automatisms have prognostic value for central nervous system integrity. Attempts to elicit them should be made only when central nervous system function is in question. Each automatism is listed here with the method of elicitation and the prognostic significance of its presence or absence. All are present at birth unless otherwise indicated. The time of disappearance is also listed.

Blinking (Dazzle) Reflex. Disappears after first year. The eyelids close in response to bright light.

Absence may indicate blindness.

Acoustic Blink (Cochleopalpebral) Reflex. Disappearance time is variable. Both eyes blink in response to a sharp loud noise.

Absence may indicate decreased hearing.

Palmar Grasp Reflex. Disappears at 3 or 4 months

With the baby's head positioned in the midline and the arms semiflexed, place your index fingers from the ulnar side into the baby's hands and press against the palmar surfaces. A positive response is one of flexion of all of the baby's fingers to grasp your fingers. This method allows for comparison of both hands. If the reflex is absent or weak, you can enhance it by offering the baby a bottle, since sucking facilitates grasping.

Persistence of the grasp reflex beyond 4 months suggests cerebral dysfunction. It should be noted that babies normally hold their hands clenched during the first month of life. Persistence of the fisted hand beyond 2 months also suggests central nervous system damage.

Light stroking of the ulnar surface of the hand and fifth finger will produce extension of the thumb and other fingers (*digital response reflex*).

Rooting Reflex. Disappears at 3 or 4 months; may be present longer during sleep

Absence of this reflex indicates severe generalized or central nervous system disease.

With the baby's head positioned in the midline and his hands held against his anterior chest, stroke with your forefinger the perioral skin at the corners of his mouth and at the midline of the upper and lower lips.

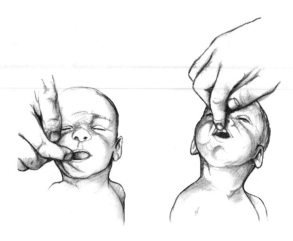

In response, the mouth will open and turn to the stimulated side. When the upper lip is stimulated, the head will retroflex; when the lower lip is stimulated, the jaw will drop. This response will also occur with stimulation of the infant's cheek at some distance from the corners of the mouth.

Trunk Incurvation (Galant's) Reflex. Disappears at 2 months

Transverse spinal cord lesions may be detected by testing for the presence of this reflex.

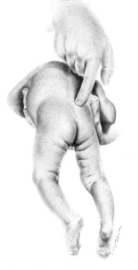

Hold the baby horizontally and prone in one of your hands. Stimulate one side of the baby's back approximately 1 cm from the midline along a paravertebral line extending from the shoulder to the buttocks. This produces a curving of the trunk toward the stimulated side, with shoulders and pelvis moving in that direction.

(Redrawn from Paine RS: Neurological examination of infants and children. Pediatr Clin North Am 7:490, 1960)

Vertical Suspension Positioning. Disappears after 4 months

While you support the baby upright with your hands under the axillae, the head is normally maintained in the midline and the legs are flexed at the hips and knees.

Fixed extension and adduction of the legs (scissoring) indicates *spastic paraplegia* or *diplegia.*

Placing Response. Best after the first 4 days. Disappearance time is variable.

Hold the baby upright from behind by placing your hands under the baby's arms with your thumbs supporting the back of the head, and allow the dorsal surface of one foot to touch the undersurface of a table top. This procedure is demonstrated in the four illustrations on the facing page.

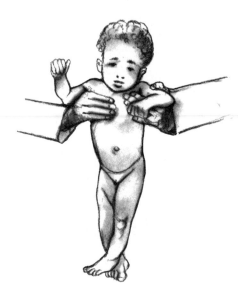

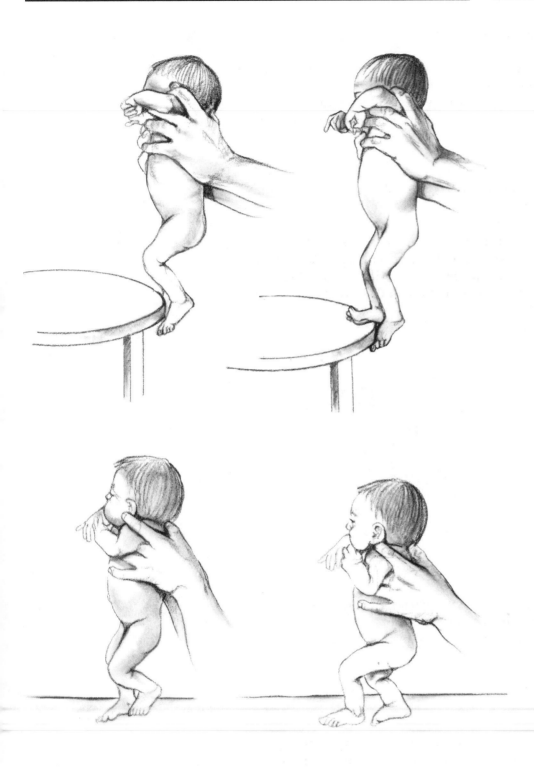

Take care not to plantar flex the foot. The baby responds by flexing the hip and knee and placing the stimulated foot on the table top. Repeat the process stimulating the other foot. With one foot placed on the table top, the opposite leg will step forward and a series of alternate stepping movements of both legs will occur as you move the baby gently forward.

These responses are absent when paresis is present and in babies born by breech delivery.

Rotation Test. Disappearance time is variable.

Hold the baby under the axillae, at arms length facing you, and rotate him in one direction and then the other. The head turns in the direction in which you turn the baby. If you restrain the head with your thumbs, his eyes will turn in the direction in which he is turned (see figure on p. 472).

The head and eyes do not move, as noted, in the presence of vestibular dysfunction. Early detection of *strabismus* may be accomplished with this maneuver.

Tonic Neck Reflex. May be present at birth but usually appears at 2 months and disappears at 6 months

With the baby in the supine position, as shown, turn the head to one side, holding the jaw over his shoulder. The arm and leg on the side to which the head is turned extend, while the opposite arm and leg flex. This response does not normally occur each time this maneuver is performed.

When this reflex is elicited each time it is evoked, it should be considered abnormal, at any age. It will persist beyond the time of expected disappearance in major cerebral damage.

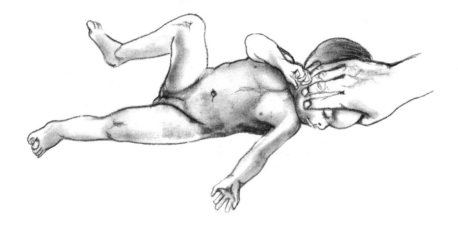

Two *mass reflexes* occur in the presence of normal subcortical mechanisms that are not yet under significant inhibitory control from higher cerebral centers. They are present at birth and disappear by the third month.

Absence of either reflex during the first 3 months of life indicates severe cerebral insult, injury to the upper cervical cord, advanced anterior horn cell disease, or severe myopathy.

Perez Reflex. **Hold the baby in a suspended prone position in one of your hands. Place the thumb of your other hand on the baby's sacrum and move it firmly toward the head along the entire length of the spine. A positive response is usually one of extension of the head and spine, flexion of the knees on the chest, a cry, and emptying of the bladder.**

The last occurs with sufficient frequency to make this reflex useful in the collection of urine specimens from neonates.

Moro Response (Startle Reflex). This response is elicited by any stimulus that suddenly moves the head in relation to the spine.

You can produce this response in several ways: by lifting the supine baby by his head at an angle approximately 30° from the examining table and suddenly releasing your grip and allowing his head to fall backward (as shown in the figure below); by holding the baby in the supine position, supporting the head, back, and legs, and then suddenly lowering the entire body about 2 feet and stopping abruptly; by holding the baby in the supine position, supporting the back and pelvis with one hand and arm and the head with the other hand, and allowing the head to drop several centimeters with a sudden, rapid, not too forceful movement; or by producing a sudden loud noise (*e.g.,* striking the examining table with the palms of your hands on either side of the baby's head).

The response itself is one in which the arms briskly abduct and extend with the hands open and fingers extended, and the legs flex slightly and abduct (but less so than the arms). The arms then return forward over the body in a clasping maneuver.

Persistence of the Moro response beyond 4 months may indicate neurologic disease; persistence beyond 6 months is almost conclusive evidence of such. An asymmetric response in the upper extremities suggests hemiparesis, injury to the brachial plexus, or fracture of the clavicle or humerus. Low spinal injury and congenital dislocation of the hip may produce absence of the response in one or both legs.

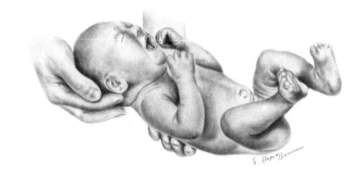

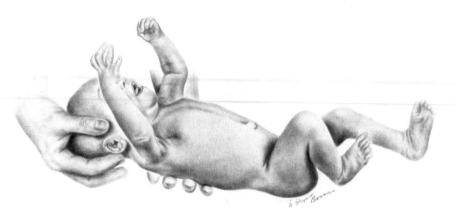

(Redrawn from Paine RS: Neurological examination of infants and children. Pediatr Clin North Am 7:494, 1960)

Neurologic screening to include assessment of positioning, spontaneous and induced movements, cry, knee and ankle jerk responses, and elicitation of the rooting, grasp, tonic neck, and Moro automatisms should be performed on all newborns. Babies showing abnormalities in these areas and those at risk should have repeated complete neurologic assessments.

In *congenital hemiplegia*, absent or diminished movement of the extremities involved plus abnormal posturing is seen rather than any changes in reflexes and muscle tone.

The following *general findings in infancy* should suggest to the clinician the presence of central nervous system disease:

1. Abnormal localized neurological findings

2. Failure to elicit expected responses

3. Asymmetry of normal responses

4. Late persistence of normal responses

5. Re-emergence of vanished responses

6. Developmental delays

Bilateral cerebral palsy produces hypotonia with normal or brisk deep tendon reflexes, delay in reaching motor milestones, and persistence of the tonic neck reflex.

The *spastic diplegias* produce variable dystonic spasms, followed by hypertonus early in infancy and persistent clenched fists coupled with scissoring after the first few months.

EARLY AND LATE CHILDHOOD

Beyond infancy, when the infantile automatisms have disappeared, the neurologic examination is conducted in much the same manner as with the adult. Samples of handwriting and figure drawing with both hands are useful in detecting fine motor defects. Stereognosis, vibration, position, two-point discrimination, number identification, and extinction are usually not testable in the child under 3 years of age, and in many under 5 years. The gait should be observed with the child both walking and running. Asymmetric movements of the arms in walking or running may indicate a hemiparesis, as may unequal wear of the soles and heels on the child's shoes (although there are localized neurologic and orthopedic conditions that may produce unequal shoe wear).

Observe the child rising from the floor from a supine position so that you can note the manner in which the muscles of the neck, trunk, arms, and legs are used to assume first the sitting position and then the standing position (see figures on facing page).

Evidence of neurologic deficits, muscular weaknesses, and orthopedic defects may be detected here that would not be noted otherwise.

In certain forms of *muscular dystrophy* with pelvic girdle weaknesses, rising from a supine to a standing position is accomplished as shown below (*Gowers's sign*).

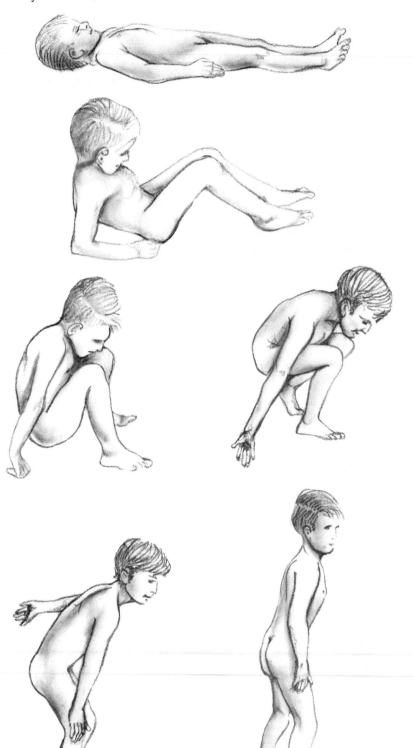

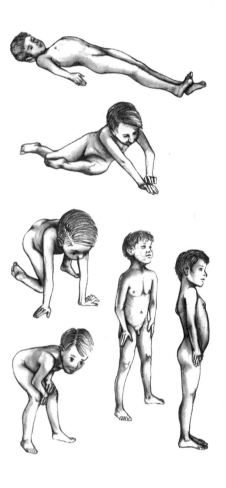

When nystagmus, unsteady gait, or history of streptomycin therapy is present, *vestibular function* should be tested. This is accomplished with the *cold caloric test*.

Inject water at 65°F temperature into the external auditory canal with an ear syringe. Observe for nystagmus, which should occur within 30 seconds.

The absence of nystagmus suggests *drug toxicity, meningitis, brain tumor,* or *labyrinthitis.*

AT ALL AGES

In essence, the complete neurologic examination in infancy and childhood includes elements of all the parts of the general physical examination as well as the specific components of the neurologic examination outlined here. The clinician is constantly assessing neurologic functioning throughout the course of every patient encounter. All of the observations made and impressions gained are used to determine the integrity of the central and peripheral nervous systems. This is equally true in the examination of adults.

Chapter 18
CLINICAL THINKING: FROM DATA TO PLAN

Like colors on an artist's palette, clinical data lack form and meaning. The clinician must not only gather data through interviewing and examination; he or she must also analyze them, identify the patient's problems, evaluate the patient's responses to his own illness, and, together with the patient, formulate a plan. This chapter describes this sequence of activities and focuses on the clinical thinking that underlies it.

FROM DATA BASE TO PLAN

Since Lawrence L. Weed introduced the problem-oriented system of record-keeping, certain terms have gained wide acceptance. Information given by the patient, or possibly by family members or significant others, is called *subjective data. Objective data* include two kinds of information: physical findings and laboratory reports. Since both physical examination and laboratory work are human activities, they too, admittedly, involve subjective elements; and, as we shall see later, all kinds of data are subject to error. A comprehensive set of subjective and objective data, such as you might gather in evaluating a new patient, makes up a *data base* for that patient.

In recording the data base you should describe your findings as accurately as possible, whether they deal with what the patient tells you or with what you observe. Although inference and interpretation inevitably affect the organization of your materials, statements in the data base should describe, not interpret. Thus, "late inspiratory crackles at the bases of both lungs" is appropriate, while "signs of congestive heart failure" is not.

In the *assessment* process, however, you go beyond perception and description to analysis and interpretation. Here you use your mind, not your senses. For example, a patient's complaint of a "scratchy throat" and "stuffy nose," together with your observations of a swollen nasal mucosa and slight redness of the pharynx, give you the subjective and objective data on which to base a presumptive diagnosis of viral naso-pharyngitis.

In order to understand a patient's problems and work out an appropriate plan with him, you will usually need to evaluate not only the patient's health problem but also his responses to it. What does he understand about his illness or about your diagnosis? What are his feelings about it? Why does he feel that way? What are his goals in seeing you? Even in a situation as apparently simple as the patient with nasopharyngitis, consider the implications of the following possibilities: (1) patient A is a student with a very important examination tomorrow; (2) patient B has just heard news of a locally severe epidemic of meningococcal meningitis; (3) patient C's eight-year-old daughter has acute lymphatic leukemia and is scheduled to come home from the hospital in two days. Probably no single plan can meet the needs of all three of these patients.

Once you have tentatively defined the patient's problems and gained at least a preliminary understanding of the patient's responses to them, you are ready to work out a *plan* with the patient. In Weed's terminology a plan has three parts: diagnostic, therapeutic, and educational. For example, you might decide on a throat culture, a decongestant for the patient's stuffy nose, cautionary advice against overfatigue, and a brief review of upper respiratory infections, their causes, and their modes of transmission.

Defining part of the plan as "educational" has one misleading connotation—that the process of communication is unidirectional. It should not be. The patient should participate in making the plan. Appropriate "education" depends on what the patient already knows and wants to know. Find out what his questions are. Other parts of the plan may well be influenced by the patient's goals, his economic means, his responsibilities, and the opinions of family or friends—to name just a few variables. Establishing a successful plan requires interviewing skills and interpersonal sensitivity, not just knowledge of diagnostic and therapeutic techniques.

The diagram below summarizes the sequence from data base to plan. The effects of the assessment process on the data base, as implied by the bidirectional arrows between them, will be discussed later in the chapter.

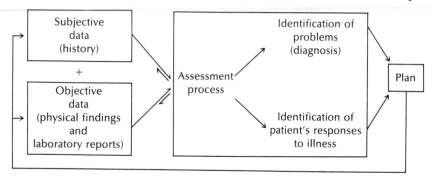

After a plan has been implemented, the process recycles. The clinician gathers more data, assesses the patient's progress, modifies the problem list if indicated, and adjusts the plan appropriately.

ASSESSMENT: THE PROCESS OF CLINICAL THINKING

Since assessment takes place in the clinician's mind, its processes often seem inaccessible, even mysterious, to the beginning student. Experienced clinicians, moreover, think so quickly, with little overt or conscious effort, that they sometimes have difficulty in explaining their own logic. They also think in different ways, with different, individualistic personal styles. Some general principles underlie this analytic process, however, and certain explicit steps may help you think constructively and purposefully about the data that you have gathered. First you must answer the questions, "What is wrong with the patient? What are the problems?" To do so, try the following steps:

1. *Identify the abnormal findings* in the patient's data base. Make a list of the *symptoms* noted by the patient, the *signs* that you observed on physical examination, and any *laboratory reports* that are available to you.

2. *Localize these findings anatomically.* This step may be easy. The symptom of scratchy throat and the sign of a reddened pharynx, for example, clearly localize a problem in the pharynx. Other data, however, present greater difficulty. Chest pain, for example, might originate in the heart, the pleural surfaces, the esophagus, or the musculoskeletal system. If the pain consistently occurs with exercise and disappears with rest, either the heart or possibly the musculoskeletal system is probably involved. If the patient notes pain only when carrying groceries with the left arm, the musculoskeletal system becomes the likely culprit. Be as explicit in your localization as your data allow, but no more so. You may have to settle for a body region (*e.g.*, the chest) or a body system (*e.g.*, musculoskeletal system), or you may be able to define the exact structure involved (*e.g.*, left pectoral muscle). Some symptoms and signs, such as fatigue or fever, have no localizing value but may be useful in the next step, interpreting probable process.

3. *Interpret the findings in terms of the probable process.* A patient's problem may stem from a *pathologic* process involving a bodily structure. There are a number of such processes, variably classified, including congenital, inflammatory, neoplastic, metabolic, degenerative, vascular, traumatic, and toxic. Other problems are *pathophysiologic*, such as increased gastrointestinal motility or congestive heart failure, while others still are *psychopathologic*, such as hallucinations or depression. Redness and pain are two of the four classic signs of inflammation, and a red, painful throat, even without the other two signs—heat and swelling— strongly suggests an inflammatory process in the pharynx.

4. *Make a hypothesis about the nature of the patient's problem.* Here you will have to draw on all the knowledge and experience you can muster, and it is here that reading will be most helpful in learning about abnormalities and diseases. Until your experience and knowledge broaden you may not be able to reach highly explicit hypotheses, but proceed as far as you can with the data and knowledge you have. The following steps should help:

   a. *Select the most specific and central findings* around which to construct your hypothesis. If a patient reports loss of appetite, nausea, vomiting, fatigue, and fever, for example, and if you find a tender, somewhat enlarged liver and mild jaundice, build your hypothesis around jaundice and hepatomegaly rather than fatigue and fever. Although the other symptoms are useful diagnostically, they are much less specific.

   b. Using your inferences about the structures and processes involved, *match your findings against all the conditions you know that can produce them.* For example, you can match your patient's red throat with a list of inflammatory conditions affecting the pharynx; or you can compare the symptoms and signs of the jaundiced patient with the various inflammatory, toxic, and neoplastic conditions that might produce this kind of clinical picture.

   c. *Eliminate those diagnostic possibilities that fail to explain the findings.* You might consider conjunctivitis as a cause of the patient's red eye, for example, but eliminate this possibility because it does not explain the dilated pupil or decreased visual acuity.

   d. *Weigh the competing possibilities* and *select the most likely diagnosis* from among those conditions that might be responsible for the patient's findings. You are looking, of course, for a *close match* between the patient's clinical presentation and a typical case of a given condition. Other clues help in this selection too. The *statistical likelihood* of a given disease in a patient of this age, sex, race, habits, lifestyle, and locality should have major impact on your selection. The *timing of the patient's illness* also makes a difference. Productive cough with purulent sputum, fever, and chest pain that develops acutely over 24 hours suggests quite a different problem than do identical symptoms that develop over 3 or 4 months. In this selection, unfortunately, you can seldom reach certainty but must often settle for the most probable explanation. Such is the real world of applied science.

   e. Finally, in considering possible explanations for a patient's problem, look not only for the most probable diagnoses but search carefully for two other kinds of problems: *potentially life-threatening conditions,* such as myocardial infarction or subdural hematoma, and *potentially treatable conditions,* such as drug-induced delirium. Here you are trying to minimize the risks of missing important, if less frequent or less probable, conditions.

5. Once you have made a hypothesis about a patient's problem, you will usually want to *test that hypothesis.* You may need further history, ad-

ditional maneuvers on physical examination, or laboratory studies to confirm or rule out your tentative diagnosis. When the diagnosis seems clear-cut—a simple upper respiratory infection, for example, or a case of hives—this step may not be necessary.

6. You should then be ready to *establish a working definition of the problem.* Make this at the highest level of explicitness and certainty that the data allow. You may be limited here to a symptom, such as "pleuritic chest pain, cause unknown." At other times you can define a problem explicitly in terms of structure, process, and cause. Examples include "pneumococcal pneumonia, right lower lobe," and "hypertensive cardiovascular disease with left ventricular hypertrophy, congestive heart failure, and sinus tachycardia."

The assessment process is not yet complete. You must next *evaluate the patient's responses to his illness* and to your diagnoses, as previously discussed. What are his understandings, his feelings, and goals? You are then ready to *work out a plan* with the patient for that problem.

DIFFICULTIES AND VARIATIONS

Limitations of the medical model. Although medical diagnosis is based primarily on identifying abnormal structures, disturbed processes, and specific causes, you will frequently see patients whose complaints do not fall neatly into these categories. Some symptoms defy analysis, and you may never be able to move beyond simple descriptive categories such as "fatigue" or "anorexia." Other problems relate to the patient's life rather than to his body. Loss of a job or loved one threatens a person, for example, and probably increases the risk of subsequent illness. Identifying such life events, evaluating a person's responses to them, and working out a plan to help him cope with them are just as appropriate as dealing with his pharyngitis or duodenal ulcer. Some people, moreover, seek health care to maintain their health, not to detect and correct a disease. For them, and most others, in fact, "health maintenance" becomes a legitimate item on a list of "problems," and plans may include, for example, immunizations, nutritional advice, explorations of feelings about an important life event, and recommendations for seat belts or exercise.

Single versus multiple problems. One of the greatest difficulties faced by the student is deciding whether to cluster the patient's symptoms into one or into several problems. The patient's *age* may help, since young people are more likely to have single diseases while older people tend to have multiple ones. Sometimes the *timing* of symptoms helps. An episode of pharyngitis 6 weeks ago is probably unrelated to fever, chills, chest pain, and cough today. Involvement of different *body systems* may be useful. You might decide, for example, to group a patient's high blood pressure and sustained thrusting apical impulse with his narrowed retinal arterioles, place them in the cardiovascular system, and label the constellation "hypertensive cardiovascular disease with hypertensive retinopathy." You will likely develop another problem around his diarrhea and left lower quadrant tenderness. None of these guidelines is foolproof, however, and the way in which you group your data will change impressively as you gain clinical knowledge and experience. Until you learn, for example, that streptococcal pharyngitis may cause acute rheumatic fever or acute glomerulonephritis several weeks later, you will not be able to cluster the past sore throat together with the present swollen joints or with the patient's darkened urine and puffy eyes.

An unmanageable array of data. In trying to understand a patient's problems, the clinician is often confronted with a relatively long list of symptoms and signs and an equally long list of potential explanations or labels. As already suggested, you can tease out separate clusters of observations and deal with them one cluster at a time.

You can also analyze a given group of observations by asking key questions, the answers to which steer your thinking in one direction and allow you to ignore others temporarily. For example, you may ask what produces and relieves a person's chest pain. If the answer is exercise and rest respectively, you can concentrate on the cardiovascular system (and possibly the musculoskeletal system as well) and put aside the gastrointestinal tract. If the pain results from eating quickly and is relieved by regurgitating the food, you logically concentrate on the upper gastrointestinal tract. A series of such discriminating questions forms a branching logic tree or algorithm and has great usefulness in solving clinical problems. The process is fundamentally a matching one, matching a single variable at a time. Most tables in Chapter 16, *Mental Status,* are based primarily on this kind of branched decision-making although they are displayed in a matching format.

Quality of the data. Virtually all the information with which the clinician works is subject to error. Patients forget symptoms, misremember the sequence in which they occurred, hide important but embarrassing facts, and shape their stories toward what interviewers seem to want to hear. Clinicians misunderstand their patients, forget some relevant information, fail to ask the one key question, identify pleural friction rubs as pulmonary crackles, or forget to examine the genitals of a patient with asymptomatic testicular carcinoma. You can avoid some of these errors and should make every effort to do so. Clinical data, however, including laboratory work, are inherently imperfect. The quality of information may be judged by its accuracy, precision, sensitivity, specificity, and predictive value.

Accuracy refers to the closeness with which a measurement reflects the true value of an object. *Precision,* on the other hand, refers to the reproducibility of a measurement. A measurement may be accurate, precise, neither, or both, as exemplified by four sets of attempts to hit a bullseye.

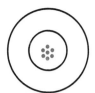

Inaccurate and imprecise	Accurate but imprecise	Inaccurate but precise	Accurate and precise

The fact that estimates of liver size vary between 2 cm and 3 cm depending on the force of percussion demonstrates that liver percussion is not an especially precise technique. The fact that percussion leads to smaller estimates of liver size than do radioisotope liver scans suggests that it is not very accurate either. Even so, percussion provides a better estimate than palpation alone.

Sensitivity of an observation refers to its ability to identify persons with a certain abnormality among a group of people all of whom have that particular abnormality. When an observation fails to identify the abnormality in a person who has it, the result is called falsely negative. A highly sensitive test or observation detects most of the people with a given abnormality and has few false negatives.

Specificity of an observation refers to its ability to identify correctly those people who do *not* have the abnormality. When it fails to do so, it produces a falsely positive result. A test that is 95% specific correctly identifies 95 out of 100 normal people. The other 5 are false positives.

Heart murmurs provide good examples of sensitivity and specificity. The vast majority of patients with significant valvular aortic stenosis have systolic murmurs audible in the aortic area. A systolic murmur is, therefore, quite a sensitive criterion for valvular aortic stenosis. Such a murmur, however, sorely lacks specificity. Many other conditions, such as increased blood flow across a normal valve or the sclerotic changes associated with aging, may also produce this kind of murmur. If you were to use an aortic systolic murmur as your sole criterion for aortic stenosis, you would falsely label many patients, thus producing many false positives. In contrast, the high-pitched decrescendo diastolic murmur heard best in the aortic area and along the left sternal border is a much more specific murmur. Most such murmurs result from aortic regurgitation, although other disorders might produce a similar sound.

The *predictive value* of an observation refers to its ability to predict correctly a certain abnormality in members of a given population. Unlike sensitivity and specificity (where populations by definition are all affected or unaffected respectively), predictive value depends heavily upon the prevalence of the abnormality within that population. Given unchanging sensitivity and specificity, the predictive value of an observation rises with prevalence.

Three examples should help to clarify these often confusing concepts. Consider three imaginary populations, A, B, and C, each consisting of 1000 people. Prevalences of an abnormality within these three groups are 40%, 10%, and 1% respectively. Each population is surveyed with an observation, or test, that has a sensitivity of 90% and a specificity of 80% for that abnormality.

Look first at population A on the opposite page. Given a prevalence of 40%, 400 out of 1000 individuals will have the abnormality. The test will correctly identify 90% of them, thus producing 360 true positives. It will miss the other 40 (400 − 360)—false negatives.

Given a prevalence of 40%, again, 600 of the 1000 people in population A do not have the abnormality. When surveyed by a test that is 80% specific, 480 (600 × 0.80) are correctly identified as normal—true negatives. But 120 (600 − 480) are falsely labelled as abnormal—false positives. Without additional information the clinician unfortunately cannot distinguish between the correctly and falsely labelled individuals, but is faced instead with 480 positives and 520 negatives. How good then is a positive test? Under these circumstances 360 of the 480 positives, or 3 out of 4 (75%), are true positives. How reassuring is a negative test under these circumstances? It is correct 92% of the time.

As prevalence of the abnormality decreases, a positive test diminishes remarkably in its predictive value while a negative test increases in this respect. Study the comparable figures for populations B and C. When the prevalence of the abnormality drops to 1%, for example, only 4% of the apparently positive cases are true positives. Ninety-six percent are false.

Because of figures such as these, your odds of being right improve when you hypothesize common abnormalities as opposed to rare ones. If a patient complains of fever, headaches, muscle pains, and cough, for example, you have a much greater chance of being correct in your diagnosis of influenza during a winter flu epidemic than you do during a quiet August. When you hear hoofbeats in the distance, according to the familiar saying, bet on horses, not on zebras, unless of course you're visiting the zoo.

Unfortunately textbooks rarely describe the accuracy and precision of measurements and rarely enumerate the sensitivity and specificity of various observations. Frequently these data do not exist. Qualitative judgments are often possible, however, and you should acquire a feel for these attributes as time goes on.

When learning a new technique, try to find out how accurate and precise it is. When evaluating a symptom or sign ask the following questions: How sensitive is this item for the diagnosis of a certain abnormality? How specific is it? In a population similar to this patient, living in a similar environment, how prevalent is the abnormality, and therefore how predictive is this item likely to be?

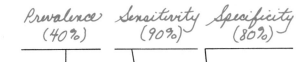

Prevalence
(40%)

Sensitivity
(90%)

Specificity
(80%)

A. Population with a 40% prevalence
of an abnormality

			Test positive	Test negative
Number with abnormality	400		360 (true)	40 (false)
Number without abnormality	600		120 (false)	480 (true)
Total	1000		480	520

Predictive value of a positive test =

$$\frac{360 \text{ true positives}}{480 \text{ total positives}} \times 100 = \boxed{75\%}$$

Predictive value of a negative test =

$$\frac{480 \text{ true negatives}}{520 \text{ total negatives}} \times 100 = \boxed{92\%}$$

B. Population with a 10% prevalence

			Test positive	Test negative
Number with abnormality	100		90 (true)	10 (false)
Number without abnormality	900		180 (false)	720 (true)
Total	1000		270	730

Predictive value of a positive test =

$$\frac{90 \text{ true positives}}{270 \text{ total positives}} \times 100 = \boxed{33\%}$$

Predictive value of a negative test =

$$\frac{720 \text{ true negatives}}{730 \text{ total negatives}} \times 100 = \boxed{99\%}$$

C. Population with a 1% prevalence

			Test positive	Test negative
Number with abnormality	10		9 (true)	1 (false)
Number without abnormality	990		198 (false)	792 (true)
Total	1000		207	793

Predictive value of a positive test =

$$\frac{9 \text{ true positives}}{207 \text{ total positives}} \times 100 = \boxed{4\%}$$

Predictive value of a negative test =

$$\frac{792 \text{ true negatives}}{793 \text{ total negatives}} \times 100 = \boxed{99 + \%}$$

THE INTERPLAY OF ASSESSMENT AND DATA COLLECTION

Beginning students have insufficient experience and knowledge to judge what parts of the data base they should emphasize and what parts they may survey quickly or safely omit. They usually end up with a much more extensive set of information than do more experienced clinicians, and at least some of it seems to lack relevance. One reason for this difference lies in the interplay between the assessment process and the collection of data.

Students have to collect comprehensive histories and perform reasonably complete physical examinations because these skills will be needed in assessing many, if not all, of their future patients. With experience, however, clinicians are guided not only by the systems they have learned but also by active assessment and thought. Experienced clinicians begin to formulate their hypotheses during the first moments of their encounter with the patient. Both the patient's appearance and his chief complaint stimulate hypotheses in the clinician's mind, and subsequent questions serve to test these hypotheses. So does each portion of the examination.

A patient with cutaneous vesicles exemplifies this point. A student may need to examine a patient thoroughly, then seek out a dermatology text, look up all the causes of vesicles and bullae, and match the patient's case against these possibilities. In contrast, the experienced clinician might make a quick series of observations: "vesicles, linear arrangement, exposed area, itchy, short duration," and offer the instant diagnosis of poison ivy.

As your experience and knowledge grow, your assessment process will increasingly affect your data collection. It should sharpen the relevance of your questions and guide you toward examining certain parts of the patient with special care and detail.

But beware of the dangers. First, initial judgments are often wrong. They allow you to overlook important data and may prevent you from entertaining other, possibly sounder hypotheses. Second, premature formulation of hypotheses may lead you to the premature asking of direct questions, and thus you may miss important parts of the patient's story. Third, focusing in on a single problem may lead you to incomplete assessment. Not every patient needs a complete evaluation, of course, but some have hypertension, some are seriously depressed, and some have cervical cancer. You cannot detect these problems unless you make the proper observations; to do so you have to be reasonably complete.

DEVELOPING A PROBLEM LIST AND PLAN

Turn now to the history and physical examination recorded for Mrs. N. in Chapter 19. Make a list of her symptoms and signs. Group these items together in a clinically rational way. Note that much of this clustering has already been done in constructing Mrs. N's present illness, since headache, nausea, vomiting, malaise, and psychological stress have all been placed together. You may or may not agree with this organization. Identify the problems insofar as you can, and assess the patient's response to her illness.

Make a tentative problem list. In the Weed system two parallel columns are used: active problems go on the left, inactive ones on the right. The problem list is placed at the front of the patient's clinical record, and all notes refer to these problems by name and number.

Date problem entered	No.	Active problems	Inactive problems
	1		

For each active problem, develop an initial plan insofar as you can. Some problems, of course, may need no immediate attention. Undoubtedly you will want more information in some areas. Make getting it part of your plan.

Chapter 19
THE PATIENT'S RECORD

The patient's clinical record documents in lasting form his history and physical findings. It shows how clinicians assessed his problems, what plans they made on his behalf, what actions they took, and how he responded to their efforts. An accurate, clear, well organized record facilitates clinical thinking. It leads to good communication among the many professionals who participate in caring for the patient, and helps to coordinate their activities. It also serves to document the patient's problems and care for medicolegal purposes.

When creating a patient's record you do more than simply make a list of what he has told you and what you have found on examination. You must review your data, organize them, evaluate the importance and relevance of each item, and construct a clear, concise, yet comprehensive report. If you are a beginner, organizing the present illness will probably constitute one of the most difficult problems because considerable knowledge is needed to recognize which symptoms and signs are related to each other. That muscular weakness, heat intolerance, excessive sweating, diarrhea, and weight loss all constitute a present illness, for example, may not be apparent to either the patient or the student who is unfamiliar with hyperthyroidism. Until your knowledge and judgment grow, the patient's story itself and the seven key attributes of symptoms listed on pages 2 and 13 are helpful guides.

Regardless of your experience, certain principles will help you organize a good record. Order is imperative. Use it consistently and obviously so that future readers, including yourself, can easily find specific points of information. Keep items of history in the history, for example, and do not let them stray into the physical examination. Make your headings clear, use indentations and spacing to accentuate your organization, and asterisk or underline important points. Arrange the present illness in chronological order, starting with the current episode and then filling in the relevant background information. If a patient with longstanding diabetes is hospitalized in coma, for example, start with the events leading up to the coma, then summarize the past history of the diabetes.

The amount of detail to be recorded often poses a vexing problem. As a student, be quite detailed, since doing so is the only way to build your descriptive skills, vocabulary, and speed—admittedly a painful, tedious process. Pressures of time, however, will ultimately force some compromises. The following guidelines may be useful in choosing what to record and what to omit:

1. *Record all the data*—both positive and negative—*that contribute directly to your assessment.* No diagnosis should be made, no problem identified, unless you have clearly spelled out the data upon which your assessment is based.

2. *Describe specifically any pertinent negative information (i.e.,* the absence of a symptom or a sign) when other portions of the history or physical examination suggest that an abnormality might exist or develop in that area. For example, if the patient has a loud, apical, pansystolic murmur, suggesting mitral regurgitation (which might have been caused by past rheumatic fever), you should specifically note the negative history for streptococcal sore throats, rheumatic fever, and arthritis in earlier life. If a patient feels depressed but not suicidal, state both facts. If the patient has no emotional problems, on the other hand, a comment on suicide is clearly unnecessary.

3. *Data not recorded are data lost.* No matter how vividly you can recall a detail today, you will probably not remember it in a few months. The phrase "neurologic exam negative," even in your own handwriting, may leave you wondering a few months hence: "Did I really do a sensory exam?"

4. On the other hand, information can be buried in a mass of excessive detail, to be discovered by only the most persistent reader. *Avoid long lists of relatively minor negative findings, as well as repetitive introductory phrases* such as "The patient reports no . . . ."

5. *Be as objective as possible.* Hostility, moralizing comments, disgust, and disapproval have no place in the patient's record, whether conveyed in words, penmanship, or punctuation. Notes such as "PATIENT DRUNK AND LATE TO CLINIC AGAIN!!" tell more about the writer than about the patient and, furthermore, might prove embarrassing in court.

Because records are scientific and legal documents, they should be understandable. Employ abbreviations and symbols only if they are commonly used and understood. Some clinicians may wish to develop an elegant style and should certainly be encouraged to do so. Time is usually scarce, however, and style may be sacrificed in favor of concise completeness. In the sample record that follows, for example, words and brief phrases substitute for whole sentences. Legibility, of course, is always a virtue. Diagrams add greatly to the speed and ease with which a record communicates its message. Two examples follow:

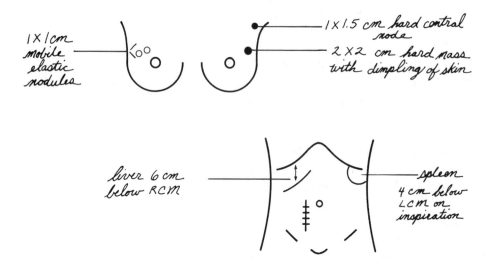

Make measurements in centimeters, not in fruits, vegetables, or nuts. "Pea-sized," "lemon-sized," and "walnut-sized" lesions vaguely convey an idea but make accurate evaluations and future comparisons impossible. How big were the lemons or peas? Did the walnut have a shell?

You should write the record as soon as possible, before the data fade from your memory. In your initial attempts at interviewing, you will probably prefer just to take notes when talking with a patient. As you gain experience, however, work toward recording in final form the past medical history, family history, and review of systems as you take them. Leave spaces for filling in later the present illness, the psychosocial history, and any other complex areas. During a physical examination it is wise to record immediately such specific measurements as the blood pressures in three positions. Recording a large number of items and descriptions interrupts the flow of the examination, however, and you will soon learn to remember your findings until you have finished.

Recording the history and physical examination is simplified, of course, by printed forms. Use them if your institution or agency provides them. You should also, however, be able to create a record without using a form. The example that follows offers one moderately complete guide. Note the difference in the statements that introduce the history and the physical examination. The basic identifying data start the history, while a descriptive paragraph that summarizes your general survey begins the physical examination.

Mrs. Audrey N., 1463 Maple Blvd., Capital City

12/13/82

Mrs. N. is a 54-year-old, widowed, white saleswoman.

Referral. None

Source. Self, seems reliable

Chief Complaint. Headaches

Present Illness. For about 3 months Mrs. N. has been increasingly troubled by headaches: bifrontal, usually aching, occasionally throbbing, mild to moderately severe. She has missed work only once because of headaches, when she felt nauseated and miserable and vomited several times. Otherwise, nausea is associated only occasionally. Headaches now average once a week, usually are there when she wakes up, and last all day. Little relief from aspirin. It helps to lie down, be quiet, use cold wet towel on head. No other related symptoms, no local weakness, no numbness or visual symptoms.

Mrs. N. first began to have headaches at age 15. "Sick headaches" recurred through her mid-20s, then diminished to one every 2 or 3 months and finally almost disappeared.

Has recently had increased pressure at work, is also worried about daughter (see psychosocial). Thinks headaches may be like those in the past, but wants to be sure because mother died of a stroke. Is concerned that they make her irritable with her family.

Past Medical History

General Health. Good

Childhood Illnesses. Only measles and chickenpox

Immunizations. Smallpox vaccination as child; oral polio vaccine, year uncertain; tetanus shots × 2 three years ago followed by a booster a year later; others uncertain

Adult Illnesses. None serious

Psychiatric Illness. None

Operations. Tonsillectomy, age 6; appendectomy, age 13

Injuries. Stepped on glass at beach 3 years ago, laceration, sutured, healed

Hospitalizations. St. Mary's, acute kidney infection, age 42

Current Medications. Aspirin for headaches, multivitamins. Has taken "water pill" for ankle swelling, but none in past several months.

*Allergies. Generalized skin rash with itching from <u>sulfa,</u> age 42

Habits

> *Diet.* Breakfast—Orange juice, two sweet rolls, black coffee
> Mid-morning—Doughnut, coffee
> Lunch—Hamburger and bun or fish sandwich, coffee
> Dinner—Meat or fish, vegetable, potato, sometimes fruit, sometimes cookies
> Snacks in evening (*e.g.*, chips, cola)
> Has almost no milk or cheese
> *Exercise.* Prolonged standing at work, little other exercise
> *Alcohol.* Rare, doesn't like it
> *Tobacco.* About one pack cigarettes per day from age 18 (36 pack years)
> *Sleep.* Generally good, average 7 hours, sometimes has trouble falling asleep, is waked by alarm

Family History. (There are two methods of recording the family history. The diagrammatic format is more helpful than the narrative in tracing genetic disorders. The negative family information follows either format.)

1. *Diagrammatic*

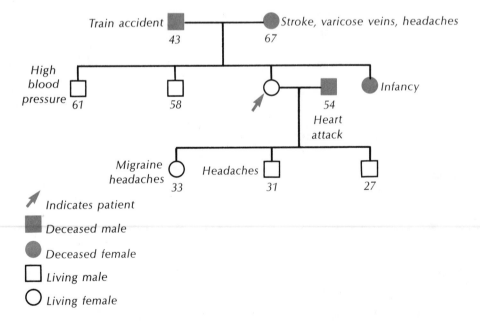

2. Narrative Outline

Father died age 43, train accident
Mother died age 67, stroke, had had varicose veins, headaches
One brother, age 61, has high blood pressure, otherwise well
One brother, age 58, apparently well but for mild arthritis
One sister, died in infancy, ? cause
Husband died age 54, heart attack
One daughter, age 33, "migraine headaches," otherwise well
One son, age 31, headaches
One son, age 27, well

No family history of diabetes, tuberculosis, heart or kidney disease, cancer, anemia, or mental illness

Psychosocial. Born and raised in Lake City, finished high school, married at age 19. Worked in store for 2 years, then moved with husband to Capital City, had 3 children. Mr. N. had steady factory job but to help with income Mrs. N. went back to work 10 years ago. Children have all married. Four years ago Mr. N. died suddenly of a heart attack. Finances now tight. Has moved to small apartment to be near daughter, Dorothy. Dorothy's husband has a drinking problem and Mrs. N.'s apartment serves as a haven for Dorothy and her two young children. Mrs. N. feels responsible for helping the family, is tense and nervous, but denies depression.

Typically up at 7:00 a.m., works 9:00 to 5:30, eats dinner alone. Dorothy or children visit most evenings and weekends. Moderate number of squabbles and considerable strain.

Review of Systems

General. Has gained about 10 pounds in the past 4 years

Skin. No rashes or other changes

Head. No head injury (see present illness)

Eyes. Reading glasses for 5 years, last checked a year ago; no other symptoms

Ears. Hearing good; no tinnitus, vertigo, infections

Nose, Sinuses. Occasional mild cold; no hay fever or sinus trouble

Mouth and Throat. Some bleeding of gums recently; last to dentist 2 years ago; occasional canker sore, has had one for 4 days

Neck. No lumps, goiter, or pain

Breasts. No lumps, pain, discharge; does breast self exams sporadically

Respiratory. No cough, wheezing, pneumonia, tuberculosis; last chest x-ray 12 years ago, St. Mary's Hospital, normal

Cardiac. No known heart disease or high blood pressure; last blood pressure taken 3 years ago; no dyspnea, orthopnea, chest pain, palpitations; no EKG

*GI. Appetite good; no nausea, vomiting, indigestion; bowel movement about once daily though sometimes has <u>hard stools, q 2–3 days, when especially tense;</u> no diarrhea or bleeding; no pain, jaundice, gallbladder, or liver trouble

*Urinary. <u>Acute kidney infection,</u> age 42, with fever and right flank pain; treated with pills, including sulfa; no recurrence; no frequency, dysuria, or hematuria; nocturia × 1, large volume; <u>occasionally loses some urine</u> when coughs hard

Genito–reproductive. Menarche at 13, regular periods, tapered off in late 40s and stopped at 49; no bleeding since; mild hot flashes and sweats then, none now

Gravida 3, para 3, living children 3; prolonged labor during first pregnancy, otherwise normal; little sexual interest now

*Musculoskeletal. Mild <u>aching low back</u> often after a long day's work; no radiation down legs; used to do back exercises, but not now; no other joint pain

*Peripheral Vascular. <u>Varicose veins</u> appeared in both legs during first pregnancy; has had swollen ankles after prolonged standing, for 10 years; wears light elastic pantyhose; tried "water pill" several months ago but it didn't help much; no history of phlebitis or leg pain

Neurologic. No faints, seizures, motor or sensory loss; memory good

Psychiatric. (see present illness and psychosocial)

Endocrine. No known thyroid trouble, temperature intolerance; sweating average; no symptoms or history of diabetes

Hematologic. Except for bleeding gums, no easy bleeding, no anemia

Physical Examination

Mrs. N. is a short, moderately obese, middle-aged woman who walks and moves easily and responds quickly to questions. She wears no makeup but her hair is neatly fixed and her clothes immaculate. Although her ankles are swollen, her color is good and she lies flat without discomfort. She talks freely but is somewhat tense, with moist, cold hands.

P 94, regular   R 18   BP 164/98 right arm, lying
                                 160/95 left arm, lying
                                 152/88 right arm, lying (wide cuff)

                                 Ht (without shoes) 157 cm (5'2")
Temp 37.1°C (oral)   Wt (dressed) 65 kg (143 lbs.)

Skin. Palms cold and moist, but color good. Scattered cherry angiomas over the upper trunk

Head. Hair of average texture. Scalp and skull normal

Eyes. Vision 20/30 in both eyes. Fields not done. Conjunctivas show good color. Scleras clear. Pupils are round, regular, equal, react to light and accommodation. Extraocular movements intact. Disc margins sharp. No arteriolar narrowing, A-V nicking, hemorrhages, or exudates

Ears. Wax partially obscures the right drum. Left canal clear and drum negative. Acuity good (to whispered voice)

Nose. Mucosa pink, septum midline. No sinus tenderness

*Mouth. Mucosa pink. Several interdental papillae red and slightly swollen. Teeth in good repair. Tongue midline, negative but for a small (3 × 4 mm), shallow, white <u>ulcer</u> on an erythematous base, located on the under surface near the tip. It is slightly tender but not indurated. Tonsils absent. Pharynx negative

Neck. Trachea midline. Thyroid isthmus barely palpable, lobes not felt

Nodes. Small (less than 1 cm), soft, nontender, and mobile tonsillar and posterior cervical nodes bilaterally. No axillary or epitrochlear nodes. Several small inguinal nodes bilaterally—soft and nontender

Thorax and Lungs. Thorax symmetrical. Good excursion. Lungs resonant. Diaphragm descends 4 cm on inspiration. Breath sounds normal with no added sounds

*Heart. Apical impulse barely palpable in the 5th left interspace 8 cm from the midsternal line. Physiologic splitting of S_2. No S_3 or S_4. A grade 2/6† medium-pitched midsystolic <u>murmur</u> heard at the aortic area; does not radiate to the neck

---

†A 2/6 murmur refers to a grade 2 murmur in a classification that has six grades.

Jugular venous pressure at the level of the sternal angle, with the patient elevated at 30°. Carotid pulses normal and symmetrical

Breasts. Large, pendulous, symmetrical. No masses. Nipples erect and without discharge

Abdomen. Obese, but symmetrical. Well-healed right lower quadrant scar. Bowel sounds normal. Except for a slightly tender sigmoid colon, no masses or tenderness. Liver, spleen, and kidneys not felt. Liver span 7 cm in the right midclavicular line. No CVA tenderness

*Genitalia. Vulva normal. On straining, a mild cystocele appears. Vagina negative. Parous cervix without redness or tenderness. Uterus anterior, midline, smooth, not enlarged. Adnexa are difficult to delineate because of obesity and poor relaxation, but there is no tenderness. Pap smears taken. Rectovaginal examination confirms above.

Rectal. Negative. Brown stool, negative for occult blood

*Peripheral Vascular
Pulses (4+ = normal)

	Radial	Femoral	Popliteal	Dorsalis Pedis	Posterior Tibial
Rt	4+	4+	4+	4+	4+
Lt	4+	4+	4+	4+	4+

2+ edema of feet and ankles with 1+ edema extending up to just below the knees. Moderate varicosities of the saphenous veins bilaterally from mid-thigh to ankles, with venous stars on both lower legs. No stasis pigmentation or ulcers. No calf tenderness

Musculoskeletal. No joint deformities. Range of motion, including hands, wrists, elbows, shoulders, spine, hips, knees, ankles, is normal.

Neurological
  Cranial nerves. See head and neck. Also—

    N_5—Sensation intact, strength good

    N_7—Facial movement good

    N_{11}—Sternomastoids and trapezii strong

Motor. No atrophy, fasciculations, tremors. Gait, heel-to-toe, heel and toe walking, knee bends, hops well done. Romberg negative. Grip and arms strong

Sensory. Pain, vibration, light touch, and stereognosis screened and intact

Reflexes. (Two methods of recording may be used, depending upon personal preference: a tabular form or a stick figure diagram, as shown below.)

	Biceps	Triceps	Sup	Abd	Knee	Ankle	Pl
Rt	2+	2+	2+	2+/2+	2+	1+	↓
Lt	2+	2+	2+	2+/2+	2+	1+	↓

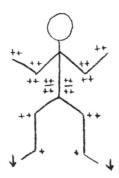

Mental Status. Tense but alert and cooperative. Thought coherent. Oriented. Cognitive testing not done in detail

Before turning the page and reading further, construct your own problem list for Mrs. N., as suggested in Chapter 18. The sequence in which problems are listed does not matter, because the importance of individual problems may be expected to change over time. One way to organize Mrs. N's problem list is shown on the following page.

Date problem entered	No.	Active problems	Inactive problems
12/13/82	1	Migraine headaches	
12/13/82	2		Acute kidney infection
12/13/82	3	Allergy to sulfa	
12/13/82	4	Tensions secondary to family situation, finances, and stress at work	
12/13/82	5	Gingivitis	
12/13/82	6	Low back pain	
12/13/82	7	Varicose veins with venous insufficiency	
12/13/82	8	Cystocele with occasional stress incontinence	
12/13/82	9	Borderline blood pressure	
12/13/82	10	Diet high in calories and carbohydrates, low in calcium	

Different clinicians often organize somewhat different problem lists for the same patient, and yours probably does not agree exactly with this one. Good lists vary in their emphases, length, and detail according to many factors, including the clinicians' philosophies, specialties, and perceptions of their appropriate roles in the care of the patient. The list illustrated here includes problems that need some attention now (such as the headaches) or may need further observation or possible future attention (such as the blood pressure and cystocele). The allergy is listed as an active problem to warn against inadvertent future prescriptions of sulfa drugs.

A few items noted in the history and physical examination, such as canker sores and constipation, do not appear in this problem list because they are relatively common phenomena that do not seem to demand attention. Such judgments are occasionally wrong, of course. Problem lists that are cluttered with relatively insignificant items, however, diminish in value. Some clinicians would undoubtedly judge this list too long; others would bring greater explicitness to problems such as "tensions," "diet," and "gingivitis." No one can specialize in everything.

When Mrs. N. was first seen, limitations of time precluded planning for all of her problems, so priority was given to the headaches. The clinician explained the nature of migraine headaches and asked her to watch for possible precipitating factors. A month later she returned for a second visit. Part of the progress notes read as follows:

1. Migraine headaches

   Subjective (S). Has had only two headaches, both mild, without associated symptoms. No longer worried about them. Cannot detect any precipitating factors

   Objective (O). Not reexamined

   Assessment (A). Improved

   Plan (P). Return as needed

9. Borderline blood pressure

   S. None

   O. BP 152/86 right arm, lying (regular cuff)
      Urinalysis, EKG normal

   A. As before

   P. Repeat BP in 3 months

Although you have insufficient information about most of Mrs. N.'s other problems, including her own priorities, try to develop an approach to them. What further data do you need?

What information do you need and how do you obtain it? These are the questions with which the book began and which continue throughout it—and long afterward. The process of learning about a patient continues far beyond the first encounter, and understanding grows in depth, complexity, and fascination. Although your knowledge of Mrs. N. is incomplete, you know a great deal about her and have the tools with which to expand your knowledge further. Needed now is repetitive practice, with supervision, in using your newly acquired tools.

Bibliography

GENERAL REFERENCES

PHYSICAL EXAMINATION

Bouchier IAD, Morris JS: Clinical Skills: A System of Clinical Examination. London, WB Saunders, 1976

Buckingham WB: A Primer of Clinical Diagnosis, 2nd ed. Hagerstown, Harper & Row, 1979

Burnside JW: Physical Diagnosis: An Introduction to Clinical Medicine, 16th ed. Baltimore, Williams & Wilkins, 1981

Clain A: Bailey's Demonstrations of Physical Signs in Clinical Surgery, 16th ed. Chicago, Year Book Medical Publishers, 1980

DeGowin EL, DeGowin RL: Bedside Diagnostic Examination, 4th ed. Philadelphia, WB Saunders, 1981

Delp MH, Manning RT: Major's Physical Diagnosis, 9th ed. Philadelphia, WB Saunders, 1981

Dunphy JE, Botsford TW: Physical Examination of the Surgical Patient: An Introduction to Clinical Surgery, 4th ed. Philadelphia, WB Saunders, 1975

Judge RD, Zuidema GD: Methods of Clinical Examination: A Physiologic Approach, 3rd ed. Boston, Little, Brown & Co, 1974

MacLeod J: Clinical Examination, 5th ed. Edinburgh, Churchill Livingstone, 1979

Morgan WL Jr, Engel GL: The Clinical Approach to the Patient. Philadelphia, WB Saunders, 1969

Patient Assessment. A series of programmed units.
Taking a patient's history. Amer J Nurs 74:293,1974
Examination of the abdomen. Amer J Nurs 74:1679,1974
Examination of the eye, Part I. Amer J Nurs 74:2039,1974
Examination of the eye, Part II. Amer J Nurs 75:105,1975
Examination of the ear. Amer J Nurs 75:457,1975
Examination of the head and neck. Amer J Nurs 75:839,1975
Neurological examination, Part I. Amer J Nurs 75:1511,1975
Neurological examination, Part II. Amer J Nurs 75:2037,1975
Neurological examination, Part III. Amer J Nurs 76:609,1976
Examination of the chest and lungs. Amer J Nurs 76:1453,1976
Examination of the heart and great vessels. Amer J Nurs 76:1807,1976

Examination of the heart, Part II. Auscultation of the heart. Amer J Nurs 77:275,1977

Abnormalities of the heartbeat. Amer J Nurs 77:647,1977

Examination of the female pelvis, Part I. Amer J Nurs 78:1717,1978

Examination of the female pelvis, Part II. Amer J Nurs 78:1913,1978

Pulses. Amer J Nurs 79:115,1979

Examination of the male genitalia. Amer J Nurs 79:689,1979

Examining joints of the upper and lower extremities. Amer J Nurs 81:763,1981

Mental status assessment. Amer J Nurs 81:1493, 1981

Prior JA, Silberstein JS: Physical Diagnosis. The History and Examination of the Patient, 6th ed. St Louis, CV Mosby, 1981

Walker HK, Hall WD, Hurst JW (eds): Clinical Methods: The History, Physical and Laboratory Examinations. Boston, Butterworth & Co, 1980

Walker WF: Color Atlas of General Surgical Diagnosis. Chicago, Year Book Medical Publishers, 1976

Zatouroff M: Color Atlas of Physical Signs in General Medicine. Chicago, Year Book Medical Publishers, 1976

ANATOMY AND PHYSIOLOGY

Anson BJ, McVay CB: Surgical Anatomy, 5th ed. Philadelphia, WB Saunders, 1971

Basmajian JV: Grant's Method of Anatomy, 10th ed. Baltimore, Williams & Wilkins, 1980

Guyton AC: Textbook of Medical Physiology, 6th ed. Philadelphia, WB Saunders, 1981

Moore KL: Clinically Oriented Anatomy. Baltimore, Williams & Wilkins, 1980

Snell RS: Atlas of Clinical Anatomy. Boston, Little, Brown & Co, 1978

Snell RS: Clinical Anatomy for Medical Students, 2nd ed. Boston, Little, Brown & Co, 1981

CHANGES WITH AGE

Adolescents

Daniel WA Jr: Adolescents in Health and Disease. St Louis, CV Mosby, 1977

Gallagher JR, Heald FP, Garell DC: Medical Care of the Adolescent, 3rd ed. New York, Appleton-Century-Crofts, 1976

Tanner JM: Growth at Adolescence, 2nd ed. Oxford, Blackwell Scientific Publications, 1962

Older Persons

Anderson WF, Caird FI, Kennedy RD et al: Gerontology and Geriatric Nursing. New York, Arco Publishing, 1982

Birren JE, Schaie KW (eds): Handbook of the Psychology of Aging. New York, Van Nostrand Reinhold, 1977

Brocklehurst JC (ed): Textbook of Geriatric Medicine and Gerontology, 2nd ed. Edinburgh, Churchill Livingstone, 1978

Brocklehurst JC, Hanley T: Geriatric Medicine for Students. Edinburgh, Churchill Livingstone, 1976

Caird FI, Judge TG: Assessment of the Elderly Patient, 2nd ed. Philadelphia, JB Lippincott, 1979

Finch CE, Hayflick L (eds): Handbook of the Biology of Aging. New York, Van Nostrand Reinhold, 1977

Mezey MD, Rauckhorst LH, Stokes SA: Health Assessment of the Older Individual. New York, Springer Publishing, 1980

Reichel W (ed): Clinical Aspects of Aging. Baltimore, Williams & Wilkins, 1978

Rossman I (ed): Clinical Geriatrics, 2nd ed. Philadelphia, JB Lippincott, 1979

MEDICINE AND SURGERY

Harvey AM, Johns RJ, McKusick VA et al (eds): The Principles and Practice of Medicine, 20th ed. New York, Appleton-Century-Crofts, 1980

Isselbacher KJ, Adams RD, Braunwald E et al (eds): Harrison's Principles of Internal Medicine, 9th ed. New York, McGraw-Hill, 1980

MacBryde CM, Blacklow RS: Signs and Symptoms: Applied Pathologic Physiology and Clinical Interpretation, 5th ed. Philadelphia, JB Lippincott, 1970

Sabiston DC Jr (ed): Davis-Christopher Textbook of Surgery: The Biological Basis of Modern Surgical Practice. Philadelphia, WB Saunders, 1981

Schwartz SI (ed): Principles of Surgery, 3rd ed. New York, McGraw-Hill, 1979

Wyngaarden J, Smith LH (eds): Cecil Textbook of Medicine, 16th ed. Philadelphia, WB Saunders, 1982

CHAPTER 1. INTERVIEWING AND THE HEALTH HISTORY

Benjamin A: The Helping Interview, 2nd ed. Boston, Houghton Mifflin, 1974

Bernstein L, Bernstein RS: Interviewing: A Guide for Health Professionals, 3rd ed. New York, Appleton-Century-Crofts, 1980

Bird B: Talking with Patients, 2nd ed. Philadelphia, JB Lippincott, 1973

Boyle WE: The pediatric history. In Hoekelman RA, Blatman S, Brunell PA (eds): Principles of Pediatrics: Health Care of the Young. New York, McGraw-Hill, 1978

Butler RN, Lewis MI: Aging and Mental Health: Positive Psychosocial and Biomedical Approaches. St Louis, CV Mosby, 1982

Daniel WA Jr: Adolescents in Health and Disease. St Louis, CV Mosby, 1977

Elling R, Whittemore R, Green M: Patient participation in a pediatric program. J Health Hum Behav 1:183, 1960

Enelow AJ, Swisher SN: Interviewing and Patient Care, 2nd ed. New York, Oxford University Press, 1979

Engel GL, Morgan WL Jr: Interviewing the Patient. Philadelphia, WB Saunders, 1973

Felman YM, Nikitas JA: Obtaining history of patient's sexual activities. NY State J Med 79:1879, 1979

Freeman MG: Sexual difficulties. In Walker HK, Hale WD, Hurst JW (eds): Clinical Methods: The History, Physical and Laboratory Examinations, 2nd ed, p 276. Boston, Butterworth & Co, 1980

Froelich RE, Bishop FM: Clinical Interviewing Skills: A Programmed Manual for Data Gathering, Evaluation, and Patient Management, 3rd ed. St Louis, CV Mosby, 1977

Green R: Taking a sexual history. In Green R: Human Sexuality: A Health Practitioner's Text. Baltimore, Williams & Wilkins, 1975

Hackett TP, Cassem NH (eds): Massachusetts General Hospital Handbook of General Hospital Psychiatry. St Louis, CV Mosby, 1978

Korsch BM, Freemon B, Negrete VF: Practical implications of doctor-patient interaction analysis for pediatric practice. Amer J Dis Child 121:110, 1971

Kübler-Ross E: On Death and Dying. New York, Macmillan, 1969

Platt WP, McMath JC: Clinical hypocompetence: The interview. Ann Intern Med 91:898, 1979

Reiser DE, Schroder AK: Patient Interviewing: The Human Dimension. Baltimore, Williams & Wilkins, 1980

Sapira JD: Reassurance therapy. What to say to symptomatic patients with benign diseases. Ann Intern Med 77:603, 1972

Starfield B, Borkowf S: Physicians' recognition of complaints made by parents about their children's health. Pediatrics 43:168, 1969

CHAPTER 3. THE GENERAL SURVEY

Nichols GA: Taking adult temperatures: Rectal measurements. Am J Nurs 72:1092, 1972

Nichols GA, Kucha DH: Taking adult temperatures: Oral measurements. Am J Nurs 72:1091, 1972

Sorlie P, Gordon T, Kannel WB: Body build and mortality: The Framingham study. JAMA 243:1828, 1980

Tanner JM: Growing up. Sci Am 229, No. 3:34, 1973

CHAPTER 4. THE SKIN

Fitzpatrick TB, Eisen AZ, Wolff K et al (eds): Dermatology in General Medicine, 2nd ed. New York, McGraw-Hill, 1979

Korting GW: Geriatric Dermatology. Curth W, Curth HO (trans): Philadelphia, WB Saunders, 1980

Melick R, Taft HP: Observations on body hair in old people. J Clin Endocrinol Metab 19:597, 1959

Moschella SL, Pillsbury DM, Hurley HJ Jr: Dermatology. Philadelphia, WB Saunders, 1975

Sauer GC: Manual of Skin Diseases, 4th ed. Philadelphia, JB Lippincott, 1980

CHAPTER 5. THE HEAD AND NECK

EYES

Arsham GM, Colenbrander A, Spivey BE: Basic Instruction in Ophthalmoscopy. Iowa City: University of Iowa, 1971. (A teaching package of 80 slides, 2 audiotape cassettes and a study guide)

Havener WH: Synopsis of Ophthalmology, 5th ed. St Louis, CV Mosby, 1979

Kornzweig AL: The eye in old age. In Rossman I (ed): Clinical Geriatrics, 2nd ed, p 369. Philadelphia, JB Lippincott, 1979

Macaraeg PVJ Jr, Lasagna L, Snyder B: Arcus not so senilis. Ann Intern Med 68:345, 1968

Michaelson IC: Textbook of the Fundus of the Eye, 3rd ed. Edinburgh, Churchill Livingstone, 1980

Newell FW: Ophthalmology: Principles and Concepts, 5th ed. St Louis, CV Mosby, 1982

Van Uitert RL, Eisenstadt ML: Venous pulsations not always indicative of normal intracranial pressure. Arch Neurol 35:550, 1978

Vaughan D, Asbury T: General Ophthalmology, 9th ed. Los Altos, CA, Lange Medical Publications, 1980

EARS, NOSE, AND THROAT

Adams GL, Boies LR Jr, Paparella MM: Boies's Fundamentals of Otolaryngology, 5th ed. Philadelphia, WB Saunders, 1978

Bull TR: Color Atlas of E.N.T. Diagnosis. Chicago, Year Book Medical Publishers, 1974

DeWeese DD, Saunders WH: Textbook of Otolaryngology, 5th ed. St Louis, CV Mosby, 1977

MOUTH

McCarthy PL, Shklar G: Diseases of the Oral Mucosa, 2nd ed. Philadelphia, Lea & Febiger, 1980

Pindborg JJ: Atlas of Diseases of the Oral Mucosa. Philadelphia, WB Saunders, 1980

Shklar G, McCarthy PL: The Oral Manifestations of Systemic Disease. Boston, Butterworth & Co, 1976

NECK

Linet OI, Metzler C: Practical ENT: Incidence of palpable cervical nodes in adults. Postgrad Med 62, No. 4:210, 1977

Solnitzky OC, Jeghers H: Lymphadenopathy and disorders of the lymphatic system. In MacBryde CM, Blacklow RS (eds): Signs and Symptoms: Applied Pathologic Physiology and Clinical Interpretation, 5th ed. Philadelphia, JB Lippincott, 1970

Werner SC: Physical examination. In Werner SC, Ingbar SH (eds): The Thyroid, p 437. Hagerstown, Harper & Row, 1978

CHAPTER 6. THE THORAX AND LUNGS

Capel LH: Lung sounds: A new approach. Practitioner 219:633, 1977

Epler GR, Carrington CB, Gaensler EA: Crackles (rales) in the interstitial pulmonary diseases. Chest 73:333, 1978

Fishman AP: Pulmonary Diseases and Disorders. New York, McGraw-Hill, 1980

Forgacs P: The functional basis of pulmonary sounds. Chest 73:399, 1978

Forgacs P: Lung Sounds. London, Baillière Tindall, 1978

Updated nomenclature for membership reaction. Reports from the ATS Ad Hoc Committee on Pulmonary Nomenclature. ATS News 7:8, Winter 1981

CHAPTER 7. THE HEART, PRESSURES, AND PULSES

Braunwald E (ed): Heart Disease: A Textbook of Cardiovascular Medicine. Philadelphia, WB Saunders, 1980

Fowler NO: Examination of the Heart, Part 2. Inspection and Palpation of Venous and Arterial Pulses. Dallas, American Heart Association, 1972

Giuliani ER, Brandenburg RO, Fuster V: Evaluation of cardiac murmurs. Cardiovasc Clin 10, No. 3:1, 1980

Hammond JH, Eisinger RP: Carotid bruits in 1,000 normal subjects. Arch Intern Med 109:563, 1962

Hurst JW, Hopkins LC, Smith RB III: Noises in the neck. N Eng J Med 302:862, 1980

Hurst JW (ed): The Heart, Arteries and Veins, 5th ed. New York, McGraw-Hill, 1982

Hurst JW, Schlant RC: Examination of the Heart, Part 3. Inspection and Palpation of the Anterior Chest. Dallas, American Heart Association, 1972

Kirkendall WM, Feinleib M, Freis ED et al: Recommendations for human blood pressure determination by sphygmomanometers. Circulation 62:1146A, 1980

Leonard JJ, Kroetz FW, Leon DF et al: Examination of the Heart, Part 4. Auscultation. Dallas, American Heart Association, 1974

O'Brien ET, O'Malley K: ABC of blood pressure measurement. Br Med J 2:795, 851, 920, 982, 1048, 1124, 1201, 1979

Perloff JK: Cardiac auscultation. DM 26, No. 9:6, 1980

Perloff JK: Innocent murmurs. In Perloff JK (ed): The Clinical Recognition of Congenital Heart Disease, 2nd ed, p 8. Philadelphia, WB Saunders, 1978

Pomerance A: Pathology of heart disease in the elderly. Br J Hosp Med 11:245, 1974

Silverberg DS, Shemesh E, Iaina A: The unsupported arm: A cause of falsely raised blood pressure readings. Br Med J 2:1331, 1977

Stefadouros MA, Little RC: The cause and clinical significance of diastolic heart sounds. Arch Intern Med 140:537, 1980

CHAPTER 8. THE BREASTS AND AXILLAE

Benedek EP, Poznanski E, Mason S: A note on the female adolescent's psychological reactions to breast development. J Am Acad Child Psychiatry 18:537, 1979

Haagensen CD: Diseases of the Breast, 2nd ed rev. Philadelphia, WB Saunders, 1974

Haagensen CD, Bodian C, Haagensen DE Jr: Breast Carcinoma: Risk and Detection. Philadelphia, WB Saunders, 1981

Harlan WR, Harlan EA, Grillo GP: Secondary sex characteristics of girls 12 to 17 years of age. The U.S. Health Examination Survey. J Pediatr 96:1074, 1980

Marshall WA, Tanner JM: Variations in pattern of pubertal changes in girls. Arch Dis Child 44:291, 1969

Stromberg M: Screening for early detection. Amer J Nurs 81:1652, 1981 (especially self-examination)

Tanner JM: Growth at Adolescence, 2nd ed. Oxford, Blackwell Scientific Publications, 1962

CHAPTER 9. THE ABDOMEN

Bonello JC, Abrams JS: The significance of a "positive" rectal examination in acute appendicitis. Dis Colon Rectum 22:97, 1979

Castell DO: The spleen percussion sign: A useful diagnostic technique. Ann Intern Med 67:1265, 1967

Castell DO, Frank BB: Abdominal examination: Role of percussion and auscultation. Postgrad Med 62:131, 1977

Castell DO, O'Brien KD, Muench H et al: Estimation of liver size by percussion in normal individuals. Ann Intern Med 70:1183, 1969

Cope's Early Diagnosis of the Acute Abdomen, 15th ed. Revised by Silen W. New York, Oxford University Press, 1979

Eipper DF, Gifford RW Jr, Stewart BH et al: Abdominal bruits in renovascular hypertension. Am J Cardiol 37:48, 1976

Harrison JH, Gittes RF, Perlmutter AD et al (eds): Campbell's Urology, Vol 1, 4th ed, p 210. Philadelphia, WB Saunders, 1978

Julius S, Stewart BH: Diagnostic significance of abdominal murmurs. N Eng J Med 276:1175, 1967

McSherry JA: The prevalence of epigastric bruit. J R Coll Gen Pract 29:170, 1979

Smith DR: General Urology, 9th ed, p 35. Los Altos, CA, Lange Medical Publications, 1978

Sullivan S, Krasner N, Williams R: The clinical estimation of liver size: A comparison of techniques and an analysis of the source of error. Br Med J 2:1042, 1976

Walzer A, Koenigsberg M: Examining the anterior right kidney: Frequent lack of appreciation in examination of the right upper quadrant. JAMA 242:2320, 1979

CHAPTER 10. MALE GENITALIA AND HERNIAS

Chapel TA, Katta T, Kuszmar T et al: Pediculosis pubis in a clinic for treatment of sexually transmitted diseases. Sex Transm Dis 6:257, 1979

Daniel WA Jr: Adolescents in Health and Disease, p 27. St Louis, CV Mosby, 1977

Felman YM, Nikitas JA: Condylomata acuminata. NY State J Med 79:1747, 1979

Felman YM, Nikitas JA: Genital herpesvirus infections. NY State J Med 79:1216, 1979

Harlan WR, Grillo GP, Cornoni-Huntley J et al: Secondary sex characteristics of boys 12 to 17 years of age. The U.S. Health Examination Survey. J Pediatr 95:293, 1979

Harrison JH, Gittes RF, Perlmutter AD et al (eds): Campbell's Urology, Vol 1, 4th ed, pp 211–212. Philadelphia, WB Saunders, 1978

Marshall WA, Tanner JM: Variations in the pattern of pubertal changes in boys. Arch Dis Child 45:13, 1970

Smith DR: General Urology, 9th ed, p 37. Los Altos, CA, Lange Medical Publications, 1978

Tanner JM: Growth at Adolescence, 2nd ed. Oxford, Blackwell Scientific Publications, 1962

U.S. Dept HEW: Syphilis. A Synopsis. Washington DC, US Government Printing Office, 1968

Wisdom A: Color Atlas of Venereology. Chicago, Year Book Medical Publishers, 1973

Zimmerman LM, Anson BJ: Anatomy and Surgery of Hernia, 2nd ed. Baltimore, Williams & Wilkins, 1967

CHAPTER 11. THE FEMALE GENITALIA

Benson RC: Current Obstetric and Gynecologic Diagnosis and Treatment, 3rd ed. Los Altos, CA, Lange Medical Publications, 1980

Danforth DN (ed): Obstetrics and Gynecology, 3rd ed. Hagerstown, Harper & Row, 1977

Felman YM, Nikitas JA: Trichomoniasis, Candidiasis, and Corynebacterium vaginale vaginitis. NY State J Med 79:1563, 1979

Gardner HL, Kaufman RH: Benign Diseases of the Vulva and Vagina, rev ed. Boston, GK Hall, 1980

Hurd JK Jr: Vaginitis. Med Clin North Am 63:423, 1979

Jones HW Jr, Jones GS: Novak's Textbook of Gynecology, 10th ed. Baltimore, Williams & Wilkins, 1981

Kreutner AKK, Hollingsworth DR (eds): Adolescent Obstetrics and Gynecology. Chicago, Year Book Medical Publishers, 1978

Magee J: The pelvic examination: A view from the other end of the table. Ann Intern Med 83:563, 1975

Marshall WA, Tanner JM: Variations in pattern of pubertal changes in girls. Arch Dis Child 44:291, 1969

Settlage DSF: Pelvic examination of women. In Green R (ed): Human Sexuality: A Health Practitioner's Text. Baltimore, Williams & Wilkins, 1975

Spiegel CA, Amsel R, Eschenbach D et al: Anaerobic bacteria in nonspecific vaginitis. N Eng J Med 303:601, 1980

Tanner JM: Growth at Adolescence, 2nd ed. Oxford, Blackwell Scientific Publications, 1962

Tunnadine P: The role of genital examination in psychosexual medicine. Clin Obstet Gynaecol 7:283, 1980

Willson JR: Obstetrics and Gynecology, 6th ed. St Louis, CV Mosby, 1979

Wisdom A: Color Atlas of Venereology. Chicago, Year Book Medical Publishers, 1973

CHAPTER 12. THE ANUS AND RECTUM

Harrison JH, Gittes RF, Perlmutter AD et al (eds): Campbell's Urology, Vol 1, 4th ed, p 212. Philadelphia, WB Saunders, 1978

Schrock TR: Diseases of the anorectum. In Sleisenger MH, Fordtran JS: Gastrointestinal Disease, 2nd ed, p 1875. Philadelphia, WB Saunders, 1978

Smith DR: General Urology, 9th ed, p 39. Los Altos, CA, Lange Medical Publications, 1978

Spiro HM: Clinical Gastroenterology, 2nd ed, p 881. New York, Macmillan, 1977

CHAPTER 13. THE PERIPHERAL VASCULAR SYSTEM

Hurst JW (ed): The Heart, Arteries and Veins, 5th ed. New York, McGraw-Hill, 1982

Juergens JL, Spittell JA Jr, Fairbairn J II (eds): Allen-Barker-Hines Peripheral Vascular Diseases, 5th ed. Philadelphia, WB Saunders, 1980

CHAPTER 14. THE MUSCULOSKELETAL SYSTEM

Brashear HR Jr, Raney RB: Shands' Handbook of Orthopaedic Surgery, 9th ed. St Louis, CV Mosby, 1978

Hoppenfeld S: Physical examination of the knee joint by complaint. Orth Clin North Am 10:3, 1979

Hoppenfeld S: Physical Examination of the Spine and Extremities. New York, Appleton-Century-Crofts, 1976

McCarty DJ (ed): Arthritis and Allied Conditions: A Textbook of Rheumatology, 9th ed. Philadelphia, Lea & Febiger, 1979

Polley HF, Hunder GG: Rheumatologic Interviewing and Physical Examination of the Joints, 2nd ed. Philadelphia, WB Saunders, 1978

CHAPTER 15. THE NERVOUS SYSTEM

Adams RD, Victor M: Principles of Neurology, 2nd ed. New York, McGraw-Hill, 1981

Ajax ET: Should the traditional hatpin be discarded? Arch Neurol 35:549, 1978

Brooke MH: Clinical examination of patients with neuromuscular disease. Adv Neurol 17:25, 1977

Chusid JG: Correlative Neuroanatomy and Functional Neurology, 17th ed. Los Altos, CA, Lange Medical Publications, 1979

Clark RG: Essentials of Clinical Neuroanatomy and Neurophysiology, 5th ed. Philadelphia, FA Davis, 1975

DeJong RN: The Neurologic Examination: Incorporating the Fundamentals of Neuroanatomy and Neurophysiology, 4th ed. Hagerstown, Harper & Row, 1979

DeMyer W: Technique of the Neurologic Examination: A Programmed Text, 3rd ed. New York, McGraw-Hill, 1980

Duvoisin R: Clinical diagnosis of the dyskinesias. Med Clin North Am 56:1321, 1972

Fahn S: Differential diagnosis of tremors. Med Clin North Am 56:1363, 1972

Jankovic J: Drug-induced and other orofacial cervical dyskinesias. Ann Intern Med 94:788, 1981

Patten J: Neurological Differential Diagnosis: An Illustrated Approach. New York, Springer-Verlag, 1977

Plum F, Posner JB: The Diagnosis of Stupor and Coma, 3rd ed. Philadelphia, FA Davis, 1980

Van Allen MW: Pictorial Manual of Neurological Tests. Chicago, Year Book Medical Publishers, 1980

CHAPTER 16. MENTAL STATUS

American Psychiatric Association: Diagnostic and Statistical Manual of Mental Disorders, 3rd ed. Washington DC, American Psychiatric Association, 1980

Birren JE, Schaie KW (eds): Handbook of the Psychology of Aging. New York, Van Nostrand Reinhold, 1977

Busse EW, Blazer DG (eds): Handbook of Geriatric Psychiatry. New York, Van Nostrand Reinhold, 1980

Jacobs JW, Bernhard MR, Delgado A et al: Screening for organic mental syndromes in the medically ill. Ann Intern Med 86:40, 1977

Kaplan HI, Freedman AM, Sadock BJ: Comprehensive Textbook of Psychiatry, III, 3rd ed. Baltimore, Williams & Wilkins, 1980

Kaplan HI, Freedman AM, Sadock BJ: Modern Synopsis of Comprehensive Textbook of Psychiatry, 3rd ed. Baltimore, Williams & Wilkins, 1981

Kolb LC: Modern Clinical Psychiatry, 9th ed. Philadelphia, WB Saunders, 1977

McEvoy JP: Organic brain syndromes. Ann Intern Med 95:212, 1981

Nicholi AM Jr (ed): The Harvard Guide to Modern Psychiatry. Cambridge, Belknap Press of Harvard University Press, 1978

Strub RL, Black FW: The Mental Status Examination in Neurology. Philadelphia, FA Davis, 1977

Thaler O, Engel I, Goldstein R: Mental status examination. Unpublished. Department of Psychiatry, University of Rochester Medical Center

CHAPTER 17. THE PHYSICAL EXAMINATION OF INFANTS AND CHILDREN

Battaglia FC, Lubchenco LO: A practical classification of newborn infants by weight and gestational age. J Pediatr 71:159–163, 1967

Burnside JW: Physical Diagnosis: An Introduction to Clinical Medicine, 16th ed. Baltimore, Williams & Wilkins, 1981

Caceres CA, Perry W: The Innocent Murmur: A Problem in Clinical Practice. Boston, Little, Brown & Co, 1967

Capraro VJ: Gynecological examination in children and adolescents. Pediatr Clin North Am 19:511–528, 1972

Chung SMK: Hip Disorders in Infants and Children. Philadelphia, Lea & Febiger, 1981

Dubowitz LV, Dubowitz C, Goldberger C: Clinical assessment of gestational age in the newborn infant. J Pediatr 77:1–10, 1970

Dynski-Klein M: Color Atlas of Pediatrics. London, Wolfe Medical Publications, 1975

Frankenberg WK, Camp BW (eds): Pediatric Screening Tests. Springfield, IL, Charles C Thomas, 1975

Fulton RT, Lloyd LL (eds): Auditory Assessment of the Difficult-to-Test. New York, RE Krieger, 1975

Goldring D, Wohltmann H: Flush method for blood pressure determinations in newborn infants. J Pediatr 40:285–289, 1952

Gorman JJ, Cogan DG, Gellis SS: An apparatus for grading the visual acuity of infants on the basis of opticokinetic nystagmus. Pediatrics 19:1088–1092, 1957

Hoekelman RA, Blatman S, Brunell PA (eds): Principles of Pediatrics: Health Care of the Young. New York, McGraw-Hill, 1978

Illingworth RS: An Introduction to Developmental Assessment in the First Year. London, National Spastics Society Medical Education and Information Unit, 1962

Lawson EE, Grand RJ, Neff RK, Cohen LF: Clinical estimation of liver span in infants and children. Am J Dis Child 132:474–476, 1978

Lowrey GH: Growth and Development of Children, 7th ed. Chicago, Year Book Medical Publishers, 1978

Lubchenco LO, Searls DT, Brazie JV: Neonatal mortality rate: Relationship to birth weight and gestational age. J Pediatr 81:814–822, 1972

Marks MB: Allergic Shiners: Dark circles under the eyes in children. Clin Pediatr 5:655–658, 1966

Nadas AS, Fyler DC: Pediatric Cardiology, 3rd ed. Philadelphia, WB Saunders, 1972

Newell FW: Ophthalmology: Principles and Concepts, 4th ed. St Louis, CV Mosby, 1978

Paine RS: Neurological examination of infants and children. Pediatr Clin North Am 7:471–510, 1960

Sweet AY: Classification of the low-birth-weight infant. In Klaus MH, Fanaroff AA (eds): Care of the High-Risk Neonate. Philadelphia, WB Saunders, 1977

Tachdjian MO: Diagnosis and treatment of congenital deformities of the musculoskeletal system in the newborn and the infant. Pediatr Clin North Am 14:307–348, 1968

Thomas A, Chesni Y, Dargassies SS: The Neurological Examination of the Infant. London, National Spastics Society Medical Education and Information Unit, 1960

Van Allen MW: Pictorial Manual of Neurological Tests. Chicago, Year Book Medical Publishers, 1980

CHAPTER 18. CLINICAL THINKING: FROM DATA TO PLAN

Brody DS: The patient's role in clinical decision-making. Ann Intern Med 93:718, 1980

Clinical disagreement, I: How often it occurs and why. Can Med Assoc J 123:499, 1980

Clinical disagreement, II: How to avoid it and how to learn from one's mistakes. Can Med Assoc J 123:613, 1980

Cutler P: Problem Solving in Clinical Medicine: From Data to Diagnosis. Baltimore, Williams & Wilkins, 1979

Feinstein AR: Clinical Judgment. Baltimore, Williams & Wilkins, 1967

Griner PF, Mayewski RJ, Mushlin AI et al: Selection and interpretation of diagnostic tests and procedures: Principles and applications. Ann Intern Med 94:553, 1981

Harvey AM, Bordley JB III, Barondess JA: Differential Diagnosis: The Interpretation of Clinical Evidence, 3rd ed. Philadelphia, WB Saunders, 1979

Koran LM: The reliability of clinical methods, data and judgments. N Eng J Med 293:642, 695, 1975

Morgan WL Jr, Engel GL: The Clinical Approach to the Patient, p 16. Philadelphia, WB Saunders, 1969

Vecchio TJ: Predictive value of a single diagnostic test in unselected populations. N Eng J Med 274:1171, 1966

Weed LL: Medical Records, Medical Education, and Patient Care. Cleveland, Press of Case Western Reserve University, 1969

Wulff HR: Rational Diagnosis and Treatment. Oxford, Blackwell Scientific Publications, 1976

CHAPTER 19. THE PATIENT'S RECORD

Hurst JW, Walker HK: The Problem-Oriented System. New York, Medcom Press, 1972

Index

Numerals followed by *t* indicate tabular material.

abdomen
    in aging, 231
    anatomy and physiology, 228–231
    auscultation of, 234–235
    hernias and bulges of, 250t
    in infancy and childhood, 492–496
    inspection of, 232–234
    involuntary rigidity of, 239
    palpation of, 238, 239
    percussion of, 235–238
    protuberant, 251t
    reflexes in, 372, 404
        in infancy, 504
    sounds in, 252t
    tenderness in, 253–254t
    wall of, masses in, 249
abducens nerve (N_6)
    examination of, 383–384
    function of, 378
abrasion of teeth, 121
abscess(es)
    adenoidal, 486
    perianal, 299
    peritonsillar, 123, 486
abstract reasoning, 429
    testing of, 437
acanthosis nigricans, 222
accommodation
    of eye, 59
    pupillary reaction to, 59, 76, 383
acne, 70
    in adolescence, 68
acoustic blink reflex, 478, 505
acoustic nerve (N_8)
    examination of, 386
    function of, 379
acrocyanosis, 462
acromegaly
    face, 95
    tongue, 90
acuity of hearing, 84–85
    in aging, 69
Addison's disease, 48, 121
adenofibroma, breast, 226

adenoiditis, 486
adenoids, 486
adenoma(s), senile sebaceous, 44–45
Adie's pupil, 102
adjustment disorder, with anxious mood, 441
adnexa
    anatomy, 274
    masses in, 295t
adolescence
    female, sexual maturity in, 212–213, 275–276, 279
    growth spurt in, 35–36
    head and neck changes in, 68
    interviewing in, 18–19
    male, sexual maturity in, 260–263
    mental functions in, 429
    musculoskeletal changes in, 338
affect, 428
    in physical examination, 41, 431
affective disorders, 439
agenesis, renal, 478
aging
    abdominal changes in, 231
    breast changes in, 214
    cardiovascular changes in, 170–171
    gait in, 419
    genitalia
        female, 276
        male, 262
    habitus in, 37
    head and neck changes in, 68–69
    hearing in, 69
    interviewing and, 19–20
    lungs and thorax in, 135
    mental function changes in, 429
    musculoskeletal changes in, 338–339
    nervous system changes in, 381
    ocular fundi in, 108–111t
    peripheral vascular changes in, 309
    skin changes in, 44–45
agoraphobia, 440
air bubble, gastric, 237
albinism, 49
Allen test, 311
ambylopia exanopsia, 474
amnestic syndrome, 444

amyloidosis, tongue, 90
anal canal, 296
anal fissure, 301
analgesia, 398
anal reflex, 504
anatomy. *See under specific body part*
anemia
    chronic hemolytic, 485
    conjunctivas in, 74
    heart murmurs in, 201
    skin color in, 49, 462
anesthesia, 399
aneurysm, aortic, 173, 234, 246
anger, in interviewing, 22
angioma(s)
    cherry, 45, 50
    spider, 50
anisocoria, 102
anisometropia, ambylopia exanopsia and, 474
ankle(s)
    anatomy, 331
    examination techniques of, 345–346
    reflexes in, 372, 406, 504
    ulcers of, 319t
ankle clonus
    in infancy, 504
    testing for, 407
ankle reflex, 372, 406
ankylosing spondylitis, 351, 368
    in neck, 356
ankylosis, 340
anorectal junction, 296
anoxia, generalized pallor in, 462
anterior horn cell disease, 374
    in infancy, 508
anus
    abnormalities of, 301–302t
    anatomy and physiology, 296–297
    examination techniques, 298–300
    inspection of, 299
anxiety(ies)
    adjustment disorder with, 441
    assessment of, 433
    and body temperature, in children, 457
    irrational, 440–441t
    of patient, in interviewing, 21

aorta
abdominal, 229
aneurysm of, 173
increased pulsation of, 234
palpation for, 246
ascending, dilation of, in heart murmur, 201
coarctation of, 186
in infancy and childhood, 489
murmur in, 490
palpation of, 246–247
recoil of, in arterial pressure, 167
aortic regurgitation
murmur of, 180, 206, 491
aortic stenosis, 173
carotid pulse in, 181
in heart murmurs, 201
midsystolic ejection murmurs in, 202t
thrill of, 173
Apgar scoring system, 449–450
aphasia, 413
testing for, 435
aphonia, 413
apical impulse, 158
assessment of, 174–176
in infancy and childhood, 490
in normal vs. enlarged left ventricle, 191t
appendicitis
abdominal palpation for, 248–249
acute, 254
in childhood, 496
aqueous humor, 57
arcus, corneal (senilis), 68, 100
areola, abnormalities of, 225t
Argyll Robertson pupil, 102
arms(s), inspection of, 310–311
arrhythmia, sinus, 192, 195
arterial pressure, factors influencing, 167
arterial pulse, 180–182
abnormalities of, 209t
blood pressure and, 166–167
arterioles, retinal, 80–81, 106
arteriovenous crossings, 106
arteriovenous shunt, intracranial, 467
artery(ies), peripheral
in aging, 309
anatomy of, 304–305
brachial, 304
carotid, 66
in aging, 171
kinking of, 171
chronic insufficiency of, 316, 318t, 319
dorsalis pedis, 305
femoral, 305, 314
iliac, 229
partial obstruction of, in abdominal auscultation, 234
popliteal, 305
posterior tibial, 305
radial, 304
superficial temporal, 54
tibial, 305
ulnar, 304
arthritis, 340–341
bacterial, 341
elbow, 360
gonococcal, 343
gouty, of feet and toes, 363
hip joint, 349
juvenile rheumatoid, 485

rheumatoid. *See* rheumatoid arthritis
spinal, 351
ascites, assessment for, 246–247
ascitic fluid, protuberant abdomen in, 251
assessment
cardiovascular, 189–190
in clinical thinking, 513–514, 515–517
interplay with data collection, 522
asterixis, 420
asthma
anterior chest in, 145
in infants and children, 458
posterior chest in, 136
sounds in, 144–145
ataxia, 388
cerebellar, 419
sensory, 419
atelectasis
diaphragmatic level in, 139, 143
in trachea examination, 92
signs in, 156
athetosis, 421
atresia
choanal, in newborn, 482
esophageal, 450
posterior nasal, 450
tricuspid, murmur in, 491
atrial fibrillation, 192, 195
first heart sound in, 196
atrial flutter, 192, 195
with regular ventricular response, 193–194
atrial gallop, 199
atrial septal defect
in infancy and childhood, 490
second heart sound in, 197
systolic murmur of, 203
atrioventricular node, 165
atrophy
of dorsal interosseous muscles, 338–339, 389
muscular, 374
optic, 105, 383
skin, 52
thenar eminence, 338–339, 359, 389
attention, 428
testing of, 434–435
attrition, of teeth, 121
auditory canal, external, 478
auricle, 60
auscultation
abdominal, 234–235
in infancy, 493
heart, 164, 176–180
of lungs, 143–144, 148
auscultatory gap, 183
Austin Flint murmur, 206
automatisms
infantile, 505–510
in neonate, 503
autonomic nerve supply, to eyes, 59
avoidance behavior(s), 440–441t
avoidant disorder of childhood and adolescence, 440

Babinski response, 407, 413
in coma, 413
in infancy, 448, 504
to plantar stimulation, 504
balanitis, 264

balanoposthitis, 264
balding, in aging, 45
Barlow's sign, 501
barrel chest, 150
Bartholin's gland
anatomy, 274
inflammation of, 287
basal cell carcinoma, 45, 98
battered child syndrome, 469
Beau's lines, 53
bed patient, examination of, 316–317
Bell's palsy, 416
benign prostatic hypertrophy, 303
biceps
muscular, tendonitis in, 362
reflexes in, 372, 402–403
bicuspid aortic valve, in heart murmurs, 201
Biot's breathing, 149
birth history, of child, 6
birth weight, classification by, 448
bismuth poisoning, gums in, 121
blacks
axillary hair in, 213
breast development in, 213
buccal mucosa in, 89
gums in, 121
ocular fundi in, 109t
bladder
distended, 229
in abdominal inspection, 233
in abdominal percussion, 235
in newborns, 493
bleeding, evidence of, in skin exam, 46, 50
blepharitis, in red eyes, 99
blind eye, 101
blind patients, interviewing of, 25
blinking reflex, 505
blood
viscosity of, in arterial pressure, 167
volume of, in arterial pressure, 167
blood pressure, 182–186
arterial pulses and, 166–167
in infants and children, 458–460
leg pulses and, 186
normal, upper limits of, 186
postural changes in, 185
body odors, in physical examination, 41
bone conduction, 85
Bouchard's nodes, 357
boutonniere deformity, 357
bowel sounds, abdominal, 234, 252
bowleg, 347, 350
bowlegged growth pattern, in infancy, 499
brachioradialis reflex, 404
bradycardia, sinus, with slow ventricular rate, 194
bradypnea, 149
brain, 380
stem of, 380
tumor of, in childhood, 512
breast(s)
adenofibroma of, 226
aging and, 214
anatomy and physiology, 210–215
asymmetry of, 214
cancer of
female, 226
male, 227
signs of, 224t

cystic disease of, 226
development of, 212–214, 488
examination techniques, 216–223
female, 216–221
lymphatics of, 214–215
male, 214, 222
of newborn, 487
nodules, differentiation of, 226t
in pregnancy, 214
sex maturity ratings in, 212, 213
supernumerary, 225
breathing, 133–134
abdominal, 488
ataxic, 149
in infancy, 483
Kussmaul, 149
obstructive, 149
paradoxical, 488
rate and rhythm, abnormalities in, 149t
rate of, in inspection, 136
breath odors, in physical examination, 41
breath sounds, 134
alterations in, 151t
auscultation of, 143–144, 148
in childhood, 489
in infancy and childhood, 488
in lung auscultation, 144
breech babies, 450
plantar reflexes in, 507
brief reactive psychosis, 442
bronchitis
breathing in, 145
breath sounds in, 144
in infants and children, 458
signs in, 155
bronchophony, 151
bronchus(i), abnormalities, physical signs
in, 154–155t
Brudzinski's sign, testing for, 408
bruit(s)
in abdominal auscultation, 234
carotid, 182
femoral artery, 314
thyroid, 94
Brushfield's spots, 473
buccal mucosa, 89
abnormalities of, 119
in childhood, 484
Buerger's disease, 310
bulge sign, in knee joint, 348, 365
bursa(e), 324
knee, 367
bursitis, 340
olecranon, 360
prepatellar, 365
shoulder, 361

calcifications, in newborns, 464
calcium
in eardrum, 114
in supraspinatus tendon, 361
callus, foot and toe, 364
cancer. See also tumor(s); specific tumors
metatastic, 369
tongue, 90
candidiasis, oral mucosa and, 119
canker sore, 119
capillary bed, fluid exchange and, 309
capillary permeability, in edema, 321
caput succedaneum, in newborns, 466

carbon monoxide poisoning, in comatose
patient, 409
caruncle, urethral, 287
carcinoma
basal cell, 45, 98
cervical, 289
lip, 118
penis, 268
prostatic, 303
rectal, 302
squamous cell, in aging, 45
tongue, 122
vulva, 286
cardiac output
in arterial pressure, 167
high, 174
cardinal fields of gaze, 59
caries, dental, 121
carotenemia, 49
carotid artery. See artery, carotid
carpal tunnel syndrome, special maneuvers
for, 352
cartilage, 66
cricoid, 66
thyroid, 66
cataract(s), 100
age factor in, 69, 82
in infancy, 473
obstructive ambylopia and, 474
central nervous system disease, in infancy,
510
cephalohematoma, 468
in newborns, 466
cerebellar system, 373
cerebellum, 380
disease of, 396
lesion of, 390
cerebral accidents, hemiplegia in, 411
cerebral palsy, bilateral, 510
cerebrum, 380
cervical disc, herniation, 355–356
cervix
in bimanual examination, 283
in bimanual rectoabdominal palpation,
498
carcinoma of, 289
cytology of, 282
ectropion of, 289
inspection of, 281–282
lacerations of, 288
nulliparous, 288
os of, 274
parous, 288
polyp of, 289
variations and abnormalities of, 288–289t
chalazion, 98
chancre, syphilitic
on lip, 117
on penis, 268
of vulva, 286
cheilitis, 117
cheilosis, 117
chest
anterior, examination of, 144–148
barrel, 150
funnel, 150
palpation of, 137–139, 145–146
percussion of, 139–143, 146–147
pigeon, 150
posterior examination of, 136–144

wall of, heart sounds and, 164–165
Cheyne-Stokes breathing, 149
chicken breast, 487
child(ren)
abuse of, 452
history, 5–6
interviewing, 18
physical examination of, 447–512
childhood
early, approach to examination in,
452–455
late, approach to examination in, 455–456
cholecystitis, acute, 254
chondrodermatitis helicis, 113
chorea, involuntary movements in, 421
chorioretinitis, 108, 473
chronic obstructive lung disease
labored breathing in, 144
posture in, 40
Chvostek's sign, in newborns, 467
ciliary injection in red eyes, 99
circumstantiality, in thought processes, 446
clanging, in thought processes, 446
clarification, in interviewing, 11
cleft palate, submucosal, 487
clinician, demeanor in interviewing, 12–13
clitoris
anatomy, 273
enlarged, 279
clubbing
of fingers, in infancy and childhood, 490
nail, 53
coarctation, aortic, 186, 459, 490
cochleopalpebral reflex, 505
cognitive functions, assessment of, 434–438
cold caloric test
in coma, 412
for vestibular function, 512
colloid bodies, in retina, 108
coloboma, in newborns, 473
colon, 229
descending, in newborns, 493
color
at birth, 450
skin, 46
variations in, 48–49t
coma, as consciousness abnormality, 413
comatose patient, examination of, 409–412
compulsions, assessment of, 433
conduction, heart, 165–166
conduction deafness, 84–85, 115
cone of light, 84
confabulation, in thought processes, 446
confrontation, in interviewing, 12
confrontation testing of visual fields, 71–72
confusion, as consciousness abnormality,
413
congestive heart failure, in edema, 320
conjugate eye movements, 59, 76, 472
conjunctiva(s), 55
physical examination of, 74
in red eyes, 99
consciousness, 380
abnormalities of, 413t
level of
in mental function, 428
in physical examination, 39, 431
consensual light reflex, 58
contractions, premature, 195
in arterial pulse, 180

contractions (*continued*)
  ventricular
    first heart sounds in, 196
    in infancy and childhood, 490
contracture
  Dupuytren's, 342, 359
  flexion, 347
conversion reaction, in sensory testing, 397–398
coordination, assessment of, 396–397
copying, testing of, 435–438
cornea, 55
  arcus of, 100
    in aging, 68
  opacity of, 100t
    obstructive ambylopia and, 474
  reflex of, 385
  scar on, 100
corns, foot, 364
corticospinal tract, 373
coryza, childhood, 484
cotton wool patches, in retina, 108–111t
cover test, eyes, 103, 474, 476
crackles, lung, 152t
cranial nerves, 380
  function of, 378–379
  examination techniques in, 382–387
  in infancy, 504
craniosynostosis, in newborns, 466
craniotabes, in newborns, 466
crepitation, 340
crescents, in optic disc, 104
cretinism
  cry in, 483
  face in, 469
cretins, in infancy, 462
cricoid cartilage, 66
crude touch, as sensation, 375
crust, skin lesions, 51
cry, quality of, in infancy, 483
cryptorchidism, 265
  in childhood, 497
cul-de-sac, anatomy of, 274
cupping
  glaucomatous, 105
  physiologic, 104
curvature, spinal, 368–369t
Cushing's syndrome
  abdominal striae in, 233
  face in, 95
  fat distribution in, 40
cutis marmorata, in infancy, 462
cyanosis, 48
  in comatose patient, 409
  congenital heart disease and, 491t
  in infancy and childhood, 490
  of lips, 89
cyclothymic disorders, 439
cystic disease, breast, 226
cyst(s)
  mucous retention, 118
  nabothian, 289
  in newborns, 493
  pilonidal, 301
  porencephalic, 467
  retention, 289
  sebaceous
    ear, 113
    scrotal, 269
    vulva, 286

thyroglossal duct, 467
cystocele, 287

dacryocystitis, 98, 473
Darwin's tubercle, 113
data
  in clinical thinking, 518–519
  collection and assessment of, 522
  in patient record, 525
dazzle reflex, 505
deaf-mute, interviewing of, 25
deafness, 84–85, 115
  selective, 482
degenerative joint disease, 339
  bony enlargement in, 341
  decreased spinal mobility in, 351
  hand, 357
  interphalangeal, 343
  knee, 347
  neck, 356
delirium, 413
  in organic brain syndrome, 444
delusions, assessment of, 433
dementia, in organic brain syndrome, 444
dental caries, 121
denture sore mouth, 89
Denver Developmental Screening Test, 503
depersonalization, feelings of, 433
depression
  assessment of, 432
  distinguishing features, 439t
  in interviewing, 22–23
  in physical examination, 40
dermatoglyphics, in newborns, 464
dermatomes, 375–377
dermis, 43
desquamation, 463
developmental history of child, 6–7
developmental levels, 448
developmental testing of children, 452
deviation(s)
  eye, 103t
  nipple, 225
  septal, 116
dextrocardia, 176
diaphragm
  level of, in pleural effusion, 139
  paralysis of, 143
diaphragmatic excursion, 143
diarrhea, bowel sounds in, 234
diastasis recti, 250
  in newborns, 492
diastole
  extra heart sounds in, 199t
  murmurs in, 205–206t
diastolic pressure, 459
digital response reflex, 505
dimpling, skin, breast, 224
diopters, 82
diphtheria, pharynx in, 123
diplegia(s)
  in infancy, 506
  spastic, 510
direct light reflex, 58
direct questions, in interviewing, 13–14
disc, optic, 79–80
diverticulitis, 254
doll's eye test, 472
dorsal interosseous muscles, atrophy of, 338–339, 389

dorsalis pedis artery
  anatomy, 305
  pulse in, 313
Douglas pouch, 274
Down's syndrome
  Brushfield's spots in, 473
  face in, 469
  in infancy, 462
dress
  mental function and, 431
  in physical examination, 40
drug toxicity, in childhood, 512
drusen, retinal, 108–111t
duct(s)
  nasolacrimal, 56, 473
  parotid (Stensen's), 64
  submaxillary (Wharton's), 64
duodenum, percussion of, 230
Dupuytren's contracture, 342, 359
dwarfism, in physical examination, 39
dysarthria, 413
dyskinesia
  oral–facial, 422
  tardive, 422
dysphasia(s), 413
  testing for, 435
dysphonia, 413
dysthymic disorders, 439
dystonia, involuntary movements in, 421
dystrophy, muscular, in childhood, 511

ear(s)
  anatomy, 60–61
  auricle, 83
  chondrodermatitis helicis, 113
  Darwin's tubercle, 113
  examination techniques, 83–85
  in infancy and childhood, 478–482
  keloids in, 113
  lymph nodes near, 113
  middle, fluid in, 84
  nodules in and around, 113t
  sebaceous cysts in, 113
eardrum, 61, 83–84
  abnormalities of, 114t
early systolic ejection sound (Ej), 162, 198
ecchymosis, 51
ectropion
  cervical, 289
  eyelid, 97
  eyelid, in aging, 68
edema, 49
  angioneurotic, of lips, 118
  areolar, 225
  leg, 314
  lymphatic, 309
  mechanisms and patterns of, 320–321t
  of nipple, 225
  orthostatic, 321–322
  periorbital, 97
  peripheral, in infancy and childhood, 490
  pulmonary, in infancy and childhood, 490
  scrotal, 270
  skin color in, 49
egophony, 151
Eisenmenger's syndrome, murmur in, 491
ejection sounds, 162
  auscultation of, 178
  distinguished from split first heart sound, 200

elbow
  anatomy, 327
  arthritis in, 360
  examination techniques of, 344
  swollen or tender, 360t
  tennis, 360
electrocardiographic waves, cardiac cycle and, 166
empathetic responses, in interviewing, 11–12
emphysema
  anterior chest and, 145
  breath sounds in, 144
  percussion in, 146
  posterior chest in, 136
  signs in, 155
entropion, 97
  in aging, 68
environment, interviewing, 9–10
epidermis, 43
epididymis
  anatomy, 259
  spermatocele of, 269
epididymitis, 270
  tuberculous, 269
epiglottis, in childhood, 487
epitrochlear node, 307
  palpation for, 311
Epstein's pearls, 483
epulis, 120
equilibrium, inner ear, 61
equipment for physical examination, xvii
erythema toxicum, 463
erythroblastosis fetalis, 485
esotropia, 474–476
examination, physical. See physical examination
excoriation, 52
exophthalmos, 72, 97
exotropia, 474–475
extinction
  in sensory testing, 401
  of vision, 383
extraocular movements, 59–60
  testing of, 383
extraocular muscles, 76–77
extrapyramidal system, 373
extremity(ies), upper, asymmetric response in, 509
exudates, hard, in retina, 108, 110–111
eye(s)
  anterior sagittal section, 55f
  autonomic nerve supply, 59
  deviations of, 103t
  examination techniques, 70–82
  extraocular movements, 59–60
  gross anatomy, 55–57
  in infancy, 471–474
  lumps and swellings, 98t
  measurement within, 82
  position and alignment, 72
  red, 99t
  visual pathways, 57–58
eyebrows, physical examination of, 73
eyelids, 55
  abnormalities of, 97t
  physical examination of, 73

face
  expression of, in physical examination, 41
  nerve of (N7), 379

examination of, 385
  paralysis of, 385, 416–417t
  physical examination of, 70, 95t
facial expression, mental function and, 431
facies, diagnostic, in childhood, 469t
fallopian tube, 274
family(ies)
  in adult history, 3
  in child history, 8
  history of, 528–529
  interviewing of, 26
fasciculations, 374, 389, 422
fatally ill, interviewing of, 25–26
fat pads, knee, 367
feelings, inquiry about, in interviewing, 12
feet
  abnormalities of, 363–364t
  anatomy, 331
  corns on, 364
  examination techniques of, 345–346
  flat, 350, 363
  in infancy, 498–499
  ulcers of, 319t
felon, 359
femoral canal, 260
femoral pulse
  in infancy and childhood, 489
  palpation of, 312
fever
  in physical examination, 41
  rheumatic, 340–341
fibroplasia, retrolental, 473
fine motor coordination testing in infancy, 503
fine touch, sensation of, 375
first heart sound (S1), 162
  in auscultation, 178
  in infancy and childhood, 490
  production of, 165
  split, 200t
  variations in, 196t
fissure
  anal, 301
  lung, 130–131
  skin, 51
  tongue, 122, 485
fistula(s)
  anorectal, 301
  thyroglossal duct, 467
  tracheoesophageal, 450, 483
fixed splitting, 197
flat feet, 350, 363
flexion
  contracture in, 347
  in hip deformity, 349
fluid wave, test for, 247
flush technique, in obtaining blood pressure, 459
fontanelles, 465
Fordyce spots, 119
foreskin, 496
fornix, 274
fourth heart sound (S4), 163
  auscultation of, 178 180, 199–200
fovea centralis, 56
fremitus, 135
  in childhood, 489
  in infants, 488
  palpation for, 138, 146
frenulum, in newborns, 483

friction rubs,
  abdominal, 235, 252
  pleural, 153
frontal release signs, 408–409
funduscopic examination, in infancy, 473
fundus ocular, 56, 109–111t
  in aging, 69
funnel chest, 150
furuncle, nose, 116

gag reflex, 386
  in childhood, 484
gait, 387–388
  abnormalities of, 418–419t
  in physical examination, 40
Galant's reflex, 506
ganglion, hand, 358
genitalia
  female
    in adolescence, 275–276
    in aging, 275–276
    anatomy, 273–276
    examination techniques, 277–285
    external, 279–280
    in infancy and childhood, 496–498
  male
    in adolescence, 260–262
    in aging, 262
    anatomy and physiology, 258–262
    examination techniques in, 263–267
genu valgum, 347
geographic tongue, 122
  in childhood, 485
gestational age, classification by, 448
gestational weight, 448–449
gibbus, 369
gingiva(e). See gums
gingivitis, 120
glans penis, 258, 496
glaucoma
  aging and, 69
  cupping in, 105
  iris in, 75
  in newborns, 464
  open-angle, 75
  in red eyes, 99
glossopharyngeal nerve (N9)
  function of, 379
  examination of, 386
"glove and stocking" sensory loss, 398
goiter, 92
  multinodular, 124
gout
  arthritis in, 340
    foot and toe, 345, 363
  chronic tophaceous, of hands, 358
Gower's sign, for muscular dystrophy, 511
grasp reflex, 408
Graves' disease, 72
great saphenous vein, 305
great vessels
  surface projections, 157–159
  transposition of, murmur in, 491
groin
  anatomy, 259
  hernias in, 271–272t
grooming, mental function and, 431
growth
  assessment of, 39, 460–462
  history of, 6–7

growth (*continued*)
  in childhood and adolescence, 35–36, 447
gums
  abnormalities of, 120–121t
  examination techniques for, 89
gynecomastia, 214, 222, 227

habitus, in physical examination, 35–37, 39
hair
  aging and, 45
  axillary
    development of, 213
    in blacks, 213
  inspection of, 47
    head, 70
    pubic, 261–262, 275–276
  secondary sexual, 498
  as skin appendage, 43
hairy tongue, 122
hallucinations
  assessment of, 434
  organic, 445
hallux valgus, 345, 363
hammer toe, 364
hand(s)
  anatomy, 325
  examination techniques of, 342–343
  swellings and deformities of, 357–359t
hard palate, abnormalities of, 119
harlequin dyschronica, in infancy, 462
head
  abnormal enlargements, in infancy, 468t
  anatomy and physiology of, 54–69
  changes with age, 68–69
  circumference, in infancy and children, 461
  in early and late childhood, 470–471
  examination techniques, 70
  in infancy, 465–467
  lymph nodes of, 67
  physical examination of, 70
hearing
  acuity of, 84–85
    in aging, 69
  impairments of, in interviewing, 25
  loss of. *See* deafness
  pathways of, 61
  testing of, in infancy, 478
heart
  anatomy and physiology, 157–171
  auscultation of, 176–180
  auscultatory areas of, 164
  block of, 192
    first heart sound in, 196
  chambers of, 160
  circulation in, 160
  congenital disease of, cyanosis and, 491t
  examination techniques of, 172–190
  extra sounds, in diastole, 199t
  extra sounds, in systole, 198t
  failure of
    edema and, 320
    in infancy and childhood, 490
    left-sided, 40
      signs in, 154
  in infancy and childhood, 489–491
  inspection of, 172–176
  murmurs of. *See* murmurs
  palpation of, 172–176
  rate of
    in auscultation, 177

  at birth, 450
  differentiation, 192–195t
  in infants and children at rest, 457t
  rheumatic disease of, murmurs in, 491
  rhythm
    in auscultation, 177
  sounds of
    differentiation, 192–195t
    in cardiac cycle, 161–163
    changes with age, 170
    relation to chest wall, 164–165
    surface projections, 157–159
    valves of, 160
Heberden's nodes, 357
Hegar's sign, 292
height
  of infants and children, 460–461
  in physical examination, 35–37
hemangioma, capillary, in newborns, 464
hematoma, subdural, 472
hemianopsia, 96
hemiparesis, 390, 417
  in newborns, 464
  spastic gait in, 418
hemiplegia, 390
  congenital, 509
  posture in, 427
  of sudden cerebral accidents, 411
hemochromatosis, 48
hemolytic anemia, chronic, 485
hemorrhage(s)
  conjunctival, in red eyes, 99
  flame-shaped, 107
  preretinal, 107
  retinal, 107, 472, 473
  splinter, 53
  subarachnoid, 408
    in comatose patient, 410
hemorrhoids, 302
hepatojugular reflux, 189
hernia(s)
  abdominal, 250t
  course and presentation, 271t
  differentiation, 272t
  femoral, 272
  function of, 259
  incarcerated, 267
  incisional, 250
  inguinal, in childhood, 496
  inspection of, 266
  linea alba, 250
  in newborns, 492
  palpation of, 266, 267
  scrotal, 269
  strangulated, 267
  umbilical, 250, 492
herniated disc
  cervical, 355–356
  intervertebral, 351
  list in, 369
  lumbar, 353
herpes, genital
  penis, 268
  vulva, 286
herpes simplex, lip eruptions in, 117
hidradenitis suppurativa, 222
hip(s)
  anatomy of, 334–335
  arthritis of, 349

  congenital dislocation of, 500
  examination techniques of, 347–350
  flexion deformity of, 349
  in infancy, 499–501
Hirschberg test, 474
Hirschsprung's disease, in newborns, 493
hirsutism, 70
history
  adult, 2–5
  child, 6–8
  confusing, in interviewing, 23–24
  family, 3
  objectives of, 1
  psychosocial, 3–4, 14
  review of systems in, 4–5
  sexual, 14–16
  transitions in, 16
hordeolum, 98
horn cell, anterior, 371
Horner's syndrome, 101, 384
Houston, valves of, 296
Hutchinson's teeth, 121
hydration, in infants' skin, 464
hydrocele, 267
  in infancy, 496
  scrotal, 269
hydrocephalus, 70, 468
  in newborns, 466
hydronephrosis, 245
hygiene, patient's personal, 40
hymen
  anatomy, 273
  imperforate, 285
hypalgesia, 398
hyperalgesia, 398
hyperesthesia, 249, 399
hyperpnea, 149
hyperpyrexia, 41
hypertension
  portal, in newborns, 492, 493
  pulmonary, 173
  renal, 234
  and second heart sound, 197
  systolic, 171
hyperthyroidism
  in childhood, 456
  convergence problems in, 77
  eyelid lag in, 77
  hair in, 70
  motor activity in, 40
  systolic bruits in, 94
hypertrophy
  prostatic, 303
  tonsillar, 123
hyperventilation, 149
hyperventilation tetany, 467
hypesthesia, 399
hypoalbuminemia, edema in, 320
hypocalcemic tetany, 467
  cry in, 483
hypoglossal nerve (N_{12})
  examination of, 387
  function of, 379
hypogonadism, 39
hypospadias, 268, 496
hypotension, 171
hypothermia, 41
hypothyroidism, ankle reflex in, 406
hypotension, 171
  orthostatic (postural), 171–185

ileus
 in infancy, 493
 paralytic, bowel sounds in, 234, 252
illusions, 434
infant, newborn
 birthweight vs gestational age of,
  448–449
 maturational categories of, 449
infant, premature, mortality rates of, 449
infancy, approach to examination in,
  448–451
information, fund of, 429
 testing of, 436
inframammary ridge, 221
inguinal canal
 anatomy of, 260
 in childhood, 496
 hernias of, 272
inguinal ring, 260
innocent murmurs. See murmurs, innocent
intellectual functions
 limited, of patient, 24
 testing of, 436–438
intention tremors, 420
interosseous dorsal muscles, 338–339,
  389
intervertebral disc, herniated, 351
interview, patient
 adolescent, 18–19
 anger and hostility in, 22
 anxiety in, 21
 of blind patient, 25
 children, 18
 closing, 16
 deaf-mute, 25
 demeanor in, 12–13
 depression in, 22–23
 of families, 26
 fatally ill, 25–26
 of hearing-impaired, 25
 language barriers in, 24–25
 literacy in, 24
 note-taking in, 16
 objectives, 1
 overtalkative patients, 20–21
 parents, 16–18
 patients with limited intelligence, 24
 patients with multiple symptoms, 21
 reassurance in, 21
 response to questions in, 26–27
 of seductive patients, 23
 setting stage for, 8–10
 silence in, 20
 special problems of, 20–27
 transitions in, 16
intestinal obstruction
 bowel sounds in, 234
 in infancy, 493
 peristaltic waves in, 234
intracranial pressure
 in infancy, 465
 in older children, 467
intrathoracic mass, 488
introitus
 anatomy of, 273
 small, 285
involuntary movements, 420–422t
iridectomy, 102
iris, 56
 examination of, 75

jaundice, 49
 in comatose patient, 409
 in infants, 463
 scleras in, 74
joint(s). See also specific joints
 degenerative disease of. See degenerative
  joint disease
 effusion in, 340
 limited motion of, describing, 354
 structure and function of, 324
 tenderness in, 340
judgment, 429, 437
jugular veins, 66
 external, unilateral distention of, 189
 pressure in, 187–190
 pulses of, 168–169, 189

keloid(s)
 ear, 113
 skin, 52
keratoses, 44
Kernig's sign, 408
kidney
 chronic disease of, 456
 enlargement of, 244–245
 neoplasms of, 245
 in newborns, 493
 palpation of, 243–245
 polycystic, 245
 right, 229
 tenderness of, 245
kinking
 carotid artery, 171
 external jugular vein, 189
Klinefelter's syndrome, 270
knee(s)
 anatomy, 332–334
 bursae and fat pad of, 367
 examination techniques of, 347–350
 local tenderness in, 366–367t
 knock, 347, 350, 499
 reflexes in, 372, 405
 stability of, 352
 swellings of, 365t
koilonychia, 53
Koplik's spots, 484
kyphoscoliosis, thoracic, 150
kyphosis, 368

labia majora, 273
labia minora, 273, 496
 fusion of, 498
labyrinthitis, 512
lacerations, cervical, 288
lacrimal apparatus, 73
lacrimal ducts, 56
lacrimal gland, enlargement of, 98
language, 429
 testing of, 435–438
lanugo, 463
lateralization test, 85
lead poisoning, gums in, 121
leg(s)
 bow, 347
 deep veins of, 305
 edema of, 314
 flaccid, in hemiplegia, 411
 inspection of, 312–316
 length of, 354

pulses of, in heart examination, 186
 shortening of, 502
lens
 examination of, 75
 opacities in, 82
lentigines, senile, 44
lesion(s)
 cerebellar, 390
 sensory cortex, 401
 skin, 46, 50–52t
  basic types, 51–52t
  vascular and purpuric, 50t
 vulvar, 286t
leukemia, dermatoglyphic patterns in, 464
leukoplakia, tongue, 122
levator palpebrae muscle, 55
lice
 in female genitalia, 279
 hair, 70
 male genital, 264
lichenification, skin, 52
ligament(s), collateral, 366
light reflex, 58, 75
limbus, 55
linea alba, hernia of, 250
lip(s)
 abnormalities of, 117–118t
 carcinoma, 118
 inspection of, 89
lipedema, 322
list, spinal, 369
liver
 in abdominal percussion, 235–237
 anatomy of, 229
 edge of, in newborns, 493
 enlarged, 255–256
 palpation of, 240–242, 495
 percussion of, 230
 span of, 236, 495t
lordosis, lumbar, 368
lower abdominal reflex, 372
lumbar curve, flattening of, 368
lumbar disc, herniation of, 353, 368
lung(s)
 abnormalities of, physical signs in,
  154–155t
 added sounds of, 152–153t
 anatomy and physiology, 125–135
 auscultation of, 143–144
 examination techniques, 136–148
 fissures, 130–131
 in infancy and childhood, 487–489
 lobes of, 129
 physical examination of, 136–148
lymphatic system, 307
 of arms, 307
 axillary, 214–215
 of breast, 214–215
 female genital, 275
 of head and neck, 67, 91–92
 of legs, 308
 male genital, 259
lymphedema, 321–322
lymph nodes, see also lymphatic system
 cervical, in adolescence, 68

macula, 56, 81
macular star, ocular fundi in, 111t
macule, skin lesions, 51
major affective disorder, 443

maladaptive nurturing, 451
malignancy, spinal, 351. *See also* cancer; tumor(s)
malingering, 442
malleus, 61, 84
malocclusion, 485
mammary souffle, 170
mandibular protrusion, 485
manner, 41, 431
manual compression test, for varicose veins, 315
Marfan's syndrome, 39
mass(es)
    adnexal, 295t
    intra-abdominal vs abdominal wall masses, 249
    intrathoracic, 488
mass reflexes, in infancy, 508
mastoiditis, 481
mastoid process, 60
match test, in assessment of pulmonary function, 148
maternal deprivation, 456
maxillary protrusion, 485
McMurray's test, 353
meatus, urethral, 259
medical models, difficulties of, 517–521
megacephaly, 466
megacolon, congenital, 493
meibomian glands, 55
memory, 428, 435
meningitis
    in childhood, 512
    in comatose patient, 410
    neck mobility in, 470–471
    testing for, 408
meniscus
    disorders in tender knees, 366
    torn, 352–353
mental function
    in aging, 429
    assessment, note on, 438
    components of, 428–429
    examination techniques in, 430–438
mental retardation, 464
mental status survey, 382
metatarsus adductus deformity, 499
metatarsus varus, 499
microaneurysms, retinal, 107
microcephaly, 466
micrognathia, 466
middle ear, 61
    fluid in, 84, 114
milia, 463
miliaria rubra, 463
miniature toy test, 477
mitral regurgitation
    first heart sound in, 196
    murmurs of, 201t, 491
    in pansystolic murmurs, 204
    thrills of, 176
mitral stenosis
    auscultation for, 180
    diastolic murmur of, 206
    first heart sound in, 196
    in infancy and childhood, 490–491
    opening snap in, 199
    thrill of, 176
mitral valve, prolapsed, 204
    systolic clicks in, 198

mobility, skin, 46
moisture, skin, 46
moniliasis, oral, 119, 483
monilia vaginitis, 290
mononucleosis, infectious, 486
mood, 428, 432
Moro response, 509
motor behavior
    in physical examination, 40
    posture and, 431
motor coordination testing, 503
motor deficit, assessment of, 374
motor dysfunctions, differentiation of, 423–424t
motor function, in infancy, 503
motor neuron, 371
    lower, paralysis of, 416
    upper, 373
        paralysis of, 417
motor pathways, 373–374
motor system, examination techniques, 387–397
mouth, 64–65
    changes in, with aging, 69
    examination techniques of, 89–90
    in newborns, 482–483
    physical examination of, 484
    trench, 120
movements, involuntary, 420–422t
mucosa
    buccal, 89
    nasal, 87
mumps, 470
murmur(s)
    of aortic regurgitation, 180, 206, 491
    of aortic stenosis, 202, 491
    Austin Flint, 206
    diastolic, 178–179, 205–206t
    functional, 202–203
    grading of, 179
    in infancy and childhood, 490
    innocent, 190, 202–203
    mechanisms of, 201t
    midsystolic murmurs, 202–203
    mitral regurgitation in, 204, 491
    of mitral stenosis, 180, 206, 491
    pansystolic regurgitant, 204t
    of pulmonic stenosis, 202, 491
    systolic, 170–171, 178–179
        cardiovascular assessment of, 190
    timing of, 178–179
    of tricuspid regurgitation, 204
    of ventricular septal defect, 204
muscle(s). *See also* specific muscles
    atrophy of, 374
    extraocular, 76–77
    flaccid, 390
    neck, spasm of, 355
    stretch reflexes, 372, 401
    testing of, 341, 390
    tone, 390
        at birth, 450
muscular dystrophy, 511
musculoskeletal system
    in aging, 338–339
    anatomy and physiology, 324–339
    examination techniques in, 340–354
    in infancy and childhood, 498–503
myasthenia gravis, 384
Mydriacyl, for ophthalmoscopic exam, 77

myoclonus, involuntary movements in, 422
myomas, uterine, 293
myopathy, 393, 508
myopia, 68
myringitis, bullous, 114
myxedema, 73, 90, 95

nails
    abnormalities and variations of, 53
    in aging, 45, 309
    as skin appendages, 43
nasolacrimal duct obstruction, 473
neck, 65–67
    changes with age, 68–69
    examination techniques for, 91–94
    lymph nodes of, 67
    musculoskeletal examination of, 342
    musculoskeletal problems in, 355–356t
    in newborn, 467
    rigidity of, 471
neoplasms. *See* tumors; *specific tumors*
nephrotic syndrome, 49, 95
nerve(s). *See also specific nerves*
    anterior root of, 371
    autonomic, to eyes, 59
    cranial, 380
    motor, 371
    peripheral, 370–371
    posterior root of, 371
    sensory fibers of, 370
    spinal, 371
nervous system
    in aging, 381
    anatomy and physiology, 370–381
    examination techniques in, 382–412
        in infancy and childhood, 503–512
neuromuscular junctions, 371–372
neuron(s)
    corticobulbar, 373
    motor, 371, 373, 416
nevus flammeus, 464
nevus vasculosus, 464
nipple(s)
    abnormalities of, 225t
    female, inspection of, 217
nits, 70
nodule(s)
    breast, 226t
    ear, 113t
    elbow, 360
    skin, 51
    thyroid, 124
nose, 62–63
    abnormalities, 116t
    in infancy and childhood, 482–487
    inspection of, 85–87
    polyps of, 116
    septum of, 62, 87
    speculum for, 85
nystagmus, 76, 414–415t
    in childhood, 512
    identification of, 383
    in infancy, 472
    opticokinetic, 474

objectivity, in patient record, 525
obligate nasal breathers, 482
obsession(s), 433
obsessive compulsive disorder, 441

obstruction
  biliary, 463
  in breathing, 149
  of external jugular vein, 189
obturator sign(s), 249, 496
ocular fundi, 56, 109–111t
  in aging, 69
oculocephalic reflex, 412
oculomotor nerve (N_3)
  examination of, 383–384
  function of, 378
  paralysis of, 101
oculovestibular reflex, 412
odors, in physical examination, 41
olfactory nerve (N_1)
  examination of, 383
  function of, 378
opacities, of cornea and lens, 100t, 474
opening snap, 163, 199
ophthalmia neonatorum, 473
ophthalmoscopic examination, 77–82
opisthotonus, 503
optical blink reflex, in newborns, 472–473
optic chiasm, in visual pathway, 58
optic disc, 56, 79–80
  abnormalities of, 105t
  normal variations of, 104t
optic nerve (N_2)
  atrophy of, 105, 383
  examination of, 383
  function of, 378
  in visual pathways, 58
optokinetic testing, 477
orange peel appearance, breast, 224–225
orchitis, 270
organic affective syndrome, 439, 445
organic brain syndrome, 442
  distinguishing features, 444–445t
organic delusional syndrome, 445
organic personality syndrome, 445
orientation, 428, 434
Ortolani's test, 500
os, cervical, 274
Osgood-Schlatter disease, 347, 366
osteoarthritis, hand, 357
osteoma(s), 83
osteomyelitis, 340
osteoporosis, spinal, 351
otitis externa, 83–84
  in childhood, 481
otitis media, 83
  acute purulent, 114
  in childhood, 481
  in comatose patient, 410
  serous, 114, 481
otoscope, 86
  pneumatic, 481
overanxious disorders, 440
overbite, 485
ovary(ies)
  anatomy, 274
  in bimanual examination, 284
  cysts of, 295
  tumors of, 233, 295

Paget's disease
  of skull, 70
  of nipple and areola, 225
pain
  sensation of, 375, 398

shoulder, 361–362t
palate, soft, paralysis of, 123, 386, 413, 487
palmar grasp reflex, in infancy, 505
palmar space infection, 358
palpation
  abdominal, 238–243
  of chest, 137–139, 145–146
  breast
    female, 219–221
    male, 222–223
  for hernias, 266–267
  hair, 47
  heart, 172–176
  kidneys, 243–245
  liver, 240–242
  penis, 265
  scrotum, 265–267
  sinuses, 87–88
  spleen, 242–243
  thyroid, 92–94
pancreas, percussion of, 230
pancreatitis, 254
panic disorder, 441
papilledema, 105, 383
  in comatose patient, 410
  in infants, 473
papule, skin lesions, 51
paradoxical breathing, 488
paradoxical pulse, 209
paradoxical splitting, in second heart
  sound, 197
paralysis
  facial, 385, 416–417t
  lower motor neuron, 416
  palatal, 386, 413, 487
  10th (tenth) cranial nerve, 123
  12th (twelfth) nerve, 122
  upper motor neuron, 417
paralytic ileus, bowel sounds in, 234
paranoid disorders, 443
paraphimosis, 264
paraplegia, 390
  spastic, 506
pansystolic regurgitant murmurs, 204t
paraurethral gland, 273–274
paravertebral spasm, 369
parent–infant interaction, observation of, 451
parents, in interview, 16–18
paresis
  plantar reflexes and, 507
  12th nerve paresis, in infancy, 504
parkinsonism, 390
  face in, 95
  gait in, 419
  speech in, 413
paronychia, 53
parotid duct, 64
parotid gland, 54
  enlargement of, face in, 95
paroxysmal auricular tachycardia, in infants
  and children, 457
patch, skin lesions, 51
patella, floating, 348
patent ductus arteriosus
  cardiovascular sounds in, 207–208
  in heart murmur, 201
pathways
  hearing, 61
  motor, 373–374
  sensory, 374–377

patient(s), aging, interviewing of, 19–20
patient record, 524–535
  example of, 527–533
pectoriloquy, whispered, 151
pectus carinatum, 487
pectus excavatum, 487
pediatric physical examination, 447–512
pelvis
  anatomy, 334–335
  inflammatory disease of, 283, 295
  tender, 253
  tilt of, 350
penis
  abnormalities, 268t
  in aging, 261
  anatomy, 259
  carcinoma of, 268
  in childhood and prepubescence, 497
  inspection of, 264
  palpation of, 265
perception, 428
  assessment of, 434
percussion
  abdominal, 235–238
    in infancy, 493
  chest, 139–143, 146–147
  notes in, 142
    in infancy, 488
Perez reflex, in infancy, 508
perforations
  eardrum, 114
pericardial friction rub, cardiovascular
  sounds in, 207–208
perineum, 273
periodontitis, 120
peripheral nerve, 370–371
peripheral resistance, in arterial pressure,
  167
peripheral vascular system
  in aging, 309
  anatomy and physiology, 304–309
  examination techniques in, 310–317
peristaltic waves, increased, of intestinal
  obstruction, 234
peritoneum metastases to, 302
peritonitis
  bowel sounds in, 234
  generalized, in childhood, 496
  light palpation in, 239
persistent posterior lenticular fibrovascular
  sheath, 473
personal hygiene, mental function and, 431
petechia(e), 50
  in newborns, 483
Peutz-Jeghers syndrome, 118
Peyronie's disease, 268
Phalen's sign, in carpal tunnel syndrome,
  352
pharyngitis
  acute exudative, 91
  streptococcal, 123
  viral, 123
pharynx
  abnormalities of, 123
  examination techniques of, 90–91
  in infancy and childhood, 483
  posterior, 64
  pheochromocytoma, 459
phimosis, 264
phlebitis, calf, 314

phobias, 440–441
  assessment of, 433
physical examination. *See also under specific area of body or specific condition*
  anatomy and physiology, 35–38
  approach and overview, 28–34
  example of, 530–534
  general survey, 35–42
  growth in, 35–37
  habitus in, 35–37, 39
  of infants and children, 447–512
  mental function and, 430–438
  motor system, 387–397
  musculoskeletal system, 340–354
  nervous system, 382–412
  ophthalmoscopic, 77–82
  rectovaginal, 284
  sensory system, 397–401
  sequence, 30–34
  techniques of, 39–42
    eyes, 70–82
    head, 70
    skin, 46–47
  temperature in, 41–42
  vital signs in, 41
pigeon chest, 150
pillars, of pharynx, 64
pilonidal cyst, 301
pilonidal sinus, 301
pinguecula, 98
placing response, 506
plagiocephaly, 466
plantar reflexes, 372, 407
  in infancy, 507
plantar wart, 364
plaque, skin lesions, 51
pleural effusion
  anterior chest in, 145
  percussion for, 143
  posterior chest in, 136
  signs in, 154
pleural rubs, 153t
PMI. *See* apical impulse
pneumonia
  lobar, signs in, 155
  right middle lobe, percussion in, 147
pneumothorax, 92
  signs in, 156
point localization, in sensory testing, 401
point-to-point testing, 396
polycystic disease, kidney, 245
polycythemia, 48
polyneuropathy, 393
  in sensory testing, 397
polyp(s)
  cervical, 289
  nasal, 116
  rectal, 302
popliteal artery
  anatomy, 305
  palpation of, 313
porencephalic cysts, 467
position
  of eyes, 72
  in male rectal examination, 298
  sense of, 375, 397, 399
  tripod, 471
positioning, vertical suspension, in infancy, 506

post-traumatic stress disorder, 441
postural tremors, 420
posture
  abnormalities of, 418–419t
  in comatose patient, 427t
  motor behavior and, 431
  in physical examination, 40
pouch, rectouterine, anatomy, 274
precocious puberty, 217
  breasts in, 217
  male sexual development in, 263
  penis enlargement in, 497
pregnancy
  breast changes in, 214
  protuberant abdomen in, 251
  ruptured tubal, 295
  uterine changes in, 292t
pregnant uterus, 229
  in abdominal inspection, 233
presbycusis, in aging, 69
presbyopia, 68, 70
present illness
  in adult history, 2
  approach to, 10–14
  in child history, 5
pressure sores, 316–317
primary teeth, 486
prism test, 474–476
pronation, of feet, 499
pronator drift, 391
prostate
  abnormalities of, 303t
  anatomy, 296
  benign hypertrophy of, 303
  carcinoma of, 303
  examination of, 300
prostatitis, 303
protuberant abdomens, 251t
pruritus ani, 299
psoas sign
  abdominal palpation for, 248
  in childhood, 496
psoriasis, scalp, 70
psychosocial history, 529
  adult, 3–4, 14
psychotic disorders, 442–443t
pterygium, 100
ptosis, 97
  obstructive amblyopia and, 474
  senile, 68
  in 3rd nerve palsy, 384
puberty
  assessment of
    female, 217, 279
    male, 263
  breast development in, 212, 213
  delayed
    female, 217, 279
    male, 263
  musculoskeletal system in, 338
  precocious
    female, 217
    male, 263, 479
  sexual development in
    female, 212, 213, 275–276
    male, 260–262
pubic hair
  in aging, 261
  in boys, sex maturity ratings in, 261–262

  in girls, sex maturity ratings in, 212–213, 275, 276
pulmonary consolidation, signs in, 154
pulmonary edema, 490
pulmonary function, clinical assessment of, 148
pulmonic ejection sound, 198
pulmonic stenosis, 173, 197, 202, 491
pulmonic systolic murmurs, 170, 203
pulsation, venous
  jugular, 169, 189
  optic disc, 80
pulse
  arterial, 180–182
    abnormalities of, 209t
    blood pressure and, 166–167
  bigeminal, 209
  bisferiens, 209
  brachial, 310
  carotid, 181
  dorsalis pedis, 313
  femoral, 312, 489
  grading of, 310
  in infants and children, 457
  leg, in heart examination, 186
  paradoxical, 209
  popliteal, 313
  posterior tibial, palpation of, 313
  radial, 310
  ulnar, 310
pulsus alternans, 209
pupils, 56
  abnormalities of, 101–102t
  accommodation, reaction to, 76
  examination of, 75–76
  fixed, 102
  inspection of, 383
  reaction to light, 75, 385
  reflexes of, in comatose patient, 410
purpura, senile, 44
purpuric skin lesions, 50t
pustule, skin, 51
pyorrhea, 120
pyramidal tract, 373
pyrexia, 41

quadrants, of abdomen, 229
quadriplegia, 390
quadruple rhythm, 199
quinsy sore throat, 123

radial artery, 304
radial pulse, 310
range of motion
  in infancy, 498
  limitations in, 340
rapid rhythm alternating movements, in assessment of coordination, 396
raspberry tongue, 485
reasoning, abstract, 429
  testing of, 437
rebound tenderness
  palpation for, 239
  referred, abdominal palpation for, 248
rectocele, 287
rectovaginal examination, 284
rectum
  anatomy and physiology, 296–297
  carcinoma of, 302

examination techniques, 298–300
  female, 300
  in infancy and childhood, 496–497
  male, 299–300
  prolapse of, 302
  temperature in, 42
red eyes, 99t
redness, in joints, 340
red reflex, 78
red spots, in retina, 107
reflex(es). *See also specific reflexes*
  examination of, 401–407
  grading of, 402
  irritability of, at birth, 450
  reflex arc, 370–372
  reflex hammer, 401
reflux, hepatojugular, 189
refractive error, 477
relationships to persons and things
  mental function and, 431
  in physical examination, 41
renal artery stenosis, in abdominal
    auscultation, 234
renal retention, of salt and water, 320
respiration
  rate of, in infancy and childhood, 458,
    488
  sighing, 149
  sounds in, 134
respiratory effort at birth, 450
resting tremors, 420
retina, 80–81
  detachment of, 473
  hemorrhages of, 107
    in infants, 472–473
  microaneurysms of, 107
  red spots in, 107
  vessels of, 56, 80–81
retinopathy, 110–111t
  hypertensive, in comatose patient, 410
retraction
  in breast cancer, 224
  eardrum, 114
  nipple, 225
  upper eyelid, 97
retroflexion, uterine, 294
retrograde filling test
  for incompetent venous valves, 323t
  for varicose veins, 316
retrolental fibroplasia, 473
retroversion, uterine, 294
rheumatic fever, 340–341
rheumatoid arthritis, 340
  foot and ankle, 345
  hand, 343, 357
  intervertebral, 351
  juvenile, 485
  muscular weakness in, 341
rheumatoid nodules
  elbow, 360
  foot and ankle, 345
  hand, 357
  subcutaneous, 341
rhinitis, 116
  perennial allergic, 469
rhythm(s)
  arterial pulse, 180
  of breathing, 136, 144, 149
  of heart, differentiation of, 192–195

rib(s), cervical, 310
rickets, in newborn, 466
right bundle branch block, 196–197
  in infancy and childhood, 490
right ventricle, 157
  enlarged, 174
rigidity
  abdominal, 239
  postural, 427
Rinne test, 85, 115
Romberg test, 388
rooting reflex, 505
rotation test, 508
rotator cuff, 361
Rovsing's sign, abdominal palpation for, 248

S$_1$. *See* first heart sound
S$_2$. *See* second heart sound
S$_3$. *See* third heart sound
S$_4$. *See* fourth heart sound
sacral promontory, 229
sacroiliac pain, 354
salpingitis, 254
salt, renal retention of, in edema, 320
saphenous veins, 305–306
scale, skin, 51
scalp, physical examination of, 70
scapula, "winging" of, 391
scar
  corneal, 100
  skin, 52
scarlet fever, tongue in, 485
Scheuermann's disease, 368
schizo-affective disorder, 443
schizophrenia, 443
  dermatoglyphic patterns in, 464
Schlemm's canal, 57
scissors gait, 418
scleras, physical examination of, 74
scleroderma, 310
scoliosis, 341, 369, 503
scrotal tongue, 485
scrotum
  abnormalities, 269–270t
  in aging, 261
  anatomy, 259
  edema of, 270
  hernia of, 269
  hydrocele of, 269
  inspection, 265
  palpation, 265–267
  transillumination in, 266
sebaceous cyst(s)
  ear, 113
  scrotal, 269
  of vulva, 286
sebaceous glands, 43–44
seborrhea, 73
second heart sound (S$_2$), 162
  in auscultation, 178
  components of, 165
  in hypertension, 197
  in infancy and childhood, 490
  physiologic splitting of, 163
  variations in, 197t
seminal vesicles, 296
senile lentigines, 44
senile macular degeneration, 81
sensations, testing of, 397–401

sensory cortex, 375
  lesions of, 401
sensory examination, in infancy, 504
sensory loss, 375
  patterns of, 425–426t
sensory nerve fibers, 370
sensory pathways, 374–377
sensory system, examination techniques in,
    397–401
separation anxiety disorder, 440
septal defects
  atrial, 197, 203, 490
  ventricular, 204
    in heart murmur, 201
septum, nasal, 87
  deviation of, 116
serials 7s or 3s, as attention test, 435
sex maturity ratings
  in boys, 261–262
  in girls, 212–213, 275–276
  in physical examination, 38
sexual attractiveness, in interviewing, 23
sexual development, 39
  female, 212–213, 217, 275–276, 279
  male, 260–263
sexual history, 14–16
shoulder(s)
  anatomy, 328–330
  examination techniques of, 344
  painful, 361–362t
silence, in interviewing, 20
sinus(es)
  arrhythmia, 192t, 195, 490
  frontal, palpation, 87
  maxillary, palpation of, 87
  paranasal, 62–63
  physical examination of, 87–89
  transillumination of, 88–89, 485
  tracts, in chest palpation, 137
sinusitis, 87–88
  transillumination in, 485
sinus node, 165
Skene's glands, 274
skin
  in aging, 44–45, 309
  anatomy and physiology, 43–45
  color of, variations in, 48–49t
  dimpling of, 224
  of head, physical examination of, 70
  in infancy, 462–464
  lesions of, 50–52t
skull
  fracture of, in comatose patient, 410
  physical examination of, 70
smell, sense of, 383
  changes of, in aging, 69
smooth tongue, 122
  in avitaminosis, 485
Snellen E chart, in visual testing, 477
snout reflex, 409
social phobia, 441
soft palate, paralysis of, 123, 386, 413, 487
sounds
  abdominal, 252t
  added, lungs, 144, 148, 152–153t
  cardiovascular, with systolic and diastolic
    components, 207–208t
  vascular in neck, 171
  voice. *See* voice sounds

spasm
of arteriolar walls, 106
paravertebral, 369
spasticity
in hemiparesis, 418
upper motor neuron, 423
speculum(a)
nasal, 85
vaginal, 278
speech
abnormalities of, 413t
mental function and, 432
in physical examination, 41
survey of, 382
spermatic cord
anatomy, 259
torsion of, 270
spermatocele, 269
sphincter, anal, 296
tightness in, 299
sphygmomanometer, 182, 459
spinal accessory nerve (N_{11})
examination of, 386
function of, 379
spinal cord, transverse lesions of, 426, 506
spinal reflex mechanisms, 504
spine
anatomy, 336–337
curvature abnormalities, 368–369t
examination techniques of, 350–352
tuberculosis of, 369
spinothalamic tracts, 374
spleen
in abdominal percussion, 237–238
enlarged, steps in, 257
in infancy, 493
palpation of, 242–243, 495
percussion of, 230
splenic percussion sign, 238
spondylitis, 351, 368
cervical, 356
spoon nails, 53
sprain(s), ligamentous, 346
squamous cell carcinoma, in aging, 45
startle reflex, 509
state of awareness, 39
stature, 39
stenosing tenosynovitis, 340
stenosis
aortic, 173, 181, 202. See aortic stenosis
mitral, 176, 180, 196, 199, 206, 490–491
pulmonic, 173, 197, 202, 491
renal artery, in abdominal auscultation, 234
Stensen's duct, 64
steppage gait, 418
stereognosis, 400
stethoscope, characteristics of, xvii
stomach, in abdominal percussion, 230, 237
stomatitis, angular, 69, 117
strabismus
ambylopia exanopsia and, 474
in infancy, 508
straight leg raising, in herniated lumbar disc, 353
strawberry tongue, 485
stress, post-traumatic, 441
striae, abdominal, 233
stridor, infantile laryngeal, 483
stupor, 409–412, 413

Sturge-Weber Syndrome, 464
sty, 98
subclavian steal syndrome, 185
subdural effusion, 467
submaxillary ducts, 64
submaxillary gland, 54
sucking reflex, 409
sudden infant death syndrome (SIDS), 458
summation gallop, 199
supinator reflexes, 372, 404
suprapatellar swelling, 365
suprapubic region, abdominal, 229
supraspinatus tendon, rupture of, 362
sutures
in infant heads, 465
premature closure of, 462
"swan neck" deformities, 357
sweat glands, 43
swellings
eye, 98t
hand, 357–359t
joint, 340
knee, 365t
synapses, spinal cord, 372
synovitis, 340
syphilis
chancre
on lip, 117
on penis, 268
of vulva, 286
craniotabes in, 466
systole
extra heart sounds in, 198t
hypertension in, 171
systolic blood pressure, in children, 458
systolic bruits, abdominal, 252

tachycardia, 192, 193
in infancy and childhood, 490
tachypnea, 149, 490
tactile fremitus, 135, 138, 146, 488, 489
talipes varus, 499
tardive dyskinesia, 422
tarsal plates, 55
taste, changes in, with aging, 69
teeth, 65
abnormalities of, 120–121t
changes in, with aging, 69
in childhood, 485–486
examination techniques for, 89
supernumerary, 482
telangiectatic nevus, 464
temperature
in infants and children, 456–457
measurement of, 41–42
sensation of, 375, 398
skin, 46
temporal artery, 54
temporomandibular joint, 325, 341
tenderness
abdominal, 253–254t
joint, 340
knee, 366–367t
tendonitis, 340
of muscle biceps, 362
tendon sheath infection, 358
tennis elbow, 360
tenosynovitis
flexor tendon, hand, 358
gonococcal, 343

stenosing, 340
testicles, undescended, 265, 497
testis
in aging, 261
anatomy of, 259
in infancy, 496
small, 270
tumor of, 269
tetanus, 467
tetany, 467, 483
tetralogy of Fallot, murmur in, 491
thalamus, 375
thenar eminence of palm, atrophy of, 338–339, 359, 389
third heart sound (S_3), 163
auscultation of, 178, 180, 199
thorax
anatomy and physiology, 125–135
deformities of, 150t
examination techniques, 136–148
in infancy and childhood, 487–489
kyphoscoliosis of, 150
physical examination of, 136–148
thought content
assessment of, 433–434
mental function and, 428
thought processes
assessment of, 432–433
mental function and, 428
variations and abnormalities in, 446t
thrills, 172
throat, 482–487
thromboangiitis obliterans, 310
thrombophlebitis, 312, 314
thrush, of oral mucosa, 119
thyroglossal duct fistula, in newborn, 467
thyroid
anatomy of, 66
bruits in, 94
cartilage, 66
enlargement of, 124
examination techniques for, 92–94
tibial artery, 305
tibial pulse, 313
tics, 421
tinea versicolor, 49
tissue(s)
joint, 341
subcutaneous, 43
in infants' skin, 464
in rheumatoid arthritis, 341
toe(s), abnormalities of, 363–364t
toenail, ingrown, 364
tongue, 64
abnormalities of, 122t
asymmetrical protrusion of, 90
in childhood, 485
in comatose patient, 410
examination techniques for, 90
12th nerve lesion of, 90
tonic neck reflex, 508
tonic pupil, 102
tonsillitis, 486
tonsils, 123, 486
tophus(i)
ear, 113
hand, 358
torsion, spermatic cord, 270
torticollis, spasmodic, 421
torus palatinus, 119

touch, as sensation, 375
trachea
  deviations of, 92
  examination techniques for, 92–94
  obstruction of, 136, 145
  rings in, 66
tracheoesophageal fistula, 450, 483
tracheomalacia, 483
tragus, skin tabs in, 478
transillumination
  scrotal, 266
  sinus, 88–89, 485
  skull, 467–468
transposition of the great vessels, murmur in, 491
tremors, involuntary, 420
trench mouth, 120
Trendelenburg's sign, 502
Trendelenburg's test, 316
triceps reflex, 372, 403, 504
trichomonas vaginitis, 290
tricuspid regurgitation, 204
trigeminal nerve (N_5)
  examination of, 384–385
  function of, 378
Trisomy 21, face in, 469
trochlear nerve (N_4)
  examination of, 383–384
  function of, 378
trunk incurvation, 506
tuberculosis, spinal, 369
tumor(s). *See also* cancer; *specific tumors*
  kidney, 245
  ovarian, 233
  protuberant abdomen due to, 251
  skin, 51
  solid, in newborns, 493
  testicular, 269
  uterine, 283
tunica vaginalis, 259
turbinates, 62, 87
12th nerve
  lesion, tongue of, 90
  paralysis of, 122
  paresis of, in infancy, 504
two-point discrimination, in sensory testing, 400–401
tympanic membrane, 478

ulcer(s)
  ankle, 319t
  aphthous, 119
  foot, 319t, 364
  skin, 51
  trophic, 319
ulnar artery, 304
  pulse in, 310
umbilical artery, single, 492
umbilicus
  abdominal region of, 229
  cord of, vessels in, 492
  hernia in, 250, 492
umbilicus amnioticus, 492

umbilicus cutis, 492
umbo, 84
underbite, in childhood, 485
unreality, feelings of, 433
uremia, 49
urethra
  caruncle of, 287
  male, 259
  meatus of, 259
  orifice in, 273–274
urethritis, 264
uterus
  abnormalities and displacements of, 293–294t
  anatomy, 274
  in bimanual examination, 283
  pregnant, 229, 292t
    in abdominal inspection, 233
uvula, 64

vagina
  anatomy, 274
  bulges and swellings of, 287t
  inflammations of and around, 290–291t
  inspection of, 282
  outlet of, 280
vaginitis, 290–291t
vagus nerve (N_{10})
  anatomy of, 379
  examination of, 386
varicocele, 269
varicose veins
  in leg, 315
  of tongue, 122
vascular skin lesions, 50t
vascular system, peripheral. *See* peripheral vascular system
vas deferens, 259
vein(s). *See also specific vein*
  abdominal hum of, 252
  anatomy of, 305–306
  cardiovascular hum of, 207–208
  communicating, 306
  deep, of leg, 305
  in edema, 321
  insufficiency of, 318t, 322
    in foot and ankle, 319
  prominence of, in breast cancer, 224
  pulsations of, in optic disc, 80
  of scalp, dilated, increased intracranial pressure and, 465
  varicose, valves in, 315
vellus hair, 43
vena cava, 159–160
  obstructed, 188, 233
venereal wart
  of penis, 268
  of vulva, 286
venous star, 50
ventricle(s), heart, 157–158
  left, apical impulse in, 191t
  right, enlargement of, 174
ventricular gallop, 199

ventricular septal defect, 204
  in heart murmur, 201
ventricular tachycardia, 193
vertical suspension positioning, 506
vesicular breath sounds, 134
vessel(s)
  great. *See* great vessels
  retinal, 56
vestibular function, 512
vestibule
  anatomy of, 273
  nose, 62
vibration, sense of, 375, 399
viscera, tender, 253–254
vision
  acuity of, 70–71
  extinction of, 383
  fields of
    confrontation testing of, 71–72
    defects in, 96t
    in infants and children, 477
  in newborn, 474
  pathways of, 57–58
  reflexes in, 58
  testing of, 70–82
vital capacity, changes with age, 135
vital signs, 41
vitiligo, 49
vitreous, opacities in, 82
vocabulary, 429
  testing of, 437
vocal cord paralysis, 386
vocal fremitus, 489
voice sounds, 135
  alterations in, 151t
  in lung auscultation, 144, 148
vulva
  anatomy, 273
  bulges and swellings of, 287t
  lesions of, 286t

wart(s)
  plantar, 364
  venereal, 268, 286
water, renal retention of, in edema, 320
Weber test, 85, 115
Weed system, 523
weight
  gestational, 448–449
  of infants and children, 461
  in physical examination, 37, 40
Wharton's ducts, 64
wheal, skin, 51
wheezes, 152–153t, 488
"winging," scapular, 391
wrist(s)
  anatomy, 325
  examination techniques of, 342–343
wrist drop, 392
writing tests, 436

xanthelasma, 98